Laparoscopic Urogynaecology

Laparoscopic Urogynaecology

Principles and Practice

Edited by

Christian Phillips
Hampshire Hospital, Basingstoke

Stephen Jeffery
Netcare Christiaan Barnard Memorial Hospital

Barry O'Reilly
Cork University Maternity Hospital

Marie Fidela R. Paraiso
Professor of Obstetrics, Gynecology, and Reproductive Biology,
Cleveland Clinic Lerner College of Medicine of Case Western Reserve University and
Vice Chair, OBGYN and Women's Health Institute
Cleveland Clinic Board of Governors
Cleveland, OH

Bruno Deval
Geoffroy St Hilaire Hospital, Paris

CAMBRIDGE
UNIVERSITY PRESS

CAMBRIDGE
UNIVERSITY PRESS

University Printing House, Cambridge CB2 8BS, United Kingdom

One Liberty Plaza, 20th Floor, New York, NY 10006, USA

477 Williamstown Road, Port Melbourne, VIC 3207, Australia

314–321, 3rd Floor, Plot 3, Splendor Forum, Jasola District Centre, New Delhi – 110025, India

103 Penang Road, #05–06/07, Visioncrest Commercial, Singapore 238467

Cambridge University Press is part of the University of Cambridge.

It furthers the University's mission by disseminating knowledge in the pursuit of education, learning, and research at the highest international levels of excellence.

www.cambridge.org
Information on this title: www.cambridge.org/9781009123174
DOI: 10.1017/9781009128377

First published 2022

Printed in the United Kingdom by TJ Books Limited, Padstow Cornwall

A catalogue record for this publication is available from the British Library.

Library of Congress Cataloging-in-Publication Data
Names: Phillips, Christian Hambro, editor. | Jeffery, Stephen (Stephen Trembarth), editor. | O'Reilly, Barry, MD, editor. | Paraiso, Marie Fidela R., editor. | Deval, Bruno, editor.
Title: Laparoscopic urogynecology : principles and practice / edited by Christian Phillips, Stephen Jeffery, Barry O'Reilly, Marie Fidela R. Paraiso, Bruno Deval.
Description: Cambridge, United Kingdom ; New York, NY : Cambridge University Press, 2021. | Includes bibliographical references and index.
Identifiers: LCCN 2021050294 (print) | LCCN 2021050295 (ebook) | ISBN 9781009123174 (hardback) | ISBN 9781009123174 (ebook)
Subjects: MESH: Gynecologic Surgical Procedures | Urologic Surgical Procedures | Laparoscopy
Classification: LCC RG104.7 (print) | LCC RG104.7 (ebook) | NLM WP 660 | DDC 618.1/0597–dc23/eng/20211101
LC record available at https://lccn.loc.gov/2021050294
LC ebook record available at https://lccn.loc.gov/2021050295

ISBN 978-1-009-12317-4 Hardback

Every effort has been made in preparing this book to provide accurate and up-to-date information that is in accord with accepted standards and practice at the time of publication. Although case histories are drawn from actual cases, every effort has been made to disguise the identities of the individuals involved. Nevertheless, the authors, editors, and publishers can make no warranties that the information contained herein is totally free from error, not least because clinical standards are constantly changing through research and regulation. The authors, editors, and publishers therefore disclaim all liability for direct or consequential damages resulting from the use of material contained in this book. Readers are strongly advised to pay careful attention to information provided by the manufacturer of any drugs or equipment that they plan to use.

Contents

In addition to the content found in this textbook, additional online resources are available to complement the book.

Videos that demonstrate lectures, surgical procedures, anatomical highlights and tips and tricks can be found by using the link below:

www.cambridge.org/phillips-resources

Contributors

Yara Abdelkhalek
Obstetrics and Gynecology Department, Hôtel-Dieu de France University Hospital, St Joseph University, Beirut, Lebanon

Igor But
Department of General Gynaecology and Urogynaecology, Clinic for Gynaecology and Perinatology, University Medical Centre Maribor, Slovenia

Rufus Cartwright
Department of Urogynaecology, LNWH NHS Trust, London, UK, and Department of Epidemiology & Biostatistics, Imperial College London, London, UK

Viviana Casas-Puig
Center for Urogynecology and Reconstructive Pelvic Surgery, Department of Obstetrics, Gynecology & Women's Health Institute, Cleveland Clinic, Cleveland, Ohio

Eric S. Chang, MD, MEng, FACOG
Urogynecology & Pelvic Reconstructive Surgery, Women's Health & Surgery Center of Advantia, Stafford, VA, USA

Olivia H. Chang, MD, MPH
Assistant Professor, Division of Urogynecology and Pelvic Reconstructive Surgery, Department of Obstetrics and Gynecology, University of Washington

Graham Chapman
Associate Professor,OB/Gyn and Women's Health Institute Section of Urogynecology and Pelvic Floor Disorders

Zhuoran Chen
Royal Brisbane and Wesley Urogynaecology, Brisbane, Australia

Patrick Culligan, MD,
Weill Cornell Department of Urology Center for Female Pelvic Health, New York, USA

Alfred Cutner, MD, FRCOG
Consultant Gynaecologist, University College London Hospitals

Emily Davidson, MD, FACOG
Assistant Professor, Department of Obstetrics and Gynecology, Urogynecology, WISH (Women's Incontinence and Sexual Health) Clinic, Medical College of Wisconsin

Siri Drangsholt, MD
Weill Cornell Department of Urology Center for Female Pelvic Health, New York, USA

Kim WM van Delft, MD, PhD
Jeroen Bosch Hospital, Department of Obstetrics and Gynaecology, Henri Dunantstraat 1, 5223 GZ 's-Hertogenbosch

Bruno Deval
Department of Functional Pelvic Surgery & Oncology, Geoffroy Saint-Hilaire, Ramsay, Générale de Santé, Paris, France

Bobby Garcia
Assistant Program Director, OB/GYN Residency Female Pelvic Medicine & Reconstructive Surgeon, New York City Health & Hospitals – Lincoln, USA

Ohad Gluck
Department of Obstetrics and Gynecology, Edith Wolfson Medical Center, Holon, Israel, affiliated with Sackler Faculty of Medicine, Tel Aviv University, Tel Aviv, Israel

Kristie A Greene, MD, FACOG
Florida Female Urology 1900 S. Tuttle Ave Sarasota FL 34239

Matt Hewitt
Consultant Gynaecological Oncologist, Cork University Maternity Hospital, Cork, Ireland, and Bon Secours Hospital, Cork, Ireland. Conflict of Interest: Intuitive Surgical Proctor

Lisa C. Hickman, MD
Division of Female Pelvic Medicine and Reconstructive Surgery, The Ohio State University Wexner Medical Center, Columbus, Ohio

Khaled M Ismail
Department of Obstetrics and Gynecology, Faculty of Medicine, Charles University, Pilsen, Czech Republic, and Biomedical Center, Faculty of Medicine in Pilsen, Charles University, Czech Republic

Matthew Izett-Kay, BM, BS, MD, MRCOG
Department of Urogynaecology, John Radcliffe Hospital, Oxford University Hospitals NHS Trust, Oxford, UK, and Nuffield Department of Women's & Reproductive Health, University of Oxford, Oxford, UK

Karl Jallad
Acting Chair Obstetrics and Gynecology, Urogynecology LAU Medical Center, Gilbert and Rose-Marie Chagoury School of Medicine, Lebanon

Swati Jha
Sheffield Teaching Hospitals NHS Foundation Trust

Vladimír Kališ
Department of Obstetrics and Gynecology, Faculty of Medicine, Charles University, Pilsen, Czech Republic; Biomedical Center, Faculty of Medicine in Pilsen, Charles University, Czech Republic; and Department of Obstetrics and Gynecology, University Hospital, Pilsen, Czech Republic

Rohna Mary Kearney, MD, FRCOG
Warrell Unit, Saint Mary's Hospital, Manchester University Hospitals NHS Trust, Manchester Academic Health Sciences Centre, Oxford Road Manchester, and Division of Developmental Biology & Medicine, School of Medical Sciences, University of Manchester

Kimberly Kenton, MD
Division of Female Pelvic Medicine and Reconstructive Surgery, Department of Obstetrics and Gynecology, Northwestern University Feinberg School of Medicine, Chicago, IL

Ilias Liapis
Birmingham Women's and Children's NHS Foundation Trust

Christopher Maher
Royal Brisbane and Wesley Urogynaecology, Brisbane, Australia

John R Miklos
Director of Urogynecology, Atlanta Urogynecology Associates, Adjunct Professor Obstetrics/Gynecology, Emory University

Robert D Moore
Director Advanced Pelvic Surgery Miklos & Moore Urogynecology and Cosmetic Vaginal Surgery Professor (Adj) OB/GYN Emory University School of Medicine Atlanta, GA USA

Tsung Mou, MD
Division of Female Pelvic Medicine and Reconstructive Surgery, Department of Obstetrics and Gynecology, Northwestern University Feinberg School of Medicine, Chicago, IL

Gemma Nightingale
Consultant Gynaecologist, Boulcott Hospital, Wellington, New Zealand

Guenter K. Noé, MD, PhD
President ISGE (Int. Soc. Gyn Endoscopy), Head of Department Obstetrics/Gynecology Rheinlandclinics Dormagen, and Assisstant Professor, University of Witten Herdecke

Marie Fidela R. Paraiso, MD, FACOG, FPMRS
Professor of Obstetrics, Gynecology, and Reproductive Biology, Cleveland Clinic Lerner College of Medicine of Case Western Reserve University, and Vice Chair, OBGYN and Women's Health Institute, Cleveland Clinic Board of Governors, Cleveland, Ohio

Christian Phillips
Department of Urogynaecology and Pelvic Floor Reconstructive Surgery, Hampshire Hospitals, Basingstoke, Hampshire, UK

Robert Pollard
Associate Professor Case School of Medicine MetroHealth Medical Center

Natalia Price
Department of Urogynaecology WAH NHS Trust, Worcester, UK

Katie Propst, MD
Assistant Professor of Surgery, Cleveland Clinic Learner College of Medicine, Cleveland Clinic, Cleveland, Ohio

Dudley Robinson
King's College Hospital NHS Foundation Trust

Anna Rosamilia
Associate Professor in Urogynaecology, Head of Pelvic floor unit, Monash Health, Melbourne, Australia

Zdenek Rusavy
Department of Obstetrics and Gynecology, Faculty of Medicine, Charles University, Pilsen, Czech Republic; Biomedical Center, Faculty of Medicine in Pilsen, Charles University, Czech Republic; and Department of Obstetrics and Gynecology, University Hospital, Pilsen, Czech Republic

Tamara Serdinšek
Department of General Gynaecology and Urogynaecology, Clinic for Gynaecology and Perinatology, University Medical Centre Maribor, Slovenia

Steven E Schraffordt Koops, MD, PhD
Meander Medical Center, Department of Urogynecology, Maatweg 3, 3813 TZ, Amersfoort, The Netherlands

Tonya N. Thomas, MD
Center for Urogynecology and Pelvic Reconstructive Surgery, Cleveland Clinic, 9500 Euclid Ave, Desk A81, Cleveland, OH, 44195, USA

Philip Toozs-Hobson
Birmingham Women's and Children's NHS Foundation Trust

Arvind Vashisht, MA, MD, FRCOG
Consultant Gynaecologist, University College London Hospitals

Nikolaus Veit-Rubin
Department of Obstetrics and Gynecology, Medical University of Vienna, Vienna, Austria

Sarah A Vogler, MD, MBA
Department of Colorectal Surgery, Digestive Disease & Surgery Institute, Cleveland Clinic, Cleveland, Ohio

Angela S Yuan, MD, FACOG
Urogynecologist, Trinity Health of New England, Hartford, CT, USA

Martino Maria Zacchè, MRCOG
Birmingham Women's Hospital, Birmingham, UK

Chapter 1

Patient Selection and Assessment for Laparoscopic Urogynaecology

Graham Chapman, Robert Pollard

Introduction

The laparoscopic approach to surgery has revolutionized modern healthcare. With advances in training and accessibility, the worldwide impact of this minimally invasive surgical modality continues to grow exponentially. High quality data continue to show advantages of laparoscopic surgery compared to open surgery in a variety of surgical fields, including lower rates of comorbidity, lower healthcare costs related to length of hospitalization, and expedited patient recovery [1,2,3]. In urogynaecology, laparoscopy can be utilized in the surgical repair of pelvic floor disorders, representing a versatile modality that can address the range from simple to the most complex cases. Adaptation of this modality greatly expands the repertoire of the urogynaecologic surgeon, and simultaneously can expand patient access to quality surgical care. The preoperative, intraoperative, and postoperative care in laparoscopy differs from that of vaginal or open surgery. This chapter will review the nuances of patient assessment and selection in urogynaecologic surgery.

General Approach to Laparoscopic Surgery

Laparoscopic surgery is used to perform abdominal surgery in a minimally invasive fashion. Limitations in laparoscopic surgery are few, particularly in the field of urogynaecology, where surgery is largely elective and non-emergent. Dependent on the skill and comfort level of the surgeon, any abdominal urogynaecologic procedure can be performed laparoscopically. Although, there are a number of factors that must be considered in the patient evaluation prior to performing laparoscopic surgery. This evaluation should be primarily centred around patient safety. Potential risks unique to laparoscopic surgery can be medical or surgical. Thus, the patient assessment must consider both medical comorbidities that increase risk related to the physiologic stressors in laparoscopic surgery, as well as surgical factors that may increase risk of injury.

Physiologic Changes in Laparoscopic Surgery

A number of physiologic changes occur that are inherent to laparoscopic surgery. Consideration of how preexisting medical comorbidities may impact the risk of these changes should be performed in conjunction with the anaesthesiology providers. The majority of intraoperative physiologic changes unique to laparoscopy are related to the synergistic effects of increased intra-abdominal pressure, carbon dioxide absorption, and the Trendelenburg position. While these factors affect patients in a variety of ways, the cardiac, vascular, and pulmonary systems are particularly impacted, placing those with significant cardiopulmonary disease at higher risk.

Cardiac Changes

Cardiovascular function changes during laparoscopic surgery in response to a combination of mechanical and endocrine changes. Upon peritoneal entry and insufflation, a vaso-vagal response resulting in severe bradycardia can rarely occur, requiring immediate release of pneumoperitoneum [4]. Typically, as pneumoperitoneum is established, mechanical pressure on the vasculature results in alterations in venous return, systemic vascular resistance, blood pressure, and cardiac output. Catecholamine release is increased. Carbon dioxide is absorbed trans-peritoneally, resulting in hypercarbia which produces acidosis, altered myocardial contractility, and sensitivity to arrhythmia [5]. Many of these effects are further exacerbated by the Trendelenburg position. In the healthy individual, these cardiovascular changes are readily compensated for, even in prolonged surgeries. Though, caution must be exercised when considering laparoscopic surgery for patients who have significant cardiac risk factors, including those with severe congestive heart failure, cardiac valvular disease, and coronary artery disease.

Pulmonary Changes

Pulmonary changes during laparoscopy also occur in response to the effects of pneumoperitoneum and patient positioning. The head-down positioning in Trendelenburg as well as increased intra-abdominal pressure from insufflation results in cephalad displacement of the diaphragm, causing decreased functional residual capacity, vital capacity, and lung compliance [4]. Extended periods in a steep Trendelenburg position can induce swelling that, when severe, can be obstructive to the airway, requiring prolonged intubation. Additionally the hypercapnic state induced by carbon dioxide absorption requires an increase in minute ventilation. While these changes can be compensated for with ventilation settings in the healthy patient, those with severe pulmonary disease may not be able to tolerate a more extensive laparoscopic surgery. Thus patients with severe asthma, chronic obstructive pulmonary disease, emphysema, pulmonary fibrosis, pulmonary hypertension, and severe obesity should be optimized and carefully considered for laparoscopic surgery. Given that open surgery presents another set of considerable risks in these patients, the implications of needing to convert to laparotomy due to an intolerance to the effects of laparoscopy should be emphasized in these patients.

Compressive Vascular Changes

Altered intra-abdominal blood flow due to compression from pneumoperitoneum is another potential risk of laparoscopy. Studies have portrayed a decrease in splanchnic blood flow to the liver and intestines, but this is not thought to be clinically significant except for in the critically ill [6]. Similarly, compression of the renal system as well as endocrine effects induced by laparoscopy have been shown to decrease renal perfusion and urine output, though urine output returns to normal shortly after surgery and renal function does not appear to be affected [7].

Neurologic Changes

Elevation in intracranial pressure is another concern during laparoscopy. As a result of the combination of head-down Trendelenburg position, increased intra-abdominal pressure, and hypercarbia, there is a notable increase in intracranial pressure [8]. Fortunately, studies have shown that cerebral blood flow and oxygenation are preserved even in prolonged laparoscopic surgeries. Though, the effects of increased intracranial pressure may be more detrimental in patients with a history of space-occupying intracranial lesions, cerebral aneurysm, and severe carotid atherosclerotic disease.

Surgical Risk Factors

In addition to an evaluation of a patient's baseline medical risk factors, one must also consider surgical risk factors that may alter the risk/benefit ratio of a laparoscopic approach. Intraoperative injuries are most likely to occur in laparoscopic surgery during initial entry, when gaining access to the peritoneal cavity. A thorough surgical history should be taken in every patient, and old operative reports reviewed meticulously. On the abdominal exam, prior scars should always be noted and explained. The prior surgical history should guide the entry location and technique. Consideration should be made to avoid entry at the location of a prior laparotomy or where intra-abdominal mesh has been placed. While individual surgeons prefer different entry techniques, data does not support one technique as clearly superior [9]. Ideally, every surgeon should be comfortable gaining access to the peritoneal cavity using multiple techniques and in multiple locations, in order to plan for the safest entry individualized to the current patient.

In addition to the impact of prior surgeries on the risk during entry, one must consider other factors that add risk to the surgery. Important information would include any history of diffuse peritonitis, extensive bowel surgery, pelvic radiation, known advanced endometriosis, pelvic inflammatory disease, history of intra-abdominal mesh placement, prior urologic surgery, inflammatory bowel disease, and any other history that may suggest a hostile abdomen. While these items rarely provide a true contraindication to laparoscopic surgery, a thorough knowledge and understanding of the individual patient's surgical risk is essential in providing safe and high-quality care.

Activity Restrictions after Laparoscopic Surgery

While laparoscopic surgery is valued for the faster recovery, there is limited consensus on postoperative activity restrictions. One survey of colorectal surgeons who performed both open and laparoscopic surgery revealed significant heterogeneity in their recommendations for activity restriction after surgery to prevent incisional hernia formation [10]. The majority of surgeons did restrict moderate activity for the first two weeks, and intense activity for six weeks postoperatively. Restrictions were significantly stricter after open surgery compared to laparoscopic surgery. In another study of patients who underwent surgery for pelvic organ prolapse, patients were randomized to lifting restrictions of no more than 10 pounds for three months after surgery, versus no restrictions [11]. The unrestricted patients had similar satisfaction scores and anatomic prolapse outcomes, and fewer pelvic floor symptoms Adverse. Outcomes after three months were not reported, nor were those related to incisional hernia. It is important to weigh the risks and benefits of postoperative activity in the individual patient, including the risk of incisional hernia and recurrent pelvic floor disorders, versus the known benefits of early activity. Non-strenuous activity should not be limited after laparoscopic surgery, and if restrictions are given in regards to lifting and other strenuous activity, there is not likely to be any benefit in extending these limitations beyond four to six weeks.

Benefits of Laparoscopic Surgery in Urogynaecology

Laparoscopy versus Open Surgery

Laparoscopy has multiple advantages in urogynaecologic surgery. Compared to the open abdominal approach, the most notable benefits of laparoscopic surgery relate to patient safety and recovery. Population-based data has illustrated this advantageous safety profile when comparing laparoscopic versus open sacrocolpopexy, with the laparoscopic group possessing reduced complication rates, lower blood loss, shorter hospital stay, and lower rates of reoperation and readmission [12]. A number of high quality, randomized controlled trials have demonstrated similar improvements in the safety profile for laparoscopic versus open approach to pelvic organ prolapse repair [13,14]. Furthermore, effectiveness of the surgical repair appears similar between the two approaches. Maher et al [14] published a large review of studies comparing open versus laparoscopic sacrocolpopexy, reporting no difference in the need for repeat prolapse surgery or quality-of-life measures, similar postoperative anterior and apical compartment support, and an improvement in postoperative posterior compartment support with the laparoscopic approach [14]. Similarly, in a systematic review of laparoscopic surgery for stress urinary incontinence, laparoscopic colposuspension had similar efficacy to open colposuspension and vaginal midurethral sling placement, and low rates of adverse events or repeat continence surgery [15]. In regards to cost, laparoscopic sacrocolpopexy is less expensive than the robotic-assisted and open approaches [16,17].

Laparoscopy versus Vaginal Surgery

The potential benefits of laparoscopy compared to vaginal surgery in urogynaecology relate to a more versatile surgical repertoire with a similar safety profile, and some evidence of improved efficacy between analogous procedures. Laparoscopy provides excellent visualization of the entire peritoneal cavity, allowing for more advanced surgery in the upper pelvis, if required during urogynaecologic procedures. This is relevant to a number of common scenarios, including the need for hysterectomy for large uterine fibroids, evaluation or removal of ovarian masses, and excision of endometriosis. Laparoscopy is beneficial in patients at risk of adhesive disease given optimal visualization. Even simple procedures, such as opportunistic salpingectomy during hysterectomy, are successfully performed at a much higher rate when performing laparoscopy compared to vaginal surgery [18].

Multiple studies have compared laparoscopic versus vaginal routes of procedures for pelvic organ prolapse [18,19,20,21,22,23,24]. Complication rates are generally similar between the two routes. Although, notably, ureteral obstruction may be lower when performing laparoscopic versus vaginal uterosacral ligament suspension [18]. In regards to prolapse-specific outcomes, some studies report no difference [19,20], while others report an advantage of laparoscopy for either subjective outcomes, anatomic results, or both [18,21,22,23,24]. While definitive conclusions cannot be made regarding the superiority of a laparoscopic compared to vaginal approach to urogynaecologic surgery, this data provokes the question. Prospective, randomized trials with long-term follow-up are needed to compare these two minimally invasive routes of urogynaecologic surgery.

Evaluation of Pelvic Floor Disorders

The preoperative evaluation prior to undergoing surgery for pelvic floor disorders requires a thorough, systematic and global approach. While the majority of laparoscopic urogynaecologic surgery is performed for pelvic organ prolapse, a full assessment must also be made of concurrent urinary incontinence or voiding dysfunction, sexual dysfunction, and defecatory disorders. Given the interrelated nature of various pelvic floor disorders, multiple issues may be addressed concomitantly during surgery if they are appropriately assessed in the preoperative period. Conversely, each of these problems has a variety of other potential aetiologies which must be fully explored to determine how surgery may or may not impact the patient's symptoms.

Vaginal Symptoms of Pelvic Organ Prolapse

The evaluation and treatment of pelvic organ prolapse should be tailored to patient symptoms, and how these symptoms impact quality of life. Symptoms such as vaginal bulge, pelvic pressure, and the feeling that something is dropping are commonly experienced by patients with prolapse. A vaginal bulge that is felt or seen by the patient is one of the most specific symptoms, with positive and negative predictive values for prolapse of >75% [25]. This complaint should elicit a targeted evaluation of further symptoms as well as risk factors for prolapse, including vaginal parity, history of perineal trauma, menopausal status, connective tissue disorders, and family history. Some risk factors are modifiable and can be addressed preventatively, such as obesity and chronic constipation [26].

Voiding Dysfunction and Urinary Incontinence

Symptoms related to voiding dysfunction should be explored thoroughly. The Urinary Distress Inventory, Short Form (UDI-6), is helpful in defining the patient's voiding symptoms as they relate to stress incontinence, overactive bladder, incomplete bladder emptying, and bladder pain. Some urinary symptoms are highly related to pelvic organ prolapse, such as urinary splinting, which has been reported to be >97% specific for anterior vaginal wall prolapse [25]. Others, such as urgency, frequency, and urge urinary incontinence are less specific but commonly seen in patients with prolapse. The evolution of symptoms as they relate to the development of prolapse should be considered. For example, if a patient has improvement in stress urinary incontinence as prolapse worsens, it can be anticipated that this issue will worsen when the prolapse is corrected. Similarly, development of incomplete bladder emptying with worsening of prolapse may likely resolve with correction of the prolapse. Urge incontinence and overactive bladder typically have a more complex aetiology. While often related to prolapse, this is rarely the most significant contributor.

Stress Urinary Incontinence

Symptoms of stress urinary incontinence should always be addressed prior to proceeding with surgery for pelvic organ prolapse, as the problems often coexist. Systematic reviews consistently identify improvement in stress urinary incontinence symptoms when a continence procedure is performed at the time of prolapse repair [27,28]. Patients who do not report symptoms of stress incontinence but then display a positive cough stress test with the prolapse reduced are termed to have de novo stress incontinence. A concomitant continence procedure at the time of prolapse repair is generally beneficial in these patients. In asymptomatic patients with negative testing for de novo stress urinary incontinence, few studies exist looking at a concomitant continence procedure at the time of prolapse surgery. Review of the existing literature in this population has not consistently reported a benefit to a preventative continence procedure, but this is an area that requires further study [27].

Overactive Bladder

Overactive bladder symptoms and incomplete bladder emptying are commonly seen in patients with pelvic organ prolapse. Overactive bladder is a complex syndrome with multiple aetiologies, though it is likely that prolapse does contribute in select patients. While there is some debate over causality, multiple theories exist as to how prolapse might induce bladder overactivity. While the most accepted theory relates to neuromuscular changes induced by prolapse-induced bladder outlet obstruction, others include bladder wall stretch inducing detrusor contraction, as well as opening of the proximal urethra leading to urine entry and subsequent detrusor contraction [29].

In a review of the effects of prolapse surgery on overactive bladder, de Boer et al [29] illustrated significant improvement in both symptoms as well as detrusor overactivity after prolapse surgery in the vast majority of studies [29]. It is likely that these effects are most prominent in patients with evidence of obstruction and incomplete bladder emptying. Given the multifactorial aetiology of overactive bladder, patients should be counselled on appropriate expectations for relief after prolapse surgery. In patients with evidence of obstruction that is relieved with prolapse reduction, some degree of improvement in overactive bladder symptoms may be expected after surgery for prolapse.

Defecatory Dysfunction

Defecatory dysfunction must be addressed in the presurgical assessment given its prevalence in patients with pelvic organ prolapse. Any symptoms of splinting, stool trapping, incomplete defecation, straining, chronic constipation, as well as fecal incontinence should be assessed. The relationship between defecatory dysfunction and pelvic organ prolapse is complex and not well understood. Obstructed defecation is often linked with a posterior wall defect. In these patients, debate exists as to whether chronic constipation and straining lead to the development of prolapse, or if prolapse is actually the cause for development of obstructed defecation and constipation. While some studies show no correlation between the stage of prolapse and the degree of constipation [30], others consistently report improvement in bowel symptoms after surgery for pelvic organ prolapse [31,32,33,34]. Interestingly, many suggest that surgical repair of the apex may be sufficient to relieve bowel symptoms, regardless of the performance of a posterior colporrhaphy. This improvement is seen across various apical repair techniques, including sacrospinous ligament suspension, uterosacral ligament suspension, and sacrocolpopexy.

Similar to overactive bladder, defecatory dysfunction can be a complex and multifactorial issue. While some patients may experience symptoms purely related to an anatomical defect that may be surgically repaired, a significant number will remain symptomatic after surgical repair. This highlights the importance of a careful and detailed evaluation of bowel symptoms prior to surgery, allowing for a discussion of the expected benefits of surgery between the patient and their physician.

Sexual Dysfunction

In addition to vaginal, bladder, and bowel-specific symptoms, one must evaluate the patient for sexual dysfunction. The relationship of sexual dysfunction with pelvic floor disorders is complex. Evidence does exist supporting a direct relationship between sexual dysfunction with both pelvic organ prolapse and urinary incontinence. Studies have reported an overall improvement in sexual function after surgery for pelvic organ prolapse [35]. Data regarding sexual dysfunction and surgery for urinary incontinence is less consistent; symptoms such as coital incontinence improve with surgery but overall sexual function is more variable [36,37]. A qualitative study on sexual function before and after surgery for pelvic organ prolapse and/or urinary incontinence reported that overall sexual function did improve after surgery, but this improvement was largely due to cure of prolapse and incontinence symptoms, as opposed to behavioural or emotional components. Patients with deterioration of sexual function after surgery attributed this to de novo dyspareunia, fear of causing damage to the surgical repair, new pelvic floor symptoms, and disappointing results of surgery [38]. This highlights the importance of a thorough sexual history and evaluation prior to surgical management of pelvic floor disorders.

Sexual dysfunction may be related to issues with sexual desire, arousal, orgasm, or pain. Patients with pelvic floor disorders including pelvic organ prolapse and urinary incontinence have been shown to be affected in each of these components. In the preoperative assessment before urogynaecologic surgery, if sexual dysfunction does exist, it is critical to determine the aetiology of the problem, and counsel the patient on the likelihood of its relationship to their surgical indication, as well as the expected impact of surgery on their specific symptoms and overall sexual well-being.

Validated Questionnaires for Evaluation of Pelvic Floor Disorders

The symptomatic profile of patients with pelvic floor disorders can be quite complex. Taking a thorough and accurate history can be difficult in these patients given the interwoven relationships between vaginal, urinary, defecatory, and sexual symptoms with pelvic organ prolapse and other pelvic floor disorders. However difficult, this history is of the utmost importance if a patient is considering undergoing an elective surgical procedure to address these issues. Their quality of life and personal goals of care must be well-understood by the physician to provide the best possible pre-surgical counselling and care. A large number of symptom- and quality-of-life-specific questionnaires exist to guide this evaluation. In 2020, the Pelvic Floor Disorder Consortium, which is an international, multidisciplinary organization of urogynaecologists, colorectal surgeons, gynaecologists, urologists, gastroenterologists, and physiotherapists, collaborated to determine the best available validated tools to utilize in the initial comprehensive evaluation of urogynaecologic patients. The final collection of validated assessment tools was combined to create the Initial Measurement of Patient-Reported Pelvic Floor Complaints Tool (IMPACT) [39]. This tool is meant for use in both women and men, and addresses the spectrum of pelvic floor disorders. The questionnaires included in this tool are summarized in Table 1.1.

Of course, in addition to a targeted urogynaecologic history, one should elicit a comprehensive history including any other gynaecologic, urologic, obstetric, medical, and surgical issues that the patient may endorse. All deliveries should be investigated, including the method of delivery, degree of perineal trauma, and any relevant complications. Medical comorbidities that may worsen pelvic floor disorders should be evaluated, such as diabetes mellitus, history of stroke or other neurologic disease, musculoskeletal issues, and pulmonary conditions causing chronic cough. The surgical history should include precise details regarding history of hysterectomy or any other pelvic surgery, pelvic radiation, abdominal surgery, and any prior surgical implants such as mesh.

Physical Evaluation of the Urogynaecologic Patient

Every patient being evaluated for surgery should undergo a similarly comprehensive physical exam. Prior to urogynaecologic surgery, this exam should focus on the abdomen, pelvis, musculoskeletal, and neurologic systems. All medical comorbidities discovered during the patient assessment should be addressed as appropriate on the physical exam. Depending on the severity of the comorbidity and the extent of the planned surgery, perioperative care of medical comorbidities should be shared with the anaesthesiology and perioperative medicine teams.

Table 1.1 Validated questionnaires recommended by the Pelvic Floor Disorders Consortium (adapted from [39])

Questionnaire	Focus	Original author	Description
Pelvic Floor Distress Inventory, Short Form (PFDI-20)	Quality of life	Barber	20 questions, quantification of degree of bother related to bowel symptoms, bladder dysfunction, and pelvic organ prolapse
Urogenital Distress Inventory (UDI-6)	Urinary incontinence	Lemack	6 questions, identifies type of urinary incontinence, type and severity of symptoms, and degree of bother
ICIQ-Female Lower Urinary Tract Symptom Questionnaire Short Form (ICIQ-FLUTS)	Lower urinary tract symptoms	Brookes	25 questions, identifies type and degree of lower urinary tract symptoms, and quality of life
Pelvic Organ Prolapse/Incontinence Sexual Questionnaire, IUGA-Revised (PISQ-IR)	Sexual function	Rogers	21 questions if sexually active, 12 if sexually inactive, identifies sexual dysfunction and inactivity in women with pelvic floor disorders
Patient Assessment of Constipation-Symptoms (PAC-SYM)	Constipation	Frank	12 and 16 questions, assesses severity of the various subsets of constipation (obstructed defecation, slow transit, irritable bowel syndrome)
Constipation Severity Instrument (CSI)	Constipation	Varma	
Cleveland Clinic Florida Incontinence Scale (CCFIS)	Faecal incontinence	Jorge, Wexner	5 and 7 questions, assesses severity of fecal incontinence, as well as the impact of urgency and constipating medications on the level of severity
St Marks Incontinence Score (MIS)	Faecal incontinence	Vaizey	

Targeted Exam for Pelvic Floor Disorders

The physical exam specific to pelvic floor disorders should generally include an evaluation of the vagina, bladder, urethra, rectum, vulva and surrounding integumentary, as well as the neurologic and musculoskeletal support of the pelvic floor [40] (Table 1.2 summarizes the steps of the exam). First an external exam should be performed, ideally with the patient in the lithotomy position. Any evidence of urinary or faecal soiling, skin irritation or breakdown, or tissue discolouration should be noted. Superficial sensation can be assessed. Severe prolapse may be noted at this time as well. The labia are then separated and an evaluation of the labia minora and clitoral anatomy, vestibule, perineal body, and urethral meatus can be performed. Evidence of hypoestrogenism should be noted. The patient should be asked to Valsalva and cough vigorously; with attention paid to evidence of stress urinary incontinence (cough stress test), proximal urethral mobility, perineal body protrusion, and vaginal prolapse. Historically, a cotton swab was placed in the urethra to measure mobility of the urethral axis, but this is no longer practised given its lack of utility and patient discomfort. The genital hiatus and perineal body are measured for the pelvic organ prolapse quantification (POP-Q) examination.

A sims retractor, or one speculum blade, should then be inserted into the vagina to assess the different compartments individually. With the posterior vagina retracted inferiorly, one can examine the urethra, bladder neck, bladder, and anterior vaginal wall. The patient should be asked to Valsalva, and the extent of anterior compartment prolapse should be measured in relation to the hymen. At this time a discrimination may also be made between central cystocele versus paravaginal defect. As described by Walters, this distinction can be made by placing a forceps in the lateral vaginal sulcus with pressure toward the ischial spine [40]. If support of a flattened or bulging lateral sulci improves the anterior prolapse, then there is presumed to be a paravaginal defect. If the anterior prolapse is unchanged with this support, it is likely due to a central cystocele without a paravaginal defect.

The retractor is then used to depress the anterior vaginal wall in order to assess the posterior compartment. With Valsalva, the extent of posterior wall prolapse should be measured in relation to the hymen. Descent of the perineal body can be assessed. A digital rectal exam at this time may be useful in delineating a rectocele versus enterocele. A full speculum may then be inserted for visualization of the cervix, and evaluation of the remaining POP-Q measurements (points C and D of the vaginal apex, and the total vaginal length).

Bimanual pelvic exam should then be performed. Attention should first be paid to uterine size, position, mass, and tenderness, as well as adnexal masses/fullness or pain. An assessment of pain or tenderness over the bladder and urethra should be made by palpation. The pelvic floor muscles are then evaluated, taking note of any evidence of muscle tenderness, tightening, or shortening. This aspect of the exam is purposefully performed at the end of the vaginal portion, as it may exacerbate patient discomfort if they have myofascial pain. An effort should be made to determine which muscles specifically are affected. Pelvic floor squeeze, or Kegel, is then assessed. Strength should be graded between 0 and 5 [40]. Digital rectal exam is then performed, with attention to any masses, resting tone, and the structure and strength of external anal sphincter with squeeze. Presence of rectal mucosal prolapse, haemorrhoids, or fissure should be noted.

Additional Evaluation

In addition to the traditional history and physical exam, a number of other analyses may be useful in the evaluation of pelvic floor disorders. Common examples include urinalysis and

Table 1.2 Comprehensive physical examination for pelvic floor disorders

Examination component	Action required	Evaluation for
External inspection	▪ Visually and superficially inspect integumentary of perineum and vulva	▪ Evidence of urinary or faecal soiling ▪ Skin discolouration, irritation, breakdown ▪ Hypoestrogenism ▪ Loss of vulvar architecture ▪ Severe vaginal or rectal prolapse ▪ Superficial sensation ▪ Vulvodynia
Superficial vaginal exam	▪ Spread labia minora to inspect urethral meatus, vestibule ▪ Perform with and without Valsalva	▪ Epithelial discolouration ▪ Loss of architecture at labia minora or clitoris ▪ Hypoestrogenism ▪ Vestibulodynia ▪ Urethral discharge, mass, prolapse ▪ Cough stress test ▪ Perineal body protrusion or descent ▪ POP-Q points PB, GH
Anterior compartment exam	▪ Retract posterior vaginal wall with Sims retractor or single speculum blade ▪ Perform with and without Valsalva	▪ Periurethral masses ▪ Proximal urethral mobility ▪ Anterior compartment prolapse ▪ Paravaginal defect versus central cystocele ▪ Prolapse of vaginal apex ▪ POP-Q points Aa, Ba, C
Posterior compartment exam	▪ Retract posterior vaginal wall in similar fashion ▪ Perform with and without Valsalva	▪ Posterior compartment prolapse ▪ Descent of perineal body ▪ POP-Q points Ap, Bp ▪ Evaluation of perineal thinning, rectocele versus enterocele (may require rectovaginal exam)
Speculum exam	▪ Insert full speculum	▪ Epithelial discolouration ▪ Cervical pathology ▪ Cervical length ▪ POP-Q point TVL
Bimanual exam	• Digital bimanual pelvic exam • Perform with and without squeeze	▪ POP-Q points C and D ▪ Uterine size, position, tenderness, masses ▪ Posterior culdesac pain ▪ Rectovaginal nodularity ▪ Adnexal fullness, masses, or pain ▪ Bladder or urethral tenderness ▪ Squeeze strength (Kegel) ▪ Pelvic floor muscle tenderness or shortening
Digital rectal exam	• External and internal rectal exam • Perform with and without squeeze	▪ External anal sphincter appearance with squeeze ▪ Anal sphincter tone at rest and with squeeze ▪ External anal sphincter defects ▪ Rectal prolapse ▪ Haemorrhoids or anal fissures

*POP-Q point definitions:

Aa: 3 cm proximal to the hymen on anterior wall

Ba: most distal point of any part of anterior wall between Aa and anterior fornix (or C if no cervix)

C: most distal point of the cervix or vaginal cuff

D: point of the posterior fornix in patients with a cervix

Ap: 3 cm proximal to the hymen on posterior wall

Bp: most distal point of any part of the posterior wall between Ap and posterior fornix (or C if no cervix)

TVL: measurement of total vaginal length

GH: measurement from urethral meatus to posterior margin of the hymen

PB: measurement from posterior margin of the hymen to mid-anal opening possible culture, measurement of post-void residual volume, voiding diaries, and validated questionnaires (see Table 1.1). Urodynamic testing, cystourethroscopy, pelvic ultrasound, anorectal manometry, and endoanal ultrasound are useful in specific situations, but are not employed as part of the routine exam. Other technology such as trans-perineal ultrasound and functional MRI are actively providing a deeper understanding of pelvic floor disorders, and their utility in clinical practice continues to be an interesting line of research.

While the use of these various testing modalities varies in clinical practice, the National Institute for Health and Care Excellence (NICE) provides evidence-based recommendations for the initial evaluation of pelvic floor disorders [41]. Urinalysis is recommended for all patients with symptoms related to urinary tract infection or incontinence. Post-void residual volume is recommended for all patients at risk of voiding dysfunction or recurrent urinary tract infection, preferably by bladder scan ultrasound as opposed to catheterization. A voiding diary detailing fluid intake, urinary symptoms, and voiding volume/frequency over at least three days is recommended in all patients with symptoms of urinary incontinence or overactive bladder. Validated questionnaires should be used routinely. Urodynamic testing does not need to be performed prior to surgery for stress urinary incontinence if the patient has pure stress incontinence or stress-predominant mixed incontinence, and demonstrates stress incontinence on exam. Though, urodynamic testing should be performed if any complicating factors exist, including anterior or apical prolapse, symptoms of voiding dysfunction, urge-predominant symptoms, or prior incontinence surgery. This recommendation is consistent with data from the Value trial, though a more comprehensive review of the utility of urodynamic testing is beyond the scope of this chapter [42].

Informed Consent

The final component of patient selection and assessment is the informed consent process. In the field of urogynaecology, this process is quite complex and nuanced. The impact of pelvic floor disorders is unequivocally dependent on patient symptoms and their impact on quality of life. Surgery is rarely an absolute necessity. A host of options exists in the management of the various pelvic floor disorders, ranging from expectant management, to conservative treatments, to a number of surgical procedures. The surgical procedures themselves vary considerably in efficacy, invasiveness, and other related outcomes. As opposed to extirpative surgery, urogynaecologic procedures are reconstructive, which places an emphasis on patient-centered outcomes and complicates the informed consent process.

The centre of any informed consent discussion in urogynaecology should be the patient's goals of care. After the decision is made to proceed with surgical care, the patient and their physician should have a clear and detailed discussion that combines their goals and priorities with the expected benefits and potential risks of the various surgical options available to them. Below is a brief description of commonly performed laparoscopic procedures in urogynaecology. Later chapters provide more extensive reviews of the surgical details and data behind each procedure.

Laparoscopic Sacrocolpopexy

In laparoscopic sacrocolpopexy, the surgeon supports the prolapsing pelvic organs by fixing a graft from the vagina to the anterior longitudinal ligament near the sacral promontory. The vaginal attachment may be to the vaginal vault in a patient who has had a hysterectomy, immediately after the performance of hysterectomy, or in a uterine-sparing fashion, as in the case of sacrohysteropexy. Graft material is most commonly a synthetic, non-absorbable mesh material, but biologic materials can be used. Vaginal graft placement varies. The mesh is typically attached to the anterior vagina, apex, and posterior vagina, though it can also be attached to the perineal body as in sacrocolpoperineopexy, or the rectal wall and pelvic floor muscles as in rectopexy. Historically considered by some to be the gold standard of surgery for pelvic organ prolapse, open abdominal sacrocolpopexy is significantly more invasive than the traditional vaginal procedures for prolapse. Though with the advent of laparoscopy, abdominal sacrocolpopexy can be performed in a minimally invasive fashion with a risk profile similar to vaginal surgery. Compared to the open approach, laparoscopic sacrocolpopexy is associated with lower rates of adverse events, shorter hospital stay, and longer operative time, with similar anatomic results [43]. In a meta-analysis comparing mesh sacrocolpopexy to native tissue vaginal procedures for apical pelvic organ prolapse, sacrocolpopexy was associated with improved anatomic outcomes, similar symptomatic improvement, and potentially higher rates of adverse events [44].

Laparoscopic Uterosacral Ligament Suspension

In laparoscopic uterosacral ligament suspension, the surgeon affixes the vagina to the proximal uterosacral ligaments, in a fashion analogous to the tradition vaginal uterosacral ligament suspension. The suture material used may be either permanent or delayed-absorbable. This procedure may be performed at the time of hysterectomy using the vaginal cuff, in the setting of remote hysterectomy by using the vaginal apex, or in a uterine-sparing fashion. Laparoscopic uterosacral ligament suspension has been compared in a retrospective fashion to the vaginal approach, with varying results. While adverse events are generally equivalent, ureteral obstruction may be lower with the laparoscopic approach [18], and may be completely avoidable as long as the ureter is visualized. For prolapse outcomes, some studies report no difference [19,20], while others report an advantage to the laparoscopic approach in regards to anatomic results [21,23] and prolapse symptoms [18,22]. Though, conclusions of these retrospective studies are quite limited and prospective randomized studies are needed to accurately compare these two operations.

Laparoscopic Moschcowitz and Halban

Both laparoscopic Moschcowitz and Halban procedures are performed in an analogous fashion to the abdominal approach, and are best used as an adjunct to a different primary procedure. In the Moschcowitz procedure, a non-absorbable suture is placed circumferentially in a purse-string fashion through the peritoneum of the posterior culdesac, obliterating this space between the posterior vagina and the serosa of the rectosigmoid colon. The Halban procedure is performed by using a series of interrupted sutures from the posterior vagina to the rectosigmoid serosa. Both of these procedures intend to treat or prevent enterocele, and are not performed as a singular operation to treat pelvic organ prolapse.

Laparoscopic Paravaginal Repair

During a laparoscopic paravaginal repair, the retropubic space is entered and dissected until the pubic symphysis, Cooper's ligaments, and the bladder neck are identified. Laterally, the obturator internus muscle, obturator foramen, and arcus tendineus fasciae pelvis are identified. The lateral vagina is affixed to the arcus tendinous fasciae pelvis using four to six stitches, starting at the level of the ischial spine and moving distally, with care to avoid the bladder neck. The efficacy of paravaginal repair has been debated. While some suggest that a paravaginal repair for treatment of a cystocele provides a more appropriate restoration of anatomy without compromising vaginal length, others argue that a vaginal approach is more appropriate as an isolated operation. In regards to apical prolapse, data is mixed, with some studies showing no difference when paravaginal repair is added to laparoscopic sacrocolpopexy or uterosacral suspension, and others touting low recurrence rates and low adverse events when the procedures are combined [45,46]. This remains an area in need of further research.

Laparoscopic Pectopexy

Laparoscopic pectopexy is a relatively new approach to the repair of pelvic organ prolapse. In this procedure, the surgeon enters the retropubic space and dissects down to identify Cooper's ligament (pectineal ligament). Permanent sutures affix a synthetic mesh from the ligament to either the anterior vaginal cuff, cervical stump, or anterior vagina and cervix in the case of hysteropexy. This procedure has been compared to vaginal sacrospinous ligament suspension [47] and laparoscopic sacropexy [48], with similar results related to anatomical outcomes and patient satisfaction, but potential advantages of pectopexy in regards to sexual and defecatory function. Conclusions cannot be made on the outcomes of this procedure given a paucity of data, but the available studies are encouraging and suggest more research is warranted.

Laparoscopic Uterine-Sparing Procedures for Prolapse

Recently, uterine-sparing procedures have been more commonly offered and performed during the surgical treatment of pelvic organ prolapse. A number of laparoscopic procedures for prolapse can be modified to perform as a uterine-sparing procedure, or hysteropexy. Common laparoscopic hysteropexy procedures include sacrohysteropexy, uterosacral hysteropexy, and pectohysteropexy. In a recent systematic review, when compared to sacrocolpopexy, sacrohysteropexy outcomes are similar in regards to prolapse recurrence, while reducing mesh exposure, operative time, blood loss, and surgical cost [49]. Compared to vaginal hysterectomy with uterosacral ligament suspension, mesh sacrohysteropexy was also associated with improvements in the C-point and total vaginal length. These outcomes are promising and suggest that uterine-sparing options should be offered to patients during counselling for pelvic organ prolapse surgery. Though, the benefits must be weighed against unknown long-term outcomes, as well as the future risk of uterine pathology after hysteropexy.

Laparoscopic Burch Urethropexy

Laparoscopic Burch urethropexy is the primary laparoscopic procedure for stress urinary incontinence. In this procedure, the surgeon enters the retropubic space, and dissects down to identify the pubic symphysis, Cooper's ligament, and the bladder neck. One to two non-absorbable stitches are placed lateral to the midurethra and bladder neck, and affixed to Cooper's ligament, using a vaginal hand for assistance in identifying the appropriate amount of bladder neck elevation. This procedure has become less common with the advent of vaginal midurethral synthetic slings. Though, given the current climate surrounding mesh use in urogynaecology, some surmise that laparoscopic colposuspension will become more commonly performed in the future. A recent systematic review supported this possibility, noting minimal differences in patient outcomes between laparoscopic Burch urethropexy when compared to either open Burch or midurethral synthetic sling [15].

Conclusion

The laparoscopic approach to urogynaecologic surgery is a rapidly evolving, contemporary approach to the treatment of pelvic floor disorders. While traditional open abdominal and vaginal procedures are more well-studied, the benefits of laparoscopy can be significant, including improved patient safety and recovery parameters, potential advantages in surgical efficacy, and the ability to perform increasingly complex surgical procedures. The basic principles of preoperative surgical assessment should be maintained in these patients, and the general nuances of risks in laparoscopic surgery should be considered. The evaluation of urogynaecologic patients should be thorough and systematic, acknowledging the complex interactions that occur amongst pelvic floor disorders, with a constant focus on improving quality of life. With the continued increase in accessibility and training in laparoscopic surgery, an increasing number of surgeons will possess the skills to improve the lives of urogynaecologic patients.

References

1. Jaschinski T, Mosch CG, Eikermann M, Neugebauer EAM, Sauerland S. Laparoscopic versus open surgery for suspected appendicitis. Cochrane Database Syst Rev 2018; 11: CD001546.
2. Hajibandeh S, Hajibandeh S, Sreh A, Khan A, Subar D, Jones L. Laparoscopic versus open umbilical or paraumbilical hernia repair: a systematic review and meta-analysis. Hernia 2017; 21(6): 905–16.
3. Bonjer HJ, Deijen CL, Abis GA, Cuesta MA, van der Pas MH, de Lange-de Klerk ES, Lacy AM, Bemelman WA, Andersson J, Angenete E, Rosenberg J, Fuerst A, Haglind E. A randomized trial of laparoscopic versus open surgery for rectal cancer. N Engl J Med 2015; 372(14): 1324–32.

4. Thompson, J. (2019). *Smith and Aitkenhead's Textbook of Anaesthesia*, 7th edn. Elsevier Limited.
5. Gutt CN, Oniu T, Mehrabi A, Schemmer P, Kashfi A, Kraus T, Büchler MW. Circulatory and respiratory complications of carbon dioxide insufflation. Dig Surg 2004; 21(2): 95–105.
6. Hatipoglu S, Akbulut S, Hatipoglu F, Abdullayev R. Effect of laparoscopic abdominal surgery on splanchnic circulation: historical developments. World J Gastroenterol 2014; 20(48): 18165–76.
7. Chiu AW, Chang LS, Birkett DH, Babayan RK. The impact of pneumoperitoneum, pneumoretroperitoneum, and gasless laparoscopy on the systemic and renal hemodynamics. J Am Coll Surg 1995; 181(5): 397–406.
8. Closhen D, Treiber AH, Berres M, Sebastiani A, Werner C, Engelhard K, Schramm P. Robotic-assisted prostatic surgery in the Trendelenburg position does not impair cerebral oxygenation measured using two different monitors: a clinical observational study. Eur J Anaesthesiol 2014; 31(2): 104–9.
9. Ahmad G, Baker J, Finnerty J, Phillips K, Watson A. Laparoscopic entry techniques. Cochrane Database Syst Rev 2019; 1: CD006583. Available at: www.cochrane.org/CD006583/MENSTR_laparoscopic-entry-techniques
10. Pommergaard HC, Burcharth J, Danielsen A, Angenete E, Haglind E, Rosenberg J. No consensus on restrictions on physical activity to prevent incisional hernias after surgery. Hernia 2014; 18(4): 495–500.
11. Mueller MG, Lewicky-Gaupp C, Collins SA, Abernethy MG, Alverdy A, Kenton K. Activity restriction recommendations and outcomes after reconstructive pelvic surgery. Obstet Gynecol 2017; 129(4): 608–14.
12. Linder BJ, Occhino JA, Habermann EB, Glasgow AE, Bews KA, Gershman B. A national contemporary analysis of perioperative outcomes of open versus minimally invasive sacrocolpopexy. J Urol 2018; 200(4): 862–7.
13. Coolen AWM, van Oudheusden AMJ, Mol BWJ, van Eijndhoven HWF, Roovers JWR, Bongers MY. Laparoscopic sacrocolpopexy compared with open abdominal sacrocolpopexy for vault prolapse repair: a randomised controlled trial. Int Urogynecol J 2017; 28(10): 1469–79.
14. Maher C, Feiner B, Baessler K, Christmann-Schmid C, Haya N, Brown J. Surgery for women with apical vaginal prolapse. Cochrane Database Syst Rev 2016; 1(10): CD012376.
15. Freites J, Stewart F, Omar MI, Mashayekhi A, Agur WI. Laparoscopic colposuspension for urinary incontinence in women. Cochrane Database Syst Rev 2019; 10(12): CD002239.
16. Paraiso MF, Jelovsek JE, Frick A, Chen CC, Barber MD. Laparoscopic compared with robotic sacrocolpopexy for vaginal prolapse: a randomized controlled trial. Obstet Gynecol 2011; 118(5): 1005–13.
17. Serati M, Bogani G, Sorice P, Braga A, Torella M, Salvatore S, … Ghezzi F. Robot-assisted sacrocolpopexy for pelvic organ prolapse: a systematic review and meta-analysis of comparative studies. Eur Urol 2014; 66(2): 303–18.
18. Houlihan S, Kim-Fine S, Birch C, Tang S, Brennand EA. Uterosacral vault suspension (USLS) at the time of hysterectomy: laparoscopic versus vaginal approach. Int Urogynecol J 2019; 30(4): 611–21.
19. Gutman RE, Rardin CR, Sokol ER, Matthews C, Park AJ, Iglesia CB, Geoffrion R, Sokol AI, Karram M, Cundiff GW, Blomquist JL, Barber MD. Vaginal and laparoscopic mesh hysteropexy for uterovaginal prolapse: a parallel cohort study. Am J Obstet Gynecol 2017; 216(1): 38.e1–38.e11.
20. Haj-Yahya R, Chill HH, Levin G, Reuveni-Salzman A, Shveiky D. Laparoscopic uterosacral ligament hysteropexy vs total vaginal hysterectomy with uterosacral ligament suspension for anterior and apical prolapse: surgical outcome and patient satisfaction. J Minim Invasive Gynecol 2020; 27(1): 88–93.
21. Lone F, Curnow T, Thomas SA. Laparoscopic sacrohysteropexy versus vaginal hysterectomy for uterovaginal prolapse using validated questionnaires: 2-year prospective study. Int Urogynecol J 2018; 29(1): 71–9.
22. Şükür YE, Dökmeci F, Çetinkaya ŞE, Seval MM. Comparison of patient-reported outcomes, pelvic floor function and recurrence after laparoscopic sacrohysteropexy versus vaginal hysterectomy with McCall suspension for advanced uterine prolapse. Eur J Obstet Gynecol Reprod Biol 2020; 14(247): 127–31.
23. Rahmanou P, Price N, Jackson SR. Laparoscopic hysteropexy versus vaginal hysterectomy for the treatment of uterovaginal prolapse: a prospective randomized pilot study. Int Urogynecol J 2015; 26(11): 1687–94.
24. Maher CF, Feiner B, DeCuyper EM, Nichlos CJ, Hickey KV, O'Rourke P. Laparoscopic sacral colpopexy versus total vaginal mesh for vaginal vault prolapse: a randomized trial. Am J Obstet Gynecol 2011; 204(4): 360.e1–7.
25. Tan JS, Lukacz ES, Menefee SA, Powell CR, Nager CW. San Diego Pelvic Floor Consortium. Predictive value of prolapse symptoms: a large database study. Int Urogynecol J Pelvic Floor Dysfunct 2005; 16(3): 203–9.
26. Carberry C, Tulikangas P, Ridgeway B, Collins S, Adam R. American Urogynecologic Society Best Practice Statement: Evaluation and counseling of patients with pelvic organ prolapse. Female Pelvic Med Reconstr Surg 2017; 23(5): 281–7.
27. van der Ploeg JM, van der Steen A, Zwolsman S, van der Vaart CH, Roovers J. Prolapse surgery with or without incontinence procedure: a systematic review and meta-analysis. BJOG 2018; 125(3): 289–97.
28. Baessler K, Christmann-Schmid C, Maher C, Haya N, Crawford TJ, Brown J. Surgery for women with pelvic organ prolapse with or without stress urinary incontinence. Cochrane Database Syst Rev 2018; 8: CD013108.
29. de Boer TA, Salvatore S, Cardozo L, Chapple C, Kelleher C, van Kerrebroeck P, Kirby MG, Koelbl H, Espuna-Pons M, Milsom I, Tubaro A, Wagg A, Vierhout ME. Pelvic organ prolapse and overactive bladder. Neurourol Urodyn 2010; 29(1): 30–9.
30. Jelovsek JE, Barber MD, Paraiso MF, Walters MD. Functional bowel and anorectal disorders in patients with pelvic organ prolapse and incontinence. Am J Obstet Gynecol 2005; 193(6): 2105–11.
31. Bradley CS, Nygaard IE, Brown MB, Gutman RE, Kenton KS, Whitehead WE, Goode PS, Wren PA, Ghetti C, Weber AM, Pelvic Floor Disorders Network. Bowel symptoms in women 1 year after sacrocolpopexy. Am J Obstet Gynecol 2007; 197(6): 642.e1–8.
32. Grimes CL, Lukacz ES, Gantz MG, Warren LK, Brubaker L, Zyczynski HM, Richter HE, Jelovsek JE, Cundiff G, Fine P, Visco AG, Zhang M, Meikle S, NICHD Pelvic Floor Disorders Network. What happens to the posterior compartment and bowel symptoms after sacrocolpopexy? Evaluation of 5-year outcomes from E-CARE. Female Pelvic Med Reconstr Surg 2014; 20(5): 261–6.

33. Lewis C, Salamon C, Priestley JL, Gurshumov E, Culligan P. Prospective cohort study of bowel function after robotic sacrocolpopexy. Female Pelvic Med Reconstr Surg 2014; 20(2): 87–9.

34. Barber MD, Brubaker L, Burgio KL, Richter HE, Nygaard I, Weidner AC, Menefee SA, Lukacz ES, Norton P, Schaffer J, Nguyen JN, Borello-France D, Goode PS, Jakus-Waldman S, Spino C, Warren LK, Gantz MG, Meikle SF; Eunice Kennedy Shriver National Institute of Child Health and Human Development Pelvic Floor Disorders Network. Comparison of 2 transvaginal surgical approaches and perioperative behavioral therapy for apical vaginal prolapse: the OPTIMAL randomized trial. JAMA 2014; 311(10): 1023–34. https://doi.org/10.1001/jama.2014.1719.

35. Jha S, Gray T. A systematic review and meta-analysis of the impact of native tissue repair for pelvic organ prolapse on sexual function. Int Urogynecol J 2015; 26(3): 321–7.

36. Jha S, Ammenbal M, Metwally M. Impact of incontinence surgery on sexual function: a systematic review and meta-analysis. J Sex Med 2012; 9(1): 34–43.

37. Duralde ER, Rowen TS. Urinary incontinence and associated female sexual dysfunction. Sex Med Rev 2017; 5(4): 470–85.

38. Roos AM, Thakar R, Sultan AH, de Leeuw JW, Paulus AT. The impact of pelvic floor surgery on female sexual function: a mixed quantitative and qualitative study. BJOG 2014; 121(1): 92–100; discussion 101.

39. Bordeianou LG, Anger JT, Boutros M et al. Measuring pelvic floor disorder symptoms using patient-reported instruments. Proceedings of the Consensus Meeting of the Pelvic Floor Consortium of the American Society of Colon and Rectal Surgeons, the International Continence Society, the American Urogynecologic Society, and the Society of Urodynamics, Female Pelvic Medicine and Urogenital Reconstruction. Female Pelvic Med Reconstr Surg 2020; 26(1): 1–15.

40. Walters MD. Evaluation of urinary incontinence and pelvic organ prolapse: history, physical examination, and office tests. In MD Walters (ed.), *Urogynecology and Reconstructive Pelvic Surgery*, 4th edn. Saunders, pp 117–29.

41. National Institute for Health and Care Excellence. Guideline 123. Urinary incontinence and pelvic organ prolapse in women: management. Published 2019. Available at: www.nice.org.uk/guidance/ng123

42. Nager CW, Brubaker L, Litman HJ et al. A randomized trial of urodynamic testing before stress-incontinence surgery. N Engl J Med 2012; 366(21): 1987–97.

43. De Gouveia De Sa M, Claydon LS, Whitlow B, Dolcet Artahona MA. Laparoscopic versus open sacrocolpopexy for treatment of prolapse of the apical segment of the vagina: a systematic review and meta-analysis. Int Urogynecol J 2016; 27(1): 3–17.

44. Siddiqui NY, Grimes CL, Casiano ER, Abed HT, Jeppson PC, Olivera CK, Sanses TV, Steinberg AC, South MM, Balk EM, Sung VW. Mesh sacrocolpopexy compared with native tissue vaginal repair: a systematic review and meta-analysis. Obstet Gynecol 2015; 125(1): 44–55.

45. Shippey SH, Quiroz LH, Sanses TV, Knoepp LR, Cundiff GW, Handa VL. Anatomic outcomes of abdominal sacrocolpopexy with or without paravaginal repair. Int Urogynecol J 2010; 21(3): 279–83.

46. Behnia-Willison F, Seman EI, Cook JR, O'Shea RT, Keirse MJ. Laparoscopic paravaginal repair of anterior compartment prolapse. J Minim Invasive Gynecol 2007; 14(4): 475–80.

47. Astepe BS, Karsli A, Köleli I, Aksakal OS, Terzi H, Kale A. Intermediate-term outcomes of laparoscopic pectopexy and vaginal sacrospinous fixation: a comparative study. Int Braz J Urol 2019; 45(5): 999–1007.

48. Noé KG, Schiermeier S, Alkatout I, Anapolski M. Laparoscopic pectopexy: a prospective, randomized, comparative clinical trial of standard laparoscopic sacral colpocervicopexy with the new laparoscopic pectopexy-postoperative results and intermediate-term follow-up in a pilot study. J Endourol 2015; 29(2): 210–15.

49. Meriwether KV, Antosh DD, Olivera CK, et al. Uterine preservation vs hysterectomy in pelvic organ prolapse surgery: a systematic review with meta-analysis and clinical practice. Am J Obstet Gynecol 2018; 219(2): 129–46.

Chapter 2 Patient Counselling and the Consent Process for Laparoscopic Urogynaecology

Swati Jha

Introduction and Background

Surgery can be distressing for many patients and lack of information is the single biggest reason for negativity around the procedure. One of the most difficult issues is fear of the unknown, and a failure to provide information regarding the risks and benefits of the surgery, as well as what to expect after the procedure, may perpetuate this. Sudden admission to hospital due to unexpected ill health can cause unpreparedness for surgery, however for elective procedures, many of the factors that result in anxiety and lack of preparation are avoidable.

Urogynaecology surgery is almost always elective and is aimed at improving quality of life usually in an already healthy patient. Patients are therefore less accepting of adverse outcomes, hence adequate preoperative preparation and counselling of patients plays an important role in meeting patient expectations. In addition, there is no justification for failing to adequately counsel and consent patients prior to urogynaecology procedures, including laparoscopic urogynaecology procedures, which are classed as major surgery and have the potential for causing considerable harm when the surgery does not go to plan.

To reach a decision regarding clinical treatment various factors are at play, including the best clinical evidence, the individual clinical expertise and the patient's values and expectations. The interplay of these factors determines patient choice in reaching a decision on how to proceed where surgery is indicated.

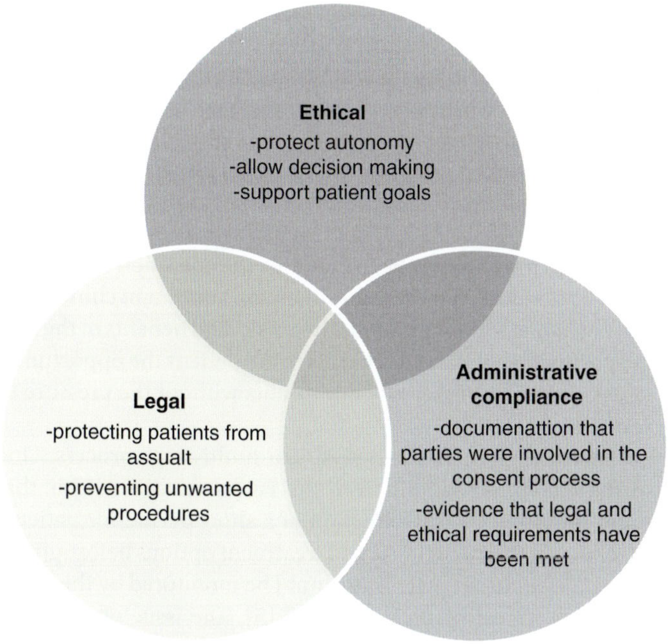

Figure 2.1 The various overlapping purposes of informed consent [23].

Informed Consent

Informed consent guides the ethical practice of medicine and is the chief paradigm for protection of the legal rights of patients. The main purpose of informed consent has three overlapping themes. These are shown in Figure 2.1.

The four principal elements required for informed consent to be valid include the clinician disclosing details of the treatment options to allow the patient to make an informed decision; the patient having the capacity to understand the information provided and make decisions leading from this; the patient demonstrating an understanding of the options provided; and finally, the patient authorizing the treatment plan. This final component of the process is the only part that is captured as a signature on the consent form.

The legal origins of written consent date back to 1914, when it was established that a patient had the 'right to determine what shall be done with their body' [1]. However, the concept of informed consent which required a physician to disclose details of the actual treatment emerged in the 1950s [2]. Informed consent protects a patient's right to autonomy, inviolability, and self-determination. The focus of informed consent in UK law is based on the standards expected by a 'reasonable patient', which has been a shift from the standards expected of a 'reasonable clinician' as stated in the *Bolam* principle.

The ethical basis of informed consent is more theoretical and is aimed at ensuring the patient's priorities, expectations and values are respected and achieved as part of the treatment. This also shifts the basis of informed consent to a more patient-centric approach. This would also imply that obtaining consent is not a one-step intervention but a process that requires the patient's expectations of treatment to be taken into account prior to the signing of the actual consent document. It is important therefore to make a distinction between the consent form and consent process. The form should merely be a validation of the process having taken place.

The administrative purpose of informed consent is to ensure this consent process has taken place. So, it would be highly unlikely that a patient would reach the operating theatre without a signed valid consent. This should not however shift the focus of the consent process from the detailed discussion to explain the procedure and its alternatives to obtaining a signature on a form.

Studies into the quality of informed consent in invasive procedures have shown half of all patients did not recall receiving explanations about risks and two thirds did not recall discussion of alternative options [3]. There was also a huge variation in the expectations about decisions, with 60% favouring shared decision-making, 20% wishing autonomous decision-making, and the remaining 20% wishing the clinician to make the decision on their behalf. A study by Geoffrion et al [4] evaluating patients' learning after an educational programme for women with incontinence and pelvic organ prolapse demonstrated that even after a 2.5 hour nurse-led workshop on pelvic floor health, knowledge scores were not 100%, though they were significantly improved from the pre-workshop knowledge scores.

Change in the Law

In 2015, the ruling of the supreme court in the case of *Montgomery v Lanarkshire Health Board* changed the practice of consent (*Montgomery v Lanarkshire Health Board* [2015] UKSC 11).

In 1999, Nadine Montgomery was pregnant with her first child, Sam. She was known to have type 1 diabetes and expressed concerns during her pregnancy that the size of her baby might lead to difficulties with a vaginal delivery. She continued to express these concerns throughout her pregnancy. There was a failure to discuss the risk of shoulder dystocia occurring and a plan was made for vaginal delivery. During her delivery, shoulder dystocia occurred with a 12-minute delay between the delivery of the head and shoulders. This resulted in a significant hypoxic injury causing brain damage and cerebral palsy in her child. The case made by Mrs Montgomery was that the consultant had failed to discuss the risks of shoulder dystocia and the potential significance of it occurring or the alternative option of a caesarean section. This impeded her ability to make a fully informed decision. The consultant accepted that the overall risk of shoulder dystocia occurring in a woman with diabetes was 10% but risks of a serious consequence such as a brachial plexus injury (0.2%) or hypoxic injury (0.1%) were relatively low. As these serious risks were felt to be small, they were not discussed. The consultant obstetrician also stated that the risks would have been mentioned if specific questions had been asked. This practice refers to the ruling of Lord Diplock in Sidaway (*Sidaway v Board of Governors of the Bethlem Royal Hospital* [1985] AC 871) who advised that if a specific question was asked, it should be answered. However, this would require a patient to have a level of knowledge that a patient without the background knowledge cannot be expected to have. The Montgomery case was heard at the UK Supreme Court in July 2014. The argument in this appeal was that it was not appropriate to use the accepted practice of a body of reasonable medical practitioners when consent is considered. It should therefore be viewed differently from the process of diagnosis or treatment where the rule of Bolam (*Bolam v Friern Hospital Management Committee* [1957] 1 WLR 582) was still standard and acceptable.

The focus of consent shifted from what the reasonable clinician would inform the patient of to what the reasonable patient would want to know. This shifted the focus of consent discussion to the specific needs of each patient.

Following the Montgomery ruling, '*The law on consent has progressed from doctor focused to patient focused. The practice of medicine has moved significantly away from the idea of the paternalistic doctor who tells their patient what to do, even if this was thought to be in the patient's best interests. A patient is autonomous and should be supported to make decisions about their own health and to take ownership of the fact that sometimes success is uncertain and complications can occur despite the best treatment.*'

Interestingly, the principles identified in this landmark ruling had already been stipulated and highlighted several years earlier by the General Medical Council (GMC) in its document on 'Good Medical Practice' [5].

Counselling for Laparoscopic Urogynaecology Procedures

One of the biggest problems in relation to counselling is that this is difficult to standardize unlike surgical procedures where a specific set of steps would be considered necessary for safe surgical practice. Consenting practices were compared between trainees and consultants with specific reference to the documentation of significant risks of surgery [6]. More often than not, patients were not provided with consistent information to make informed choices. This study suggested preprinted consent forms in an attempt to standardize the process of consent.

The issue of informed consent is contentious and a patient's signature on a consent form is not valid evidence of this. Though it may demonstrate that the patient has given consent to carry out the procedure, it is not proof that this is informed consent. As previously discussed, for consent to be informed and therefore valid, it must be given voluntarily and freely, without pressure or undue influence, by an appropriately informed person who has the capacity to consent to the intervention in question.

In the context of surgery, the patient should be competent to take the particular decision, have received sufficient information to make an informed decision, and should not be acting under duress. This third issue may be pertinent if consent is obtained on the day of surgery. The GMC recommends a cooling-off period between obtaining consent and the surgical procedure. This is because even though a majority of patients will be clear about their intentions to proceed with surgery, some may have doubts if new information comes to light that was not previously discussed. Having these doubts arise on the day of surgery may induce the patient to make a decision under duress, as all plans have already been made for the operation to proceed.

It is therefore more sensible to obtain consent in clinic at the time of listing for surgery and when risks and benefits of the surgery are being explained. This gives the patient the opportunity to ask questions and clarify any doubts without the pressure to proceed.

Increasingly, consent is seen as a multi-stage process. One of the recommendations from the Peterson report [7] is that there should be an 'introduction of a short period for patients to reflect on their diagnosis and treatment options before giving their consent to surgery. This should be monitored by the GMC as part of 'Good Medical Practice' [5]. The issue of duress to proceed with surgery was mentioned by patients in the enquiry too. Even in cases where surgery is scheduled very soon after the decision has been made, there should be adequate time for a patient to reflect on their diagnosis and treatment options to ensure they are giving informed consent for their treatment.

A study aimed at investigating how well women understand their condition and treatment alternatives when agreeing to a sacrocolpopexy showed some worrying results [8]. Despite detailed preoperative discussions, women had deficiencies in their understanding and this study recommended better ways of educating patients and ensuring their comprehension prior to such major surgery. Interestingly, the variation in the patient's knowledge scores was not surgeon-dependent. The authors recommend that preoperative education and discussion to allow realistic expectations of the surgery is essential.

Informed consent once obtained remains valid for an indefinite period. For surgical procedures therefore, provided the patient's condition has not changed, and/or new information concerning the proposed intervention or alternative treatments have not come to light in the intervening period, the consent still stands. It would however be expected that if consent was obtained in advance, the details mentioned are checked again on the day of surgery.

The common complications a patient should be informed of prior to laparoscopic urogynaecology surgery are shown in Table 2.1.

Table 2.1 Complications of laparoscopic urogynaecology procedures

Infection
Bleeding and need for blood transfusion
Clots in legs and lungs (thrombosis)
Injury to bladder, bowels and ureters
Need for open surgery (laparotomy)
Failure
Recurrence
Failure to achieve the desired result
Chronic pain
Sexual problems
For continence procedures, additional risks of voiding problems, need for self-catheterization, and overactive bladder should be discussed.
Where mesh is used, additional risks of mesh exposure and extrusion into adjacent organs and the need for further surgery to deal with these complications should be discussed.

Patient Information Leaflets

Patient information leaflets (PIL) should be provided in all cases and constitute a legal requirement. The use of PIL has been shown to enhance a patient's understanding of their condition and proposed treatment. They are also helpful in making patients feel more involved in the surgical decision-making process; however, they do not influence overall outcome or satisfaction metrics [9,10]. PIL are widely used as a source of information but should be clear and easy to understand. They should allow the patient sufficient understanding to act on it and should be used to compliment not substitute for face to face discussion with the patient. It is recommended that when producing a PIL, the language is kept simple and a reading age of 11 years is advisable. Jargon and medical terminology should be avoided, and it should be tested in the population in which it is going to be used. Organizations such as the International Urogynaecology Association (IUGA) and the British Society of Urogynaecology (BSUG) have produced valid leaflets for most of the laparoscopic urogynaecology procedures. Problems may however arise in non-English-speaking women when consent needs to be obtained. Whereas IUGA have translated several of their leaflets, this is not feasible for every language, and this is a limitation which is difficult to address.

Procedure-specific Consent Forms

Procedure-specific consent forms (PSCF) have been identified as a means of standardizing the consent process for surgery. Studies into the use of PSCF suggest that the list of complications should be agreed by national regulating bodies to ensure that all nationally standardized lists of complications are captured in the form [11,12]. Otherwise, there can be huge variations in the contents of these forms. This form can then be used as a prompt for the discussion and documentation of risk rather than being the sole tool used.

Patient Decision Aids

Patient decision aids (PDA) allow for shared decision-making, allowing patients to make decisions about their healthcare that take into account their personal values and preferences [13]. They make it easier for patients and clinicians to discuss treatment options [14–16]. A PDA has the following objectives:

- Encourage active participation by the patient in the decision-making process
- Inform patients of the evidence base to the available options
- Enable patients to identify what is important to them so that their choices reflect their preferences and values.

In a recent study [17] investigating the role of PDA in the clinical management of women with urinary incontinence it was shown that 'The use of a PDA in the surgical treatment of stress urinary incontinence reduces decision conflict and ensures patients are sure of their decision, understand the information provided as well as the risk-benefit ratio of the various options, and feel they have adequate support and advice to make a choice.'

The National Institute for Health and Care Excellence (NICE) [18], in its guidance on the management of urinary incontinence and prolapse, have recommended the use of PDA when consenting women for incontinence and prolapse procedures. NICE have developed PDAs for women with uterine prolapse (which includes comparative data for sacrohysteropexy), vault prolapse (which includes comparative data for sacrocolpopexy), and urinary incontinence (which includes comparative data for laparoscopic colposuspension). These commonly performed laparoscopic urogynaecology procedures are therefore included as part of the NICE PDAs. Comparative data for other procedures performed for the same condition are also available in these PDAs based on existing research and evidence.

For some of the less commonly performed laparoscopic urogynaecology procedures, such as paravaginal repairs, there are no existing PDAs and therefore it is important that patients are adequately counselled and a detailed discussion of the procedure, together with the alternatives as well as their risks, takes place. In addition, the existing evidence for these procedures is more limited, making it more difficult to counsel, and clinician bias and preferences may play a role. The lack of evidence and long-term data should be made explicitly clear to the patient as part of the consent process, so that they are aware of this.

Duty of Candour

The word candour describes a quality of being honest and open. In 2015, the GMC document *'Openness and honesty when things go wrong: the professional duty of candour'* was published and sent to doctors with a license to practice [19]. This lays out the responsibilities of individuals when things go wrong, but duty of candour (DoC) would also extend to being honest and open with patients.

There is an obvious learning curve for laparoscopic urogynaecology procedures [20,21]. When training to perform these procedures, they take longer to complete but no difference in the success of the procedure was noted. Though complications were higher in the training phase, these did not reach statistical significance [22]. Therefore, when trainee surgeons are going to perform this procedure, it is incumbent on the surgeon to make the patient aware of this.

Duty of Candour has now become a legal requirement and is a contractual duty imposed on all NHS organizations.

Conclusion

Inherently, laparoscopic urogynaecology procedures are quite complex, hence difficult for a patient to comprehend. The patient is required to understand the anatomy of the pelvic floor and how their own anatomy is different from the normal. In addition, use of medical terminology may add to the confusion. In laparoscopic urogynaecology procedures, more than one clinical visit is to be highly recommended, to allow an improvement in the level of understanding of the proposed interventions through multiple patient contacts and preoperative education. The first clinical consultations should be utilized to make a provisional diagnosis and, where surgery is an option or likely, to introduce the concept of this surgery, with a view to further review and discuss these surgeries in more detail at a subsequent visit once the patient has had an opportunity to read the PIL on the procedure. Consideration should be given to the use of PDA and PSCF to aid the counselling and preoperative discussions.

In conclusion, when counselling and obtaining informed consent for laparoscopic urogynaecology procedures, the discussion should include the diagnosis, options and various alternatives for treatment, the proposed treatment, risks and benefits of all options, and the risks and benefits of declining surgical treatment. Only when all these components of the consent process have been achieved and understood should a signature be obtained on the consent form, as this is the final step of the consent process. This ensures our legal, ethical and administrative obligations as clinicians consenting patients for complex surgery are fulfilled.

References

1. N.Y.125 1NE9. *Schloendorff v Society of New York Hospital*. Vol 211. 1914.
2. Berg JW, Appelbaum PS, Lidz CW, Parker LS. The legal requirements for disclosure and consent: history and current status. In: *Informed Consent: Legal Theory and Clinical Practice*, 2nd edn. Oxford University Press; 2001, p. 41–74.
3. Brezis M, Israel S, Weinstein-Birenshtock A, Pogoda P, Sharon A, Tauber R. Quality of informed consent for invasive procedures. Int J Qual Health Care 2008; 20(5): 352–7.
4. Geoffrion R, Robert M, Ross S, et al. Evaluating patient learning after an educational program for women with incontinence and pelvic organ prolapse. Int Urogynecol J Pelvic Floor Dysfunct 2009; 20(10): 1243–52.
5. General Medical Council. Good Medical Practice: Consent: patients and doctors making decisions together. Published 2008.
6. Chen AM, Leff DR, Simpson J, Chadwick SJ, McDonald PJ. Variations in consenting practice for laparoscopic cholecystectomy. Ann R Coll Surg Engl 2006; 88(5): 482–5.
7. Jones G. Report of the Independent Inquiry into the Issues raised by Paterson. Published 2020. Available at: https://assets.publishing.service.gov.uk/government/uploads/system/uploads/attachment_data/file/863211/issues-raised-by-paterson-independent-inquiry-report-web-accessible.pdf
8. Adams SR, Hacker MR, Merport MA, Rosenblatt PL, Elkadry EA. Informed consent for sacrocolpopexy: is counseling effective in achieving patient comprehension? Female Pelvic Med Reconstr Surg 2012; 18(6): 352–6.
9. Ashraff S, Malawa G, Dolan T, Khanduja V. Prospective randomised controlled trial on the role of patient information leaflets in obtaining informed consent. ANZ J Surg 2006; 76(3): 139–41.
10. Bayram JM, Lawson GM, Hamilton DF. The impact of a preoperative information leaflet on expectation management, satisfaction and patient outcomes in patients undergoing knee arthroscopy. Knee 2019; 26(5): 1026–31.
11. Courtney MJ, Royle TJ. Current use of procedure-specific consent forms for laparoscopic cholecystectomy. Ann R Coll Surg Engl 2018; 100(6): 446–9.
12. Courtney MJ, Royle TJ. Pre-made consent for elective inguinal hernia repair: the need for standardisation –a survey of all UK NHS Trusts. Hernia 2018; 22(3): 549–53.
13. McAlpine K, Lewis KB, Trevena LJ, Stacey D. What is the effectiveness of patient decision aids for cancer-related decisions? A systematic review subanalysis. JCO Clin Cancer Inform 2018; 2: 1–13.
14. Reder M, Kolip P. Does a decision aid improve informed choice in mammography screening? Study protocol for a randomized controlled trial. BMC Womens Health 2015; 22(15): 53.
15. Stacey D, Legare F, Lewis K, et al. Decision aids for people facing health treatment or screening decisions. Cochrane Database Syst Rev 2017; 12(4): CD001431.
16. Stacey D, Legare F, Lewis KB. Patient decision aids to engage adults in treatment or screening decisions. JAMA 2017; 318(7): 657–8.

17. Jha S, Duckett J. Utility of patient decision aids (PDA) in stress urinary incontinence surgery. Int Urogynecol J 2019; 30(9): 1483–6.
18. National Institute for Health and Care Excellence. Urinary incontinence and pelvic organ prolapse in women: management [NG123]. Published 2019.
19. General Medical Council. Openness and honesty when things go wrong: the professional duty of candour. Published 2015.
20. Claerhout F, Verguts J, Werbrouck E, Veldman J, Lewi P, Deprest J. Analysis of the learning process for laparoscopic sacrocolpopexy: identification of challenging steps. Int Urogynecol J 2014; 25(9): 1185–91.
21. Mowat A, Maher C, Pelecanos A. Can the learning curve of laparoscopic sacrocolpopexy be reduced by a structured training program? Female Pelvic Med Reconstr Surg 2018; 24(4): 272–6.
22. Vandendriessche D, Giraudet G, Lucot JP, Behal H, Cosson M. Impact of laparoscopic sacrocolpopexy learning curve on operative time, perioperative complications and short-term results. Eur J Obstet Gynecol Reprod Biol 2015; 191: 84–9.
23. Hall DE, Prochazka AV, Fink AS. Informed consent for clinical treatment. CMAJ 2012; 184(5): 533–40.

Chapter 3

Measuring Outcomes in Urogynaecologic Surgery

Philip M Toozs-Hobson, Dudley Robinson, Ilias Liapis

Introduction

> When I operate almost all my patients are cured. You know what I mean
>
> Jerry Blaivas famously wrote this in an editorial in *Neurourology and Urodynamics* and with this statement he opened the debate about measuring outcomes in pelvic floor medicine.

The measurement of outcome is essential in clinical practice, although traditionally has often been subjective and based on the views, and inherent prejudices, of both patients and surgeons. Whilst the importance of robust outcome measures has long been acknowledged in clinical research, it is only more recently that the importance in clinical practice has been acknowledged as the realization that 'big data' and routine data collection is important [1].

The need for measuring outcome has been driven within urogynaecology by a need to understand, and define success, in terms of improvement in symptoms of pelvic floor dysfunction and is also regarded as important by those who commission and pay for urogynaecological services. More recently, given the concerns regarding the use of synthetic mesh for incontinence and urogenital prolapse it has also been important in terms of clinical governance and potential litigation.

Outcomes may be measured objectively or subjectively, and this chapter will focus on the subjective outcomes used within urogynaecological surgery, with a particular focus on laparoscopic procedures.

Limitations in Research in Pelvic Floor Surgery

Current recommendations in prolapse surgery are that patients should be followed up for five years [2], but in practice, trials are expensive and patient drop-out or incomplete data may compromise the power and hence the significance of longer-term outcomes. As such, powering for primary endpoints at a time of more than a year is seldom attempted as it is impractical. Currently, being sufficiently powered for a two-year follow-up would be exceptional and viewed as excellent.

This point is highlighted with the Ward and Hilton randomized controlled trial looking at tension-free vaginal tape (TVT) versus colposuspension. Whilst this study and its resultant papers are often cited, the actual recruitment was in the end under that required and so the study conclusions become clinically less robust. This point was recently highlighted as the 'shrinking denominator effect' [3] quoting the 17-year follow-up of 90 women having undergone a TVT [4]. Hennigan, in this analysis, highlights the results being per protocol or 'best fit' based on patients available rather than intention to treat or 'assuming' all absent as failures. Interestingly Hennigan, in this article, offers no further advice and as such highlights the difficulty in longer-term follow-up and also makes no comment where it is known that the patients remained well in terms of their surgery at the time of their death or where they became lost to follow-up.

Garry Leach, a renowned urologist from the US, in many ways was the first person to highlight the need for longer-term follow-up when he presented his long-term data in a retrospective series of endoscopic bladder neck suspensions at the International Continence Society (ICS) meeting in 1995 [5]. The remarkable thing about this presentation was that it was unique in presenting a series with negative or poor long-term outcomes (in this case average of 10 years), reinforcing the bias to publication of positive outcomes [6] and potentially publication bias [7]. The introduction of guidelines that all randomized controlled trials (RCTs) should be registered prospectively now allows investigators to search for trials rather than publication [8]. The second influence in trials is ownership of the data. In commercial trials where a company owns the data, the drive to publish where results do not endorse the company's product is substantially reduced. An example within urogynaecology would be with the porcine acellular matrix small-intestinal submucosal (SIS) mesh which was used in a company-sponsored randomized controlled trial against native tissue repair. The results did not show any advantage (in fact showed a negative outcome). The trial was reported in abstract form, but never as a full peer-reviewed publication [9].

At a similar time to the Leach presentation, a seminal paper by Gerry Jarvis was published in the *BJOG* on surgery for stress incontinence. This was one of the first structured attempts to assess surgical outcomes [10]. The Jarvis paper at the time was widely applauded and quoted, but by today's standards failed to assess many of the parameters that would now be seen as critical in assessing the validity of trials included in a review, in that it was unsystematic, did not comment on the quality of publications, and offered no meta-analysis; yet it did highlight the flaws in then contemporary continence surgery, namely how poorly endoscopic bladder neck suspensions and anterior repair performed in anything other than short-term follow-up.

The following year, Black and Downs [11] published the first systematic review of continence surgery which analysed 31 trials.

They concluded that 'There is an urgent need for some large, rigorous, prospective studies of high quality. Until such studies have been completed, recommendations as to the best clinical practice cannot be based on scientific evidence. Studies need to define cases according to widely accepted criteria, including standard measures of the severity of stress incontinence, and surgical terminology for the procedures performed needs to be standardized and outcomes need to be clearly defined, valid and reliable, not confined to short-term assessment and include patients' views along with the surgeon's assessments.' In particular, they highlighted the variation and poor quality of outcome measures. At this time, the first published long-term outcomes of case series began to appear [12,13]. It is interesting that this has been castigated by Hannigan as discussed above, reinforcing the gap between the theoretical ideal and the practicalities of collecting trial data longer term. As such, this highlights the need for prospective data collection outside the auspices of the gold standard of an RCT using real life data sets.

To these ends the Black and Downes paper highlighted a number of issues around the use of RCTs, which require closer consideration. One of the key points of this work concentrated on the contrast between comparing a treatment and the patient. As such, whilst RCTs are 'standardized', they do not consider the patient variation (in fact look to minimize differences between patients) but compare treatments (and their effectiveness as a proof of concept against placebo). Hence the wider interpretation may be limited by the population included (and by whom is excluded) so that the results truly can only be applied to a limited population. However, once published, they are inappropriately extrapolated to a wider population. This in part can be considered part of the Hawthorn effect [14], which in its truest form represents a change of behaviour in trials and can also be considered when inclusion criteria cherry-pick patients for trials. This is often seen as a limitation and why elderly (co-morbid) patients are often excluded and why trials in the elderly are less often done (despite them often being the 'target population' for drug therapy) [15]. Such limitations in trial strategies and narrowing of populations for studies result in the increasing request for 'real-life data' and highlight that RCTs may have removed the 'decision-making' from the process. Such data may provide evidence of efficacy of the procedure, but not the appropriateness to the patient.

Furthermore, whilst studies have been done looking at patients' and clinicians' thoughts into participating in surgical trials [16], little work has been done to look at the impact of investigations on outcome. There are limited and conflicting data on urodynamics [17–19] which demonstrate how the process of an investigation or its results may affect the patient's or clinician's decision-making.

The second issue highlighted, with regards to studies into incontinence, is the need to quantify or grade leakage on entry into a study. As of yet, no reliable method currently exists, and hence results have to be interpreted carefully.

The third issue about randomized studies is how should outcome measures be assessed? This is an issue addressed by Blaivas [20], after his editorial in 1998, yet remains unsolved [21]. As such, we await the outcomes of the COMET initiative on this [22]. This issue has, however, been partly addressed for prolapse in the International Urogynecological Association/International Continence Society (IUGA/ICS) standardization document, but worthy of greater consideration. In the previously mentioned Ward and Hilton study, dealing with the outcome of colposuspension and TVT [23], they compared various outcome measures and revealed markedly different results. Based on the measure chosen, this led to the conclusion that the TVT could be better, the same or worse than colposuspension. This was a conclusion that drew criticism [24] and highlighted the need for a standardized approach to reporting outcomes. The study did however highlight that a patient measure of satisfaction (with all its limitations of potential bias) may be the most important measure, but this does raise the issue of reporting bias based on how the question is asked (and by whom), and also how the patient responds (and to whom). In an ideal world the question posed should be asked in a standardized way and by an independent third party.

Finally, as Ward and Hilton demonstrated in their five-year study, there were three late complications in the tape group, which highlighted the need for longer-term results and large series surveillance. Again, this highlights why larger (non-randomised) data sets have an important role, highlighting the point from Hannigan's paper about diminishing denominators.

Patient Outcome Measures

Whilst objective measures have traditionally been used to assess outcome following pelvic floor surgery, more recently there has been a shift towards more subjective outcome assessment, including Health Related Quality of Life (HRQoL), Patient Reported Outcome Measures (PROMs) and Patient Reported Expectation Measures (PREMs).

Health Related Quality of Life

There are two types of Health Related Quality of Life (HRQoL) measures: generic and condition-specific.

Generic measures are designed to assess outcomes in a broad range of populations and are generally multidimensional, assessing the physical, social and emotional dimensions of life. An example of this type of instrument is the Medical Outcomes Study SF-36 Health Status Profile [25].

A second type of measure is condition-specific (e.g., instruments designed to assess the impact of specific diseases, conditions, age groups, or ethnic groups). Condition-specific measures can be similar to generic instruments in that they assess multiple outcome dimensions, but condition-specific measures also include items more specific to the particular condition or population being studied. Examples of condition specific instruments in urology and urogynaecology include the Incontinence Impact Questionnaire [26], the King's Health Questionnaire [27], and the OAB-q [28].

Grade A HRQoL Questionnaires: Lower Urinary Tract Symptoms

Pelvic Floor Distress Inventory (PFDI) [29]

Pelvic Floor Impact Questionnaire (PFIQ) [29]

Prolapse Quality of Life Questionnaire (P-QoL) [30]

Pelvic Organ Prolapse Urinary Incontinence Sexual Questionnaire (PISQ) [31],

(PISQ 12) [32]

Pelvic Organ Prolapse Urinary Incontinence Sexual Questionnaire – IUGA Revised (PISQ-IR) [33]

ICIQ Vaginal Symptoms Questionnaire (ICIQ-VS) [34]

Grade A HRQoL Questionnaires: Lower Urinary Tract Symptoms

B-FLUTS- Bristol Female Lower Urinary Tract Symptom Questionnaire [35]

ICIQ-SF – International Consultation on Incontinence Questionnaire [36]

IIQ – Incontinence Impact Questionnaire [37]

I-QoL – Incontinence Quality of Life Questionnaire [38]

KHQ – Kings Health Questionnaire [38]

LUTSS – Lower Urinary Tract Symptom Score [39]

N-QoL – Nocturia Impact Diary [40]

OAB-q – Overactive Bladder Questionnaire [41]

PFDI – Pelvic Floor Distress Inventory

PFIQ – Pelvic Floor Impact Questionnaire

UISS – Urinary Incontinence Severity Score [42]

Grade A HRQoL Questionnaires: Faecal Incontinence

ICIQ – Bowel [43]

Faecal Incontinence QoL Scale [44]

Birmingham Bowel and Urinary Symptom Questionnaire [45]

Questionnaire for the Assessment of Faecal Incontinence and Constipation [46]

International Consultation on Incontinence Modular Questionnaire

The International Consultation on Incontinence Modular Questionnaire (ICIQ) has more recently been developed to meet the need for a universally applicable standard guide for the selection of questionnaires for use in clinical practice and clinical research for lower pelvic dysfunction [47,48]. The ICIQ has a number of different modules allowing assessment of different aspects of pelvic floor dysfunction which may be used in combination or as a standalone measure. Each module also has a short form and long form questionnaire allowing the clinician to decide which is more appropriate for the patient population.

In general, it is now common to include condition-specific outcome measures in clinical practice due to their enhanced sensitivity to change and the need to minimize participant burden. Importantly, the type of instruments selected for use will depend on the aims of the intervention and the specific outcomes to be addressed.

Patient Reported Outcome Measures

Patient Reported Outcome Measures (PROMs) are questionnaires measuring the patient's views regarding their own health status and allow the efficacy of a clinical intervention to be measured from the patient's own perspective. They may be used to measure the patient's perceptions of their general health as well as their health related to a specific disease process. In addition, they may be used to measure clinical effectiveness and safety. PROMs may be divided into generic measures and disease-specific measures.

A specific type of PROM is the use of patient-orientated goals [49] which may be used to investigate the patient's expectations regarding their treatment and the treatment outcome. Long-term follow-up studies have revealed that goal achievement is related to general QoL measures [50] and hence they would appear to be a valid measure of outcome.

The use of patient-orientated goals has been described as a more sensitive approach to counselling women and also assessing outcome [51]. In addition, there is considerable evidence that there may be a discrepancy between patient satisfaction and objective outcome measures, meaning that a patient-goal-driven approach is more clinically meaningful. This is further supported by the significant association between Quality-of-Life assessment and goal achievement. Long-term follow-up of patients has demonstrated that achievement of patient-reported goals persists for one to three years following surgery for pelvic floor dysfunction and is related to, but not identical to, other measures of pelvic floor disorders such as HRQoL assessment [50]. Goal attainment has also been shown to correlate with Quality-of-Life evaluation in both surgical and medical management of patients with lower urinary tract symptoms and urogenital prolapse [52].

Patient-orientated goals may also be used to assess overall patient satisfaction following pelvic floor surgery. In a one-year follow-up of patients following surgery, there was a significant association between satisfaction and objective cure of urogenital prolapse but no association between the objective cure of incontinence and patient satisfaction [53]. This may of course reflect the fact that women might suffer complications following continence surgery such as de novo urgency and urge incontinence and this has been shown to reduce goal achievement and patient satisfaction [54].

Grade A Patient Reported Outcome Measures

PGII – Patient Global Impression of Improvement [55]

PGIS – Patient Global Impression of Severity [32]

PPBC – Patient Perception of Bladder Condition [56]

UDI – Urogenital Distress Inventory [57]

Patient Reported Experience Measures

The overall concept of patient experience was first described using the acronym EGGS which related to Expectations, Goal setting, Goal attainment and Satisfaction. Subsequently this concept of a global experience of a patient's interaction with the healthcare system has been measured using Patient Reported Experience Measures (PREMs).

Patient Reported Experience Measures (PREMs) measure the patient's perceptions of their experience whilst receiving care. Whilst they are an indicator of the quality of care, they do not measure it directly. In contrast to PROMs, PREMs do not look at the outcomes of care but the impact of the process of care on the patient's experience. PREMs may be classified as either relational or functional. The former identifies the patient's experience of their relationships during treatment whilst the latter examines more practical aspects such as the environment and practicalities of their care.

There were several studies undertaken looking at qualitative outcomes and decision-making by patients (CARPET [58] and Katharine Loane [59]) which highlighted the bias from surgeons. Simply put, women expected surgeons to know what was the right operation and wanted to be confident in the surgeon. These studies demonstrated how difficult surgical trials are and the need for independent counselling, as patients did not understand surgical equipoise from the surgeon.

At this time there was a huge rise in the interest in outcome measures based on the Bristol heart scandal [60] which was the start of the process for the NHS in the UK looking at better objective outcome measures. In surgery such as cardiothoracic surgery, the hard endpoint of death made measurement easier. Despite this, the development of risk adjustment for case selection remained a major challenge. In cardiac surgery this resulted in the RACHS adjustment [61]. The use of crude mortality rates has however more recently been criticized [62]. The development of outcome measures in areas such as female urology and urogynaecology have been even more complex, since absolute hard endpoints are, as the Ward and Hilton paper suggest, far more difficult to define.

Why Measure Outcomes?

The drivers for measuring outcomes can be on several levels and much is set out in the editorial in the *International Urogynecology Journal* (IUJ) [63]. With increased scrutiny and annual appraisal, individual clinicians may wish to present their data. If this is positive, it gives reassurance and as such is helpful. If negative, then this gives an opportunity to address any underlying issues. Potential factors, other than performance, affecting outcome include data quality (including completeness) and case selection. Data completeness is affected by return rates to clinic and also uploading of data, both of which are addressed later. As demonstrated earlier, there may be identifiable criteria for quality (in the case of TVT perforation rate). Knowing data is also helpful in informing (defending) one's position. During an investigation into an adverse outcome, one of the authors was able to pull similar cases from the database and defend the decision to operate, based on previous outcomes (and the outcomes of their colleagues). On a larger scale, 'rare' events, which may be more common in some procedures, may be picked up earlier with the combined data of larger numbers and this is the driver of the national joint registry. Finally, with the increasing drive towards personalized medicine, having a large personal series means that individuals can counsel patients with 'national' or 'research' results in standardized leaflets and also quote personal series, to give individual clinician outcomes. Likewise, contributing to a larger series allows comparators and analysis of practice. As such, the British Society of Urogynaecology (BSUG) database now has information over a longer period of time (more than 10 years) on a large series (approaching 200,000 procedures) assisting patients in informed decision-making (with the use of individualized tools).

Difference between Registries and Databases

Database is a generic term which is defined as 'a structured set of data held in a computer, especially one that is accessible in various ways' and a registry as 'a place where official records are kept'. Registries tend to be more specific, for example the national joint registry [64], which was set up in 2003 and became mandatory in 2011. This records all artificial joints inserted in the UK but not comparative operations. As such, their main objective is to look at safety data relating to these procedures and act as a warning system rather than to give comparative data between procedures.

Databases are more complete and look at practice but are still currently procedure based. As such, comparing surgeons will continue to have the limitations which the risk adjustment in paediatric cardiac surgery has, as there is an assumption that all surgeries are carried out at the same point in the disease process.

The UK and Denmark were the first countries to attempt national databases in urogynaecology, with the setup of the Danish Urogynaecological Database (DUGAbase) and BSUG database. Both were launched in 2006. DUGAbase [65] became a mandatory national database in 2008, whereby recording of all urogynaecological procedures was mandated by government. Despite this, it possibly missed up to 10% of cases. Its publications have been mainly limited to individual PhD theses [66]. The BSUG database was originally set up 'nationally' as a standardized audit tool for individual consultants where data was uploaded. 2008 saw the launch of the online version and this, to date, has collected nearly 200,000 procedures. Early publications gave reassurance of efficacy and also helped validate outcome measures [67,68]. It was also helpful in calculating risks of complications [69]. Subsequent publications began to look in more detail at factors affecting outcome [70–72] which potentially allow the surgeon to modify and individualize risks based on patient factors and hopefully will lead to the development of a risk and success calculator.

Larger series do also potentially overcome some of the issues of missing data and so can also assess quality of surgery [73]. Using a dataset of nearly 19,000 we demonstrated a statistical association between bladder perforation and poorer clinical outcome. As the event rate was so small (significantly less than 10%), the numbers needed become exponentially greater to demonstrate a size effect. Whether the actual perforation led to a poorer clinical outcome is debatable, as under a duty of candour surgeons are obliged to tell patients. Likewise, where a catheter has been left in, patients may perceive a poorer outcome. Further questions were raised, as the study highlighted that perforations occurred more frequently with trainees than seniors, and also that perforations were associated with a U-shaped form together with BMI, where very high and very low BMIs had a greater perforation rate. As such it also raises a question as to the ethics of how patients should be counselled and about rights to choose a surgeon.

Preliminary data are starting to emerge from various sources, including national audits of data [77], databases on comparative procedures such as bulking versus retropubic tapes [74,75], as well as an overview of niche areas such as surgery for recurrent incontinence[76].

Limitations of Databases

Most current databases have three major flaws; firstly, completion of data, and in Europe, GDPR regulations stipulate the need for consent, so that patients have the right not to be included, and those that do consent need to give written consent. In the UK this was previously covered by the best interest (Caldecott guardianship, which meant each Trust dealt with matters differently). Secondly, who owns the data? The latter is important and may yet present legal issues based on whether the data is deemed to be the individual patient's, the operating clinician, or the administrating body with control of the database. Lastly, as already highlighted, completeness of data based on patient attendance and subsequent administrative support to upload results. As such, the amount of available data may be far from complete and often is dependent on individual clinicians to ensure outcomes. Again, with this there is potential for selection bias which may also be significant in terms of missing data potentially being more likely to be negative. These factors have been overcome to a point in Denmark with the DUGAbase (in urogynaecology) and the national joint registry (in the UK) by mandating completion (references to DUGAbase results). Many of the limitations have been highlighted in the recent HQIPP appraisal as part of the Cumberlege enquiry into mesh complications in the UK [78].

Factors Affecting Outcome

As highlighted above, whilst databases and registries are important, it is important to understand their limitations so that data may be interpreted appropriately. Greater granularity on outcomes would require understanding of decision-making and where patients are on the disease process when they have surgery. As such, the decision-making which occurred prior to the surgery has been ignored by the data collection methodology (based on surgery rather than disease). One potential solution is to adopt the International Consortium of Healthcare Outcome Measures (ICHOM) (www.ichom.org) set to follow decision-making and disease process, which inform on where and when procedures are most appropriate. This idea is based on the Boston consulting group suggestion of value-based healthcare [79], which is encouraging healthcare professionals to routinely collect pre-defined assessments at pre-defined points in the patient journey from presentation to treatment. This would preclude erroneous conclusions; an example would be the recent meta-analysis [80] for risk factors for recurrence of prolapse (after surgery) correctly predicting the higher recurrence rate on higher order prolapse, but failing to take into account time from the index prolapse occurring. For example, if a prolapse takes five years to progress from stage II to stage III. The women with stage III will already be five years ahead of the women with stage II. If the recurrence for stage II occurs at year 4 and year 2 for stage III, the women with the stage III will have in fact had the better outcome (age matched); as such, understanding when and why a woman opts for surgery is critical in assessing the outcome.

The Future

In a world where data is increasingly measured, Big data is becoming important. Big data describes data volume, variety, and velocity, and may be used to create greater value. It includes structured data (such as databases), unstructured data (such as emails), and rich content such as video [2] and offers the opportunity for patient collected data (via smart apps/devices) to be automatically uploaded and to feed into outcome measurement.

Currently, national bodies (such as NICE in the UK) do not consider data from databases or registries as important or of high enough quality to influence decision-making in policy decisions, which is an area that needs to be addressed, as merely dismissing non-randomized data means that the whole picture can never be seen. Expressly in the UK, the National Institute of Clinical Excellence (NICE) looks at cost effectiveness but not quality. A simple example is that ring pessaries are not discussed as a simple treatment for stress incontinence, merely on the absence of data rather than on efficacy or risk assessment.

Increasingly, the option of self-reporting is being considered, particularly using apps. The challenge here is to work out how to standardize how the question is asked and therefore reported. In the future undoubtedly these will be increasingly linked to electronic databases in the same way as biometric data are already widely collected and reported through devices such as Fitbit.

What has become evident is that many trials collect large volumes of data, much of which is never used for publication. The use of Delphi techniques to narrow down data sets in large series achieves several objectives. Firstly, and most importantly, it makes the data entry easier and therefore in theory increases compliance. It also allows the data set to be changed periodically to allow particular focus. Undoubtedly, moving forwards, databases will be used to drive firstly the research question and also the answers to supplement randomized controlled trials. As such investment in database design will help design trials databases.

Personalized Medicine

The concept of individualized care is also increasingly being recognized and in order to look at the wider issues (what is MY chance of success) such as co-morbidities, BMI, urodynamic diagnosis and age will require much larger data sets. Part of this may also involve patient choice of clinician, and so the use of published outcome measures for clinicians is also becoming important.

Other factors which may need to be considered in assessing outcome include the concept of Hardiness [81,82] and in the future, integration of data from different sources (Big data) may allow for correction or weighting of outcomes. This has been highlighted with Botox [83].

Work on these factors has already begun and the move towards population datasets rather than procedures has already started. The International Consortium on Healthcare Outcome Measurement (ICHOM) have been driving this work for a number of years and have already developed standards, using the 'best' available assessment tools, and defined when in a patient journey they should be used. As such, they potentially can start to look at the optimum time or person for an intervention. Within pelvic floor medicine, these protocols are already available for overactive bladder (OAB) [84] and childbirth [85].

Conclusions

Currently, the role of randomized trials should be recognized, but as with any tool, identifying and acknowledging the limitations is important. Defining outcomes are only useful if the population they are applied to is properly understood. As such, trials in pelvic floor medicine should conform to the published IUGA standardization papers. We are expecting new incontinence outcome datasets from the COMET criteria.

There is an ethical obligation to routinely collect data and understand both the strengths and weaknesses of the data collected. Efforts should be made to improve data collection using value-based healthcare [86] methodology rather than procedure-based methodology. Future consideration should consider multi-source feedback and wider metrics of patient modifiable elements, including how these data should be collected, as in the future we will be using multi-source data (Big data) to help deliver choices through personalized medicine.

References

1. Toozs-Hobson P, Toozs-Hobson N, Kelley T. Big data: why ignorance is no longer acceptable. Int Urogynecol J 2018; 29: 1235–7.
2. Toozs-Hobson P, Freeman R, Barber M, Maher C, Haylen B, Athanasiou S, et al. An International Urogynecological Association (IUGA)/International Continence Society (ICS) joint report on the terminology for reporting outcomes of surgical procedures for pelvic organ prolapse. Int Urogynecol J 2012; 31(4): 415–21.
3. Heneghan, C. TVT: seventeen-year follow up and the shrinking denominator effect. BMJ EBM Spotlight (Online) 2018. Available at: https://blogs.bmj.com/
4. Nilsson CG, Palva K, Aarnio R, Morcos E, Falconer C. Seventeen years' follow-up of the tension-free vaginal tape procedure for female stress urinary incontinence. Int Urogynecol J 2013; 24(8): 1265–9
5. Trockman BA, Leach GE, Hamilton J, Sakamoto M, Santiago L, Zimmern PE. Modified Pereyra bladder neck suspension: 10-year mean follow-up using outcomes analysis in 125 patients. J Urol 1995; 154(5): 1841–7.
6. Devito NJ, Goldacre B. Catalogue of bias: Publication bias. BMJ Evidence-Based Medicine 2019; 24(2): 53–4.
7. Kirkham JJ, Dwan KM, Altman DG, Gamble C, Dodd S, Smyth R, et al. The impact of outcome reporting bias in randomised controlled trials on a cohort of systematic reviews. BMJ (Online) 2010; 340: c365.
8. ISRCTN Registry. Available at: www.isrctn.com/?gclid=CjwKCAiAs92MBhAXEiwAXTi2559Ooxsqhi59kgqsGICyJx28Q49PNaqGNwC8v-JIhTchKzpsua8W0hoC9uAQAvD_BwE
9. Mouritsen L, Glavind K, 2009 KB-I, 2009 undefined. Results after vaginal repair of recurrent prolapse with and without xenograft reinforcement: a randomized study. forskningsdatabasen.dk.
10. Jarvis GJ. Surgery for genuine stress incontinence. BJOG 1994; 101(5): 371–4.
11. Black NA, Downs SH. The effectiveness of surgery for stress incontinence in women: a systematic review. Br J Urol 1996; 78: 497–510.
12. Alcalay M, Stanton SL, Monga A. Burch colposuspension: a 10–20 year follow up. BJOG 1995; 102(9): 740–5.
13. Nilsson CG, Palva K, Aarnio R, Morcos E, Falconer C. Seventeen years' follow-up of the tension-free vaginal tape procedure for female stress urinary incontinence. Int Urogynecol J 2013; 24(8): 1265–9. doi: 10.1007/s00192-013-2090-2
14. McCambridge J, Witton J, Elbourne DR. Systematic review of the Hawthorne effect: new concepts are needed to study research participation effects. J Clin Epidemiol 2014; 67: 267–77.
15. Shenoy P, Harugeri A. Elderly patients' participation in clinical trials. Perspect Clin Res 2015; 6(4): 184.
16. Jackson CJ, Dixon-Woods M, Eborall H, Kenyon S, Toozs-Hobson P, Tincello DG. Women's views and experiences of a patient preference trial in surgery: a qualitative study of the CARPET1 trial. J Clin Trials 2010; 7(6): 696–704.
17. Toozs-Hobson P, Majundar A, Robb K, Powles K. How does urodynamics affect subsequent patient behaviour? Int J Pelvic floor Dysfunct 2007 Suppl. 1 93: 66.
18. Jha S, Toozs-Hobson P, Parsons M, Gull F. Does preoperative urodynamics change the management of prolapse? J Obstet Gynaecol 2008; 28(3): 320–2.
19. Agarwal A, Rathi S, Patnaik P, Shaw D, Jain M, Trivedi S, et al. Does preoperative urodynamic testing improve surgical outcomes in patients undergoing the transobturator tape procedure for stress urinary incontinence? A prospective randomized trial. Korean J Urol 2014; 55(12): 821–7.
20. Blaivas JG. Outcome measures for urinary incontinence. J Urol 1998; 51(2): 11–9.
21. Lim R, Liong ML, Leong WS, Yuen KH. Which outcome measures should be used in stress urinary incontinence trials? BJU Int 2018; 121(5): 805–10.
22. Doumouchtsis SK. COMET Initiative. Developing a core outcome set for female pelvic floor disorders (urinary incontinence, pelvic organ prolapse, childbirth perineal trauma and pelvic pain syndromes). Available at: www.comet-initiative.org/Studies/Details/981
23. Ward KL, Hilton P. Tension-free vaginal tape versus colposuspension for primary urodynamic stress incontinence: 5-Year follow up. BJOG 2008; 115(2): 226–33.
24. Ward K, Hilton P. Prospective multicentre randomised trial of tension-free vaginal tape and colposuspension as primary treatment for stress incontinence. Br Med J 2002; 325(7355): 67–70.
25. Ware JE, Kosinski M, Bayliss MS, McHorney CA, Rogers WH, Raczek A. Comparison of methods for the scoring and statistical analysis of SF-36 health profile and summary measures: summary of results from the Medical Outcomes Study. Med Care 1995; 33(4Suppl).

26. Wyman JF, Harkins SW, Choi SC, Taylor JR, Fantl JA. Psychosocial impact of urinary incontinence in women. Obstet Gynecol 1987; 70: 378–81.
27. Kelleher CJ, Cardozo LD, Khullar V, Salvatore S. A new questionnaire to assess the quality of life of urinary incontinent women. BJOG 1997; 104(12): 1374–9.
28. Coyne K, Revicki D, Hunt T, Corey R, Stewart W, Bentkover J, et al. Psychometric validation of an overactive bladder symptom and health-related quality of life questionnaire: The OAB-q. Qual Life Res 2002; 11(6): 563–74.
29. Barber MD, Kuchibhatla MN, Pieper CF, Bump RC. Psychometric evaluation of 2 comprehensive condition-specific quality of life instruments for women with pelvic floor disorders. Am J Obstet Gynecol 2001; 185(6): 1388–95.
30. Digesu GA, Khullar V, Cardozo L, Robinson D, Salvatore S. P-QOL: a validated questionnaire to assess the symptoms and quality of life of women with urogenital prolapse. Int Urogynecol J 2005; 16(3): 176–81.
31. Rogers RG, Kammerer-Doak D, Villarreal A, Coates K, Qualls C. A new instrument to measure sexual function in women with urinary incontinence or pelvic organ prolapse. Am J Obstet Gynecol 2001; 184(4): 552–8.
32. Rogers RG, Coates KW, Kammerer-Doak D, Khalsa S, Qualls C. A short form of the Pelvic Organ Prolapse/Urinary Incontinence Sexual Questionnaire (PISQ-12). Int Urogynecol J 2003; 14(3): 164–8.
33. Rogers RG, Rockwood TH, Constantine ML, Thakar R, Kammerer-Doak DN, Pauls RN, et al. A new measure of sexual function in women with pelvic floor disorders (PFD): The Pelvic Organ Prolapse/Incontinence Sexual Questionnaire, IUGA-Revised (PISQ-IR). Int Urogynecol J 2013; 24(7): 1091–103.
34. Price N, Jackson SR, Avery K, Brookes ST, Abrams P. Development and psychometric evaluation of the ICIQ Vaginal Symptoms Questionnaire: The ICIQ-VS. BJOG 2006; 113(6): 700–12.
35. Jackson S, Donovan J, Brookes S, Eckford S, Swithinbank L, Abrams P. The Bristol female lower urinary tract symptoms questionnaire: development and psychometric testing. Br J Urol 1996; 77(6): 805–12.
36. Avery K, Donovan J, Peters TJ, Shaw C, Gotoh M, Abrams P. ICIQ: a brief and robust measure for evaluating the symptoms and impact of urinary incontinence. Neurourol 2004; 23: 322–30.
37. Hagen S, Hanley J, Capewell A. Test-retest reliability, validity, and sensitivity to change of the Urogenital Distress Inventory and the Incontinence Impact Questionnaire. Neurourol 2002; 21(6): 534–9.
38. Wagner TH, Patrick DL, Bavendam TG, Martin ML, Buesching DP. Quality of life of persons with urinary incontinence: development of a new measure. Urology J 1996; 47(1): 67–71; discussion 71–2.
39. Blaivas JG, Tsui JF, Mekel G, Benedon MS, Li B, Friedman FM, et al. Validation of the lower urinary tract symptom score. Can J Urol 2015; 22(5): 7952–8.
40. Holm-Larsen T, Andersson F, Meulen E van der, Yankov V, Rosen RC, Nørgaard JP. The nocturia impact diary: a self-reported impact measure to complement the voiding diary. Value Health 2014; 17(6): 696–706.
41. Coyne KS, Thompson CL, Lai JS, Sexton CC. An overactive bladder symptom and health-related quality of life short-form: validation of the OAB-q SF. Neurourol 2015; 34(3): 255–63.
42. Stach-Lempinen B, Kujansuu E, Laippala P, Metsänoja R. Visual analogue scale, urinary incontinence severity score and 15 D – Psychometric testing of three different health-related quality-of-life instruments for urinary incontinent women. Scand J Urol 2001; 35(6): 476–83.
43. Cotterill N, Norton C, Avery KNL, Abrams P, Donovan JL. Psychometric evaluation of a new patient-completed questionnaire for evaluating anal incontinence symptoms and impact on quality of life: the ICIQ-B. Dis Colon Rectum 2011; 54(10): 1235–50.
44. McLeod RS. Fecal Incontinence Quality of Life Scale: quality of life instrument for patients with fecal incontinence. Dis Colon Rectum 2000; 43(1): 16–17.
45. Bugg GJ, Kiff ES, Hosker G. A new condition-specific health-related quality of life questionnaire for the assessment of women with anal incontinence. BJOG 2001; 108(10): 1057–67.
46. Österberg A, Graf W, Karlbom U, Påhlman L. Evaluation of a questionnaire in the assessment of patients with faecal incontinence and constipation. Scand J Gastroenterol 1996; 31(6): 575–80.
47. Abrams P, Avery K, Gardener N, Donovan J. The international consultation on incontinence modular questionnaire: www.iciq.net. J Urol 2006; 175(3): 1063–6.
48. Avery K, Donovan J, Peters TJ, Shaw C, Gotoh M, Abrams P. ICIQ: a brief and robust measure for evaluating the symptoms and impact of urinary incontinence. Neurourol 2004; 23: 322–30.
49. Hullfish KL, Bovbjerg VE, Gibson J, Steers WD. Patient-centered goals for pelvic floor dysfunction surgery: what is success, and is it achieved? Am J Obstet Gynecol 2002; 187(1): 88–92.
50. Hullfish KL, Bovbjerg VE, Steers WD. Patient-centered goals for pelvic floor dysfunction surgery: Long-term follow-up. Am J Obstet Gynecol 2004; 191(1): 201–5.
51. Elkadry EA, Kenton KS, FitzGerald MP, Shott S, Brubaker L. Patient-selected goals: a new perspective on surgical outcome. Am J Obstet Gynecol 2003; 189(6): 1551–7; discussion 1557–8.
52. Hullfish KL, Bovbjerg VE, Gurka MJ, Steers WD. Surgical versus nonsurgical treatment of women with pelvic floor dysfunction: patient centered goals at 1 year. J Urol 2008; 179(6): 2280–5.
53. Mahajan ST, Elkadry EA, Kenton K, Fitzgerald MP, Shott S, Brubaker L. Non-oral poster 99: patient selected goals: perspectives on surgical outcomes one year after surgery. J Pelvic Med Surg 2004; 10: S57–8.
54. Mahajan ST, Elkadry EA, Kenton KS, Shott S, Brubaker L. Patient-centered surgical outcomes: the impact of goal achievement and urge incontinence on patient satisfaction one year after surgery. Am J Obstet Gynecol 2006; 194(3): 722–8.
55. Yalcin I, Bump RC. Validation of two global impression questionnaires for incontinence. Am J Obstet Gynecol 2003; 189(1): 98–101.
56. Coyne KS, Matza LS, Kopp Z, Abrams P. The validation of the patient perception of bladder condition (PPBC): a single-item global measure for patients with overactive bladder. Eur Urol 2006; 49(6): 1079–86.
57. Hagen S, Hanley J, Capewell A. Test-retest reliability, validity, and sensitivity to change of the Urogenital Distress Inventory and the Incontinence Impact Questionnaire. Neurourol 2002; 21(6): 534–9.
58. Jackson CJ, Dixon-Woods M, Eborall H, Kenyon S, Toozs-Hobson P, Tincello DG. Women's views and experiences of a

patient preference trial in surgery: a qualitative study of the CARPET1 trial. M Clinical Trials 2010; 7(6): 696–704.

59. Loanne K, Toozs-Hobson PHC. Women's experiences of stress incontinence surgery. Neurourol 2009; 28(7): 581.

60. Butler P. The Bristol Royal infirmary inquiry: the issue explained. Published 17 January 2002. Available from: www.theguardian.com/society/2002/jan/17/5

61. Thiagarajan RR, Laussen PC. Risk adjustment for congenital heart surgery -1 (RACHS-1) for evaluation of mortality in children undergoing cardiac surgery. In: *Pediatric and Congenital Cardiac Care, Volume 1: Outcomes Analysis*. Springer-Verlag Ltd; 2015, 327–36.

62. Spence RT, Mueller JL, Chang DC. A novel approach to global benchmarking of risk-adjusted surgical outcomes: beyond perioperative mortality rate. JAMA Surg 2016; 151: 501–2.

63. Abdelrahman A, Moore A, Trochez R. Editorial: use of surgical databases in urogynaecology. Int Urogynecol J 2019; 30: 851–2.

64. National Joint Registry. About the NJR [Internet]. Available from: http://www.njrcentre.org.uk/njrcentre/About-the-NJR

65. DugaBase. Dansk Urogynækologisk Database [Internet]. Available from: http://dugabase.dk/

66. Hansen UD, Gradel KO, Larsen MD. Danish Urogynaecological Database. Clin Epidemiol 2016; 8: 709–12.

67. Sinha D, Blackwell A, Moran PA. Outcome measures after TVT for mixed urinary incontinence. Int Urogynecol J 2008; 19(7): 927–31.

68. Elbiss HM, Thomson AJM, Moran PA. How useful are the BSUG database outcome criteria: validation using the MESA questionnaire. J Obstet Gynaecol 2010; 30(7): 716–20.

69. Assassa P, Moran P, Duckett J. Stress incontinence surgery in the UK (1). Pre-operative work up and intra-operative complications. Analysis of the British Society of Urogynaecology Database. BSUG NUU 2010; 29(6): 809–10.

70. Aslam N, Moran PA, Assassa R. Does BMI affect the results of continence surgery? An analysis of the British Society of Urogynaecology (BSUG) database. IUJ 2011; 22.

71. Toozs-Hobson P, Devani P, Pick J, Moran PA, Assassa P, Burton C. Does age affect the outcome of suburethral tape surgery? The importance of national registries in answering bigger questions. Int Urogynecol J 2016; 27(10): 1541–5.

72. Bach F, Hill S, Toozs-Hobson P. The effect of body mass index on retropubic midurethral slings. Am J Obstet Gynecol 2019; 220(4): 371.e1–371.e9.

73. Bach F, Toozs-Hobson P. What can we learn from large data sets? An analysis of 19,000 retropubic tapes. Int Urogynecol J 2017; 28(4): 629–36.

74. Bach F, Toozs-Hobson P, Duckett J. What can we learn from large data sets? When we use bulking procedures and comparison to mid urethral slings (MUS). IUJ 2017; 28(1).

75. Daly C, Mathew J, Aloyscious J, Tyagi V, Guerrero K. Macroplastique and Bulkamid-experience of bladder neck injections over 8 years. BJOG 2019; 126: 230–1.

76. Tincello D, Toozs-Hobson P. Surgery for recurrent stress incontinence in the UK 2007–2015. IUJ 2017; 28(1).

77. Jha S, Hillard T, Monga A, Duckett J. National BSUG audit of stress urinary incontinence surgery in England. Int Urogynecol J 2019; 30(8): 1337–41.

78. Interim Database Feasibility Report: Urogynaecological Surgical Mesh. HQIP 2019: 1–102.

79. Porter ME. What is value in health care? New Engl J Med; 2010; 363(26): 2477–81.

80. Vergeldt TFM, Weemhoff M, IntHout J, Kluivers KB. Risk factors for pelvic organ prolapse and its recurrence: a systematic review. Int Urogynecol J 2015; 26(11): 1559–73.

81. Perkins K, Randall D, Toozs-Hobson P, Sitch A, Ismail KMK. Hardiness and Outcome of Self-catheterisation Training (HOST): Protocol for an observational study exploring the effects of personality traits in women on ability to learn clean intermittent self-catheterisation. BMJ Open 2014; 4(1): e003986.

82. Israfil-Bayli F, Lowe S, Spurgeon L, Toozs-Hobson P. Managing women presenting with urinary incontinence: is hardiness significant? Intl Urogynecol J 2015; 26(10):1437–40. Available from: www.ncbi.nlm.nih.gov/pubmed/25986233

83. Tincello D, Owen R, Slack M, Toozs-Hobson P, Mayne C, Abrams K. Patient factors influencing the likelihood of cure or improvement after treatment with botulinum toxin for refractory detrusor overactivity: secondary analysis of data from a randomised trial. IUJ 2014; 25(S1): 215.

84. Overactive Bladder Archives – ICHOM – International Consortium for Health Outcomes Measurement [Internet]. Available from: www.ichom.org/resource-library/category/condition-specific-resources/overactive-bladder/

85. ICHOM – International Consortium for Health Outcomes Measurement. Pregnancy and childbirth standard set. Measuring outcomes [Internet]. Available from: www.ichom.org/portfolio/pregnancy-and-childbirth/

86. Gray M. Value based healthcare. BMJ (Online) 2017; 356.

Chapter 4

Surgical Set-up, Ergonomics, Entry Techniques, Port Placement and Instrumentation for Laparoscopic Urogynaecology

Gemma Nightingale, Christian Phillips

Surgical Set-up

Operating theatres have advanced significantly since the nineteenth century when paying members of the public used to attend operations and observe from a viewing gallery. In attempts to minimize infection, theatre spaces, ventilation, sterilization, clothing, equipment, and surgical techniques have seen huge developments, but the fundamentals remain unchanged.

With the dawn of minimal access surgery and the huge advances in equipment, operating theatres now face different challenges, namely adequate space.

Most hospitals do not have integrated theatres designed to house all the specialist equipment required for operative laparoscopic surgery. As a result, the operative theatre becomes a crowded workspace. This can lead to operative inefficiency and potential injury to the patient and surgeon, but to date there is insufficient evidence that integrated theatres improve ergonomics and reduce stress, so the surgical team are required to adapt the current working environments [1].

As well as maximizing the space available for equipment and wider members of the surgical team, there are factors that the surgeon should consider in terms of ergonomics; the position of monitors, the height of the operating table, and the choice of equipment. These are explored further below. Some theatre teams will work regularly together, making theatre set up more routine. If there is any variation in the team, then the World Health Organization (WHO) team brief should be adapted to incorporate a discussion about theatre set-up as well as patient and surgery specifics. The effect of theatre set-up should not be overlooked, as when done badly, it can directly impact patient safety.

A suggested theatre set up is shown in Figure 4.1.

Ergonomics

Originally derived from the Greek words '*ergon*' and '*nomos*', meaning 'work' and 'arrangement' respectively, ergonomics can be considered as 'the science of best suiting the worker to his job' [2]. Applied to laparoscopic surgery, this is focused on the surgeon's posture, the surgical environment, visual displays, and instrument design [3].

Laparoscopic surgery differs from open surgery in many ways. Although the benefits to patients are well documented, there are several challenges facing the surgeon. Visual and motor axes are decoupled, tactile feedback is reduced, the range of motion is limited, and physical barriers such as an insufflated abdomen and steep Trendelenburg require the surgeon to adapt their standing position.

These adaptations by the surgeon come at a personal cost. Studies looking at musculoskeletal disorders in laparoscopic surgeons found that 73% to 87% report regular pain [4,5]. Surgeons performing high volume laparoscopic work report pain in their neck, lower back, shoulders and thumbs. Although the physical strain of laparoscopic surgery cannot be completely

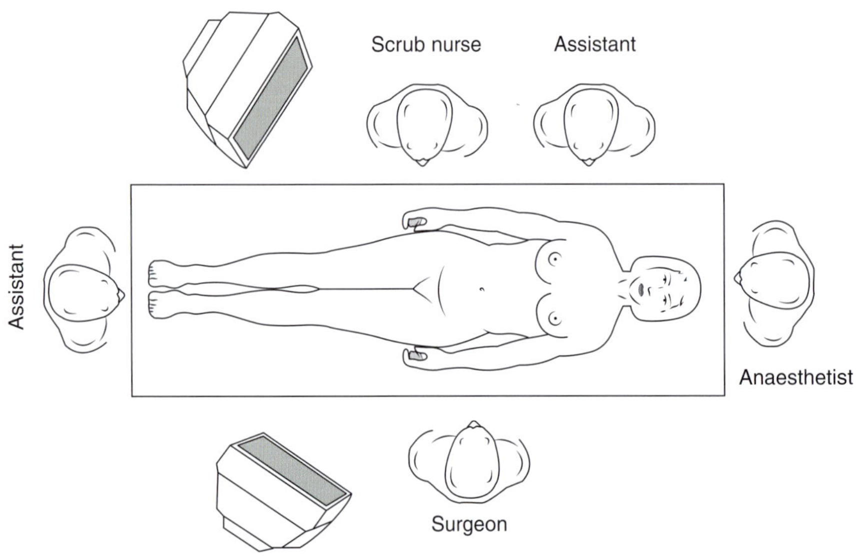

Figure 4.1 Typical set-up of a laparoscopic theatre.

avoided, measures can be taken to minimize the risk and this should be a routine consideration for all gynaecologists.

The advancement and mainstay of laparoscopic surgery for incontinence and prolapse is coupled with increased operating time and increased levels of mental and physical stress on the surgical team [6]. As well as reducing the physical side effects for the surgeon, improved ergonomics have been shown to improve task performance, particularly suturing [7] which is paramount for most laparoscopic urogynaecology surgeries.

Physical and environmental factors such as body posture, position and number of monitors, operating table height, foot pedals and instrumentation are considered below. Each surgeon can also improve their personal ergonomics and surgical efficiency by maintaining a good level of core strength and fitness. Improved economy of movement will reduce operating time and complex tasks such as laparoscopic suturing should be perfected on a box trainer prior to entering the operating theatre [8].

Body Posture

Compared to open surgery, a surgeon interacts with the operating field completely differently in laparoscopic surgery. This is manifested as a change in body posture and movement, mainly of the upper limbs. There are 36 degrees of freedom in open surgery and this is severely restricted to four in laparoscopic surgery. Any deviation from the neutral position leaves a surgeon at risk of musculoskeletal disorders.

Laparoscopic surgery results in the surgeon holding a more static, forced and awkward posture, often maintained for several hours [9]. Studies have shown that surgeons move a lot less during laparoscopic surgery which leads to the build-up of lactic acid, reducing precision and efficiency as well as causing physical harm to the operator [1,10,11].

There are several factors which can be manipulated to improve a surgeon's body posture; height of the operating table, port placement, surgical instruments and the use of foot pedals.

The ideal position for laparoscopic surgery is: [3,12,13]

- Arms slightly abducted, retroverted and rotated inward at the shoulder level
- Elbow bent at 90–120-degree angle (see Figure 4.2)
- Hands grasping the instruments with the wrist slightly extended
  - Distal interphalangeal joints almost extended
  - Metacarpophalangeal and proximal interphalangeal joints flexed at 30–50 degrees
  - Fingers abducted and thumb opposed to the index finger

One study by Haramis et al found that placing a gel mat under the surgeon's feet resulted in less back, knee and foot pain, and also reduced fatigue and surgical errors [14].

The Monitor

The laparoscopic screen or monitor relays the visual information from the surgical scenario to the surgeon and is paramount to laparoscopic surgery. To avoid undesirable postures for a long period of time, it should be positioned prior to surgery. Both the horizontal and longitudinal plane should be considered as well as the distance from the surgeon.

Surgical performance is best when the monitor is placed directly in front of the surgeon [1]. In the horizontal plane, it should be straight ahead of the surgeon in line with the forearm-instrument motor axis. Longitudinally, it should be positioned lower than the surgeon's eye level to avoid neck extension. A 15-degree downward angle has been suggested as optimal by van Det et al [15]. More practically, this could be achieved by

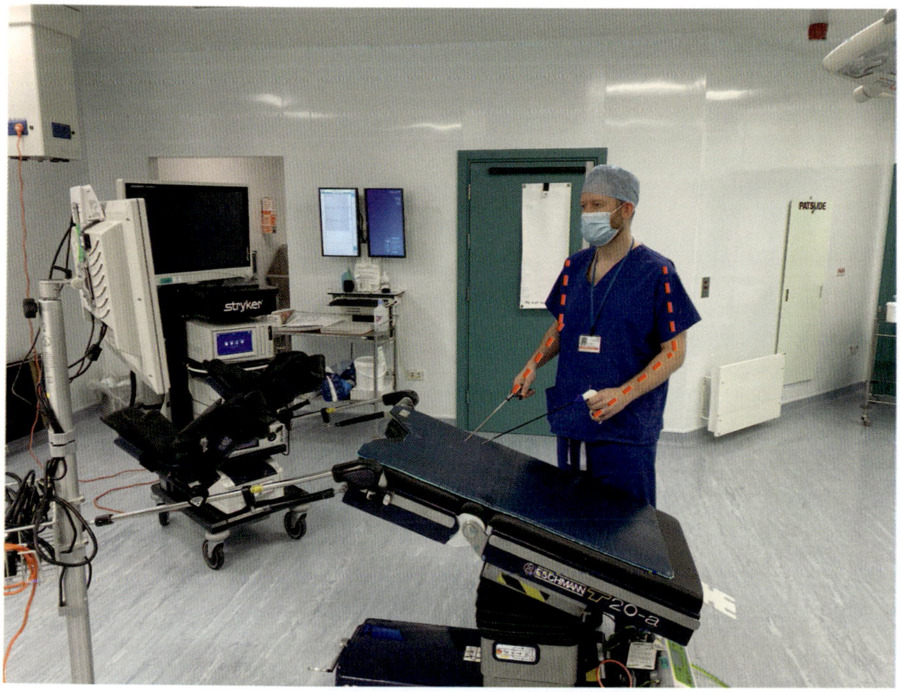

Figure 4.2 The ideal position for laparoscopic surgery, with arms slightly abducted, retroverted and rotated inward at the shoulder level and elbow bent at 90–120-degree angle.

ensuring the middle of the monitor is 20 cm below the height of the surgeon [1,16]. The viewing distance will be dictated by the size of the screen, but should be far enough away to avoid extensive accommodation of the eyes while being close enough to avoid staring and loss of detail. A distance of 80–120 cm is suggested [17] (see Figure 4.3).

The strain on surgical assistants must also be considered, particularly during lengthy operations. It is essential to adopt the use of a slave screen(s): a secondary or tertiary screen for the surgical assistants.

Operating Table

The height of the operating table is particularly important to avoid musculoskeletal problems and to allow the surgeon to perform optimally. When the table is too high, greater muscle contraction is required to raise and hold the shoulders and elevate the elbows. Holding this position for any length of time leads to muscle fatigue and poor neck posture.

Laparoscopic surgery is easier and causes less discomfort if instrument handles are at, or up to, 5 cm above the elbow height of the surgeon. This corresponds to an approximate table height of 64–77 cm above floor level [18,19]. Alternatively, the table height can be set so that the patient's umbilicus (after insufflation) is 70–80% of the surgeon's ground-to-elbow distance [1,20].

Many surgical tables are designed for open surgery and may not lower sufficiently for the surgeon. In this situation a step or raised platform can be useful, although maintaining balance and placement of foot pedals must be considered.

Gynaecologists often require a steep Trendelenburg position to assist with keeping bowel out of the surgical field. Various non-slip mats, bean bags and suction mattresses are available to support the patient on the surgical bed and reduce movement during surgery [21]. Care must be taken when positioning the patient to prevent prolonged pressure on peripheral nerves which can cause neuropathy. Figure 4.4 demonstrates a gel non-slip matt.

In addition to the height and longitudinal tilt of the table, the horizontal position can also be altered to aid surgery. When using contralateral ports for suturing, applying a horizontal tilt towards the side of the operator can reduced shoulder strain and improve efficiency.

Foot Pedals

Most operative laparoscopy requires some form of electrocautery for dissection or haemostasis. Modern instruments are controlled by the surgeon with finger switches located on the instrument handle, but many reusable instruments still require activation with a foot pedal. If the pedals are not positioned

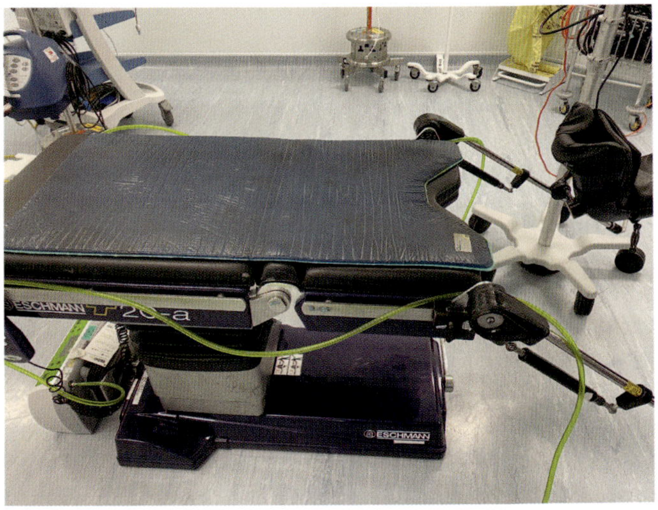

Figure 4.4 A theatre table with gel non-slip matt to prevent patient slipping cephaloid when placed in steep Trendelenburg.

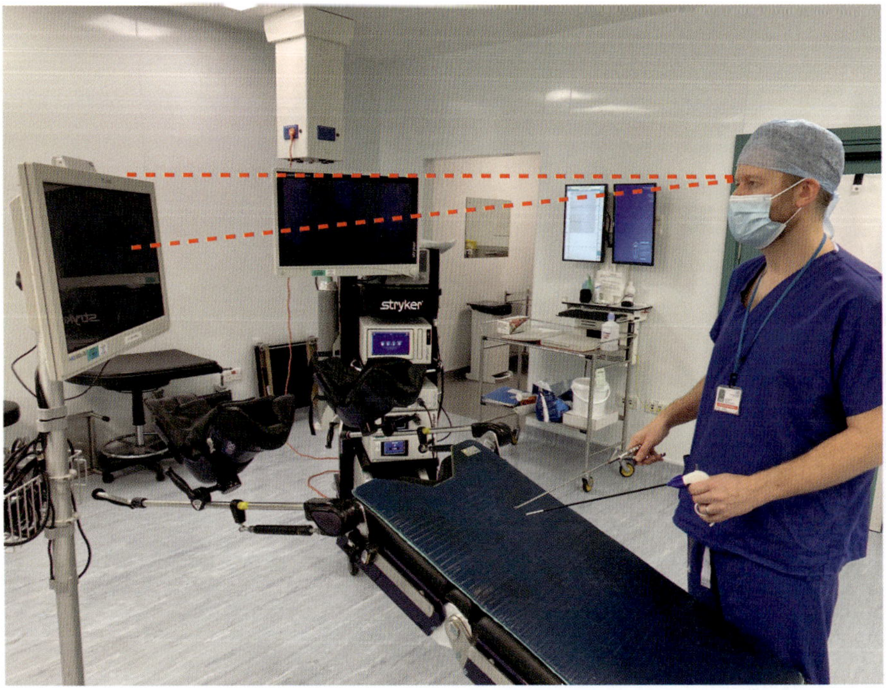

Figure 4.3 Ideal monitor position showing a 15-degree downward angle from eye height and 80–120 cm distance away from the surgeon.

correctly, they demand awkward and unnatural postures for activation. This can lead to reduced visual control and an unbalanced position. Pedals should be placed near the foot and aligned in the same direction as the instruments.

Surgical Instruments

The position and performance of a surgeon is highly dependent on the design of surgical instruments. Straight stick instruments and fixed access ports limit movement and tactile feedback, in turn worsening surgical performance and demanding greater muscular activity [3]. Laparoscopic instruments require three to five times the muscle contraction force to open instruments compared to open surgery, meaning the surgeon works harder for the same outcome [22–24]. This has necessitated advances in ergonomic laparoscopic equipment to relieve pressure-related chronic pain among surgeons [25].

The shape and length of the handle should be considered to allow the surgeon to minimize wrist flexion, rotation and ulnar deviation. Typically handles are either pistol-type, best for tasks requiring force, or axial-type which are often favoured for suturing and precision work [11,22,26]. Both can cause harm to the surgeon following prolonged use (see Figures 4.5 and 4.6).

Many companies produce laparoscopic instruments with slight variations in their weight, style, grip, and length. Individuals should try different instruments to test which ones are more comfortable for them; differences in surgeon sex, size, and height mean that one instrument does not fit all.

Entry Techniques

The majority of laparoscopic injuries are related to entry into the abdominal cavity [27]. There is a risk of visceral (bladder, bowel) or vascular (major abdominal blood vessel or abdominal wall vasculature) injury, which have the potential to cause long-term morbidity or rarely, mortality. For gynaecological surgery, the rate of laparoscopic complications related to entry is quoted as 0.3% [28,29].

There are fundamentally two ways to enter the abdominal cavity for laparoscopic procedures; open entry and closed entry. Closed entry can be achieved using a Veress needle which is passed into the abdomen and used to create the pneumoperitoneum prior to primary port insertion. This is generally preferred by gynaecologists worldwide [30,31]. The Royal College of Obstetricians and Gynaecologists in the UK released guidance regarding laparoscopic entry [32] but there is a wide variation in practice [33]. Another closed entry technique is direct trocar entry. This is thought to allow immediate recognition of any vascular or visceral injury and save time. Open entry techniques are traditionally used by general surgeons and were first described by Hasson in 1971 [34]. This involves cutting down to the peritoneum and inserting a blunt trocar into the abdominal cavity under direct vision.

Although the evidence is of low quality, a Cochrane review in 2019 found insufficient evidence to support one laparoscopic entry technique over another in terms of mortality, vascular injury rates, or visceral injury rates [35]. Evidence did suggest a reduced rate of failed entry into the abdomen with direct trocar entry. Ultimately, each surgeon should use an entry technique that they have been trained to perform safely and regularly review their own complication rates.

Additional ports should be inserted under direct vision after achieving a pneumoperitoneum with carbon dioxide. When deciding on additional port placement, care should be taken to avoid the obliterated umbilical artery and other superficial blood vessels. Blunt, or radially expanding trocars have been found to be safer and cause less port site bleeding and pain [36].

Port Placement

There is no uniform consensus about port placement for advanced laparoscopic procedures. Practice is largely dictated by surgeon preference and individual experience. However, there are several factors to take into consideration when working in the pelvis, the retroperitoneal space or when access to the sacral promontory is needed.

Port placement should be chosen to allow adequate visualization with the camera and facilitate smooth instrument manipulation in the area needed. Triangulation is used by many surgeons to allow optimal access and view (see Figure 4.7). This generates a 60–90-degree angle for instruments to work with the target tissue [2]. Whenever possible, surgeons should place ports to minimize extreme horizontal or vertical displacement of their hands away from a neutral position [23]. The

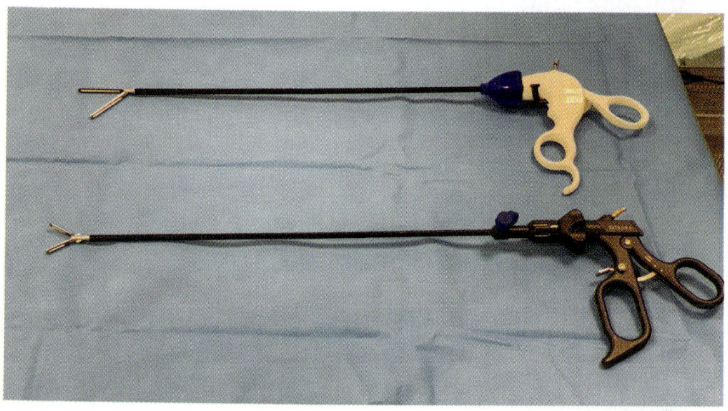

Figure 4.5 Examples of laparoscopic graspers with pistol grip and rotation cog.

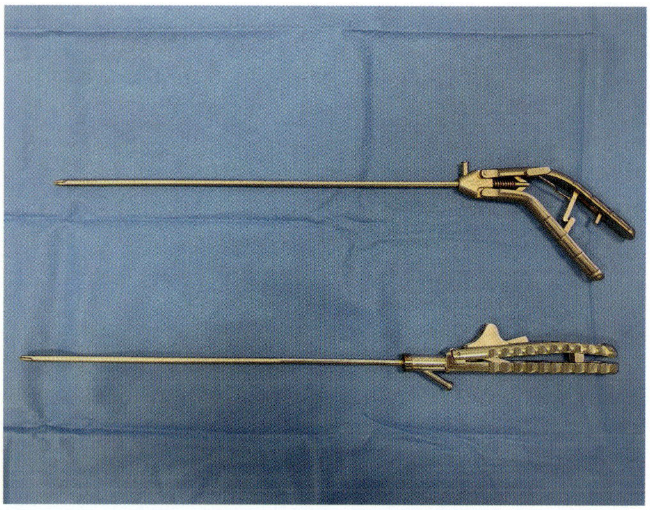

Figure 4.6 Examples of pistol grip and axial laparoscopic needle holders for suturing.

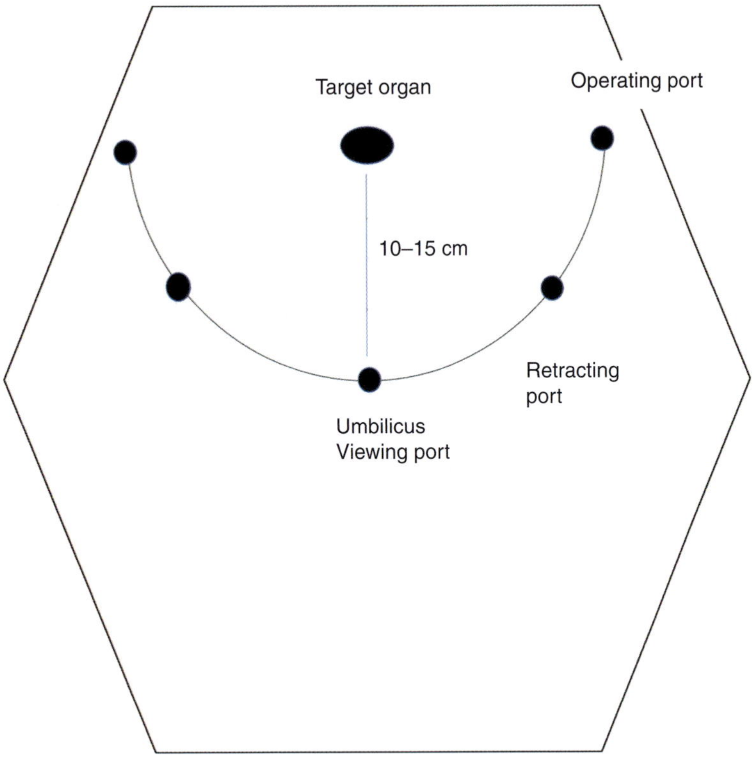

Figure 4.7 Port placement showing triangulation to allow optimal access and view and generates a 60–90-degree angle for instruments to work with the target tissue.

positioning of ports on the ipsilateral side of the patient to the surgeon reduces strain on the surgeon's shoulders and improves posture but may reduce triangulation and axis into the pelvis.

Instrumentation

Straight stick instruments have limited movement through fixed ports. Laparoscopic instruments typically have four degrees of freedom; rotation, up and down angulation, left and right angulation, and in or out movement. Over time, instrument quality, ergonomics, and function have been improved, meaning that surgeons now have a large armamentarium available to meet their operative needs.

Laparoscopic instruments are usually made of high-quality stainless steel and all have a very narrow shaft so that they can fit inside laparoscopic ports. Various tips are available for manipulating tissues, and the handle styles allow ergonomic rotation, grasping, and locking. Instruments used for grasping or cutting tend to be at right angles to the shaft, but needle holders usually have a straight axial design to allow greater manoeuvrability and a more natural motion of the wrist when suturing. Needle holders require a ratcheted locking mechanism in the handle, but this must be easy to operate considering the surgeon must grasp and release the needle repeatedly whilst suturing (see Figure 4.6). The jaws of a needle holder can be straight, curved right, curved left, or self-righting. Each surgeon will have individual preferences for the style of tip, handle, and grip. Instrumentation involving energy has also been rapidly developed. This will be discussed further in another chapter, but the use of monopolar, bipolar, or ultrasound and the expansion of instruments available has revolutionized minimal access surgery.

Single-incision laparoscopic surgery (SILS) has been developed to reduce the number of skin incisions, in turn reducing the risk of bleeding, hernia formation, and improving cosmetics [37]. SILS uses articulating or bent instruments with specialized multi-lumen ports. Such developments with instrumentation obviate the need for trocar triangulation on the abdomen. Another route being utilized is natural-orifice transluminal endoscopic surgery (NOTES) and for gynaecological procedures, transvaginal NOTES (vNOTES) can be used. Studies looking at total laparoscopic hysterectomy (TLH) versus hysterectomy performed via vNOTES, found vNOTES was non-inferior for conversion to laparotomy and actually allowed more women to be treated in a day-care setting [38,39].

Robotic surgery is also an increasingly expanding technology that uses human–machine interfaces to provide solutions to laparoscopic constraints. Articulated instruments can enhance dexterity, manoeuvrability, stability, and accuracy, but must be balanced with the significant increase in costs [40].

Whether using 'straight stick', SILS, NOTES, or robotics, a variety of laparoscopes are available: zero-degree, 30-degree, or even articulated (although these have not become popular). Angulated laparoscopes can aid better visualization of the surgical field. For pelvic surgery, a 30-degree laparoscope can be helpful.

It is essential that the competent laparoscopic surgeon be well versed in the various options for different equipment as well as the set-up, utilization, and trouble-shooting of each instrument. The WHO theatre checklist and preoperative briefing are essential in ensuring all theatre staff are aware of theatre set-up, necessary equipment, as well as any critical steps anticipated in the procedure. With adequate equipment, theatre ergonomics, and a well-trained/informed team, laparoscopic surgery can be effective and safe for both surgeon and patient.

References

1. Quinn D, Moohan J. Optimal laparoscopic ergonomics in gynaecology. Obstet Gynaecol 2015; 17: 77–82. https://doi.org/10.1111/tog.12176
2. Supe A, Kulkarni G, Supe K. Ergonomics in laparoscopic surgery. J Minim Access Surg 2010; 6: 31. https://doi.org/10.4103/0972-9941.65161
3. Sánchez-Margallo FM, Sánchez-Margallo JA. Ergonomics in laparoscopic surgery. In: A Malik (ed.), *Laparoscopic Surgery*. InTechOpen Book Series.
4. Sari V, Nieboer TE, Vierhout ME, et al. The operation room as a hostile environment for surgeons: physical complaints during and after laparoscopy. Minim Invasive Ther Allied Technol 2010; 19: 105–9. https://doi.org/10.3109/13645701003643972
5. Park A, Lee G, Seagull FJ, et al. Patients benefit while surgeons suffer: an impending epidemic. J Am Coll Surg 2010; 210: 306–13. https://doi.org/10.1016/j.jamcollsurg.2009.10.017
6. Vereczkei A, Bubb H, Feussner H. Laparoscopic surgery and ergonomics: it's time to think of ourselves as well. Surg Endosc Other Interv Tech 2003; 17: 1680–2.
7. Joice P, Hanna GB, Cuschieri A. Ergonomic evaluation of laparoscopic bowel suturing. Am J Surg 1998; 176: 373–8. https://doi.org/10.1016/S0002-9610(98)00202-5
8. Molinas CR, Binda MM, Campo R. Dominant hand, non-dominant hand, or both? The effect of pre-training in hand-eye coordination upon the learning curve of laparoscopic intra-corporeal knot tying. Gynecol Surg 2017; 14 (online). https://doi.org/10.1186/s10397-017-1015-3
9. Nguyen NT, Ho HS, Smith WD, et al. An ergonomic evaluation of surgeons' axial skeletal and upper extremity movements during laparoscopic and open surgery. Am J Surg 2001; 182(6): 720–4.
10. Kant IJ, de Jong LCGM, van Rijssen-Moll M, Borm PJA. A survey of static and dynamic work postures of operating room staff. Int Arch Occup Environ Health 1992; 63: 423–8. https://doi.org/10.1007/BF00386939
11. Berguer R, Rab GT, Abu-Ghaida H, et al. A comparison of surgeons' posture during laparoscopic and open surgical procedures. Surg Endosc 1997; 11: 139–42.
12. Matern U, Waller P. Instruments for minimally invasive surgery: Principles of ergonomic handles. Surg Endosc 1999; 13: 174–82. https://doi.org/10.1007/s004649900934
13. Matern U. Ergonomic deficiencies in the operating room: examples from minimally invasive surgery. Work 2009; 33: 165–8. https://doi.org/10.3233/WOR-2009-0862
14. Haramis G, Rosales JC, Palacios JM, et al. Prospective randomized evaluation of FOOT gel pads for operating room staff COMFORT during laparoscopic renal surgery. Urology 2010; 76: 1405–8. https://doi.org/10.1016/j.urology.2010.01.018
15. van Det MJ, Meijerink WJHJ, Hoff C, et al. Ergonomic assessment of neck posture in the minimally invasive surgery suite during laparoscopic cholecystectomy. Surg Endosc 2008; 22: 2421–7. https://doi.org/10.1007/s00464-008-0042-6
16. Zehetner J, Kaltenbacher A, Wayand W, Shamiyeh A. Screen height as an ergonomic factor in laparoscopic surgery. Surg Endosc Other Interv Tech 2006; 20: 139–41. https://doi.org/10.1007/s00464-005-0251-1
17. Van Det MJ, Meijerink WJHJ, Hoff C, et al. Optimal ergonomics for laparoscopic surgery in minimally invasive surgery suites: a review and guidelines. Surg Endosc 2009; 23: 1279–85.
18. Berquer R, Smith WD, Davis S. An ergonomic study of the optimum operating table height for laparoscopic surgery. Surg Endosc Other Interv Tech 2002; 16: 416–21. https://doi.org/10.1007/s00464-001-8190-y
19. Manasnayakorn S, Cuschieri A, Hanna GB. Ergonomic assessment of optimum operating table height for hand-assisted laparoscopic surgery. Surg Endosc 2009; 23: 783–9. https://doi.org/10.1007/s00464-008-0068-9
20. Van Veelen MA, Kazemier G, Koopman J, et al. Assessment of the ergonomically optimal operating surface height for laparoscopic surgery. J Laparoendosc Adv Surg Tech – Part A 2002; 12: 47–52. https://doi.org/10.1089/109264202753486920
21. Das D, Propst K, Wechter ME, Kho RM. Evaluation of positioning devices for optimization of outcomes in laparoscopic and robotic-assisted gynecologic surgery. J Minim Invasive Gynecol 2019; 26: 244–52.e1. https://doi.org/10.1016/j.jmig.2018.08.027
22. Berguer R, Gerber S, Kilpatrick G, Beckley D. An ergonomic comparison of in-line vs pistol-grip handle configuration in a laparoscopic grasper. Surg Endosc 1998; 12: 805–8. https://doi.org/10.1007/s004649900717
23. Berguer R, Forkey DL, Smith WD. The effect of laparoscopic instrument working angle on surgeons' upper extremity workload. In: GB Hanna, MA Talamini, *Surgical Endoscopy*. Springer: pp. 1027–9.
24. Berguer R. Surgical technology and the ergonomics of laparoscopic instruments. Surg Endosc 1998; 12: 458–62. https://doi.org/10.1007/s004649900705
25. Van Veelen MA, Meijer DW. Ergonomics and design of laparoscopic instruments: results of a survey among laparoscopic surgeons. J Laparoendosc Adv Surg Tech A 1999; 9: 481–9. https://doi.org/10.1089/lap.1999.9.481
26. Berguer R, Forkey DL, Smith WD. Ergonomic problems associated with laparoscopic surgery. Surg Endosc 1999; 13: 466–8. https://doi.org/10.1007/PL00009635
27. Alkatout I. Complications of laparoscopy in connection with entry techniques. J Gynecol Surg 2017; 33: 81–91.
28. Jansen FW, Kapiteyn K, Trimbos-Kemper T, et al. Complications of laparoscopy: a prospective multicentre observational study. BJOG 1997; 104: 595–600. https://doi.org/10.1111/j.1471-0528.1997.tb11539.x
29. Jansen FW, Kolkman W, Bakkum EA, et al. Complications of laparoscopy: an inquiry about closed- versus open-entry technique. Am J Obstet Gynecol 2004; 190: 634–8. https://doi.org/10.1016/j.ajog.2003.09.035
30. Lalchandani S, Phillips K. Laparoscopic entry technique – A survey of practices of consultant gynaecologists. Gynecol Surg 2005; 2: 245–9.
31. Vilos GA, Ternamian A, Dempster J, et al. Laparoscopic entry: a review of techniques, technologies, and complications. J Obstet Gynaecol Canada 2007; 29: 433–47. https://doi.org/10.1016/S1701-2163(16)35496-2
32. Royal College of Obstetricians and Gynaecologists. Preventing Entry-related Gynaecological Laparoscopic Injuries. Green-top Guideline No. 49. Published 2008.
33. Ahmad G, Duffy JMN, Watson AJS. Laparoscopic entry techniques and complications. Int J Gynecol Obstet 2007; 99: 52–5. https://doi.org/10.1016/j.ijgo.2007.04.042

34. Hasson HM. A modified instrument and method for laparoscopy. Am J Obstet Gynecol 1971; 110: 886–7. https://doi.org/10.1016/0002-9378(71)90593-X

35. Ahmad GWA. Cochrane Database of Systematic Reviews: Laparoscopic entry techniques (Review). https://doi.org/10.1002/14651858.CD006583.pub5

36. Bhoyrul S, Payne J, Steffes B, et al. A randomized prospective study of radially expanding trocars in laparoscopic surgery. J Gastrointest Surg 2000; 4: 392–7. https://doi.org/10.1016/S1091-255X(00)80018-9

37. Raman JD, Cadeddu JA, Rao P, Rane A. Single-incision laparoscopic surgery: initial urological experience and comparison with natural-orifice transluminal endoscopic surgery. BJU Int 2008; 101: 1493–6.

38. Baekelandt J, De Mulder P, Le Roy I, et al. Hysterectomy by transvaginal natural orifice transluminal endoscopic surgery versus laparoscopy as a day-care procedure: a randomised controlled trial. BJOG2019; 126: 105–13. https://doi.org/10.1111/1471-0528.15504

39. Housmans S, Noori N, Kapurubandara S, et al. Systematic review and meta-analysis on hysterectomy by vaginal natural orifice transluminal endoscopic surgery (vNOTES) compared to laparoscopic hysterectomy for benign indications. J Clin Med 2020; 9: 3959. https://doi.org/10.3390/jcm9123959

40. Judd JP, Siddiqui NY, Barnett JC, et al. Cost-minimization analysis of robotic-assisted, laparoscopic, and abdominal sacrocolpopexy. J Minim Invasive Gynecol 2010; 17: 493–9. https://doi.org/10.1016/j.jmig.2010.03.011

Chapter 5

Surgical Dissection and Mesh Attachment Techniques for Laparoscopic Sacrocolpopexy

Olivia H Chang, Katie Propst, Tonya N Thomas

Introduction

Sacrocolpopexy is a durable treatment option for women with symptomatic pelvic organ prolapse. The success rates associated with sacrocolpopexy range from 74% to 94% depending on the definition of success [1,2].

In the past two decades, various innovations have taken place including a transition to minimally invasive surgery with the use of lighter weight mesh for sacrocolpopexy. While the steps of a sacrocolpopexy are standardized, there are variations as to the techniques for dissection, and for attachment of the mesh to the vagina and to the anterior longitudinal ligament.

While innovative techniques may reduce operative time and simplify certain steps of the procedure, it is important to remember that the goals of surgery remain to improve pelvic organ prolapse symptoms while minimizing intraoperative and postoperative adverse events. Nygaard et al summarized key aspects of the attachment of mesh during a sacrocolpopexy [3].

1. Use a graft to affix the vagina/uterus to the sacrum
2. Avoid excessive tension on the anterior vaginal graft to minimize the risk of stress urinary incontinence postoperatively
3. Decrease the risk of massive presacral haemorrhage by placing sutures through the anterior longitudinal ligament closer to the sacral promontory
4. Avoid placing layers of synthetic graft material on a denuded vagina
5. Place multiple sutures over the vaginal portion of graft to spread out tension

This chapter will review the relevant anatomy for a sacrocolpopexy dissection, tools for dissection, and various ways for securing mesh to the vagina and sacral promontory during minimally invasive sacrocolpopexy.

Relevant Anatomy for Sacrocolpopexy

Anterior Vaginal Wall

The anterior portion of the mesh is attached to the pubocervical fascia. The bladder is dissected off the anterior vagina to reveal this tissue. Normally, the bladder and the vagina are connected by the vesicovaginal adventitia, or endopelvic fascia [4].

Clinical Implications

In a patient who is undergoing a concurrent hysterectomy, this plane can be created during the dissection of the bladder and creation of bladder flap. The round ligament is transected and the anterior leaf of the broad ligament is opened anteriorly. The bladder is then dissected off of the anterior vagina with a combination of blunt and sharp dissection. With adequate dissection, the vagina appears 'white', suggesting the correct plane. (See Video 5.1: 'Dissection of anterior bladder flap'). In our practice, we perform the anterior dissection prior to amputation of the uterus. We find that the uterine manipulator provides excellent counter-traction for successful and safe dissection of this space.

In a patient undergoing sacrocolpopexy with a history of a prior hysterectomy, we place an end-to-end anastomosis (EEA) sizer into the vagina for manipulation and counter-traction. In these patients, the anterior dissection is often more difficult as there may be adhesions from the hysterectomy. It may be useful to fill the bladder with fluid to delineate the border of the bladder. Once the bladder is visualized, the bladder can be dissected off the vagina with a combination of sharp and blunt dissection.

The anterior dissection should extend to the level of the bladder neck so that the mesh can be attached distally. To facilitate this dissection, using a transurethral catheter, the bladder neck and urethra can be identified with concurrent vaginal exam.

Posterior Vaginal Wall

The posterior portion of the mesh is attached to the vagina between the vagina and the rectum in the rectovaginal space. A layer of adventitia separates the rectum from the rectovaginal septum [5].

Clinical Implications

For the posterior vaginal dissection, we place an EEA sizer into the vagina to better delineate the posterior vaginal wall. With tension placed on the rectum, we can identify a safe space for entry into the rectovaginal space. (Video 5.2 – 'Dissection of the rectovaginal space'). Typically, this space is relatively free of adhesions and the space can be opened bluntly. If there is uncertainty with regards to the proximity of the rectum, a second EEA sizer can be placed in the rectum to clearly show the rectovaginal space.

Sacral Promontory

The anatomy of the sacral promontory is complex with the close proximity of major vasculature, ureter and sacral nerves. The goal of the dissection and mesh attachment is to secure the sacral mesh arm to the anterior longitudinal ligament at the level of the S1 vertebra. Thorough understanding of the anatomy in this region is needed to avoid major vascular, nerve, or ureteral complications (see Figure 5.1). Anatomic studies demonstrate average distances of relevant anatomic structures from the sacral promontory. The first sacral nerve is found to be 25 mm below the midpoint of the sacral promontory and about 20 mm to the right of the midline [6]. The average distance of the midsacral promontory to the aortic bifurcation is 61 mm with a range of 45–71 mm. The left common iliac vein is an average of 22 mm to the left of the promontory (range 15–27 mm). On the right side, the common iliac vein and artery were roughly 21–23 mm from the midsacral promontory [6]. In cadaveric studies, the average distance between the sacral promontory to the right ureter was 27 mm (range 16–38 mm) [7].

In cadaveric studies, the anterior longitudinal ligament is the thickest at roughly 2 cm above the sacral promontory. As it descends caudally towards the sacrum, the ligament significantly decreases in thickness [8]. The thickness of the anterior longitudinal ligament has been measured to be roughly 2 mm [6,8].

Clinical Implications

Attachment of mesh is achieved by first dissecting the presacral space to allow visualization of the anterior longitudinal ligament. As described, the structures in the presacral space are vital and their relationships must be well understood to allow for dissection and mesh fixation without injury or complication. Many of the available innovations are intended to allow mesh attachment to the anterior longitudinal ligament with minimal dissection of the presacral space. It is thought that with minimal dissection of this space, risk of presacral haemorrhage is minimized. In our practice, we believe the contrary. A thorough familiarity of the anatomy in this area, along with careful dissection of the presacral space, is paramount to reducing presacral haemorrhage, ensuring precise attachment of the sacral mesh arm, and to managing haemorrhage, should it occur.

Surgical Dissection

During a sacrocolpopexy, there are four areas which require dissection: anterior vaginal wall for anterior mesh attachment, posterior vaginal wall for posterior mesh attachment, sacrum for sacral mesh attachment, and peritoneum for retroperitonealizing mesh. Meticulous dissection is needed to avoid injury to the ureter, nerves, blood vessels, bladder and to the rectum. With the use of the right instrument, dissections can be achieved with accuracy with minimal blood loss and complications.

Dissection without Energy

Cutting/Blunt Dissection

Endoshears

Endoshears are useful during a sacrocolpopexy as the fine tips allow for precise dissection and tissue cutting. The curve of the scissor tip can be used for blunt dissection by pushing the 'back' of the scissors against the tissue. With the addition of monopolar energy, hemostasis can be achieved with appropriate use of the tissue vaporization and cutting ability. In our practice, we use endoshears for the majority of the dissection of the anterior vagina, posterior vagina, peritoneum, and the sacrum. For all of these dissections, use of countertraction is a vital component of use of the endoshears.

Laparoscopic Dissectors

Laparoscopic dissectors are disposable blunt-tip instruments which can be useful during the sacral dissection. Typically, after identifying the common iliac vessels and palpating the sacral promontory, we cut open the peritoneum overlying the sacral promontory. Laparoscopic dissectors (also known as a Kittner or 'peanut') are then used to atraumatically dissect off any tissue overlying the anterior longitudinal ligament once the majority of presacral fat is cleared using endoshears.

Hydrodissection

Hydrodissection can be performed with a suction irrigator. In our practice, we typically use pneumodissection as the CO_2 gas can separate tissue planes to facilitate dissections. However, in scarred planes or tissues, this same effect can be achieved with hydrodissection by instilling small amounts of fluid into the tissue plane. We find that this technique is most useful in patients

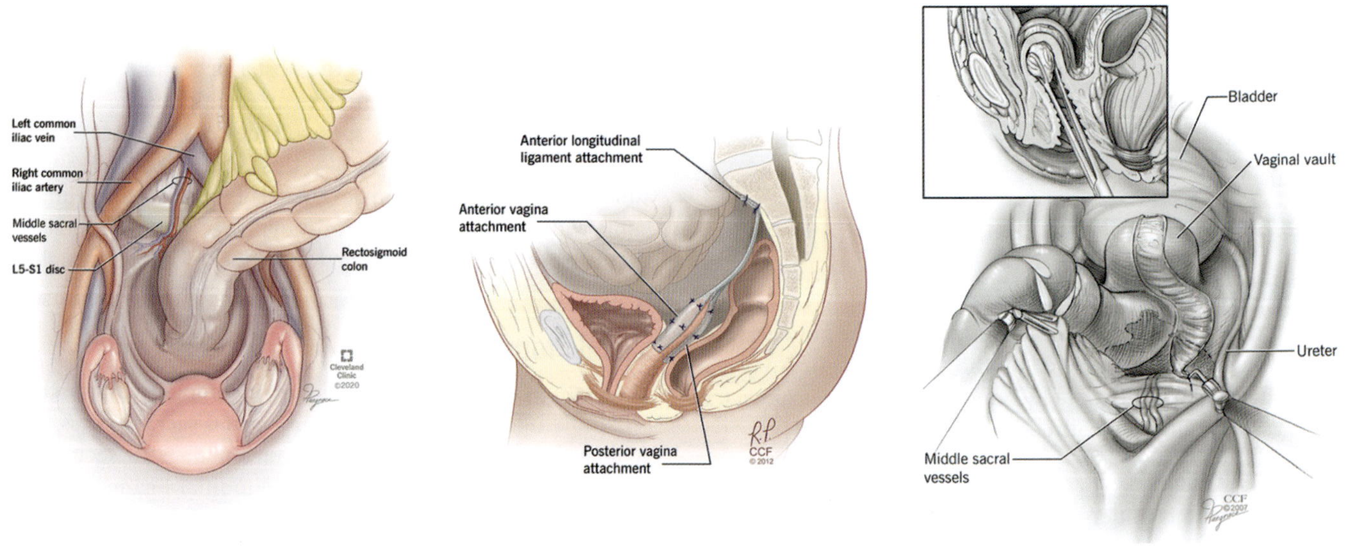

Figure 5.1 Anatomy of the sacral promontory.

with a prior caesarean delivery where there may be scarring between the lower uterine segment and bladder, or in cases where the bladder is scarred to the top of the vaginal cuff.

Peritoneal Tunnelling

After dissection of the sacrum, the peritoneal incision is extended inferiorly toward the medial edge of the right uterosacral ligament. The dissection of the peritoneum is needed so that the sacral mesh arm can be reperitonealized. One technique described in the literature is the peritoneal tunnelling technique. After the sacral promontory is exposed, a tunnel is dissected in the right pararectal space between the rectum and right ureter. This dissection is continued until the posterior dissection is reached (Video 5.3 – Peritoneal tunnelling by Guan et al) [9].

Dissection with Energy Sources

Monopolar Energy

Monopolar energy is typically delivered via scissor tips in both laparoscopic and robotic-assisted laparoscopic surgery. The fine tip concentrates the current and power to allow for tissue vaporization and cutting [10]. Because the current is concentrated and delivered via a fine tip, there is high power density resulting in tissue vaporization. During a sacrocolpopexy, accurate and meticulous dissection of planes is needed to ensure both hemostasis and safe placement of the sacrocolpopexy mesh. When using monopolar energy, one consideration is the collateral coagulation or spread of the monopolar energy. A low voltage energy, or pure 'cut', has minimal spread whereas high voltage energy, or 'coag' has increased spread [10]. With the use of monopolar energy, because its function is reliant on a dispersive electrode, the energy may arc to another instrument causing unintended damage.

In our practice, for laparoscopic sacrocolpopexies, we deliver monopolar energy through disposable scissors which allows for the flexibility of sharp dissection without energy, targeted dessication, and precise coagulation. In robotic sacrocolpopexies, we typically deliver monopolar energy to scissors for the same reasons. Overall, monopolar energy can be very useful during sacrocolpopexy, particularly for dissecting the bladder off of the vagina, and to dissect open the rectovaginal space. Surgeons must be cautious to ensure that instruments do not arc, and that thermal energy is used judiciously.

Bipolar Energy

Bipolar energy can be delivered via a variety of instruments including Maryland tip graspers, fenestrated graspers, or blunt graspers. Energy is delivered so that the tissue temperature is raised to achieve coagulation and dessication [10]. During a sacrocolpopexy, bipolar energy may be useful to precisely target the area of interest by delivering the electrical current only between the two tips of the instrument. This allows for targeted tissue sealing/hemostasis, and unlike monopolar energy, bipolar energy can be used in 'wet' surgical fields. The major limitation of bipolar energy is its limited ability to cut and vaporize. In our experience, bipolar energy is not crucial for a laparoscopic sacrocolpopexy. However, it is useful when there are concurrent procedures such as hysterectomy, salpingectomy. and oophorectomy where major vessels will need to be coagulated. In robotic sacrocolpopexies, we typically deliver bipolar energy via Maryland tip graspers.

Ultrasonic Scalpels

Ultrasonic scalpels are novel devices that were introduced in 1994. This technology converts electrical energy to mechanical energy. In other words, there is a transducer that vibrates at a high frequency to generate frictional heat to seal vessels. Ultrasonic scalpels come with two settings with the MAX and the MIN. The MAX setting is suitable for tissue cutting but is less suitable for achieving hemostasis as it has less thermal spread. The MIN setting has more thermal spread and a better ability to achieve hemostasis [10]. Certain ultrasonic scalpels have an additional vessel sealing capability [11]. The major disadvantage of the ultrasonic scalpels is that it can retain its heat for 20–45 seconds. In our practice, we do not typically use ultrasonic scalpels if an endoshear with monopolar energy is available.

Attachment of Mesh to the Anterior and Posterior Vagina

Transvaginal Mesh Attachment

Indications and Steps

When a total hysterectomy is indicated at the time of sacrocolpopexy, surgeons have the option of attaching the mesh laparoscopically or vaginally. In our practice, if a total hysterectomy is needed at the time of sacrocolpopexy, we elect to proceed with transvaginal hysterectomy to avoid the use of electrocautery on the vaginal cuff. We then proceed with vaginal dissection of the anterior and posterior vagina, followed by either vaginal or laparoscopic attachment of mesh.

We begin the hysterectomy by completing a circumferential colpotomy with a scalpel. A vaginal hysterectomy is performed in the usual manner. To perform the anterior and posterior dissections, Allis clamps are placed on the edges of the vagina. We use injectable saline or diluted lidocaine with epinephrine for hydrodissection. The bladder and rectum are then sharply dissected off of the vagina. Anteriorly, the dissection is performed until the urethrovesical junction is reached, this is confirmed by palpating the transurethral catheter balloon. Posteriorly, the dissection is performed at least 5 cm distal to the vaginal cuff. The distance of this dissection is determined based on vaginal length, size of the genital hiatus, and the patient's defecatory symptoms. If a posterior colporrhaphy is needed to treat a wide genital hiatus or defecatory dysfunction, adequate distal posterior vaginal length is maintained for posterior colporrhaphy and perineorrhaphy. A rectal exam is indicated at the completion of this dissection to ensure that no injury has been made.

Once the dissection is completed, we then proceed with double layer vaginal cuff closure if the mesh is to be attached laparoscopically. If the mesh is to be attached vaginally, we proceed with attachment using interrupted sutures. The proximal ends of the mesh are then guided intraperitoneally. At this point, we then close the vaginal cuff in two layers with absorbable suture. The remaining portion of the sacrocolpopexy – dissection of the sacrum, attachment of the mesh to the sacrum, and the reperitonealization of the mesh – are then performed laparoscopically.

In a retrospective study of 392 patients with a median follow-up time of 26 weeks (3–210 weeks), the authors found that the incidence of mesh exposure was higher when the vaginal cuff was opened either at the time of a total hysterectomy or post-hysterectomy sacrocolpopexy. In this cohort, transvaginal mesh was attached vaginally at the time of total hysterectomy in 81% of cases. For patients with a prior hysterectomy, the vaginal cuff was opened for vaginal attachment of the mesh in 15% of cases. The authors found that total hysterectomy had a mesh exposure rate of 4.9% compared to 0% at the time of supracervical hysterectomy (p=0.032). When a total hysterectomy was performed, there was higher incidence of mesh exposure with laparoscopic attachment of the mesh 14.3% compared to transvaginal attachment 2.7% (N=5/35), p=0.013, with a relative risk of mesh exposure of 5.4 [12]. This finding was similarly demonstrated in another retrospective cohort with a 32% of mesh or suture erosion with laparoscopic attachment of mesh compared to 14% of vaginal mesh attachment; however, these findings were not significant [13].

When looking at operative time, vaginal hysterectomy with sacrocolpopexy with vaginal mesh attachment decreased the total operative time by about an hour [14,15]. This is not surprising, as direct suturing with vaginal mesh attachment is less time-consuming than intracorporeal or extracorporeal knot-tying.

Laparoscopic/Robotic Mesh Attachment

Indications and Steps

In patients undergoing minimally invasive sacrocolpopexy for post-hysterectomy vaginal vault prolapse, or when a colpotomy is not indicated during a supracervical hysterectomy, mesh can be attached to the vagina laparoscopically or via robotic-assisted laparoscopy. With this method, the mesh is introduced abdominally and then secured to the anterior and posterior vagina after the dissection has been completed (Figure 5.2). In this next section, we review the different methods for securing mesh to the anterior and posterior vagina.

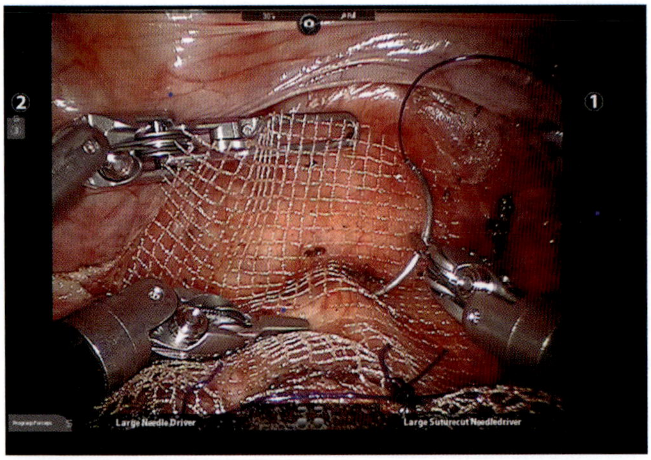

Figure 5.2 Placement of monofilament delayed absorbable sutures onto the anterior vaginal wall.

Type of Sutures Used

When it comes to attachment of the mesh arms to the vagina, there are many implications with the selection of suture ranging from permanent to delayed absorbable and traditional sutures to barbed sutures. Selection of suture material raises multiple questions. Theoretically, permanent sutures may decrease risk of prolapse recurrence by providing a permanent mesh anchoring to the vaginal tissue. Despite this theoretical benefit, there is concern for increased incidence of vaginal suture exposure. Data from porcine models demonstrates that tissue grows into polypropylene mesh by two weeks after implantation, questioning for the need for permanent sutures [16]. Infectious questions are relevant as well. There is the theoretical risk that if a full-thickness purchase is taken to attach the mesh vaginally, this may serve as a channel for the mesh to be colonized by vaginal bacteria, which may be more pronounced with multifilament sutures. Case reports of postoperative vertebral osteomyelitis suggest that a full-thickness purchase of the vagina may have resulted in a fistulous tract and ascending infection resulting in osteomyelitis [17–19].

In the next section, we review the advantages and disadvantages of the different sutures available for a sacrocolpopexy.

Permanent versus Delayed Absorbable Sutures

In a cadaveric study by Pilkinton et al, the authors compared three non-barbed sutures: 2–0 polydioxanone suture (PDS II®; Ethicon, Somerville, NJ), CV-2 polytetrafluoroethylene suture (GORE-TEX®; W. L. Gore & Associates, Newark, DE), and 2–0 polypropylene suture (Prolene™; Ethicon, Somerville, NJ) and two barbed sutures (2–0 unidirectional V-Loc™ 180 wound closure device (Covidien, Mansfield, MA) and 3–0 bidirectional Quill™ SRS polydioxanone barbed suture device [20]. Strips of polypropylene mesh were attached to the rectus abdominus fascia of the three cadavers with the sutures listed above. A pulley system was then used to grasp the mesh strip, and the pull-out force of a suture was measured. In this study, there were no differences in mesh pull-out force, except for the 3–0 bidirectional Quill suture. The Quill suture had the lowest pull-out force. The authors postulated that perhaps the smaller calibre of the Quill suture may have resulted in the difference in pull-out force.

Linder et al evaluated the use of dissolvable sutures (Vicryl®; Ethicon, Somerville, NJ) for the placement of mesh on the vagina and on the sacrum [21]. In this retrospective review of 132 robotic-assisted sacrocolpopexies with a median follow-up time of 33 (IQR 15.7–57) months, the authors looked at incidence of prolapse recurrence requiring retreatment with repeat surgery or pessary. Ten patients required surgical retreatment (7.6%) with recurrences found in the anterior compartment (n=2), distal anterior compartment (n=4), and posterior compartment (n=2). In one patient who underwent repeat sacrocolpopexy, the sacral portion of the mesh completely detached from the sacrum. In this cohort, the vaginal mesh exposure rate was 6.1%, and the majority of cases were treated with surgical excision. There were no cases of suture erosion into the bladder or osteomyelitis.

When delayed absorbable monofilament sutures were compared to permanent monofilament for vaginal attachment of mesh, there were no differences in apical failure rates between the two groups [22]. Suture erosions were found in two patients in the permanent monofilament group (2/148, 1.4%), while no patients in the delayed absorbable monofilament group had any suture erosions. In both patients with suture erosions, there was evidence of permanent suture in the bladder with one resulting in a vesicovaginal fistula. There were no statistically significant differences between the two groups for vaginal mesh erosion (17% for permanent versus 13% in delayed absorbable suture group, p=0.385).

Permanent Monofilament versus Braided Sutures

In the secondary analysis of the Colpopexy and Urinary Reduction Efforts (CARE) trial looking at risk factors for mesh or suture exposure, Cundiff et al noted a mesh or suture erosion rate of 6.6% (95% CI = 4.0–9.5%) of the 322 patients at two years [23]. There was no difference in the rates of mesh erosion by the three types of sutures used – polypropylene suture (Prolene™; Ethicon, Somerville, NJ), braided polyester (Ethibond; Ethicon, Somerville, NJ), and polytetrafluoroethylene suture (GORE-TEX®; W. L. Gore & Associates, Newark, DE). In another retrospective study of 415 patients, the authors compared the incidence of mesh and suture erosion at their institution when Ethibond was used for mesh attachment, to a later time period when 2–0 PDS was exclusively used. The authors noted a significantly higher rate of mesh and suture erosion rate for Ethibond sutures when compared to PDS (3.7% versus 0% for PDS, P=0.002) [24]. There was no significant differences in the prolapse recurrence rate between the two groups. While this study was a large cohort over the span of 10 years, there were limitations to this paper. The follow-up time difference may have contributed to the difference in mesh and suture exposure rates. Furthermore, as surgeons continually evolve their skills for sacrocolpopexy, this may have been another variable which limits the conclusion of this paper.

Interrupted versus Barbed Self-anchoring Delayed Absorbable Suture

A study by Tan-Kim et al compared women undergoing laparoscopic and robotic sacrocolpopexy to either six 0-polydioxanone (PDS®; Ethicon, Somerville, NJ) interrupted sutures or 1 PDS barbed suture (Quill™) to secure the polypropylene mesh to the anterior and posterior vagina. The Quill™ suture is a bidirectional, barbed, self-anchoring delayed absorbable suture. The barbs anchor to the tissues at fixed intervals and can secure the polypropylene mesh without the use of suture knots [25]. This study's primary outcome was to determine whether using barbed suture would be faster than the standard placement of interrupted sutures. A total of 64 patients were included with 32 patients in the barbed suture arm and 32 patients to the PDS arm. The authors found that the barbed suture technique was 11–16 minutes faster in attaching mesh to the vagina, which was significantly faster than the use of interrupted sutures, with the mean suturing time for barbed sutures ranging from 27.3–30 minutes [26]. In a small retrospective study of 20 patients also using another type of barbed delayed absorbable suture (V-loc 180 Wound Closure Device), the mean mesh suturing time was 33.7 minutes (SD =17.3). Interestingly, there was evidence of a learning curve as the suturing times for the first 10 cases were 46.9 +/− 12.6 minutes versus 20.5 +/− 9.3 minutes [27].

With anatomic recurrence defined as prolapse beyond the hymen, there were no differences in anatomic failure at 12 months (10.7% versus 7.4%, barbed versus non-barbed) [26]. In a retrospective cohort study, it was shown that patients who had mesh attached with a barbed suture had significantly higher rates of anatomic success at three months (defined as POP-Q <0) when compared to the interrupted suture group at 12 months (98% versus 62%, p <0.0001) [28]. However, this result should be interpreted with caution as there was a nine-month difference in follow-up time between the two groups.

For complications, there were generally no significant differences between the two groups when it comes to mesh erosion. In the study by Tan-Kim et al, there were two cases of mesh erosion in each group which were conservatively managed with the use of vaginal estrogen. No significant difference was seen in the retrospective study by Bazzi et al [28].

Other complications included that one patient in the study by Tan-Kim et al was found to have suture tails perforating the bladder epithelium postoperatively in the interrupted suture group, which was also managed conservatively. The authors did note that the 'appearance' of the mesh attachment in the barbed suture group 'was significantly less satisfying' though this did not result in a difference of anatomic outcomes.

In summary, current studies do not demonstrate a statistically significant difference between prolapse recurrence rates when comparing different suture materials. The use of barbed sutures does decrease the total suturing time. Current studies seem to demonstrate a higher rate of vaginal suture exposure when permanent monofilament or permanent braided sutures are used. In our practice, despite the shorter suturing time with barbed sutures, we prefer placing interrupted sutures as this allows for precise placement of the mesh according to the patient's anatomy. We use delayed-absorbable, monofilament sutures to attach mesh to the anterior and posterior vagina.

New research is underway which may answer whether there is a difference in composite success and adverse events between mesh attached with polytetrafluoroethylene (Goretex TM) versus polydioxanone (PDS). The Permanent versus Absorbable Colpopexy Trial (PACT) [29] is a randomized controlled trial conducted across five institutions to evaluate prolapse outcomes and adverse events associated with absorbable versus delayed absorbable sutures placed at the time of sacrocolpopexy. The findings from this study may offer high-quality evidence to guide management.

Attachment of Mesh to the Anterior Longitudinal Ligament of the Sacral Promontory

The dissection of the sacrum and attachment of mesh to the anterior longitudinal ligament are arguably the most difficult parts of the surgery and require surgical expertise. The ideal location of sacral mesh attachment is at the level of the S1 vertebra in the anterior longitudinal ligament. The sacral promontory is the result of the difference in angle between L5 and S1; the average angle, or 'slope' in between is roughly 60.5 degrees in cadavers [30]. Because of this 60-degree difference at the sacral promontory, direct visualization of S1 may be difficult. In our practice, we routinely use a 30-degree laparoscope to facilitate direct visualization of the relevant anatomy of the presacral space. All the major vasculature, nerves, and right ureter are within 3 cm of the ideal location for mesh attachment at the level of S1. Furthermore, regardless of the method used for attachment, the mesh must not be secured or anchored deeply at the sacral promontory as that may increase the risk of vertebral osteomyelitis or discitis.

In this section, we review the various tools available for the attachment of the sacral arm of the mesh.

Location and Orientation of Suture Placement

Based on cadaveric studies, the sutures for the sacral promontory are most secure when they are placed at the level of the sacral promontory or 1 cm above it [8]. The authors report that there is no difference between vertically and horizontally placed sutures as they have similar pull-out forces at the level of the sacral promontory [8]. Nonetheless, the preferred location of sacral mesh attachment is *at the level of the S1 vertebra*. Because of this, sutures should be placed horizontally, or in the direction from 'right-to-left' for a right-handed surgeon, as the anterior longitudinal ligament becomes thinner as it descends caudally.

Method of Attachment

As mentioned early in the chapter, the sacral dissection is crucial as it allows visualization of the proper location of mesh attachment and avoidance of injury to vital structures. Proponents of securing mesh to the sacrum with anchors and tacks argue that these devices reduce the risk of haemorrhage as they limit need for sacral dissection and also allow for more precise anchoring compared to suturing.

Sutures

The most traditional way of securing mesh to the anterior longitudinal ligament is with sutures, with permanent sutures being the mainstay (see Figure 5.3) [31]. Most studies on the different techniques of sacral promontory attachment use permanent sutures as the existing standard for comparison.

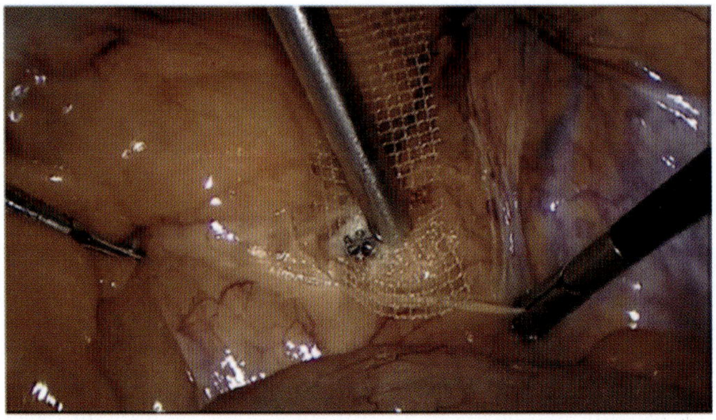

Figure 5.3 Fixation of the mesh to the anterior longitudinal ligament with Spider Fasteners™.
Reprinted with permission from Figure 2 of Braun et al. Safety and efficacy of spider anchoring device for apical repair in laparoscopic sacrocolpopexy: retrospective cohort study. Eur J Obstet Gynecol Reprod Biol 2019; 235: 88–92.

One study has reported outcomes of sacrocolpopexy with the technique of using an absorbable suture for fixation of the sacral mesh. Of the two patients (1.5%, n= 2/132) with apical recurrence, one patient was confirmed to have sacral detachment of the mesh at the time of her repeat sacrocolpopexy [21].

The use of suture is highly dependent on the operating surgeon for three reasons. First, the surgeon must be aware of the anatomy of the sacral promontory to reduce complications, and to ensure that the suture is placed into the anterior longitudinal ligament at the level of S1. Second, the surgeon must have excellent handling of the needle to ensure that only the anterior longitudinal ligament is included, and not the vertebral disc. Furthermore, the surgeon must have spatial awareness to ensure that the needle tip does not exit into the middle sacral artery or other surrounding structures. Lastly, the surgeon must be able to perform either intracorporeal or extracorporeal knot-tying to ensure that the sutures are tied down securely. For these reasons, it is crucial that surgeons have expertise in laparoscopic suturing and knot tying.

Because of the technical challenges of the sacral dissection and mesh attachment with sutures, a variety of innovative techniques have been introduced. Below, we review some of the techniques described in the literature.

Titanium Suture Anchors/Tacks

One study reported the use of a bone anchor screw at the time of laparoscopic sacrocolpopexy. In this study, the authors used a self-tapping titanium Corkscrew Suture Anchor (AR1925S, Arthrex, Naples, Florida, USA) [32]. The authors first dissected the presacral space until the avascular plane is developed. Then, the screw was used to penetrate the midline of the sacral segment with the bone anchor inserter followed by the titanium screw via a suprapubic port. Prolene sutures attached to the screw were then threaded through the mesh arm. In this cohort, one patient reported a neurological adverse event (2%). The authors reported that the patient had 'irritation of the left sacral plexus', which then resolved spontaneously in six months.

The authors report a median operative time of 120 minutes (range 60–240) for their cohort. With a follow-up time of six months looking at anatomic and subjective outcomes, the anatomic success rate was 98%. In regards to adverse events, neurologic complication rate was 2% as noted above, and mesh exposure rate also was 2%.

There are other systems available such as the Vesica PRESS IN suture Anchor System which is a titanium anchor (2 mm in diameter and 7.2 mm long) that is placed into the L5 or S1 vertebral body then attached through the mesh [33]. For the placement of anchor and tacks, a suprapubic port is often needed.

Anchoring Device

In 2019, the authors Braun et al report the use of the EndoFast Reliant ™ sacrocolpopexy. The novelty of this technology is the use of IBI Medical Systems' Spider Fastener ™. These fasteners are introduced via 5 mm trocars to secure the mesh to the sacral promontory [34]. The mean surgical time was 78 minutes (+/– 21 minutes).

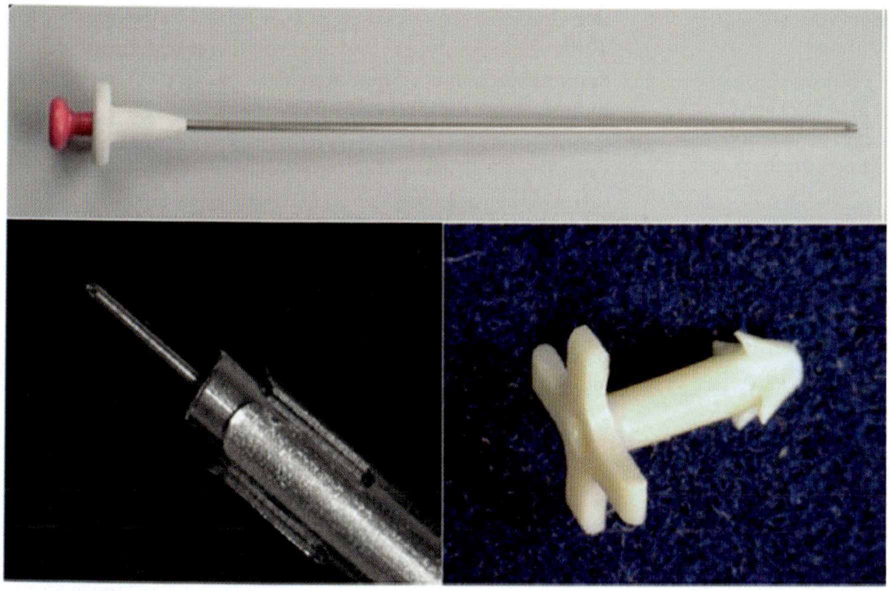

Figure 5.4 Polyether ether keton (PEEK) harpoon inserter, showing the extended needle without the loaded harpoon and the harpoon.
Reprinted with permission from Figure 5.1 of Vilarmau et al. Peek's harpoon: a new device for treatment of laparoscopic sacropexy. Prelimnary study in unembalmed cadavers. Int Urogynecol J 2017; 28(6): 881–5.

The authors reported one case of intraoperative haemorrhage and one case of postoperative vaginal bleeding, though the authors did not elaborate on the source of bleeding. Two patients (2.3%) reported chronic abdominal pain after this surgery.

Because this technology is relatively new, at this point, more studies are warranted to determine the adverse events associated with the Spider Fasteners ™ found in the EndoFast Reliant™.

Other Technology: Peek's Harpoon

Peek's harpoon is a biosynthetic material made with polyether ether ketone (PEEK) (see Figure 5.4) [35]. This device was tested in cadaveric studies by placing the harpoon into four locations – to the left or to the right of the middle sacral vessels and 0.5 cm or 1 cm above the sacral promontory into the anterior longitudinal ligament, and compared it to 0 silk sutures. The median tensile strength was comparable between the two groups. The authors' hypothesis was that because the harpoon is made of biocompatible material, it has a lower risk of rejection and extrusion when compared to other tacking devices. More studies are needed before making definite conclusions on this new technology.

Summary/Conclusions

Minimally invasive sacrocolpopexy is a safe and effective surgery to anatomically correct pelvic organ prolapse. A thorough familiarity with the relevant anatomy, particularly of the sacral promontory, is needed to reduce complications. Compared to the traditional way of performing minimally invasive sacrocolpopexy with the attachment of mesh with interrupted sutures, new innovative techniques promise shorter operating time and ease of use. Prospective studies are needed to compare these tools to the existing standard of using interrupted sutures to evaluate prolapse outcomes, adverse events, and cost. Finally, even with new innovation, surgeons must remain meticulous and careful while performing this surgery.

References

1. Hilger WS, Poulson M, Norton PA. Long-term results of abdominal sacrocolpopexy. Am J Obstet Gynecol 2003; 189(6): 1606–10; discussion 1610–11.
2. Culligan PJ, Murphy M, Blackwell L, et al. Long-term success of abdominal sacral colpopexy using synthetic mesh. Am J Obstet Gynecol 2002; 187(6): 1473–80; discussion 1481–2.
3. Nygaard IE, McCreery R, Brubaker L, et al. Abdominal sacrocolpopexy: a comprehensive review. Obstet Gynecol 2004; 104(4): 805–23.
4. Walters MD, Karram MM. *Urogynecology and Reconstructive Pelvic Surgery*, 4th edn. Elsevier; 2015.
5. Walters MD, Karram MM. *Urogynecology and Reconstructive Pelvic Surgery*, 4th edn. Elsevier; 2015.
6. Florian-Rodriguez ME, Hamner JJ, Corton MM. First sacral nerve and anterior longitudinal ligament anatomy: clinical applications during sacrocolpopexy. Am J Obstet Gynecol 2017; 217(5): 607.e1–607.e4.
7. Good MM, Abele TA, Balgobin S, et al. Vascular and ureteral anatomy relative to the midsacral promontory. Am J Obstet Gynecol 2013; 208(6): 486.e1–486.e7.
8. White AB, Carrick KS, Corton MM, et al. Optimal location and orientation of suture placement in abdominal sacrocolpopexy. Obstet Gynecol 2009; 113(5): 1098–1103.
9. Guan X, Ma Y, Gisseman J, et al. Robotic single-site sacrocolpopexy using barbed suture anchoring and peritoneal tunneling technique: tips and tricks. J Minim Invasive Gynecol 2017; 24(1): 12–13.
10. Feldman L, Fuchshuber P, Jones DB (eds.). *The SAGES Manual on the Fundamental Use of Surgical Energy (FUSE)*. Springer; 2012.
11. JNJ Medical Devices. Ethicon Product Catalogue.
12. Warner WB, Vora S, Hurtado EA, et al. Effect of operative technique on mesh exposure in laparoscopic sacrocolpopexy. Female Pelvic Med Reconstr Surg 2012; 18(2): 113–17.
13. Tan-Kim J, Menefee SA, Luber KM, et al. Prevalence and risk factors for mesh erosion after laparoscopic-assisted sacrocolpopexy. Int Urogynecol J 2011; 22(2): 205–12.

14. Nosti PA, Carter CM, Sokol AI, et al. Transvaginal versus transabdominal placement of synthetic mesh at time of sacrocolpopexy. Female Pelvic Med Reconstr Surg 22(3): 151–5.
15. Von Pechmann WS, Aungst MJ, Gruber DD, et al. A pilot study on vaginally assisted laparoscopic sacrocolpopexy for patients with uterovaginal prolapse. Female Pelvic Med Reconstr Surg 2011; 17(3): 115–19.
16. Majercik S, Tsikitis V, Iannitti DA. Strength of tissue attachment to mesh after ventral hernia repair with synthetic composite mesh in a porcine model. Surg Endosc Other Interv Tech 2006; 20(11): 1671–4.
17. Hart SR, Weiser EB. Abdominal sacral colpopexy mesh erosion resulting in a sinus tract formation and sacral abscess. Obstet Gynecol 2004; 103(5 Pt 2): 1037–40.
18. Downing KT. Vertebral osteomyelitis and epidural abscess after laparoscopic uterus-preserving cervicosacropexy. J Minim Invasive Gynecol 2008; 15(3): 370–2.
19. Propst K, Tunitsky-Bitton E, Schimpf MO, et al. Pyogenic spondylodiscitis associated with sacral colpopexy and rectopexy: report of two cases and evaluation of the literature. Int Urogynecol J 2014; 25(1): 21–31.
20. Pilkinton ML, Levine GC, Bennett L, et al. Comparison of strength of sacrocolpopexy mesh attachment using barbed and nonbarbed sutures. Int Urogynecol J 2018; 29(1): 153–9.
21. Linder BJ, Anand M, Klingele CJ, et al. Outcomes of robotic sacrocolpopexy using only absorbable suture for mesh fixation. Female Pelvic Med Reconstr Surg 2017; 23(1): 13–16.
22. Tan-Kim J, Menefee SA, Lippmann Q, et al. A pilot study comparing anatomic failure after sacrocolpopexy with absorbable or permanent sutures for vaginal mesh attachment. Perm J 2014; 18(4): 40–4.
23. Cundiff GW, Varner E, Visco AG, et al. Risk factors for mesh/suture erosion following sacral colpopexy. Am J Obstet Gynecol 2008; 199(6): 688.e1–5.
24. Shepherd JP, Higdon HL, Stanford EJ, et al. Effect of suture selection on the rate of suture or mesh erosion and surgery failure in abdominal sacrocolpopexy. Female Pelvic Med Reconstr Surg 2010; 16(4): 229–33.
25. Surgical Specialities Corporation. Quill | Barbed Suture helps reduce closure time by 50%.
26. Tan-Kim J, Nager CW, Grimes CL, et al. A randomized trial of vaginal mesh attachment techniques for minimally invasive sacrocolpopexy. Int Urogynecol J 2015; 26(5): 649–56.
27. Borahay MA, Oge T, Walsh TM, et al. Outcomes of robotic sacrocolpopexy using barbed delayed absorbable sutures. J Minim Invasive Gynecol 2014; 21(3): 412–16.
28. Bazzi AA, Osmundsen BC, Hagglund KH, et al. Anatomical outcomes based on suturing technique during vaginal mesh attachment in robotic sacrocolpopexy. Female Pelvic Med Reconstr Surg 2019; 25(2): 105–8.
29. ClinicalTrials.gov. Permanent versus Absorbable Colpopexy Trial. Available at: https://clinicaltrials.gov/ct2/show/NCT02277925
30. Good MM, Abele TA, Balgobin S, et al. Preventing L5-S1 discitis associated with sacrocolpopexy. Obstet Gynecol 2013; 121: 285–90.
31. Nygaard IE, McCreery R, Brubaker L, et al. Abdominal sacrocolpopexy: a comprehensive review. Obstet Gynecol 2004; 104(4): 805–23.
32. Withagen MI, Vierhout ME, Mannaerts GH, et al. Laparoscopic sacrocolpopexy with bone anchor fixation: short-term anatomic and functional results. Int Urogynecol J 2012; 23(4): 481–6.
33. Sanz LE, Verosko J. Modification of abdominal sacrocolpopexy using a suture anchor system. J Reprod Med 2003; 48(7): 496–500.
34. Braun NM, Andraos W, Bettin S. Safety and efficacy of spider anchoring device for apical repair in laparoscopic sacrocolpopexy: retrospective cohort study. Eur J Obstet Gynecol Reprod Biol 2019; 235: 88–92.
35. Girvent Vilarmau M, Ojeda Pérez F, Canto Rivera MJ, et al. Peek's harpoon: a new device for the treatment of laparoscopic sacropexy. Preliminary study in unembalmed cadavers. Int Urogynecol J 2017; 28(6): 881–5.

Chapter 6

Surgical Anatomy for Laparoscopic Urogynaecology

Eric S Chang, Kristie A Greene

The Abdominal Wall

The abdominal wall is comprised of several layers, through which access to the peritoneal cavity and gynaecologic organs can be obtained. Beneath the skin lies the subcutaneous fat, followed by the Camper's and Scarpa's fascia which merge into a single layer at the linea alba in the midline. Practically, these two layers of fascia are typically indistinguishable from each other in surgery, and appear as a single layer of white collagenous tissue [1]. The umbilicus typically lies at a vertical level between the L3 to L5 vertebrae and is used to separate the abdominal wall into quadrants. The umbilicus contains a dense, fibrous umbilical ring which arises through the linea alba, and is traditionally the thinnest part of the abdominal wall. Because of this, the umbilicus is often used as the first site of entry into the abdominal cavity for laparoscopic surgery [2]. Running parallel to, and on either side of the linea alba, are the rectus abdominis muscles which extend from the pubic symphysis and pubic crest inferiorly to the xiphoid process of the sternum and costal cartilages of the ribs superiorly and laterally. The rectus muscle is enveloped in the rectus sheath, which itself is the aponeurosis of the lateral abdominal muscles which, from superficial to deep, are comprised of the external oblique, the internal oblique, and the transversus abdominis muscles. Inferiorly, the pyramidalis muscle originates from the pubic crest inferiorly, and inserts into the linea alba superiorly and at the midline [1]. The arcuate line is a horizontal demarcation across the abdomen exiting at a vertical level, approximately halfway between the umbilicus and pubic symphysis. Above the arcuate line, the rectus sheath is split into an anterior and posterior sheath, which exit superficial and deep to the rectus abdominis muscles, respectively. Below the arcuate line, we find the anterior rectus sheath [3]. The transversalis fascia lies beneath the transversus abdominis muscle and extends across the entirety of the anterior abdominal wall. Beneath this fascia lies a layer of preperitoneal fat, then the peritoneum which is a serous membrane that envelops most of the intra-abdominal organs [1].

Nerves

Afferent sensory peripheral nerves supply sensation to the abdominal wall, with dermatomes representing the sensory coverage of a single peripheral nerve. Of note, the T6 to L1 dermatomes contain the nerves supplying the anterior abdominal wall and are the target for performing a transversus abdominis plane block for analgesia after lower abdominal wall surgery. The T10 dermatome is notable as it contains the umbilicus, and this dermatome can be more specifically targeted for a peripheral block [4].

The L1 spinal nerve branches into the ilioinguinal and iliohypogastric nerves. The ilioinguinal nerve provides sensation to the mons pubis, medial thigh, and labia majora and courses laterally across the quadratus lumborum muscle of the lower back, crosses the iliacus muscle at the iliac crest, then wraps anteriorly and crosses through the transversus abdominis and internal oblique muscles before entering the inguinal canal and exiting through the superficial inguinal ring [5]. On average, the proximal end enters the abdominal wall 3 cm medial and 4 cm inferior to the anterior superior iliac spine (ASIS), then travels superiorly, terminating approximately 2 cm superior and 3 cm lateral to the midline [6].

The iliohypogastric nerve courses through the transversus abdominis muscle and along the external oblique aponeurosis traveling approximately 2 cm medial and 1 cm inferior to ASIS and terminating 5 cm superior to ASIS and 4 cm lateral to the midline. It provides motor innervation to the transversus abdominis and external oblique muscles, and sensory input for the skin overlying the mons pubis as well as an anterior cutaneous branch providing sensory innervation to upper and lateral thigh [6].

Blood Vessels

Three vessels supply a majority of the anterior abdominal wall. The superficial epigastric artery provides blood supply to the superficial structures of the abdominal wall and branches off the femoral artery below the level of the inguinal ligament, then courses between Camper's and Scarpa's fascia cephalad, parallel to and along the lateral border of the rectus muscle, to approximately the level of the umbilicus [1,7]. The superior and inferior epigastric arteries run along the deep surface of the rectus abdominis muscle and provide the blood supply to the muscles of the anterior abdominal wall (Figure 6.1). The superior epigastric branches off the internal thoracic artery, and the inferior epigastric branches off the external iliac above the level of the inguinal ligament. The two epigastric vessels then anastomose at approximately the level of the umbilicus [7]. The inferior epigastric vessels are approximately 4 cm lateral to midline at the level of the ASIS, and lateral to the rectus muscles at a level 2 cm superior to the pubic symphysis [7].

Landmarks for Port Placement and Avoiding Vascular and Nerve Injuries

For pelvic surgery, the peritoneal cavity is typically entered at the umbilicus as this is usually the thinnest portion of the anterior abdominal wall and lacks major nerves or vessels [8]. The

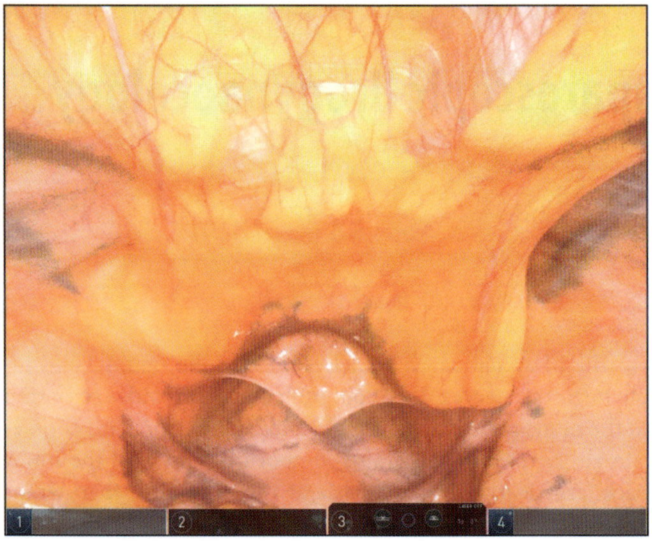

Figure 6.1 Laparoscopic surgical photo demonstrating transperitoneal visualization of the inferior epigastric vessels traversing along the anterior abdominal wall.

umbilicus is typically located at the level of the L3 to L4 vertebrae, and the aortic bifurcation is at L4 to L5. With obese patients, the umbilicus can shift caudad and can actually be at a level below the aortic bifurcation [9,10,11]. As such, in thin women, the umbilical trocar should be placed with an angle towards the pelvis, whereas in obese women, the trocar can be inserted more perpendicular to the abdominal wall.

An alternate entry point is in the left upper quadrant known as Palmer's point. Palmer's point is located in the midclavicular line approximately 3 cm inferior to the left costal margin. This entry point may be useful if patient has a prior surgical history, which may predispose to adhesions at the level of the umbilicus [12,13].

Port placement can vary based on surgeon preference, but awareness of key anatomic structures is critical to avoid neurovascular injury. One example of typical port placement for pelvic surgery is depicted in Figure 6.2. Both the ilioinguinal and iliohypogastric nerves are susceptible to potential injury with port placement sites that are inferior to the level of the anterior superior iliac spine. Therefore, the lower quadrant ports are typically placed 2 cm medial to and either at the level of or superior to the ASIS [7].

The superficial epigastric artery branches off the femoral artery and runs cephalad, parallel to and along the lateral border of the rectus muscle to approximately the level of the umbilicus. This artery can be transilluminated to delineate its course along the anterior abdominal wall. The inferior epigastric arteries run along the deep surface of the rectus abdominis muscle and can be traced intra-abdominally coursing lateral to the medial umbilical folds but medial to the deep inguinal ring. Care should be taken to place lower quadrant ports lateral to these vessels. The superior epigastric artery is rarely encountered in laparoscopic pelvic surgery. However, the inferior epigastric artery can be accidentally entered with lower quadrant port placement.

Incisions are typically made in a horizontal orientation parallel to a patient's natural Langer's lines, which are the naturally occurring skin lines traversing horizontally across the abdomen and associated with the distribution of collagen and elastin fibres of the skin. This is thought to allow closures with less tension and improved cosmesis [14].

Laparoscopic View of the Pelvis

In pelvic laparoscopy, the pelvis is viewed in a cephalad to caudad direction. Within the visualized abdomino-pelvic space lie the reproductive organs, gastrointestinal organs, parts of the urinary system, and important blood vessels, nerves, and muscles. The laparoscopic urogynaecologist must be familiar with this anatomy in order to minimize the risk of complications during surgery.

The internal surface of the anterior abdominal wall contains several important structures, commonly used as landmarks in laparoscopic pelvic and urogynaecologic surgery. The single median umbilical ligament runs longitudinally along the midline and is the remnant of the obliterated urachus, with overlying peritoneum forming the medial umbilical fold. Lateral to this are the paired medial umbilical ligaments, which are the remnants of the obliterated umbilical arteries and run deep to the rectus muscles in a longitudinal fashion. Peritoneum overlying these ligaments forms the medial umbilical folds. Lateral to these structures are the inferior epigastric arteries [15,16]. Care to avoid these vessels must be taken when placing ports in the lower quadrants. Knowledge of the anatomy of these peritoneal folds is important in accessing the retroperitoneal space laparoscopically so as to avoid injury to the epigastric vessels.

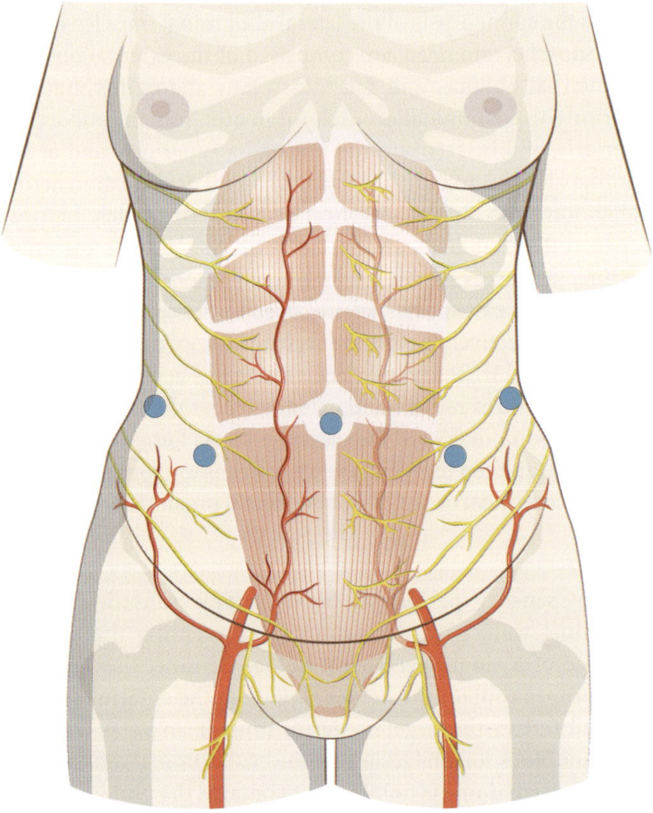
Figure 6.2 Anterior abdominal wall nerves and blood vessels in relation to port placement locations for laparoscopic pelvic surgery.

The Reproductive Organs

On laparoscopy, the female reproductive organs that can be visualized are the uterus, fallopian tubes, ovaries, and vagina. The uterus is comprised of the fundus, the corpus, and cervix. It is located midline deep in the pelvis and can vary in size depending on the patient's menstrual status as well as with presence of any pathology such as leiomyoma or adenomyosis [17].

The uterus is typically larger than the cervix in a premenopausal woman but in the postmenopausal population, the two can be similar in size. Laparoscopically, the cervix cannot be directly visualized. However, with use of a colpotomizer device placed vaginally around the cervix and pushing cephalad into the vaginal fornicies, the transition point between the vagina and the uterine cervix can be delineated more clearly on laparoscopic view [18]. Beyond the colpotomizer is the vaginal tube. If the patient has undergone a prior hysterectomy, the vaginal tube can be visualized more clearly with a vaginal stent such as an EEA sizer. This is useful in situations where vesicovaginal or rectovaginal space dissection is necessary on a post-hysterectomy patient [19].

The fallopian tubes appear as long tubular structures arising from the uterine cornua bilaterally. The parts of the fallopian tube from proximal to distal in relation to the uterus are the isthmus, ampulla, infundibulum, and fimbriae. The blood supply to the fallopian tubes includes both the uterine and ovarian arteries. The fallopian tube is attached to the mesosalpinx which is the portion of the broad ligament stretching between the ovary and fallopian tube [17].

The ovaries are located lateral and posterior to the uterus and fimbriae of the fallopian tubes and are suspended by the utero-ovarian ligament, which attaches the ovary to the uterus, and the infundibulopelvic ligament, which attach the ovaries to the pelvic sidewall. The ovaries derive a majority of their blood supply from the ovarian arteries which traverse through the infundibulopelvic ligament. Ovarian size can vary greatly depending on the patient's menstrual status as well as the presence of pathology [17].

Levels of Support

The structures that support the uterus and vagina can be separated into three different levels as originally described by DeLancey in 1992 [20] (see Figure 6.3). Each level of support is comprised of connective tissue attachments that stabilize different portions of the uterus and vagina, with Level I comprising the cardinal ligament and uterosacral ligaments, Level II comprising the paravaginal attachments along the length of the vagina, and Level III comprising the perineal membrane and perineal body [3]. Although this description suggests a separation of function, Levels I, II, and III exist as a continuous part of the endopelvic fascia. Defects on an individual level, or a combination thereof, can lead to specific pelvic floor conditions such as pelvic organ prolapse or urinary incontinence.

Level I support, comprising the cardinal ligament/uterosacral ligament complex, is considered the most cephalad level of support for the pelvic structures, specifically suspending the uterine cervix and vaginal apex. The cardinal ligament and uterosacral ligaments are parametrial condensations of connective

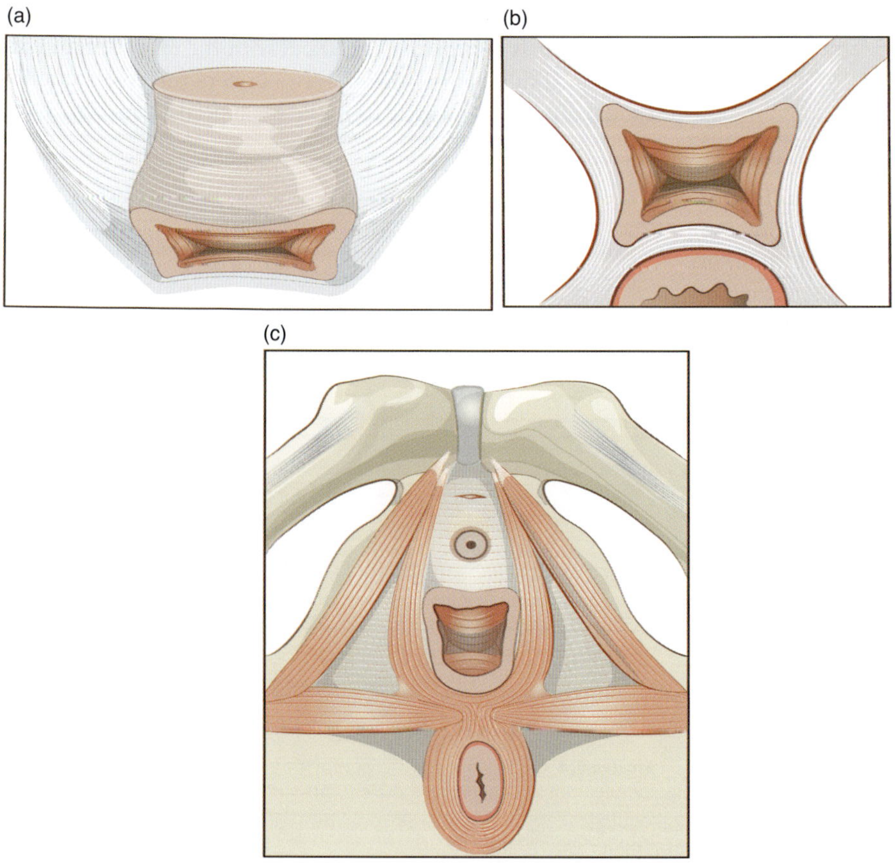

Figure 6.3 Pelvic levels of support. (a) Level I is comprised of the cardinal ligament and uterosacral ligaments and supports the cervix and vaginal apex. (b) Level II is comprised of paravaginal attachments that serve to support the mid-vagina. (c) Level III is comprised of the perineal membrane and perineal body and provides support for the distal vagina.

tissue that fuse at the posterior lower uterine segment at the level of the internal cervical os [21]. The cardinal ligaments continue laterally to the pelvic sidewall near the origin of the internal iliac artery, fusing with the obturator fascia of the obturator internus muscle, and are surrounded by the blood vessels supplying the uterus and vagina. The uterosacral ligaments continue posteriorly to attach to the sacrum and ischial spines [20]. In the standing position, Level I fibres are oriented vertically, suspending the uterine cervix and upper vagina, and maintaining the vaginal axis nearly horizontal [22]. Manifestations of Level 1 support defects include uterovaginal prolapse or post-hysterectomy vaginal apical prolapse.

Restoration of vaginal apical support defects using structures native to Level , include uterosacral ligament suspension which can be performed both vaginally and laparoscopically with laparoscopic route demonstrating benefit in regard to perioperative blood loss, ureteral obstruction, and patient recovery as compared to vaginal route [23,24]. Laparoscopic visualization of the uterosacral ligaments can be facilitated by manipulation of the uterus or vaginal cuff in a post-hysterectomy patient towards the anterior abdominal wall. This places the uterosacral ligaments on tension and can make for easier identification of the ligaments.

Level II support is comprised of paravaginal visceral connective tissue that extend from the midportion of the vagina to the lateral pelvic sidewall at the arcus tendinous fascia pelvis anteriorly, and the arcus tendinous rectovaginalis posteriorly [22]. These supports form a 'hammock' upon which the midvagina orients, and maintains the vagina at midline. The arcus tendinous fascia pelvis is the consolidation of the endopelvic fascia originating at the ischial spine and inserting on the inferior aspect of the superior pubic ramus. The arcus tendinous fascia pelvis supports and creates the anteriorlateral vaginal sulci. These attachments maintain the upper vagina in a near horizontal position and resist caudal movement of the upper vagina and urethra with Valsalva when in standing position [25]. The arcus tendinous rectovaginalis is the consolidation of the levator ani fascia extending from the perineal body to the midpoint of the arcus tendineus fascia pelvis and is approximately 4 cm in length [26]. This connection creates the postero-lateral vaginal sulci and changes the orientation of the distal vagina to a more vertical axis. Manifestations of Level II support defects include anterior or posterior vaginal wall prolapse, paravaginal defects, and stress urinary incontinence [27]. Laparoscopic operations developed to address pelvic floor conditions involving Level II support include laparoscopic paravaginal repair, Burch urethropexy, and historically the Marshall-Marchetti-Krantz procedure [28,29].

Level III support is comprised of the perineal membrane and perineal body and provides support and orientation for the distal vagina [20]. The perineal membrane involves a continuation of the endopelvic fascia, which dorsally attaches the distal lateral wall of the vagina and perineal body to the ischiopubic ramus. Ventrally, the perineal membrane is closely associated with the sphincter mechanism of the urethra and is continuous with the insertion of the arcus tendineus fascia pelvis [30]. The perineal body is a fibromuscular structure located at the junction of the anus and urogenital triangle at the midline and provides attachments to the paired bulbospongiosus and superficial transverse perineal muscles, as well as the external anal sphincter. Together, the perineal membrane and perineal body play an important role in maintaining the integrity of the pelvic floor. Disruption of the perineal membrane or separation of the perineal body can result in posterior vaginal wall prolapse, perineocele, defecatory dysfunction, and anal incontinence.

Muscles and Connective Tissue of the Pelvic Floor

The levator ani complex is comprised of the paired iliococcygeous, pubococcygeus, and puborectalis muscles which originate from the arcus tendineus fascia pelvis and meet at the midline, inserting into the anococcygeal raphae [31]. The levator ani complex is typically described as a 'bowl' of muscles forming part of the pelvic floor (Figure 6.4), which is more representative of the pelvic floor in its relaxed state. These muscles are typically tonically contracted in order to support pelvic organs such as the bladder, uterus, and rectum. Dysfunction of the levator ani complex can lead to pelvic floor dysfunction such as prolapse, incontinence, or myofascial pain syndrome [32,33].

The endopelvic fascia provides connective tissue support for the pelvis. It exists as a continuation of the transversalis fascia and lines the levator ani complex, coccygeus, obturator internus, and piriformus muscles before fusing with the periosteum of the pelvic bones [34].

Ureter, Bladder, and Urethra

Ureter

The ureter is a paired long tubular conduit through which urine passes from the renal collecting system to the bladder. In adults, each ureter is approximately 30 cm with the exact length correlating to the woman's height. The ureters traverse a craniocaudal direction and arise from the renal pelvis, coursing in the

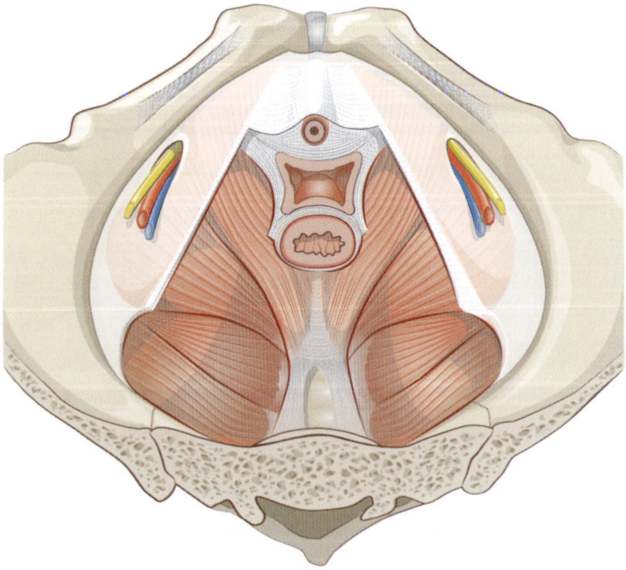

Figure 6.4 Cephalad to caudad view of the levator ani. The levator ani is formed from three separate muscle components. From lateral to medial, the components are the iliococcygeus muscle, the pubococcygeus muscle, and the puborectalis muscles.

retroperitoneal space on the anterior surface of the psoas muscle and passing medial to the sacroiliac joints. The ureters enter the pelvis lying anterior to, and at the level of the bifurcation of the common iliac vessels, continuing lateral to the internal iliac vessels along the pelvic sidewall peritoneum. The ureters will turn in a medial direction, passing lateral to the uterosacral ligaments at the level of the ischial spines, then underneath the uterine artery while entering the endopelvic fascia of the parametrium. The ureters will then continue to course medially over the lateral vagina to enter the bladder trigone [35].

The ureter is lined by transitional urothelium overlying the lamina propria, a connective tissue layer containing blood vessels, lymphatics, and nerves. These layers are surrounded by irregular layers of smooth muscle fibres oriented in multiple directions which rhythmically contract to propel urine from the kidneys to the bladder. Distally, the ureter is surrounded by the fibromuscular Waldeyer's sheath which serves to fix the ureter as it enters the bladder, and links the ureter to the detrusor muscle [35].

The vascular supply of the ureter is derived from the vessels it passes on its caudal course. The upper ureters receive blood supply from the renal arteries, the mid-portion of the ureter is supplied by the ovarian arteries, and the distal ureter is supplied by branches of the common iliac, internal iliac, and vesical arteries [31,35].

In laparoscopic urogynaecology, the most commonly encountered portion of the ureter is within the pelvis [36]. Identification of the course of the ureters is of utmost importance when performing dissections in the deep pelvis or pelvic sidewall such as with hysterectomy, vesicovaginal space dissection for sacrocolpopexy, or laparoscopic uterosacral ligament suspension. Often, the ureter can be identified in a transperitoneal approach by visualizing the intermittent rhythmic vermiculation of the ureter along the pelvic sidewall. When transperitoneal identification of the ureter cannot be accomplished quickly, we recommend identification of the common iliac bifurcation where the ureter can typically be seen crossing medially over the bifurcation to enter the pelvis. Alternatively, the peritoneum of the pelvic sidewall can be carefully opened and the ureter can be identified in the retroperitoneal space coursing along the medial leaf of the peritoneum [37]. The course of the ureter can be helpful in identification of other landmarks within urogynaecologic surgery. For example, the right ureter lies approximately 3 cm lateral to the sacral promontory at the level of the pelvic brim [38], which can be helpful in beginning the dissection for a sacrocolpopexy over a promontory that is obscured by significant presacral fat.

Bladder

The bladder is an extraperitoneal hollow, muscular viscus whose purpose is to store urine. The bladder is collapsed when empty but compliance of its walls allows for distention of the reservoir as it fills. The capacity of the adult bladder is typically 400–500 ml [35]. When empty, the bladder is typically wholly intrapelvic and situated behind the pubic symphysis. When full, the bladder can extend into the lower abdomen and can often be palpated on abdominal examination.

The anterior bladder is located immediately behind the pubic bones within the retropubic space (of Retzius). In this space lies loose areolar tissue, adipose tissue, pubovesical ligaments, and the venous plexus of Santorini. The superior and upper posterior aspects of the bladder are covered by peritoneum that extends onto the lower uterine segment forming the vesico-uterine pouch. The remainder of the posterior bladder rests upon the lower uterine segment and anterior vagina with the endopelvic fascia separating the organs. The median umbilical ligament is a fibrous cord that extends from the dome of the bladder to the umbilicus and represents the obliterated urachus. The paired ureters enter the bladder postero-inferiorly and together with the urethral orifice, form the bladder trigone. Between the two ureteral orifices is the raised interureteric ridge. The urethral orifice is located in the bladder neck where smooth muscle fibres of the detrusor muscle converge and continue as smooth muscle of the urethra [31,35].

The bladder is internally lined by transitional urothelium, which sits atop a submucosal layer comprised of connective and elastic tissue. Overlying the submucosal layer is the detrusor muscle containing smooth muscle fibres arranged in irregular and random orientation except at the bladder neck where three discernible layers of inner longitudinal, middle circular, and outer longitudinal smooth muscle can be identified [35].

The vascular supply of the bladder is derived from the superior, middle, and inferior vesical arteries, which arise from the anterior division of the internal iliac artery, as well all branches off the uterine, vaginal, obturator, and inferior gluteal arteries.

Manipulation of and close dissection around the bladder is required in many laparoscopic urogynaecologic surgeries such as with hysterectomy, Burch colposuspension, paravaginal repairs, and vesicovaginal space development for sacrocolpopexy. For these, and other similar procedures, it is important to demarcate the exact borders of the bladder to minimize the risk of potential bladder injury. When adhesive disease or scarring, such as in patients with a prior history of caesarean delivery, impedes the clear visualization of the bladder limits, we recommend retrograde filling of the bladder with a urinary catheter.

Urethra

The female urethra is approximately 3–4 cm long and 6–8 mm in diameter [35]. The urethra lies beneath the pubic symphysis and anterior to the vagina in the retropubic space (of Retzius). The urethra is lined by stratified squamous epithelium, except for near the bladder where it becomes transitional urothelium. Overlying the connective and elastic tissue submucosa layer of the urethra is a longitudinal layer of smooth muscle continuous with the inner longitudinal layer of the bladder encircled by circular smooth muscle fibres comprising the involuntary intrinsic urethral sphincter. External to these muscle layers is circular striated muscle in the proximal two-thirds of the urethra comprising the sphincter urethrae, and the compressor urethrae and urethrovaginal sphincter, whose striated fibres form a sling underneath the distal third of the urethra. Together, these three striated muscles comprise the voluntary extrinsic urethral sphincter mechanism [40].

Except in Burch colposuspension and paravaginal repair, the urethra is rarely encountered in laparoscopic urogynaecology. In these procedures, the retropubic space (of Retzius) is entered and the bladder is dissected away from the pubic symphysis. The dissection is carried to the level of the bladder neck and urethra which can be visualized resting atop the anterior vagina.

Sigmoid Colon, Rectum, Anus

Sigmoid Colon

The sigmoid colon is the terminal portion of the large intestine starting as a continuation of the descending colon at the level of the pelvic brim and reaching the rectum at the level of the third sacral vertebrae. This portion of the colon is named after the Greek letter sigma as it usually takes on a characteristic curved 'S' shape. The primary function of the sigmoid colon is to reabsorb water and nutrients from the stool prior to its passage into the rectum for storage prior to defecation. The sigmoid colon stretches an average of 25 to 40 cm and typically resides in the pelvis, though as a mobile structure with a mesentery, it can be wholly displaced into the abdomen. The sigmoid colon is surrounded by peritoneum and is thus an intraperitoneal structure unlike the descending colon and rectum, which are both retroperitoneal [41].

The sigmoid colon derives its blood supply from the sigmoid branches of the inferior mesenteric artery as well as collateral blood supply from the left colic artery and superior rectal arteries, both of which also originate from the inferior mesenteric artery. These vessels travel through the sigmoid mesocolon which is a peritoneal fold attaching the sigmoid colon to the posterior pelvic wall. The apex of the mesocolon is near the division of the left common iliac vessels and medial to the left ureter as it crosses the pelvic brim into the pelvis [41].

In laparoscopic urogynaecology, the sigmoid colon is typically a structure that must be manipulated by the surgeon to optimize visualization of the surgical field. A large, distended, or redundant sigmoid colon can often block access to pelvic structures such as the uterus and adnexa, the bladder, and the sacral promontory, even when the patient is placed in steep Trendelenburg positioning. In these cases, blunt laparoscopic graspers can be first used to attempt to flip the sigmoid leftward towards the pelvic sidewall and superiorly into the abdomen. If this does not achieve adequate retraction and additional assistance is available, a laparoscopic retractor such as an articulating fan can be used to hold the sigmoid. Alternatively, a suture can be carefully placed through an epiploic appendage of the sigmoid colon, then through the left anterior abdominal wall peritoneum and loosely tied for retraction. When robotic assistance is utilized, a wide blunt grasping instrument may be utilized in the left-most port to assist in retraction of the rectosigmoid colon. In manipulation of the sigmoid colon, care must be taken to not place excessive traction on the mesocolon as its blood supply and lymphatics course through this area. Additionally, direct repeated manipulation of the colon, especially with sharp instruments, should be avoided to minimize the risk of bowel injury. It is important to remember to only apply the minimum amount of retraction necessary to visualize the target anatomy as, unlike the small intestine and more proximal portions of the large intestine, the sigmoid colon will oftentimes not completely retract into the abdomen. If injury or devascularization to the sigmoid colon is suspected, intraoperative colorectal surgery consultation is recommended.

Rectum and Anus

The rectum is a retroperitoneal structure beginning at the termination of the sigmoid colon at the level of the third sacral vertebrae and continuing to the anal orifice. The primary purpose of the rectum is a reservoir for storage of faecal matter prior to defaecation. The rectal musculature consists of an inner circular and outer longitudinal layer of smooth muscle. However, unique to the rectum is a thickening of the inner circular layer at the level of the perineal flexure forming the internal anal sphincter (IAS) [42]. The internal anal sphincter is under autonomic control and is tonically contracted, accounting for 85% of the resting tone of the anus [43]. As the rectum distends with stool or gas, the IAS will relax temporarily during a process known as the anorectal inhibitory reflex (RAIR) reflex. This is thought to help in rectal sampling or distinguishing between gas and stool [44]. The external anal sphincter is comprised of striated muscle and has somatic innervation from the pudendal nerve. It can be voluntarily contracted and often functions in conjunction with the puborectalis muscle to aid in continence of stool. The puborectalis muscle, which is a component of the levator ani complex, forms a sling originating from the pubic bone on one side, wrapping around the rectum and then back on the pubic bone on the contralateral side. The puborectalis muscle creates an anorectal angle that acts as a physical barrier to stool and assists in maintaining continence. As the puborectalis muscle is relaxed during defaecation, the anorectal angle widens, and allows passage of rectal contents.

The dentate line is a line in the rectal epithelium that divides the rectal canal into the upper two-thirds and lower third. Above the dentate line, the mucosa is comprised of columnar epithelium similar to much of the rest of the digestive tract. Here, the superior rectal artery provides blood supply. Below the dentate line, the mucosa is comprised of non-keratinized stratified squamous epithelium until the anal verge merges with keratinized stratified squamous epithelium of the perineal skin. Below the dentate line, the middle and inferior rectal arteries provide blood supply [42].

Knowledge of the location of the rectum is particularly important during laparoscopic sacrocolpopexy. Aggressive dissection into the rectovaginal space such as with posterior dissection of the vagina holds potential for injury to the rectum. As such, it is important to perform any sharp dissection of the rectovaginal space with instrument tips pointing away from the rectum and towards the vaginal wall. Additionally, wide dissection of this space should be avoided as injury to the rectal pillars laterally can cause bleeding and obscuring of the space. Should the location or extent of the rectum be unclear, a rectal stent such as an EEA sizer can be inserted into the rectum to aid in visualization. If injury or devascularization to the rectum is suspected, intraoperative colorectal surgery consultation is recommended.

Major Blood Vessels of the Pelvis

Many of the surgeries performed in laparoscopic urogynaecology may require dissection close to major blood vessels. As such, a careful understanding of the blood vessels of the pelvis is important to minimize the risk of vascular injury.

The abdominal aorta branches into the common iliac arteries at the level of L4 to L5 and then branches again into the internal and external iliac arteries at the level of the sacral promontory at L5 to S1 [45]. The middle sacral artery is a direct branch of the aorta that traverses caudad in the midline across L4 and L5, the sacrum, and the coccyx before terminating in the coccygeal gland [46]. This vessel is commonly encountered with dissection of the sacral promontory and should be avoided or cauterized to prevent bleeding and loss of visualization of the space.

The ovaries receive blood supply from the ovarian arteries, which are direct branches of the infrarenal abdominal aorta. These vessels pass through the infundibulopelvic ligament, tethering the ovaries to the pelvic sidewall. The ureters run in close proximity to the base of the infundibulopelvic ligaments and thus, should be identified prior to clamping and cauterization of the ovarian vessels.

Transperitoneal visualization of the external iliac arteries and their paired veins along the pelvic sidewall is usually possible, though overlying fat or scar tissue from prior surgery may make these large vessels difficult to see. The internal iliac arteries course through the pelvic sidewall in the retroperitoneal space, eventually branching into the anterior and posterior divisions. Branches of the posterior division provide blood supply to the buttocks, as well as several muscles of the deep pelvis. Branches arising from the anterior division provide blood supply to the buttocks, bladder, rectum, and uterus. The uterine artery travels through the cardinal ligament in a lateral to medial direction and crosses anterior to the juxtavesical ureter before reaching the uterine isthmus.

Nerves of the Pelvis

The nerves of the pelvis originate from sympathetic, parasympathetic, and somatic nerves. The sympathetic elements originate from T5 through L2 and reach the pelvis through the superior hypogastric plexus, continuing on as the sacral splanchnic nerves. These elements promote relaxation of the bladder and rectum, and contraction of smooth muscle components of the urethral and anal sphincters to promote storage.

The parasympathetic elements originate from S2 through S4 and are known as the pelvic splanchnic nerves. These elements cause contraction of the detrusor muscle and relaxation of the smooth muscle components of the urethral and anal sphincters to promote voiding and defaecation.

Somatic innervation is derived from roots L4 through S4, which form the sacral plexus, and is comprised of afferent fibres carrying sensory information and efferent fibres carrying motor information to innervate the pelvis and lower extremities. The muscles of the levator ani are innervated by a nerve originating from the S3 and S4 travelling on the intrapelvic surface of the muscles. The sciatic nerve, originating from L4 through S3, and the gluteal nerves, originating from L4 through S2, provides innervation to the lower limbs and buttocks. The pudendal nerve originates from S2 through S4 and its many branches supply sensation to the clitoris, labia, and perineum, as well as motor function to the bulbospongiosus and ischiocavernosus muscles as well as the external urethral sphincter and external anal sphincters [47].

Avascular Spaces

The pelvis contains several avascular spaces, which are used as surgical landmarks important to many gynaecologic, urologic, and colorectal surgeries (Figure 6.5). These avascular spaces are potential spaces filled with loose areolar tissue and devoid of blood vessels and nerves that allow for separation between the urinary, reproductive, and defaecatory systems [31,45,48].

Retropubic Space

The retropubic space is also called the space of Retzius after the nineteenth century Swedish anatomist Anders Retzius. This space holds a particularly important place in laparoscopic urogynaecology as procedures such as retropubic midurethral sling placement, Burch colposuspension, and paravaginal repair, among others, all require an intimate understanding and dissection of this space. The retropubic space is the avascular potential space between the pubic symphysis and the urinary bladder (Figure 6.6). The anatomic bounds of the space are the pubic bone and muscles of the anterior abdominal wall anteriorly, the urinary bladder and peritoneum posteriorly, and the arcus tendinous fascia pelvis and ischial spines forming the lateral borders. Aside from loose areolar tissue and adipose tissue, this space contains several important structures to be aware of during laparoscopic dissection. The dorsal clitoral nerve and

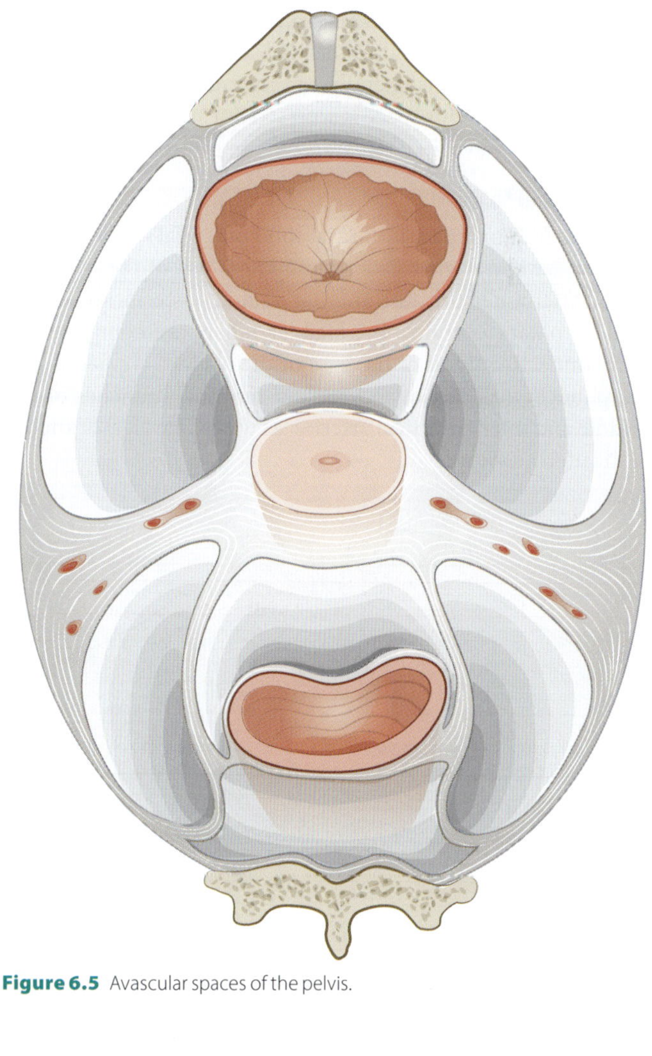

Figure 6.5 Avascular spaces of the pelvis.

vessels lie midline within the space. Laterally, the obturator nerve and vessels can be encountered as they enter the obturator canal. Along the posterior wall of the space, the tissue surrounding the bladder neck and urethra contains the venous plexus of Santorini which drains into the internal iliac vein and can cause brisk bleeding if entered.

The retropubic space is entered laparoscopically by pulling with downward traction on the peritoneum overlying the median umbilical ligament at the level of the superior edge of the bladder and making an incision in the peritoneum sharply. To aid in visualization of the bladder edge, the bladder may be backfilled with a urinary catheter. Once the peritoneal incision is made, it is carried bilaterally in a horizontal manner towards the medial umbilical ligaments. Using dissection with a blunt instrument such as a laparoscopic Kittner, the bladder and urethra are mobilized downward. Visualization of the pubic ramus and the pectineal (Cooper's) ligaments is accomplished by dissecting the preperitoneal fat and loose areolar tissue away from the bone. Laterally, the arcus tendineus fascia pelvis can be visualized as a white fibrous band of tissue overlying the pubococcygeus and obturator internus muscles running from the lower edge of the pubic symphysis towards the ischial spine. Care must be taken to avoid the obturator nerve and vessels during lateral dissection in this space.

The paravesical space is the avascular potential space located within the retropubic space. This space is located anterior to the cardinal ligaments, lateral to the bladder pillars, and bounded by the pelvic sidewalls laterally and the medial umbilical ligaments superiorly. This space is accessed during Burch colposuspension and paravaginal repairs.

Vesicovaginal Space

The vesicovaginal space is the avascular potential space between the bladder and vagina. The anatomic bounds of the space are the bladder anteriorly, the anterior vagina posteriorly, and the bladder pillars laterally. The bladder pillars are comprised of fibroconnective tissue at the base of the bladder connecting to the pubocervical fascia, and contain terminal branches of the middle and inferior vesical arteries, as well as cervical branches of the uterine artery.

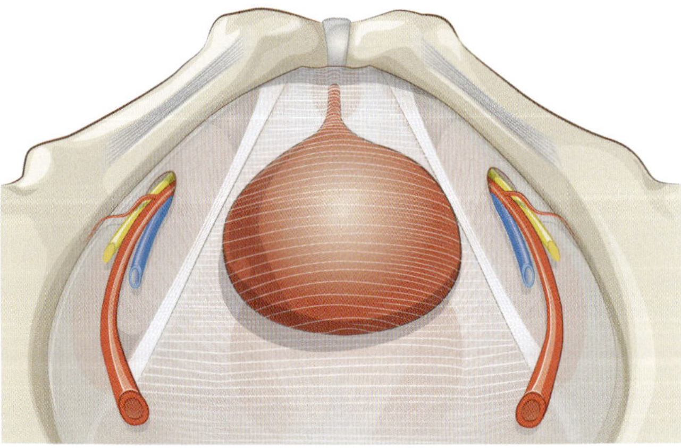

Figure 6.6 Anatomic bounds of the retropubic space and associated neurovascular structures within the space.

The vesicovaginal space is entered by elevating the bladder with a blunt grasper, then making an incision along the peritoneal reflection at the superior bladder border. The space can then be developed by using a blunt instrument to dissect the loose areolar tissue downward onto the bladder. The place along which the space opens should not bleed. If bleeding is encountered, then either accidental dissection into the bladder or vaginal muscularis should be suspected. Identification of the lattice-like pattern of the interwoven detrusor muscle fibres suggests proximity to the bladder.

This space is familiar to gynaecologists as it is entered when performing a bladder flap during hysterectomy to bring the bladder off the lower uterine segment and decrease the risk of inadvertent cystotomy. For sacrocolpopexy, this space is entered and dissection can be carried to the level of the bladder trigone. It is within this space that the anterior leaflet of a sacrocolpopexy mesh is placed and sutured to the pubocervical fascia along the anterior vaginal wall. It is important to stay midline and open the space wide enough to just fit the mesh, as dissecting laterally into the bladder pillars can result in bleeding and obscuring of the space.

Rectovaginal Space

The rectovaginal, also called the pouch of Douglas after the eighteenth century Scottish physician James Douglas, is the avascular potential space between the vagina and the rectum. The anatomic bounds of the space are the posterior vagina anteriorly, the rectum posteriorly, the posterior cul-de-sac superiorly, the internal margin of the perineal body inferiorly, and the rectal pillars laterally. The rectal pillars are structures derived from the cardinal-uterosacral ligament complex and are comprised of fibroconnective tissue, within which the middle rectal arteries run.

During sacrocolpopexy, the rectovaginal space is dissected to allow for attachment of the posterior mesh leaflet to the pubocervical fascia of the posterior vaginal wall. Laparoscopic entry into the space is accomplished by first placing a stent in the vagina to visualize the vaginal tube, then grasping and retracting the midline peritoneum overlying the posterior vagina downward. The stretched peritoneum is then incised sharply at midline. Further downward traction on the cut peritoneal edge will allow for pneumoperitoneum to enter this space and further delineate the dissection plane. The loose areolar tissue may then be bluntly separated, or sharply dissected with instrument tips pointing away from the rectum. The dissection can be carried distally to the extent of the posterior compartment prolapse, or all the way down to the perineal body. It is important to stay midline and open the space wide enough to just fit the mesh, as dissecting laterally into the rectal pillars can result in bleeding and obscuring of the space.

Pararectal Space

The pararectal space is the avascular potential space anatomically bounded by the cardinal ligament anteriorly, the sacrum posteriorly, the rectum medially, and the internal iliac artery and pelvic sidewall laterally. In urogynaecology, the pararectal space is typically entered vaginally when performing a sacrospinous ligament fixation. In laparoscopic urogynaecology, the pararectal space may need to be accessed when adhesions have obliterated the posterior cul-de-sac in order to ensure safe access to the rectovaginal space, or when a sacrocolpopexy mesh is reperitonealized by tunnelling the mesh underneath the pelvic sidewall peritoneum. The space can be entered by opening up the peritoneum at the midpoint between the right ureter and colon [49].

Other Noteworthy Spaces

Sacral Promontory

The sacral promontory is an important landmark in laparoscopic urogynaecology. The promontory demarcates the upper limit of the pelvic brim posteriorly, and is comprised of the anterior superior edge of the sacrum, which articulates with the last lumbar vertebrae (Figures 6.7 and 6.8). This articulation forms the sacrovertebral angle, which can be palpated transabdominally to assist with laparoscopic entry, or visualized transpertioneally as a landmark to start the presacral dissection for sacrocolpopexy. Along the anterior surface of the promontory runs the anterior longitudinal ligament, which is a band of fibrous tissue running along the anterior surface of the spine. It is within the ligament that sutures for attachment of sacrocolpopexy mesh are placed. The middle sacral artery is a direct branch of the aorta that traverses cauded in the midline across the fourth and fifth lumbar vertebrae, the sacrum, and the coccyx before terminating in the coccygeal gland [46,50]. This vessel is commonly encountered with dissection of the sacral promontory and should be avoided to prevent bleeding and loss of visualization of the space. Ligation or cauterization of this vessel may also be performed to decrease risk of vascular injury to this artery.

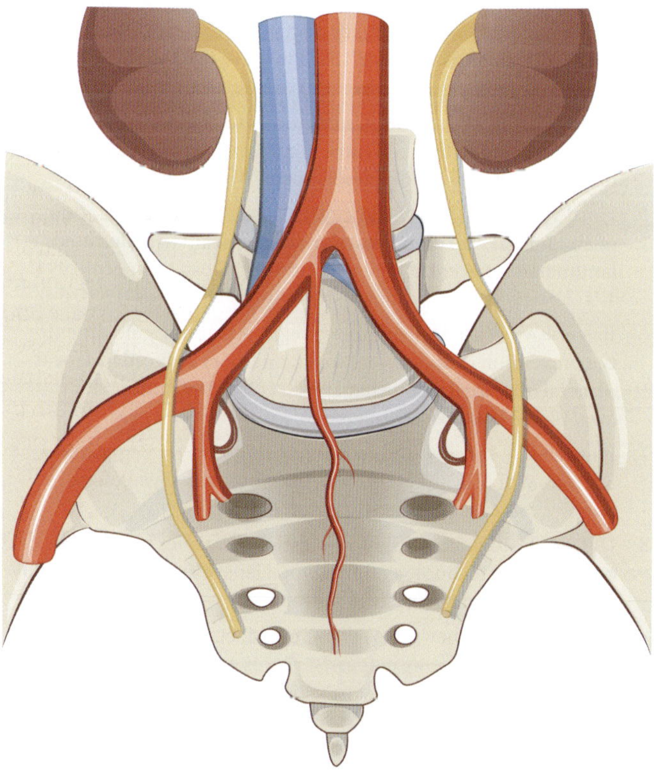

Figure 6.7 Anteroposterior view of the sacral promontory demonstrating its relationship to the ureters and surrounding blood vessels.

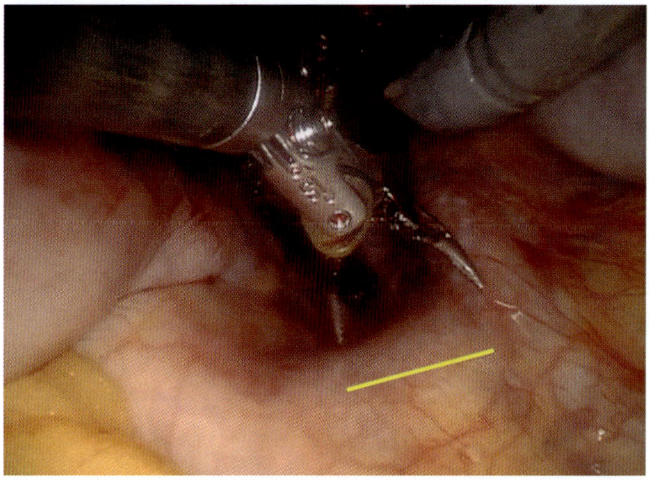

Figure 6.8 Laparoscopic surgical photo demonstrating visualization of the sacral promontory.

The sacral promontory rests below the aortic bifurcation and between the right and left common iliac vessels. In a prior cadaveric and imaging studies, the closest cephalad vessel to the promontory was the left common iliac vein with average distance being 2.7 cm. To the right, the internal iliac artery was found to be 2.5 cm away from the promontory. The average distance from the promontory to the aortic bifurcation cephalad was found to be 5–6 cm [50,51]. Anatomic variation of this vasculature exists, so it is important to identify these large vessels prior to dissection of this space.

Dissection of the sacral promontory first requires adequate visualization of the sacrovertebral angle. During laparoscopy, steep Trendelenburg positioning will allow for small bowel to slide cephalad in the abdomen. A large rectosigmoid colon can be retracted off the promontory with use of a laparoscopic blunt grasper or fan, or by placing a retraction suture through an epiploic appendage of the sigmoid colon and affixing the rectosigmoid colon to the left pelvic sidewall peritoneum. When robotic assistance is utilized, a wide blunt grasping instrument may be utilized in the left-most port to assist in retraction of the rectosigmoid colon. Once an adequate view of the sacrovertebral angle is ascertained, gentle palpation of the promontory with a laparoscopic instrument can be performed to ensure that the dissection will be performed over bone. However, in robotic surgery, there is no haptic feedback and careful observation of the instrument tip must be performed to determine if a hard surface is being palpated. The peritoneum overlying the promontory is then grasped, retracted upwards, and incised. Further upward retraction of the cut peritoneal edge will then allow for pneumoperitoneum to enter the retroperitoneal space to enable further dissection. Blunt dissection should be carefully performed in the opened retroperitoneal space to clear away any presacral fat and avoid vascular injury. This dissection should be carried downwards until the glistening white of the anterior longitudinal ligament is visualized. Typically, only a 1–2 x 1–2 cm opening through which the anterior longitudinal ligament can be clearly visualized is necessary to place two sutures for suspension of sacrocolpopexy mesh.

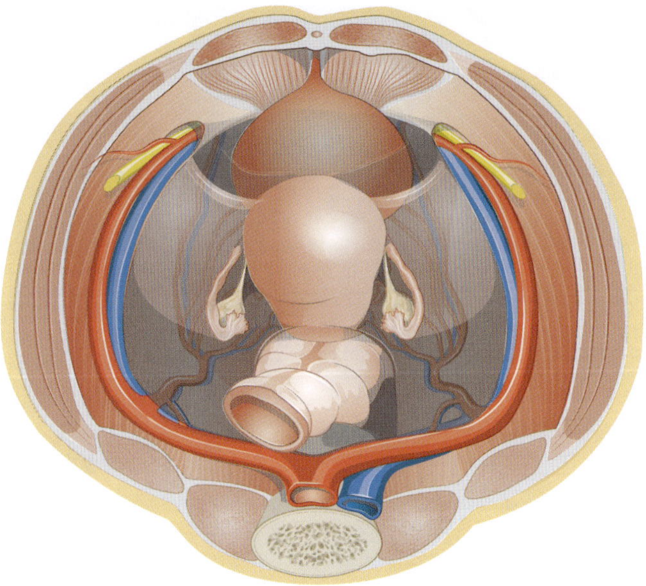

Figure 6.9 Pelvic sidewall anatomy.

Pelvic Sidewall

The pelvic sidewall is notable for containing several key structures (Figures 6.9). Knowledge of these structures is important in minimizing potential complications when performing pelvic laparoscopy. Along the pelvic sidewall, the common iliac vessels can be found bifurcating into the internal and external iliac vessels at the level of the pelvic brim. The paired external iliac vessels are typically seen rising in an anterior-caudal direction along the pelvic sidewall whereas the internal iliac vessels course deeper into the pelvis, eventually branching into the anterior and posterior divisions [52].

The ureter enters the pelvis in the retroperitoneum superficial to the bifurcation of the common iliac vessels. It then traverses along the medial leaf of the broad ligament in a lateral to medial fashion until crossing underneath the uterine artery and inserting into the bladder trigone. Ureteral vermiculation can typically be seen through the peritoneum allowing for the surgeon to distinguish between the ureter and vascular structures [52].

Opening the pelvic sidewall can be accomplished in an area of clear peritoneum and may be safely accomplished once the iliac vessels and ureter is identified. The retroperitoneum is entered safely along the medial leaf of the broad ligament near the pelvic brim and retraction of the peritoneum away from the pelvic sidewall prior to incising the peritoneum will bring the layer away from the underlying retroperitoneal structure.

References

1. Flynn W, Vickerton P. Anatomy, abdomen and pelvis, abdominal wall. In: *StatPearls*. StatPearls Publishing; 2020.
2. Alkatout I, Mettler L, Maass N, et al. Abdominal anatomy in the context of port placement and trocars. J Turk Ger Gynecol Assoc 2015; 16(4): 241–51. https://doi.org/10.5152/jtgga.2015.0148
3. Loukas M, Myers C, Shah R, et al. Arcuate line of the rectus sheath: clinical approach. Anat Sci Int 2008; 83(3): 140–4. https://doi.org/10.1111/j.1447-073X.2007.00221.x
4. Tsai HC, Yoshida T, Chuang TY, et al. Transversus abdominis plane block: an updated review of anatomy and techniques. Biomed Res Int 2017: 8284363. https://doi.org/10.1155/2017/8284363
5. Klaassen, Z, Marshall, E, Tubbs, RS, et al. Anatomy of the ilioinguinal and iliohypogastric nerves with observations of their spinal nerve contributions. Clin Anat 2011; 24: 454–61. https://doi.org/10.1002/ca.21098
6. Whiteside JL, Barber MD, Walters MD, Falcone T. Anatomy of ilioinguinal and iliohypogastric nerves in relation to trocar placement and low transverse incisions. Am J Obstet Gynecol 2003; 189(6): 1574–8. https://doi.org/10.1016/s0002-9378(03)00934-7
7. Rahn DD, Phelan JN, Roshanravan SM, et al. Anterior abdominal wall nerve and vessel anatomy: clinical implications for gynecologic surgery. Am J Obstet Gynecol 2010; 202(3): 234.e1–234.e2345. https://doi.org/10.1016/j.ajog.2009.10.878
8. Thepsuwan J, Huang KG, Wilmarta M, et al. Principals of safe abdominal entry in laparoscopic gynecologic surgery. Gyn and Min Inv Therapy 2013; 2(4): 105–9. https://doi.org/10.1016/j.gmit/2013.07.003
9. Hurd WW, Bude RO, DeLancey JO, Pearl ML. The relationship of the umbilicus to the aortic bifurcation: implications for laparoscopic technique. Obstet Gynecol 1992; 80(1): 48–51.
10. Hurd WH, Bude RO, DeLancey JO, et al. Abdominal wall characterization with magnetic resonance imaging and computed tomography. The effect of obesity on the laparoscopic approach. J Reprod Med 1991; 36(7): 473–6.
11. Nezhat F, Brill AI, Nezhat CH, et al. Laparoscopic appraisal of the anatomic relationship of the umbilicus to the aortic bifurcation. J Am Assoc Gynecol Laparosc 1998; 5(2): 135–40. https://doi.org/10.1016/s1074-3804(98)80079-0
12. Palmer R. Safety in laparoscopy. J Reprod Med 1974; 13(1): 1–5.
13. Childers JM, Brzechffa PR, Surwit EA. Laparoscopy using the left upper quadrant as the primary trocar site. Gynecol Oncol 1993; 50(2): 221–5. https://doiorg/10.1006/gyno.1993.1196
14. Wong VW, Bhatt KA, Vial IN, et al. Beyond Langer's lines: manipulating wound mechanical forces to control hypertrophic scar formation in the red Duroc pig. Plast Surg 2010; 211(3 S77). https://doi.org/10.1016/j.jamcollsurg/2010.06.202
15. Hurd WW, Bude RO, DeLancey JO, Newman JS. The location of abdominal wall blood vessels in relationship to abdominal landmarks apparent at laparoscopy. Am J Obstet Gynecol 1994; 171(3): 642–6. https://doi.org/10.1016/0002-9378(94)90076-0
16. Balzer KM, Witte H, Recknagel S, et al. Anatomic guidelines for the prevention of abdominal wall hematoma induced by trocar placement. Surg Radiol Anat 1999; 21(2): 87–9. https://doi.org/10.1007/s00276-999-0087
17. Baggish MS. Intra-abdominal pelvic anatomy. In: Baggish MS, Karram MM (eds), *Atlas of Pelvic Anatomy and Gynecologic Surgery*, 3rd edn. Saunders Elsevier: 2011, p 179.
18. Jackson T, Advincula AP. Optimization strategies for colpotomizer technology during total laparoscopic hysterectomy. Surg Technol Int 2012; 22: 183–8.
19. Brueseke T, Matthews C, Willis-Gray M, et al. Analysis of robotic procedural times using colpassist versus end-to-end anastomosis sizer for robotic-assisted sacrocolpopexy: a randomized controlled trial. Female Pelvic Med Reconstr Surg 2019; 25(2): e12–e17. https://doi.org/10.1097/SPV.0000000000000692
20. DeLancey JO. Anatomic aspects of vaginal eversion after hysterectomy. Am J Obstet Gynecol 1992; 166(6 Pt 1): 1717–28. https://doi.org/10.1016/0002-9378(92)91562-o

21. Ramanah R, Berger MB, Parratte BM, DeLancey JO. Anatomy and histology of apical support: a literature review concerning cardinal and uterosacral ligaments. Int Urogynecol J 2012; 23(11): 1483–94. https://doi.org/10.1007/s00192-012-1819-7
22. Corton MM. Anatomy of the pelvis: how the pelvis is built for support. Clin Obstet Gynecol 2005; 48(3): 611–26. https://doi.org/10.1097/01.grf.0000170578.24583.64
23. Szymczak P, Grzybowska ME, Wydra DG. Comparison of laparoscopic techniques for apical organ prolapse repair – a systematic review of the literature. Neurourol Urodyn 2019; 38(8): 2031–50. https://doi.org/10.1002/nau.24115
24. Turner LC, Lavelle ES, Shepherd JP. Comparison of complications and prolapse recurrence between laparoscopic and vaginal uterosacral ligament suspension for the treatment of vaginal prolapse. Int Urogynecol J 2016; 27(5): 797–803. https://doi.org/10.1007/s00192-015-2897-0
25. Pit MJ, De Ruiter MC, Lycklama A et al. Anatomy of the arcus tendineus fasciae pelvis in females. Clin Anat 2003; 16(2): 131–7. https://doi.org/10.1002/ca.10102
26. Leffler KS, Thompson JR, Cundiff GW, et al. Attachment of the rectovaginal septum to the pelvic sidewall. Am J Obstet Gynecol 2001; 185(1): 41–3. https://doi.org/10.1067/mob.2001.116366
27. Arenholt LTS, Pedersen BG, Glavind K, et al. Paravaginal defect: anatomy, clinical findings, and imaging. Int Urogynecol J 2017; 28(5): 661–73. https://doi.org/10.1007/s00192-016-3096-3
28. Chinthakanan O, Miklos JR, Moore RD. Laparoscopic paravaginal defect repair: surgical technique and a literature review. Surg Technol Int 2015; 27: 173–83.
29. Miklos JR, Kohli N. Laparoscopic paravaginal repair plus Burch colposuspension: review and descriptive technique. Urology 2000; 56(6 Suppl 1): 64–9. https://doi.org/10.1016/s0090-4295(00)00510-0
30. Stein TA, DeLancey JO. Structure of the perineal membrane in females: gross and microscopic anatomy. Obstet Gynecol 2008; 111(3): 686–93. https://doi.org/10.1097/AOG.0b013e318163a9a5
31. Netter FH. *Atlas of Human Anatomy*, 6th edn. Elsevier Saunders: 2014.
32. Kearney R, Sawhney R, DeLancey JO. Levator ani muscle anatomy evaluated by origin-insertion pairs. Obstet Gynecol 2004; 104(1): 168–73. https://doi.org/10.1097/01.AOG.0000128906.61529.6b
33. Lawson JO. Pelvic anatomy. I. Pelvic floor muscles. Ann R Coll Surg Engl 1974; 54(5): 244–52.
34. Otcenasek M, Baca V, Krofta L, Feyereisl J. Endopelvic fascia in women: shape and relation to parietal pelvic structures. Obstet Gynecol 2008; 111(3): 622–30. https://doi.org/10.1097/AOG.0b013e3181649e5c
35. Tanagho EA, Lue TF. Anatomy of the genitourinary tract. In: McAninch JW, Lue TF (eds), *Smith and Tanagho's General Urology*, 18th edn. McGraw Hill Lange: 2013, pp 7–8.
36. Teeluckdharry B, Gilmour D, Flowerdew G. Urinary tract injury at benign gynecologic surgery and the role of cystoscopy: a systematic review and meta-analysis. Obstet Gynecol 2015; 126(6): 1161–9. https://doi.org/10.1097/AOG.0000000000001096
37. Chan JK, Morrow J, Manetta A. Prevention of ureteral injuries in gynecologic surgery. Am J Obstet Gynecol 2003; 188(5): 1273–7. https://doi.org/10.1067/mob.2003.269
38. McCullough M, Valceus J, Downes K, Hoyte L. The ureter as a landmark for robotic sacrocolpopexy. Female Pelvic Med Reconstr Surg 2012; 18(3): 162–4. https://doi.org/10.1097/SPV.0b013e3182544e17
39. Tanagho EA, Lue TF. Anatomy of the genitourinary tract. In: McAninch JW, Lue TF (eds), *Smith and Tanagho's General Urology*, 18th edn. McGraw Hill Lange: 2013, pp 15.
40. Colleselli K, Stenzl A, Eder R, et al. The female urethral sphincter: a morphological and topographical study. J Urol 1998; 160(1): 49–54. https://doi.org/10.1016/s0022-5347(01)63025-8
41. Harkins JM, Sajjad H. Anatomy, abdomen and pelvis, sigmoid colon. In: *StatPearls*. StatPearls Publishing: 2020.
42. Ahmed A, Qureshi WA. Anatomy, abdomen and pelvis, anal canal. In: *StatPearls*. StatPearls Publishing: 2020.
43. Stepp KJ, Walters MD. Anatomy of the lower urinary tract, pelvic floor, and rectum. In: Walters MD, Karram MM (eds), *Urogynecology and Reconstructive Pelvic Surgery*, 4th edn. Elsevier Saunders: 2015, p 27.
44. Taylor BM, Beart RW Jr, Dozois RR, et al. The endorectal ileal pouch-anal anastomosis. Current clinical results. Dis Colon Rectum 1984; 27(6): 347–50. https://doi.org/10.1007/BF02552994
45. Selçuk İ, Ersak B, Tatar İ, et al. Basic clinical retroperitoneal anatomy for pelvic surgeons. Turk J Obstet Gynecol 2018; 15(4): 259–69. https://doi.org/10.4274/tjod.88614
46. Zilberlicht A, Molnar R, Pal-Ohana H, et al. Characterization of the median sacral artery course at the sacral promontory using contrast-enhanced computed tomography. Int Urogynecol J 2017; 28(1): 101–4. https://doi.org/10.1007/s00192-016-3074-9
47. Spence KT, Forro SD. Anatomy, bony pelvis and lower limb, nerves. In: *StatPearls*. StatPearls Publishing: 2020.
48. Kostov S, Slavchev S, Dzhenkov D, et al. Avascular spaces of the female pelvis: clinical applications in obstetrics and gynecology. J Clin Med 2020; 9(5): 1460. https://doi.org/10.3390/jcm9051460
49. Walid SM, Heaton RL. Laparoscopic dissection of the pararectal space. J Minim Access Surg 2011; 7(3): 190–1. https://doi.org/10.4103/0972-9941.83513
50. Good MM, Abele TA, Balgobin S, et al. Vascular and ureteral anatomy relative to the midsacral promontory. Am J Obstet Gynecol 2013; 208(6): 486.e1–486.e4867. https://doi.org/10.1016/j.ajog.2013.02.039
51. Giraudet G, Protat A, Cosson M. The anatomy of the sacral promontory: how to avoid complications of the sacrocolpopexy procedure. Am J Obstet Gynecol 2018; 218(4): 457.e1–457.e3. https://doi.org/10.1016/j.ajog.2017.12.236
52. Delancey JO. Surgical anatomy of the female pelvis. In: Rock JA, Jones III HW (eds), *Te Linde's Operative Gynecology*, 10th edn. Lippincott Williams & Wilkins: 2011, pp 99–105.

Chapter 7

Learning Curve in Laparoscopic Urogynaecologic Surgery: Strategies to Optimize Training and Acquire Competence

Claire M McCarthy, Barry O'Reilly, Orfhlaith O'Sullivan

Introduction

Medical education has rapidly expanded as a topic over the past 20 years. A wide variety of teaching concepts have been described, illustrated, and become part of undergraduate and postgraduate medical education.

The traditional Halstedian concept from the 1890s of 'See one, Do one, Teach one' was the core of medical and surgical education through the nineteenth and twentieth centuries. However, with time, the realization was that this model is inadequate to train surgeons to the highest level without impacting on patient care [1]. While there still may be a role for this dictum, the concept has been adapted and moulded to fit modern medical education models and needs.

Teachers of medical education not only focus on the topics of education, but also more holistically on areas such as patient safety, practitioner fatigue, and, as technology enhanced learning (TEL) rapidly advances, the application of this to improve training and outcomes.

Similar to other medical and surgical subspecialties, urogynaecologic surgery has had to rapidly adapt over the past number of decades. Traditional 'bread and butter' open procedures of the speciality have been superseded by the newer techniques of traditional straight stick laparoscopy and more recently by robotic surgery, leading to a drastic reduction in open procedures to treat the common urogynaecological conditions. This is clear from figures from the British Society of Urogynaecology, showing that laparoscopic vaginal vault suspension procedures have increased nearly 20-fold in the past 12 years [2]. As laparoscopic surgery advances, with additional techniques such as robotic surgery becoming a routine part of the surgical armoury, including the potential of remotely controlled surgery, medical education has again had to evolve to match the pace of surgical evolutions. The surgical technique between surgeons and centres can vary widely, and highlights the importance of evaluating the effect of surgical technique on outcome [3]. Equally, it has been shown that newer techniques can be as safe as others, with robotic surgery for example being shown as being effective for the management of apical prolapse [4].

Initially, we describe the learning curve as it applies to laparoscopic urogynaecologic surgery, followed by an exploration of training in this rapidly advancing subspeciality, the techniques which can be utilized in educating the surgeons of the future, as well as examine successes, pitfalls, and medical education pearls that can be applied to this niche area of gynaecology.

The Learning Curve

The Wright Learning Curve

The concept of 'The Learning Curve' was first coined in 1936 by TP Wright, and referred to processes in aircraft manufacturing [5]. The term was then extrapolated to medicine in the 1980s after the successful introduction of minimal access surgerysurgery (see Figure 7.1).

Wright utilized the term to describe the basic theory for costing the repetitive production of airplane assemblies. The underlying hypothesis of the learning curve states that the direct man-hours necessary to complete a unit of work decreases by a defined amount each time the production quantity is doubled. Thus, in manufacturing, factors such as time and cost are considered. The learning curve refers to a process or system leading to an improvement in performance over time, and can be plotted as a curvilinear relationship with respect to time.

Factors Affecting the Learning Curve in Surgery

The Learning Curve in Surgery

While the term 'learning curve' is in common parlance in medical education, there is no standardization of the term, with a number of groups attempting to provide this [6]. Given it was originally extrapolated from the manufacturing world and adapted into medicine, it is difficult to determine what factors the surgical learning curve may refer to. Some authors have utilized it to refer to time taken to perform a procedure, the number of procedures that are performed, or the length of time in training [7]. However, in surgical practice, tasks are performed

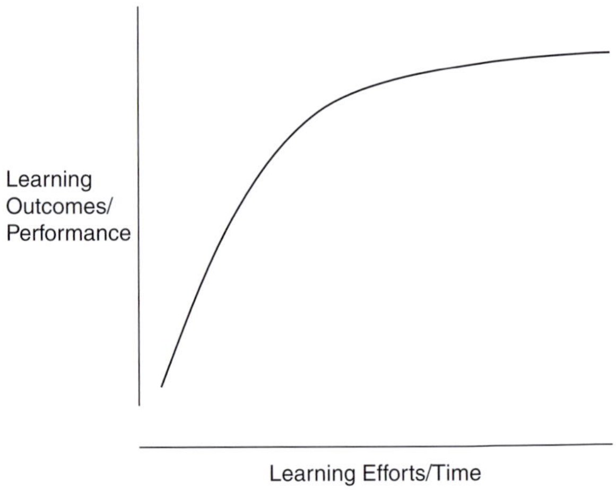

Figure 7.1 The Learning Curve as applied to surgery.

manually and not by a computer process, which is a reflection of the manufacturing learning curve. Thus, it does not take into account a number of integral variables to the procedure, nor outcomes.

There are three main features that a learning curve possesses to describe surgical performance [8]. Firstly, the starting point refers to the initial stage of an individual performance. Secondly, the rate of learning measures how quickly the surgeon will reach a certain level of performance, and thirdly, the asymptote or expert level measures where and when the surgeon's performance stabilizes.

Learning curves can be constructed using a variety of methods [9]. Typically, the Cartesian method was utilized, plotting the learning series on the x-axis, with response characteristics on the y-axis. More recently, the Cumulative Sum method has been successfully utilized in the assessment of anaesthetic procedures. Alternative methods include the multimode learning curve, or the moving average method, which are useful when plotting different outcomes, such as time in the case of the latter.

Level of Skill Acquisition

Surgical skill is an important component of the learning curve; for example, it may be easy for a large number of surgeons to obtain competency at a simple procedure; however, a more difficult procedure will be more difficult to obtain competency in, and thus less surgeons are able to perform this procedure.

Outcome Measures

The evaluation of any health-related outcomes can be divided into two categories of outcome measures – measures of the clinical process and task efficiency, which examines operating time, number of procedures performed or measures of patient outcome, and quality assurance, which can refer to complication rates, conversion rates, or cure rates [8]. This reflects that attaining a certain number of procedures in medicine does not equate with competency, and thus professional bodies can examine competency and ability utilizing characteristics such as outcomes, cure rates, complication rates, or length of stay.

The way outcome measures are collected can influence the learning curve, for example a faster operative time can be examined with a smaller number of cases compared to complication rates; this can influence the scientific interpretation of trials examining the surgical learning curve.

The ideal learning curve evaluation would comprise of a multi-dimensional evaluation of outcome measures [10].

Surgeon Characteristics

Baseline knowledge of the surgeon is an integral component of the learning curve [7], and those with prior experience have a shorter learning curve than those with less surgical experience.

Cost

The introduction of new procedures can have negative economic implications on healthcare environments [12]. There can be a reduction in operating time owing to off-site training, as well as longer operating times associated with the learning curve. A reduction in cases can reduce productivity, increase theatre time, and increase waiting lists. Also, there is the potential for increased complications, or the anticipation of complications, lengthening hospital stay, and potentially increased readmission rates.

Negative Characteristics Associated with the Learning Curve

The concept of the learning curve and a surgeon not automatically having competence at a procedure can be exploited in the case of adverse outcomes [13]. It has been highlighted that while surgeons are on a learning curve, a higher death rate is inevitable, which the legal profession and the public can use against the medical profession [14]. It also caught the attention of the public and the legal profession when a surgeon told a public enquiry in Britain that a high death rate was inevitable while surgeons were on a learning curve.

The Learning Curve in Urogynaecology

As discussed, all surgical procedures are associated with learning curves; these curves represent the phases of learning a surgeon achieves prior to gaining proficiency in the technique. Teaching laparoscopic surgery is also significantly different to the teaching of other surgical skills. In contrast to open surgery, there is limited direct control over the trainee's actions, and a lack of depth perception, altered visuospatial awareness, and the lack of tactile feedback make it a more complex trainer–trainee relationship.

As with other surgical education models, the classic master–apprentice model is seen in the teaching of laparoscopic urogynaecology [15]. This has advanced over the past decade, with technology enhanced learning (TEL) providing a critical learning technique. TEL can reduce patient exposure prior to competency, through models such as video-assisted education and high-fidelity simulation [16]. These models all adapt concepts from medical education – namely vertical and horizontal integration [17].

Laparoscopic urogynaecology encompasses a wide range of procedures, which have largely superseded open procedures, the most common of which are laparoscopic sacrocolpopexy and hysteropexy. The first laparoscopic urogynaecological procedure (laparoscopic retropubic urethropexy) was performed in 1991, thus giving us a relatively short time period to study the evolution of this advance in urogynaecology [18].

Laparoscopic Urogynaecology

The expansion of laparoscopic urogynaecology to include robotic surgery has led to the provision of a wider range of information on the learning curve for urogynaecologists. In particular, the procedure of laparoscopic sacrocolpopexy has been studied in depth. Conventional laparoscopic surgery competence can be obtained following 20–25 procedures [19], as well as reduced operating times being correlated with between 18 and 24 surgeries [20]. It is felt that competency in robotic surgery can be achieved in in as few as 10 robotic procedures [21]. Pulliam demonstrates a shorter robotic learning curve in surgeons with prior laparoscopic surgery operating experience [22].

The shorter robotic learning curve trend is explained by a number of factors [23]. Firstly, surgeons typically have prior experience with laparoscopic surgery, so are familiar with the principles of the surgery. The technique has many of the advantages of laparoscopic surgery, but also minimizes the technical difficulties associated with straight stick surgery. This includes having the provision of haptic feedback, three-dimensional visualization, being more ergonomically sound, and allowing seven degrees of motion versus the four degrees in traditional surgery. For example, the skill of intracorporeal knot tying can be a stumbling block for some surgeons, due to limited freedom of motion and difficulty controlling suture tension [24]; however, this can be overcome in robotic surgery due to the presence of additional operating arms and a wider range of motion [25]. In addition, instrument grip strength sutures can be tightened effectively in robotic surgical procedures [26].

In order to shorten the learning curve, suggestions have been made to improve performance during the early learning period. It is recommended that a designated theatre team are allocated for the initial 20 procedures [27]. Secondly, patient positioning should be standardized for all cases. All members of the surgical team should be familiar with the instruments set, and deviation from standard practice only considered once these initial procedures have been successfully performed [8].

Comparison with Other Surgical Procedures

Learning curves in other gynaecological specialties have also been examined, with competency being deemed attained in 20 cases for hysterectomy and pelvic lymphadenectomy for endometrial cancer [26], but ranging up to 75 cases for benign hysterectomies [29]. A recent study assessing the learning curves associated with robot-assisted laparoscopic colorectal surgery revealed that it consisted of three distinct phases [30]. The first phase or the initial phase occurred over the first 15 cases; during this phase the operating time decreased. The second phase or plateau phase occurred over the next ten cases; during this phase the operator becomes more competent with the robotic technology. The third phase or the mastery phase occurred for the subsequent cases. During the mastery phase the complexity of the cases undertaken increased.

When the learning curve in robot-assisted laparoscopic radical prostatectomy was examined, it was deemed that challenges were often multi-factorial, and the actual learning curve could be surgeon dependent [31]. They concluded that an educated support team had a positive effect on the achievement of competency and proficiency.

Strategies to Optimize Training

Throughout a surgeon's working life, continual professional development and skill improvement is integral to providing the best possible outcomes for patients and the health services that they work in. Lifelong learning requires a motivated provider of teaching, as well as a motivated learner, or recipient of teaching. Liberman, with respect to robotic urological surgery, notes that a clear curriculum with access to training facilities optimizes this journey [32]. The teacher can provide appropriate supervision, allowing the learner to obtain graduated responsibility and real-time feedback. This learning can be then measured against a standardized training programme and set of mandatory procedures.

Over recent decades, there has been an increased focus placed on patient safety, particularly after public inquiries such as the Francis Report [33]. This has allowed topics such as communication, patient safety, and quality improvement to be included in medical curricula at an undergraduate and postgraduate level. Teaching styles have also adapted, moving from didactic to self-directed, the utilization of TEL, and the introduction of simulation training. These training adjuncts can be echoed in the field of aviation, with simulators frequently utilized to train fighter pilots prior to taking the controls of a plane in flight [34].

In addition to these changes in education, there has also been the addition of a number of types of assessments [35]. These are typically criterion-referenced, against a fixed standard. Within a trainee's career progression, ipsative assessment is also utilized to show a progression through the complexity of training activities. In order to progress in assessment, with the ultimate aim of achieving competency, there are a number of pre-requisites that trainees need to achieve [36]. For surgical trainees, these include the acquisition of cognitive knowledge, the development of surgical technical expertise, as well as clinical knowledge and acumen; all contributing to the maturation of a competent surgeon [37]. Miller designed a Prism of Clinical Competence which clearly demonstrates the steps needed for a clinician to move from novice to expert status (Figure 7.2).

The development of surgical technical expertise can take a number of forms, which can be classified as either experiential learning, in that it is based on experience, or observation/

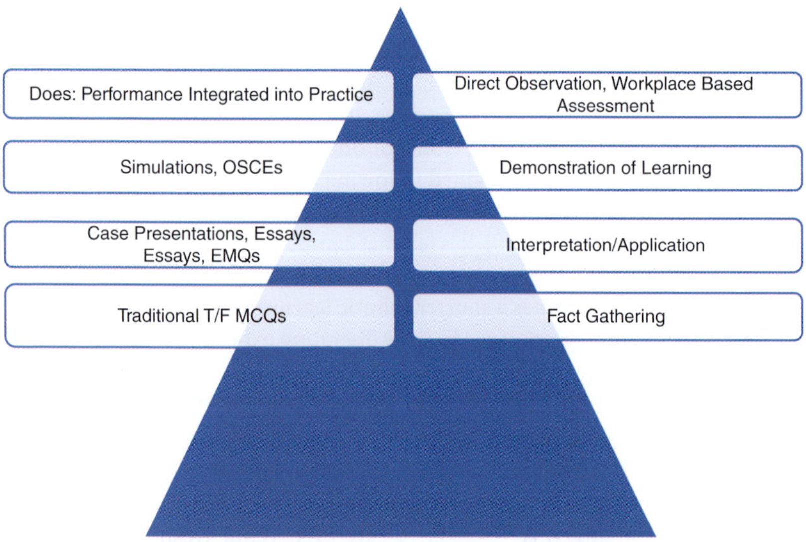

Figure 7.2 Miller's Prism of Clinical Competence, which clearly demonstrates the steps needed for a clinician to move from novice to expert status.

simulation, which has been catapulted into the realms as the optimal surgical training preference in the twenty-first century [38].

Experiential Training

The traditional Halstedian model of 'See one, do one, teach one' was the mainstay of surgical training over many decades, and was widely accepted and practised. It allows a surgical trainee 'the orderly exposure to graduated clinical experience ... during several years of residency under the close tutelage of dedicated seniors attending surgeons.'

However, a number of developments have led to this model of surgical training being superseded by other models. This includes a number of factors such as an increase in litigation, increased productivity and time-pressures, as well as limitations to surgical training time, such as those placed by the European Working Time Directive [39].

The theory of experiential training, proposed by David Kolb [38], is defined as 'the process whereby knowledge is created through the transformation of experience ... combinations of grasping and transforming the experience'. The former occurs through having a concrete experience and abstract conceptualization with the latter focussing on reflective observation and active experimentation.

The application of this to urogynaecology is seen in Figure 7.3.

Simulation

In order to address some of the pitfalls of the traditional models of surgical teaching, surgical education programmes have drawn on experience from aviation, music, and sports industries and have begun to utilize simulation training [40]. Simulation training is included in the curriculum of a number of surgical specialties, as well as in gynaecological surgical training. It has been described as the 'passport to a successful future in medicine', helping to counter some of the challenges placed by modern medical training [41]. The European Society for Gynaecological Endoscopy have developed a competency programme (Gynaecological Endoscopic Surgical Education and Assessment programme) with five skill sets over three levels of expertise; this, however, is not widely utilized or a mandatory part of laparoscopic surgical training [42].

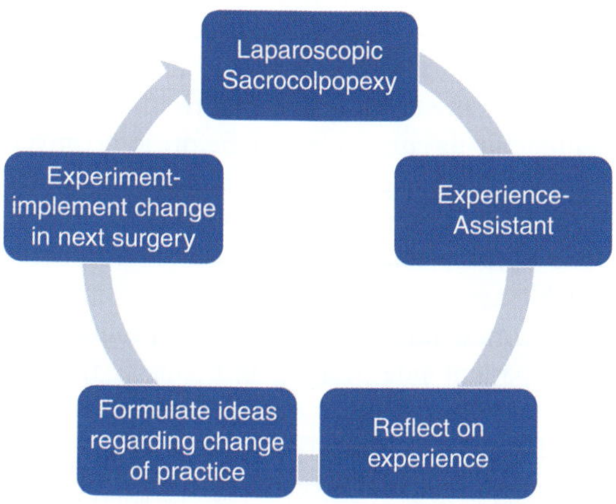

Figure 7.3 Experiential training as applied to laparoscopic sacrocolpopexy.

Within urogynaecology, simulation training has been utilized in both open and laparoscopic training, with international training programmes, such as the Surgical Masterclass in Urogynaecology and Urology conducted in Cork, Ireland [43], and more general programmes like the Anatomy of Complications workshop conducted throughout the world [44]. Internationally, the International Urogynaecological Association have investigated the potential of simulation training to conduct laparoscopic sacrocolpopexy, successfully showing that after five one-hour training sessions, the surgeon was able to successfully complete a laparoscopic sacral colpopexy in a live operative setting [45].

There are a number of categories of simulation training that can be utilized in gynaecological surgical training.

Low-fidelity Training

At a basic level, low-fidelity training can be utilized on a wide-scale level [46]. This can utilize cost effective surgical box trainers, but also include trainers with higher quality materials or those connected to computer equipment.

High-fidelity Training

High fidelity simulation utilizes more life-like mannequins and can be adapted to include cadaveric models in order to provide more tactile feedback, which may not be as readily available with low fidelity models [47].

Online Training

Online simulation can additionally be utilized to aid the acquisition of some technical skills relevant to surgical training. This can allow ongoing, interactive education which may provide opportunities for education prior to hands-on training, as well as consolidate that which has been taught in sessions [48]. This consolidation is an essential factor in the maintenance of skills and ensuring that skill attrition does not occur.

Furthermore, with advances in technology, it is possible to utilize both video-based instruction in the form of theoretical training, as well as practical training. This can take the form of application on mobile phones, allowing those in training to utilize down-time to practice skills essential to laparoscopic surgery.

There is a large amount of interest in addition to video gaming, as it applies to laparoscopic surgical aptitude, with those who have this experience performing superiorly to their non-gaming counterparts in laparoscopic simulation trainers [40]. Those who utilize video games have learned to dissociate their motor commands with the vision of their actions (for example can use a controller without looking at it). This adjunct to surgical education continues to be explored.

Cadaveric Training

Cadaveric models provide a realistic learning model that is comparable to live surgery [49], and allows trainees to complete full procedures in real-time [50]. However, these are less cost-effective and a sparse commodity, with moral and ethical objections a potential complicating factor. Fresh-frozen cadavers are the preferred specimen and are considered essential learning for surgeons who deliver care [51]. While fresh cadavers offer the most authentic tissue-handling fidelity, they deteriorate rapidly and require a rapid turn-around in laboratories. Animal cadavers, such as ewe and porcine cadavers, can also allow the successful demonstration and practice of laparoscopic surgical techniques, which has been shown to translate to the live theatre setting [52].

The Future of Laparoscopic Surgery

With the roll-out of fifth generation (5G) wireless technology, telerobotic surgery is now being conducted in countries such as China, with potential expansion internationally over the next few years [53]. 5G technology allows surgeons to operate on patients in another hospital, in another part of the country or world. This has the potential to allow access to surgical procedures and expertise which are not otherwise available. Additionally, the training potential of 5G surgery can also be capitalized, particularly in the setting of limited international travel which has occurred in the recent past owing to disease pandemics. This still allows surgeons to continue training and improving their skills under the directions of skilled mentors.

Assessing, Acquiring, and Evaluating Competency

Assessment Methods

As with other learned skills, assessment is a crucial part of ensuring competency as much as possible. Assessment can ensure that certain proficiencies have been met, and allow progression to additional stages of learning, in the path towards competency. Objective summative assessment has long been utilized in medical and surgical training, in the form of objective structured assessment of technical skills (OSATS); however, this is utilized primarily as a marker of improvement and progress rather than certifying competency [40]. Assessing and certifying proficiency in laparoscopic surgery has been performed by the expert assessment of serial unedited videos, but has not been assessed utilizing simulators. Some training curricula (such as Gynaecological Endoscopic Surgical Education and Assessment programmes) have utilized box simulators and demonstrate feasibility, construct validity, and transfer of skill to the operating room [40].

Acquisition of Competency

It is important to assess what combination of educational tools can be used to both attain and assess competency Skill acquisition is an area with many psychological theories described [40]; however, two principles are commonly found in these:

- Changes in performance proceed in a non-linear fashion
- As learning advances the trainee proceeds through qualitatively different phases.

Evaluation and Certification of Competency

Robust quality assurances are essential to ensure the retention and maintenance of high-quality skills once they have been acquired [54]. This can involve compiling logbooks of cases performed, refresher courses, or periodic supervision of the competent surgeon by a mentor [55]. In addition, the provision of a mentor–mentee relationship could be crucial in troubleshooting problems as the mentee progresses along the learning curve.

However, the failure to meet competency is also a challenge that needs to be tackled. While the competency-based model has its successes, the flaws occur when there is a failure to deliver these opportunities [56]. This can be related to workload or failure to individualize learning to the learner, and occurs when problems are encountered such as workforce planning, unexpected leave from training, and infrastructural issues.

Therefore, a combination of the traditional apprenticeship model, supported by a competency-based framework with room for adaptation may prove a more accessible concept for surgical trainees going forward. This has been echoed by consensus group models finding that a framework for minimally invasive surgery curriculum consists of multimodal learning, clinical proctorship, and competency-based assessment, all as integral related elements, without one showing superiority [57].

Robotic Urogynaecology Surgery – Training Optimization and Competency – A Case Study

Brief History of Robotic Surgery

The development of robotic surgery was in part due to work by the Defense Advanced Research Projects Agency (DARPA), which funded research into the possibility to perform minimally invasive surgery in the battlefield utilizing remote control [58]. The Da Vinci robotic system retains the main market share in robotic urogynaecology, yet as the twenty-first century progresses, other companies are beginning to venture into the field of robot-assisted surgery. Thus, robot-assisted surgery has the potential in the future to replace conventional laparoscopy throughout many fields of surgery [59]. However, in a relatively short period of time, robotic surgery has catapulted itself from a figment of a surgeon's imagination, to being at the forefront of a surgeon's armoury in complex urogynaecological care.

Training Courses

As with the adoption of any new technique, there is a period of education and learning to reach satisfactory surgical ability and proficiency. Given the recent introduction of robotic surgery, there was a need to train surgeons in its use and the nuances associated with the technique. Initial training courses were held by manufacturing companies, but before long university- and institution-affiliated groups commenced structured robotic training. With its exponential increase, there have been successful robotic surgery fellowships, educational courses, and curricula established to allow acquisition of basic robotic skills, followed by more complex skills. Training programmes typically consist of patient side training and console training and can involve the multi-disciplinary team. Online modules have been provided by the da Vinci surgery community in basic concepts, and advanced console skills can be pursued in virtual reality simulators (which are evaluated for face, content, and construct validity), dry labs, or wet labs [59]. Structured curricula can allow the safe and stepwise accumulation of these skills over a relatively short learning curve [61].

Training courses on robotic surgery are typically performed using inanimate, animal, or cadaver models. The length of the course varies from several hours to several days, sometimes even weeks in a mini-fellowship situation. The content depends on the attendees at the course. Inanimate exercises offer a cost-effective and robot-agnostic approach to training surgeons [62]. They can be designed to target specific (or a subset of) technical skills needed to understand the basic functionality of a robotic system [63]. With various levels of difficulty, a continuum of inanimate exercises can guide surgeons of different abilities through their initial learning curves. Inanimate exercises for learning the fundamentals of laparoscopic surgery can be expanded to effectively target robot-specific skills [64]. In order to be useful training tools, inanimate exercises must challenge both specific technical skills of using a robotic surgical system and have validated metrics so that surgeons can accurately track their performance [65].

It is certain that the advent of excellent surgical simulators and structured inanimate exercises has provided tools for novice surgeons to acquire console skills in a safe and structured environment. This will enhance their operating performance and reduce aspects of the learning curve such as operating time; however, the lack of availability of *in vivo* training opportunities greatly limits the applicability of this method of surgical training [66].

Introduction of the da Vinci Si system has given surgeons a second robotic console, facilitating collaboration between proctor and trainee. The mentoring console has two collaborative modes: (1) the swap mode allows the mentor and trainee to operate simultaneously and actively swap control of the robotic arms; (2) The nudge mode allows them to have control simultaneously, sharing the two robotic arms.

Live case observation remains an important component of a robotic training programme [67] and allows the trainee to become familiar with the steps of a specific robotic procedure. Proctoring is defined as direct supervision by an expert during the initial phase of training and the learning curve. It provides a safe environment during the introduction of a new technique and prevents surgeons from performing procedures before they have mastered the technique.

Proctorship

The concept of proctorship has become an essential part of robot-assisted surgery training, providing efficient and rapid progression of the learning curve amongst surgeons [68]. Typically, in surgical training, the trainer–trainee relationship is one of preceptorship, that is stepping in when required. However, with the majority of robotic surgery training, candidates have attained competency at open or laparoscopic surgery or both. Thus, a proctoring relationship, where a trainer supervises and allows the trainee opportunity to operate, is more beneficial and allows a trainee to reach competence at a faster pace. In addition, the proctor is able to provide off-site advice and education if needed as the trainee advances past competency to mastery.

Adjuncts to the Robotic System Facilitating Education

Education, training, and support for all members of the multidisciplinary team is essential when introducing new technology to the operating environment. Teamwork is an essential component to success in all operative procedures, and focus should be placed on the provision of ongoing professional development for all members of the operative team in all phases of the patient's operative journey (i.e. preoperative assessment, intraoperative and postoperative care).

The introduction of robotic surgery to urogynaecology provides a unique opportunity to examine the learning curve of a new technique to surgery which can be adapted to laparoscopic surgery. When we examine the learning curve of a robotic procedure with respect to apical prolapse surgery, it has been shown to be as short as 10 to 20 procedures [69], but more recently has been demonstrated to be up to 60 cases [70]. However, given that there is significant heterogeneity in what is reported as the learning curve, and who is considered, it is difficult to secure a definite figure for specific procedures at this juncture without bias.

As newer models consist of additional consoles, this allows training to be pursued in a formal clinical setting, an essential adjunct to the operators.

However, notwithstanding its advantages, robot-assisted surgery has created new challenges to ensure proper training and avoid subjecting patients to unnecessary risk. Increased scrutiny of credentialing and medico-legal aspects of robotic surgery have reinforced the importance of training and have led to a number of papers outlining pathways to facilitate this [71]. Learning tools for robotic surgery can include simulators, dual consoles, robotic courses, and proctoring.

The reality is that simulators, dual consoles, and robotic courses should play an important role in bridging the gap between early surgical skills and effective performance using the robot in a clinical setting without subjecting patients to unnecessary risk. It is also important to have tools that provide an objective means by which to evaluate a trainee's performance in anticipation of their ultimate graduation [72]. Physicians in training can acquire robotic surgery competency. Participants who acquire skills faster regain robotic skills faster after a training hiatus, but, on retraining, all participants can regain equivalent competence. This information provides a benchmark for a simulator training programme [72]. One institution has incorporated a graduated programme of resident and fellow console involvement based on level of training. They found this approach did not significantly hinder operating room efficiency [73]. However, once acquired, robotic surgical skills deteriorate without use; in one study, robotic surgical skills degraded significantly within four weeks of inactivity in newly trained surgeons [74]. The University of Toronto, in a pilot study assessing robotic skill training, concluded that the implementation of a multi-disciplinary, simulation-based, robotic surgery basic skills training curriculum revealed significantly improved basic robotic skills among novice trainees, regardless of specialty or level of training. Competency-based training was associated with significantly better acquisition of basic robotic skills.

Research and Conducting Research into the Learning Curve of Laparoscopic Urogynaecological Surgery

Research in medicine and surgery are integral to inform practice. Given the dynamic changes that can occur in medicine, it is essential to both keep abreast of current developments, but also contribute to these by engaging in research in the field.

A number of institutions and groups have conducted research into the learning curve of laparoscopic procedures.

In the case of laparoscopic urogynaecology, Mowat et al showed that with the introduction of a structured training programme, operative time was reduced, with subjective and patient-determined success at over 95% [75]. Researchers are also continuing to innovate, introducing learning aids to help reduce the long learning curve of laparoscopic urogynaecological procedures [76]. In general gynaecology, virtual reality simulation has successfully been used in the early portion of the learning curve, and aids in the acquisition of reflex movements associated with laparoscopic surgery [77].

However, we need to consider the optimum way to assess the learning curve and competency, and ensure this is consistent. We also need to examine the feasibility of randomized controlled trials in the area of medical education, where patients are the subject. Therefore, constant innovation is required, as well as maximizing use of augmented reality and cadaveric training.

Specifically, in laparoscopic urogynaecology, this means utilizing and expanding current training courses such as the Anatomy of Complications workshops, and making these available to those in all geographical areas of the world, as well as taking advantage of advances in technology generally (e.g. utilization of 5G networking) to allow those seeking to excel in their field to capitalize on resources which may not be easily accessible to them.

Conclusion

Laparoscopic urogynaecological surgery continues to adapt and gain momentum as the population of women that we serve grows, and conditions which may pre-dispose women to urogynaecological issues increases. Thus, it is integral that the learning and education surrounding laparoscopic surgery increases.

We have examined the context of the learning curve as it is applied to urogynaecology, and examined factors that are relevant in its adaptation, as learning advances within the confines of modern surgical practice.

Through utilizing robotic surgery as a model, we can examine the learning curve trajectory that this has undergone, and the trajectory that has underpinned its success in a relatively short period of time. This model can then be applied to laparoscopic urogynaecology and its performance as we train a new generation of surgeons who will manage the increasing workload of the urogynaecologist.

Training should be optimized through a number of modalities of training, utilizing the most up-to-date techniques, and adapting already utilized services (such as the Internet) to optimize this. Formal assessment techniques can ensure the achievement of competency, which needs to be assessed on an ongoing basis.

Through formal training programmes, the learning curve of urogynaecological laparoscopic surgery can be summited, and lead to a new cohort of successful surgeons entering the workforce to competently care for women.

References

1. Rodriguez-Paz JM, et al. Beyond 'see one, do one, teach one': toward a different training paradigm. Qual Saf Health Care 2009; 18(1): 63–8.
2. BSUG Audit and Database Committee 2019. Vaginal Vault Suspension Surgery in the UK 2008–2017.
3. O'Sullivan OE, Matthews CA, O'Reilly BA. Sacrocolpopexy: is there a consistent surgical technique? Int Urogynecol J 2016; 27(5): 747–50.
4. van Zanten F, Schraffordt Koops SE, O'Sullivan OE, et al. Robot-assisted surgery for the management of apical prolapse: a bi-centre prospective cohort study. BJOG 2019; 126(8): 1065–73. https://doi.org/10.1111/1471-0528.15696.
5. Wright TP. Factors affecting the cost of airplanes. J Aeronaut Sci 1936; 3(4): 122–8.
6. Subramonian K, Muir G. The 'learning curve' in surgery: what is it, how do we measure it and can be influence it? BJU Int 2004; 93(9).
7. Hopper AN, Jamison MH, Lewis WG. Learning curves in surgical practice. Postgrad Med J 2007; 83(986): 777–9. http://doi.org/10.1136/pgmj.2007.057190
8. Murnaghan JJ, Hutchinson C, Moreai G, Gofton W. *The Learning Curve and the Practicing Surgeon: Integrating a New Skill/Procedure into Your Practice*. Orthogate.
9. Shaw RE, Allet TR. How to draw learning curves: their use and justification. In: Ed TD Johnson, AT Pietrewicz (eds), *Ecological Study of Learning*. Erlbaum: 1985.
10. Goddard M, Davies HT, Dawson D, et al. Clinical performance measurement: part 1–getting the best out of it. J R Soc Med 2002; 95(10): 508–10. https://doi.org/10.1258/jrsm.95.10.508
11. Tekkis PP, Senagore AJ, Delaney CP, Fazio VW. Evaluation of the learning curve in laparoscopic colorectal surgery: comparison of right-sided and left-sided resections. Ann Surg 2005; 242(1): 83–91. https://doi.org/10.1097/01.sla.0000167857.14690.68
12. Varabyova Y, Rudolf Blankart C, Schreyogg J. The role of learning in health technology assessments: an empirical assessment of endovascular aneurysm repairs in German hospital. Health Econ 2017; 26(51).
13. Dyer C. Bristol case surgeon claimed to have been on 'learning curve'. BMJ 1999; 319: 1456.
14. Morgenstenn L. Warning! Dangerous curve head: the Learning Curve Surgical Innovation. Surg Innov 2005; 12(1): 101–3.
15. Rashid P. Surgical education and adult learning: integrating theory into practice. F1000Res 2017; 6: 143. https://doi.org/10.12688/f1000research.10870.1
16. Cagiltay NE, Berker M. Technology-enhanced surgical education: attitudes and perceptions of the endoscopic surgery community in Turkey. BMJ STEL 2017; 5 (1).
17. de Cates P, Owen K, Macdougall CF. Warwick Medical School: a four dimensional curriculum. Med Teach 2018; 40(5): 488–94. https://doi.org/10.1080/0142159X.2018.1435857
18. Vancaillie T, Schuessler W. Laparoscopic bladder neck suspension. J Laparoendosc Surg 1991; 1: 169.
19. Akladios CY, et al. Laparoscopic sacrocolpopexy for female genital organ prolapse: establishment of a learning curve. Eur J Obstet Gynecol Reprod Biol 2010; 149(2): 218–21.

20. Akladios CY, et al. Laparoscopic sacrocolpopexy for female genital organ prolapse: establishment of a learning curve. Eur J Obstet Gynecol Reprod Biol 2010; 149(2): 218–21.
21. Akl MN, et al. Robotic-assisted sacrocolpopexy: technique and learning curve. Surg Endosc 2009; 23(10): 2390–4.
22. Pulliam SJ, Weinstein MM, Wakamatsu MM. Minimally invasive apical sacrocolpopexy: a retrospective review of laparoscopic and robotic operating room experiences. Female Pelvic Med Reconstr Surg 2012; 18(2): 122–6.
23. Soomro NA, Hashimoto DA, Porteous AJ, et al. Systematic review of learning curves in robot-assisted surgery. BJS Open 2020; 4(1): 27–44. https://doi.org/10.1002/bjs5.50235
24. Elliott DS. Assessment of the durability of robot-assisted laparoscopic sacrocolpopexy for treatment of vaginal vault prolapse. J Robotic Surg 2007; 1: 163–8.
25. Thiyagarajan M, Ravindrakumar C. A comparative study in learning curves of two different intracorporeal knot tying techniques [published correction appears in Minim Invasive Surg 2018 May 20; 2018: 7646831]. Minim Invasive Surg 2016; 2016: 3059434. https://doi.org/10.1155/2016/3059434
26. Muffly T, et al. An evaluation of knot integrity when tied robotically and conventionally. Am J Obstet Gynecol 2009; 200(5): e18–20.
27. Maruthappu M, Duclos A, Lipsitz SR, et al. Surgical learning curves and operative efficiency: a cross-specialty observational study. BMJ Open 2015; 5: e006679. https://doi.org/10.1136/bmjopen-2014-006679
28. Seamon LG, et al. A detailed analysis of the learning curve: robotic hysterectomy and pelvic-aortic lymphadenectomy for endometrial cancer. Gynecol Oncol 2009; 114(2): 162–7.
29. Terzi H, Biler A, Demirtas O, et al. Total laparoscopic hysterectomy: analysis of surgical learning curve in benign conditions. Int J Surg 2016; 35: 51–7.
30. Bokhari MB, et al. Learning curve for robotic-assisted laparoscopic colorectal surgery. Surg Endosc 2011; 25(3): 855–60.
31. Lebeau T, et al. The role of a well-trained team on the early learning curve of robot-assisted laparoscopic procedures: the example of radical prostatectomy. Int J Med Robot 2011; 8(1): 67–72.
32. Liberman D, et al. Training and outcome monitoring in robotic urologic surgery. Nat Rev Urol 2012; 9(1): 17–22.
33. Francis R. Report of the Mid Staffordshire NHS Foundation Trust Public Inquiry. London: The Stationery Office; 2013.
34. Lenihan JP Jr. Navigating credentialing, privileging, and learning curves in robotics with an evidence and experienced-based approach. Clin Obstet Gynecol 2011; 54(3): 382–90.
35. Isaacs T, Zara C, Herbert G, et al. *Key Concepts in Educational Assessment*. SAGE Publications; 2013.
36. Paydar S, Ghahramani Z, Bolandparvaz S, et al. Learning operational strategies in surgery training. J Adv Med Educ Prof 2014; 2(2): 92–4.
37. Shemin RJ. Postgraduate experiential learning is essential for surgical maturation. J Thoac Cardiovasc Surg 2015; 150: 1069–70.
38. Kolb DA. Experiential learning: experience as the source of learning and development. Prentice Hall; 1983.
39. Schimmack S, Hinz U, Wagner A, et al. Maximizing time from the constraining European Working Time Directive (EWTD): The Heidelberg New Working Time Model. Health Econ Rev 2014; 4: 14. https://doi.org/10.1186/s13561-014-0014-6
40. White C, Rodger MWM, Tang T. Current understanding of learning psychomotor skills and the impact on teaching laparoscopic surgical skills. TOG 2016; 18: 53–63.
41. McCarthy CM, O'Sullivan OE, O'Reilly BA. Simulation training: our passport to a successful future in medicine. BMJ STEL 2020; 6: 67–8.
42. The Gynaecological Endoscopic Surgical Education and Assessment (GESEA) programme. The European Academy of Gynaecological Surgery. Accessed at: https://europeanacademy.org/about/
43. Surgical Masterclass in Urogynaecology and Urology at the ASSERT Centre, University College Cork. Accessed at: https://assert.ucc.ie/surgical-masterclasses-in-urogynaecology-and-urology/
44. The Anatomy of Complications Workshop. Accessed at: https://acworkshop.com/workshops/laparoscopic/
45. Tunitsky-Bitton E, King CR, Ridgeway B, et al. Development and validation of a laparoscopic sacrocolpopexy simulation model for surgical training. J Minim Invasive Gynecol 2014; 21(4): 612–18. https://doi.org/10.1016/j.jmig.2013.12.124
46. Ellinas H, Denson K, Simpson D. Low-cost simulation: how-to guide. J Grad Med Educ 2015; 7(2): 257–8. https://doi.org/10.4300/JGME-D-15-00082.1
47. La Cerra C, Dante A, Caponnetto V, et al. Effects of high-fidelity simulation based on life-threatening clinical condition scenarios on learning outcomes of undergraduate and postgraduate nursing students: a systematic review and meta-analysis. BMJ Open 2019; 9: e025306. https://doi.org/10.1136/bmjopen-2018-025306
48. Mandler AG. Touch surgery: a twenty-first century platform for surgical training. J Digit Imaging 2018; 31(5): 585–90. https://doi.org/10.1007/s10278-018-0102-y
49. Salameh FT, O'Reilly BA, Balta JY. The cadaver is not dead. Anat Sci Int 2020; 95(4): 571–2.
50. Gilbody J, Prasthofer AW, Ho K, Costa ML. The use and effectiveness of cadaveric workshops in higher surgical training: a systematic review. Ann R Coll Surg Engl 2011; 93(5): 347–52. https://doi.org/10.1308/147870811X582954
51. Hughes JL. The development of cadaveric simulation for core surgical trainees. Bull Roy Coll Surg Engl 2018; 101: 38–43.
52. Stefanidis D, Yonce TC, Green JM, Coker AP. Cadavers versus pigs: which are better for procedural training of surgery residents outside the OR? Surgery 2013; 154(1): 34–7. https://doi.org/10.1016/j.surg.2013.05.001
53. Tian W, Fan M, Zeng C, et al. Telerobotic spinal surgery based on 5G network: the first 12 cases. Neurospine 2020; 17(1): 114–20. https://doi.org/10.14245/ns.1938454.227
54. Blencowe NS, Skilton A, Gaunt D, on behalf of the ROMIO Study team, et al. Protocol for developing quality assurance measures to use in surgical trials: an example from the ROMIO study. BMJ Open 2019; 9: e026209. https://doi.org/10.1136/bmjopen-2018-026209
55. Platz J, Hyman N. Mentorship. Clin Colon Rectal Surg 2013; 26(4): 218–23. https://doi.org/10.1055/s-0033-1356720
56. Sonnadera RR, Mui C, McQueen S, et al. Reflections on competency-based education and training of surgical residents. J Surg Educ 2014; 71(10): 151–8.
57. Awad M, Awad F, Carter F, et al. Consensus views on the optimum training curriculum for advanced minimally invasive surgery: a Delphi study. Int J Surg 2018; 53: 137–42.

58. Martinic G. Glimpses of future battlefield medicine – the proliferation of robotic surgeons and unmanned vehicles and technologies. J Mil Vet Health 2014; 22()3.

59. Schwaibold H, Wiesend F, Bach C. The age of robotic surgery - Is laparoscopy dead? Arab J Urol 2018; 16(3): 262–9.

60. Seixas-Mikelus SA, Kesavadas T, Srimathveeravalli G, et al. Face validation of a novel robotic surgical simulator. Urology 2010; 76(2): 357–60.

61. Ahmed K, Khan R, Mottrie A, et al. Development of a standardised training curriculum for robotic surgery: a consensus statement from an international multidisciplinary group of experts. BJU Int 2015; 116(1): 93–101.

62. Dutto L, O'Reilly BA. Robotic repair of vesico-vaginal fistula with perisigmoid fat flap interposition: state of the art for a challenging case. Int Urogynecol J 2013; 24(12): 2029–30.

63. van Iersel JJ, de Witte CJ, Verheijen PM, et al. Robot-assisted sacrocolporectopexy for multicompartment prolapse of the pelvic floor: a prospective cohort study evaluating functional and sexual outcome. Dis Colon Rectum 2016; 59(10): 968–74.

64. Nitti VW. Complications of midurethral slings and their management. Can Urol Assoc J 2012; 6(5 Suppl 2): S120–2.

65. Nitti VW. Miduretharal sling erosion; NYU Case of the Month. Rev Urol 2017; 19(3): 185–6.

66. Lo TS, Tan YL, Khanuengkitkong S, Dass AK. Delayed intravesical mesh erosion in a midurethral sling following further mesh-augmented pelvic prolapse surgery. J Obstet Gynecol Res 2014; 40(3): 862–4.

67. Lee KS, Choo MS, Doo CK, et al. The long term (5 year) objective TVT success rate does not depend on predictive factors at multivariate analysis: a multicentre retrospective study. Eur Urol 2008; 53(1): 176–82.

68. Santok GD, Raheem AA, Kim LHC, et al. Proctorship and mentoring: its backbone and application in robotic surgery. Investig Clin Urol 2016; 57(Suppl 2): S114–S120.

69. Serati M, Bogani G, Sorice O, et al. Robot-assisted sacrocolpopexy for pelvic organ prolapse: a systematic review and meta-analysis of comparative studies. Eur Urol 2014; 66(2): 303–18.

70. Linder BJ, Anand M, Weaver AL, et al. Assessing the learning curve of robotic sacrocolpopexy. Int Urogynecol J 2016; 27(2): 239–46.

71. Rey D, Helou E, Oderda M, et al. Laparoscopic and robot-assisted continent urinary diversions (Mitrofanoff and Yang-Monti conduits) in a consecutive series of 15 adult patients: the Saint Augustin technique. BJU Int 2013; 112(7): 953–8.

72. Vallabh-Patel V, Salamon C. Case series: removal of sacrocolpopexy mesh. J Urol Res 2016; 3(7): 1076.

73. Tijdink MM, Vierhout ME, Heesakkers JP, Withagen MIJ. Surgical management of mesh-related complications after prior pelvic flood reconstructive surgery with mesh. Int Urogynecol J 2011; 22(11): 1395–404.

74. Kilic OF, Börgers A, Köhne O, et al. Effects of steep Trendelenburg position for robotic-assisted prostatectomies on intra- and extrathoracic airways in patients with or without chronic obstructive pulmonary disease. Br J Anaesth 2015; 114(1): 70–6.

75. Mowat A, Maher C, Pelecanos A. Can the learning curve of laparoscopic sacrocolpopexy be reduced by a structured training programme? Female Pelvic Med Reconstr Surg 2018; 24(4): 272–6.

76. Serdinšek T, Andrić BŽ, But I. A new affordable and easy-to-make pelvic model for training in complex urogynecological laparoscopic procedures. Int Urogynecol J 2019; 30(9): 1497–501. https://doi.org/10.1007/s00192-018-3803-3

77. Lamblin G, Thiberville G, Druette L, et al. Virtual reality simulation to enhance laparoscopic salpingectomy skills. J Gynecol Obstet Hum Reprod 2020; 49(3): 101685. https://doi.org/10.1016/j.jogoh.2020.101685

Chapter 8

Prevention and Management of Complications in Laparoscopic Urogynaecologic Surgery

Martino Zacchè, Rohna Kearney

Introduction

Laparoscopy is widely applied in gynaecology, with evident patient benefits compared with open abdominal surgery, including reduced intraoperative blood loss, shorter hospital stay, and faster recovery. The potential risks of laparoscopic surgery should be well known to urogynaecologists who wish to offer this approach to treat pelvic floor disorders. Complications can be encountered even in a potentially straightforward diagnostic laparoscopy. These include laparoscopic entry injuries to bowel and major blood vessels, which can result in serious morbidity or death. Guidelines aiming to minimize injuries during laparoscopic procedures have been developed by professional bodies [1–3]. Thus, prior to commencing training in laparoscopic urogynaecology, it is advisable that surgeons have already achieved the required skills needed to safely perform more basic laparoscopic procedures, such as surgical management of ectopic pregnancies or tubal sterilization.

This chapter will give an overview of the complications related to laparoscopic surgery and their incidence, with a focus on laparoscopic urogynaecology. We will describe potential injuries specific to the most commonly performed laparoscopic urogynaecology procedures (colposuspension and sacrocolpopexy), including critical steps which can be taken to minimize risks. Finally, we will discuss recognition and management of complications, as a good prognosis often results from a prompt diagnosis and institution of appropriate treatment.

Epidemiology

The complication rate of gynaecological laparoscopy is estimated between 0.3% and 0.6%, and up to 50% are related to the initial laparoscopic access [4]. In 2019, a Cochrane review of 57 randomized controlled trials (RCTs) concluded that there is no evidence to support the use of a specific entry technique [5]. Life-threatening complications include vascular injuries of major intra-abdominal vessels (common iliac artery, vena cava, aorta) and bowel perforation, with a respective incidence of 0.01–0.64% [6] and 0.03–0.39% [7]. Early diagnosis is mandatory, as the mortality rate increases up to 5% when a bowel injury is missed or diagnosed late. Overall, the estimated mortality rate associated with laparoscopy is of 4 cases per 100,000 procedures, with the degree of surgical complexity playing a major role. Although not life-threatening, other complications associated with the initial entry may cause significant morbidity, with a prolonged recovery and a potential reoperation risk. Insertion of lateral trocars can cause injury to the inferior epigastric arteries, with a reported incidence of 0.2–2% [8]. Inadequate closure of the rectus sheath for port sites ≥ 10 mm may predispose to hernia. However, this may also result from smaller incisions. A review of 22 studies, including a minimum of 300 patients each, reported a pooled prevalence of 0.5% for trocar site hernia in any laparoscopic procedure [9]. Finally, there are some minor complications related to the insufflation of CO_2, such as subcutaneous emphysema and postoperative shoulder pain. On occasion, if subcutaneous emphysema causes anaesthetic difficulty, the laparoscopic approach may need to be abandoned.

With regard to pelvic surgery, gynaecologists are well aware of complications involving the lower urinary tract, as this is in close anatomical relationship with the reproductive system. An increase in the rate of ureteric injuries in gynaecology has been reported since the introduction of minimally invasive surgery [10]. A recent systematic review evaluated bladder and ureteric injuries occurring during laparoscopic gynaecological procedures for benign conditions. Out of 140,444 cases, a total of 458 injuries were counted, with an overall incidence of 0.33% [11]. The incidence for bladder and ureteric injury was 0.24% and 0.08%, respectively. This confirms previous studies, which reported that the rate of bladder injury is three-fold higher compared to ureteric injury [12]. Interestingly, endometriosis resection was found to be the procedure with the highest incidence of ureteric injury (0.4%). On the other hand, bladder injury was more commonly described during laparoscopic hysterectomy, followed by laparoscopically assisted vaginal hysterectomy, with an incidence of 1.6% and 0.8%, respectively. Of note, ureteric injuries are often overlooked and most of the diagnoses are achieved postoperatively. The role of intraoperative cystoscopy following major gynaecological surgery has been largely debated, however its routine use does not appear to be cost-effective [13].

Data regarding complications in laparoscopic urogynaecology are somewhat limited. Initial trials were published at the end of the last century for both surgical management of stress urinary incontinence (laparoscopic colposuspension) and apical prolapse (laparoscopic sacrocolpopexy and sacrohysteropexy). Laparoscopic urogynaecology in the UK has been mainly concentrated in tertiary centres, with most laparoscopic surgeons performing apical prolapse procedures. Also, with the introduction of mid-urethral slings (MUS) in early 2000, a significant drop in the numbers of traditional incontinence surgery has been reported [14]. As a result, few surgeons had the opportunity to be trained in colposuspensions. Of these, a minority will be able to offer a laparoscopic approach. With regard to apical procedures, the learning curve has been often described as steep. Deprest et al showed that it takes 60 laparoscopic sacrocolpopexies to effectively limit the number of complications [15]. In 2019, a Cochrane meta-analysis summarized the available evidence regarding laparoscopic colposuspension, but adverse events were not included in all of the 26 trials considered [16]. Table 8.1 summarizes the complications reported by two large RCTs comparing laparoscopic versus open colposuspension.

Fewer data are available regarding laparoscopic sacrocolpopexy. A large French single-centre retrospective study included 464 cases performed between January 2003 and December 2013, with a mean follow-up of four years [17]. Adverse perioperative events requiring reoperation occurred in 21 cases (4.5%), including bladder (1.9%) and vaginal (1.5%) perforation and epigastric vessels injury (1.1%). Blood transfusion was needed in only one patient (0.2%) following epigastric vessel injury and hemoperitoneum. Mesh complications were reported in 11 cases (2.8%), of which vaginal exposure was the most common (n=6). Comparable results were recently published by Sato et al, who retrospectively analysed 46 cases performed in a single Japanese centre between August 2015 and July 2017 [18]. A 2.2% incidence for bladder, ureteric, and vaginal injury was reported. Data from prospective studies carried out in the US [19] and in the Netherlands [20] are presented in Table 8.2. Rare but life-threatening complications may occur during a sacrocolpopexy. Presacral vessels may be injured during dissection and attachment of the mesh to the sacral promontory. Also, the risk of rectal injury increases if surgeons perform a deep dissection in order to attach the mesh at the level of the levator ani muscle.

Urogynaecologists should also consider long-term mesh complications, such as vaginal exposure, mesh infection, bladder and bowel perforation. In many cases, surgical management is required. The reoperation rate for mesh complication has been reported between 2.8% and 7% [17,21]. The pathogenesis of long-term mesh complications is still poorly understood, and their surgical treatment can be challenging. In fact, the mesh may be in close anatomic relationship with important structures (including major vessels and nerves). Advanced laparoscopic skills are often required to achieve complete removal. In a recent case-series considering 56 complete laparoscopic removals of retropubic MUS, the risk of postoperative retropubic haematoma was highlighted. Out of 56 cases, two (3.5%) required return to theatre for surgical evacuation within the first two weeks [22]. Other complications involving mesh include osteomyelitis (following sacrocolpopexy) and nerve injuries (following sacrocolpopexy and MUS). In such cases, complete mesh removal may require the expertise of a multi-disciplinary team, including colorectal and plastic surgeons, to deal with potential bowel involvement and nerve reconstruction, respectively.

Table 8.1 Complication rate in the laparoscopic colposuspension group of two randomized controlled trials

Study	Complications		
	Urinary tract	Vascular	Bowel
Carey [48]	Sutures through the bladder: 5.2% (5/96) – 2 cases were converted to open surgery to re-site the sutures	Laceration of the obturator vein: 1% (1/96)	0
Kitchener [49]	Bladder injury: 2.8% (4/144)	Haemorrhage > 500 ml: 0.7% (1/144)	Bowel injury: 0.7% (1/144)

Table 8.2 Complication rate in the laparoscopic sacrocolpopexy group of two randomized controlled trials

Study	Complications		
	Urinary tract	Vascular	Bowel
Maher [19]	Bladder injury: 1.8% (1/53)	Blood transfusion: 1.8% (1/53)	Bowel injury: 1.8% (1/53)
Coolen [20]	Bladder injury: 2.7% (1/36) – requiring laparotomy	Bleeding: 2.7% (1/36) – requiring laparotomy	0

Prevention of Complications

In the senior author's experience, appropriate patient selection is critical to achieving good results and avoiding serious complications. Preoperative counselling should inform regarding available treatments, including non-surgical options. The discussion must include benefits and risks of each approach. A vaginal procedure may be more appropriate to reduce the risk of serious complications when the anatomy is likely to be altered by previous abdominal surgery, endometriosis, pelvic inflammatory disease, malignancy, and radiotherapy. Below, we describe steps that can be taken to avoid complications in two commonly performed laparoscopic urogynaecology procedures: colposuspension and sacrocolpopexy.

Laparoscopic Colposuspension

This is a retropubic urethropexy, originally described by Burch in the 1960s and subsequently modified [23]. It can be performed by an extraperitoneal or intraperitoneal approach. The authors adopt the intraperitoneal approach and will discuss this technique. The urethra and bladder neck are elevated by placing two sutures through each side of the paravaginal fascia and the ipsilateral iliopectineal (Cooper's) ligament. Knowledge of the prevesical space (or space of Retzius) and its anatomy is of paramount importance. Commonly reported complications are lower urinary tract injuries and bleeding from the perivesical venous plexus and obturator veins.

- Entry into the prevesical space is aided by placing lateral ports at the level of the lower margin of the umbilicus and applying downwards traction on the median umbilical ligament. A distance of at least 8 cm from the midline is recommended in order to avoid injury of the epigastric vessels. Identification of the bladder dome is improved with 150 ml of methylene blue mixed with sterile water. If retropubic dissection is carried out too laterally, the inferior epigastric artery, the neurovascular obturator bundle, and external iliac vessels may be injured. The accessory (or aberrant) obturator artery or vein crossing the iliopectineal ligaments should be identified, as injury can result in haemorrhage.

- The bladder is emptied before exposing the paravaginal fascia to allow easier access. A 10–12 mm port is placed suprapubically to facilitate mobilization of the bladder medially with a small pledget, while the paravaginal fascia is elevated at the level of the midurethra with the index finger of the surgeon's non-dominant hand. The authors pass a Vicryl suture tie (see Figure 8.1) through the gauze pledget so that it can be easily found if released from the grasper, as otherwise it is difficult to identify when blood stained. A 10–12 mm Hegar dilator replaces the index finger of the surgeon's hand before suturing. It is important to avoid overelevation as this can result in vaginal perforation and long-term voiding difficulty.
- If vaginal perforation occurs, a 2-0 Vicryl suture can be used to close the defect. It is important to perform the fewest possible manoeuvres to identify the paravaginal tissue, as venous bleeding can result from excessive dissection. Sutures should be placed lateral to the urethra at the level of the bladder neck. If sutures are placed too high, there is an increased risk of ureteric kinking, resulting in ureteric obstruction. If bleeding occurs while passing sutures through the paravaginal fascia, the surgeon can either tie a knot onto the fascia or expedite elevation of the vagina and tie an extra-corporeal knot leaving a 2 cm 'suture bridge' to prevent voiding dysfunction due to excessive elevation. If complete haemostasis has not been achieved and there is a minimal amount of bleeding or 'ooze' in the retropubic space, a small drain can be inserted via a lateral 5 mm trocar port and left in situ for 24 hours (Figure 8.2).
- We recommend performing a cystoscopy (ideally with a 70-degrees cystoscope) at the end of the procedure to ensure that there are no sutures inadvertently placed in the bladder (Figure 8.3). Patency of the ureteric orifices can also be confirmed by visualizing efflux of urine. If a suture is seen in the bladder, this can simply be removed laparoscopically, and another suture placed followed by a repeat cystoscopy.

Laparoscopic Sacrocolpopexy

Prolapse of the apical compartment can be treated laparoscopically with suspension of the vault to the sacral promontory with a polypropylene mesh. Common complications reported during this procedure are bladder and bowel injury. Although uncommon, bleeding from laceration of presacral vessels (left common iliac vein, middle sacral artery, presacral venous plexus) can be life-threatening.

- A Trendelenburg position can help to move the bowel out of the pelvis. Atraumatic forceps, such as Johann grasping forceps, should be used when handling bowel loops to minimize the risk of injury. The peritoneum is initially opened at the level of the sacral promontory. Upwards traction before incising reduces the risk of injuring a vessel on the promontory.
- The peritoneum is divided parallel and medial to the right utero-sacral ligament up to the level of the vaginal vault. The right ureter must be visualized throughout and a minimum of 2 cm distance should be kept between the surgical plane and the ureter. The peritoneum is opened posteriorly close to the attachment of the utero-sacral ligaments.
- With a rectal and a vaginal probe, the rectum can be mobilized posteriorly and the vagina anteriorly in order to identify the rectovaginal space. Care needs to be taken that probes are inserted under vision, so that inadvertent perforation does not occur. In the event of a rectal injury, the procedure should be abandoned, as to continue with mesh placement would increase the risk of mesh infection and rectal perforation (Figure 8.4). The bladder is emptied with a Foley catheter, reducing the risk of injury while it is dissected from the vaginal vault and anterior vaginal wall. The vaginal

(a)

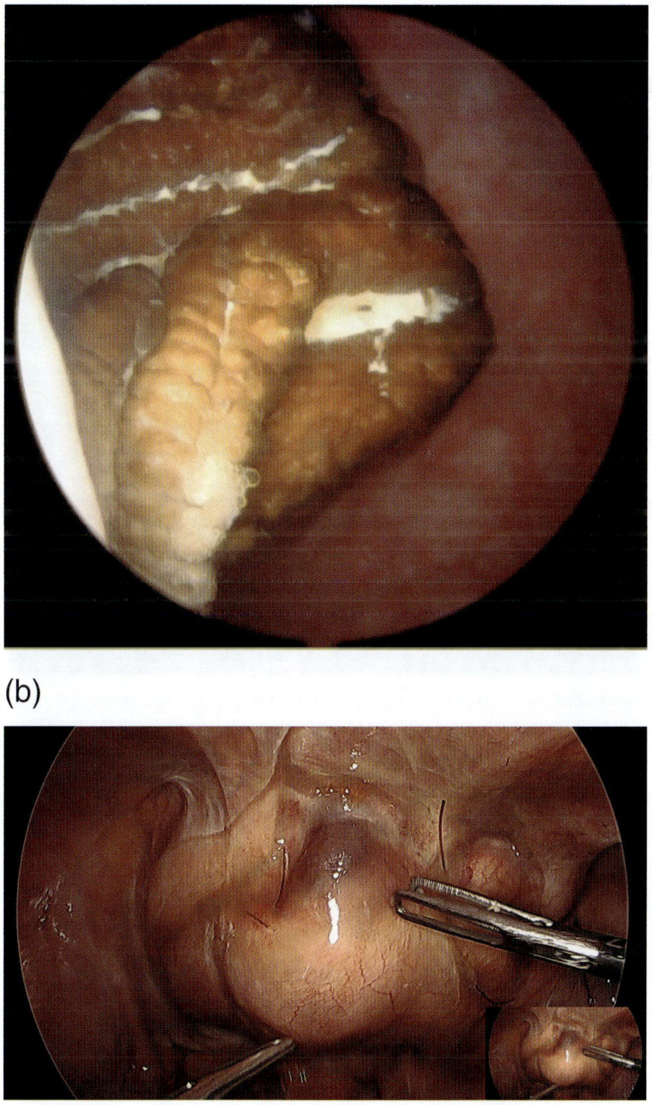

(b)

Figure 8.1 A small swab with suture tie migrated in the bladder. (a) Cystoscopic and (b) laparoscopic findings in a patient who previously underwent a laparoscopic colposuspension (with permission of Mr Alfred Cutner, University College Hospital, London, UK).

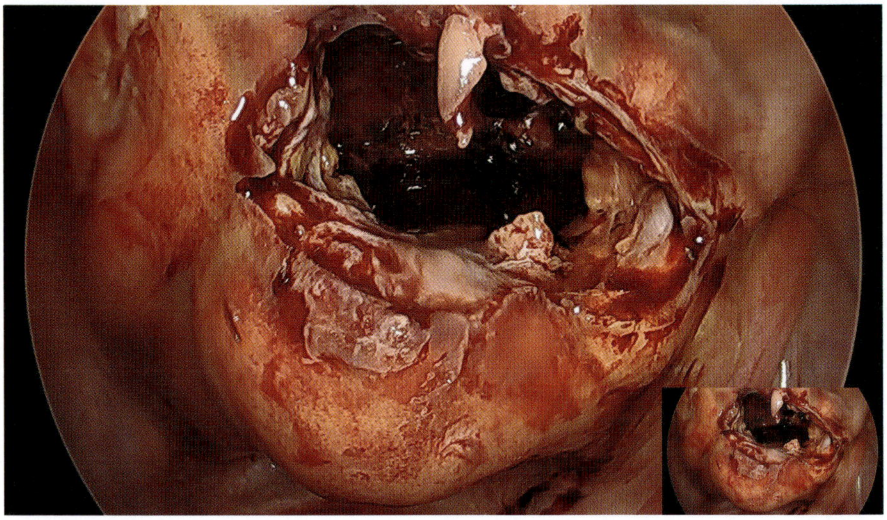

Figure 8.2 Drainage of haematoma in the prevesical space following laparoscopic colposuspension (with permission of Mr Alfred Cutner, University College Hospital, London, UK).

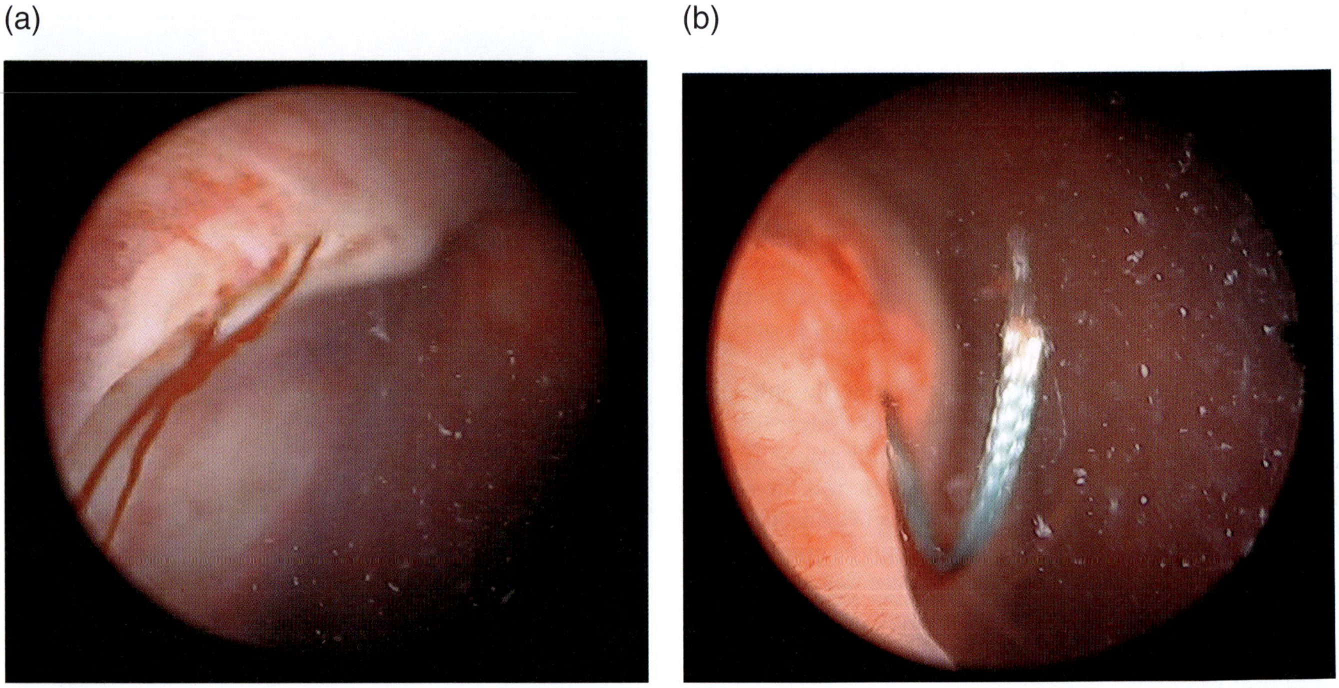

Figure 8.3 Cystoscopic check during laparoscopic colposuspension. (a) The right bladder wall appears 'hitched-up' with distortion of the anatomy and absent ipsilateral ureteric jet. Thus, colposuspension sutures were removed and re-inserted laparoscopically. (b) Small residual portion of suture (Ethibond) is visualized in the bladder and removed cystoscopically.

probe should be gently pushed towards the head of the patient and posteriorly in order to facilitate dissection. If a bladder injury occurs, surgeons may continue with the procedure, provided that the mesh is not in contact or close to the bladder repair [24]. Surgeons should be mindful that a deep dissection into the vagina may eventually cause a vaginal laceration. This can be closed with sutures, however, if mesh is attached in close proximity to the suture line, the risk of vaginal mesh exposure is increased.

- Reperitonealization will reduce the risk of bowel adhering to the mesh. In fact, bowel adhesions may be a cause for postoperative chronic pain and repeat surgery. This can be accomplished either with interrupted sutures or a continuous barbed suture. However, the latter has been reported to cause small bowel obstruction secondary to adhesions [25]. Consequently, it is the authors' preferred technique to close the peritoneum with interrupted absorbable sutures. Of note, small 'bites' of peritoneum should be taken in order to minimize the risk of ureteral kinking.
- Careful exposure of the sacrum is essential prior to mesh attachment. The sacral promontory can be 'explored' using a blunt probe which provides good tactile feedback. Mesh can be attached to the promontory using either non-absorbable sutures or titanium tacks (Protac™).

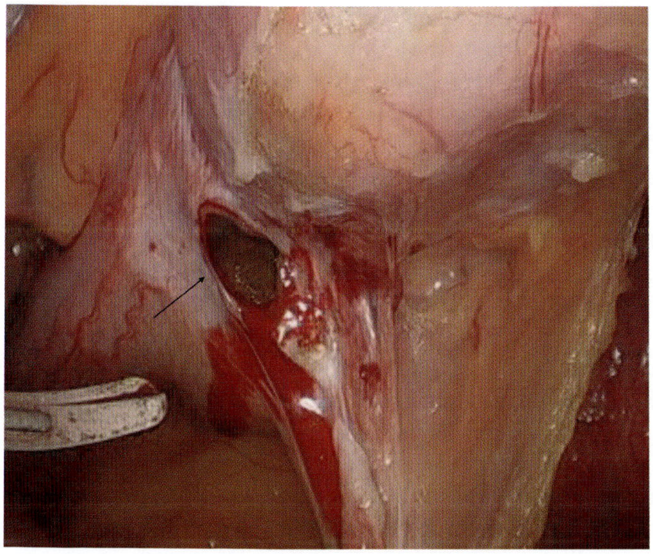

Figure 8.4 Rectal injury (see black arrow) during dissection of the rectovaginal space prior to insertion of sacrocolpopexy mesh. A laparoscopic repair was performed and the procedure abandoned.

Recognition and Management of Complications

Bladder Injury

A Foley catheter should always be inserted during laparoscopic urogynaecology procedures. Common intraoperative signs of bladder injury include laparoscopic visualization of the catheter, haematuria, and presence of CO_2 gas in the catheter bag. However, a bladder injury may also be less obvious and should be suspected even in the presence of slight haematuria. To confirm the diagnosis, a cystoscopy should be performed to rule out any breaching of the bladder wall or the presence of sutures within the urothelium. Alternatively, the bladder can be filled with diluted methylene blue while the surgeons look for any spillage into the pelvis.

Cystostomies more commonly occur at the bladder dome, away from the trigone and ureteric orifices. These can be repaired in one or two layers with either a continuous or interrupted 2-0 Vicryl suture. If the surgeon is inexperienced in bladder repair, there are multiple bladder defects, or there is any risk of ureteric involvement (e.g. the defect is within 2–3 cm of the ureteric orifice), the assistance of a urologist should be requested. In fact, inadequate closure or a ureteric injury can have significant long-term consequences. Intracorporeal knots are generally preferable to extracorporeal sutures for bladder closure, as correct tensioning can be ensured. If the injury occurs close to the trigone, both ureteric orifices should be identified and ureteric stent(s) inserted. The patient can be discharged home with a Foley catheter on free drainage for two weeks. A leg bag can be used to facilitate patient mobilization postoperatively. A cystogram should be arranged two weeks following the repair and, if bladder integrity is confirmed, a trial without catheter can be considered. The ureteric stents are usually left in situ for two to six weeks, depending on the severity of the injury. Intraoperative recognition and management carries the best chances of success, reducing the risk of fistula formation.

Ureteric Injury

A ureteric injury is often identified postoperatively. Thus, a high index of suspicion is mandatory to achieve prompt diagnosis and management. A delay can cause significant morbidity (urinoma, stricture, hydronephrosis, genitourinary fistula, ipsilateral kidney failure) and is a common cause of medicolegal litigation.

Intraoperatively, visualization of ureteric peristalsis does not exclude ureteric injury. Cystoscopy can be performed to visualize urine efflux from ureteric orifices. A 'sluggish' or absent jet is a sign of ureteric kinking until proven otherwise. The assistance of a urologist will be helpful in ascertaining whether further intervention is required, such as retrograde pyelography and stent insertion. If ureteric efflux is not seen following colposuspension, ipsilateral sutures should be removed to see if this results in efflux. Sutures can then be replaced followed by repeat cystoscopy. At sacrocolpopexy, the ureter may be injured while developing the retroperitoneal space, therefore it is important to visualize the right ureter prior to beginning dissection and, again, prior to mesh fixation to the promontory. Reperitonealization can result in ureteric kinking or obstruction. Thus, care should be taken to identify the right ureter during closure of the peritoneum. Also, if thermal injury is suspected, it is prudent to ask for the assistance of a urologist to consider stenting the ureter, as this may develop a stricture or a fistula over the first few postoperative weeks. If retrograde stenting is unsuccessful, antegrade stenting can be attempted. Of note, catheters and stents not only facilitate urine drainage, but also prevent stenosis, protecting the ureter during healing. Partial or complete ureteric laceration require surgery. However, in case immediate repair can't be performed, placement of a percutaneous nephrostomy tube may be required as an interim measure.

Postoperatively, close monitoring of urinary output, renal function, and electrolytes is essential when a ureteric injury has been repaired. A ureteric obstruction may present in day 1 with a markedly reduced urinary output (<25 ml/kg/hr). In this scenario, clinicians should have a low threshold to arrange appropriate investigations. Initially, common causes such as dehydration, bleeding, sepsis, and chronic kidney failure must be ruled out. An input/output chart is essential to manage fluids and prevent overload. Missed ureteric perforation and thermal injuries may present respectively two to three days and 10–14 days after surgery. In patients readmitted with pyrexia, leukocytosis, abdominal and flank pain, dysuria, palpable pelvic mass, haematuria, and increased vaginal discharge, it is important to look for a lower urinary tract injury (bladder and ureter). A renal ultrasound study may be obtained initially to exclude hydronephrosis and urinoma. However, further anatomical details, such as site and severity of urine leak, can be obtained through retrograde pyelography or computed tomography with contrast. If a small lesion is noted, ureteric stenting should be attempted and, in case of failure, a percutaneous nephrostomy must be placed to drain urine and prevent ipsilateral renal failure. If definitive surgery is required, this should be performed either in an early postoperative phase (within the first five days) or at a later stage (after six weeks) as postoperative inflammation is a risk factor for surgical failure.

In urogynaecology, ureteric injuries mainly involve the lower third, which is the portion from the pelvic brim to the ureteral orifice. In case of partial transection, a primary repair with fine absorbable sutures can be attempted. If a complete transection or a thermal injury are identified, a ureteroneocystostomy is required. Injuries in the middle segment of the ureter (near the iliac vessels) are typically treated with ureteroureterostomy. In complex cases, in order to reduce the tension on the anastomosis, the bladder can be mobilized (psoas hitch), extended (Boari flap), or a segment of ileum can be interposed between the ureter and the bladder (ureteroileal interposition). When surgery is performed, a ureteric stent should always be left in situ. At follow-up, in order to confirm ureteric integrity, repeat imaging is mandatory prior to considering stent removal. It is the authors' view that all urinary tract injuries, with the exception of a simple bladder dome injury, should be repaired by a urologist with appropriate expertise.

Bowel Injury

Bowel injury is a potentially lethal complication, which can occur at the time of entry into the peritoneal cavity. The antimesenteric border of the small intestine is more frequently damaged, in particular if adhesions are present to the anterior peritoneum. Different techniques are available to gain access into the abdomen. Gynaecologists have traditionally used the closed entry, with establishment of the pneumoperitoneum with Veress needle. Interestingly, this was originally developed by János Veres(s) in 1932 as a treatment strategy for pulmonary tuberculosis ('collapse therapy'). Subsequently, its use to induce pneumoperitoneum in laparoscopy was developed in 1947 by Raoul Palmer, who was the first to publish data regarding its safety in 1974 [26]. Open technique was described by Hasson in 1971, with the aim to reduce gas embolism, preperitoneal insufflation, and visceral injury [27]. This is the preferred entry method of general surgeons, but it has also been adopted by some gynaecologists, in particular if retrieval of a surgical specimen through the umbilicus is planned. More recently, single-use optical trocars have been marketed, but their superiority in avoiding visceral injury has not been demonstrated.

Surgeons should use the entry technique they have been trained in. There is insufficient evidence to state whether one method of laparoscopic entry is better than another. Patient's characteristics should also be taken into consideration. A previous transverse suprapubic incision is associated with a 19.8% risk of periumbilical adhesions. This increases to 51.7% in the case of a previous midline incision. In the latter scenario, an alternative site entry may be considered, such as the left upper quadrant or Palmer's point (3 cm below the left subcostal border in the midclavicular line).

Once the laparoscope is introduced in the peritoneal cavity, a 360-degree view should be obtained to rule out any visceral injury during the entry. A bowel injury provoked with Veress needle may be difficult to detect as its external diameter measures 2 mm only. However, this may not need formal repair, unless it is associated with bleeding or leaking stools. Optical trocars may cause a more obvious injury, in particular if the laparoscope is inserted directly into the bowel lumen. When injury occurs during open entry, leakage of stools is invariably detected. Injuries to the bowel with trocar or during open entry can be mostly repaired in a primary fashion in two layers with delayed absorbable sutures. However, in case of complicated laceration, segmental resection is recommended, with or without stoma formation. A minilaparotomy is often performed to address this complication, although a laparoscopic repair is feasible but advanced skills are required. The assistance of a general surgeon should always be requested when a bowel injury is diagnosed or suspected (Figure 8.5).

In a sacrocolpopexy, intraoperative bowel injury may occur during dissection of the rectovaginal space. A vaginal and rectal probe can facilitate the identification of the correct surgical plane. Also, exposure of the sacral promontory may be challenging in patients with high body mass index or significant intra-abdominal adhesions (e.g. previous surgery or peritonitis). In high-risk cases, we recommend thorough preoperative counselling and consideration of alternative routes of surgery, such as sacrospinous fixation or colpocleisis. In case laparoscopy reveals adhesions or a difficult anatomy is unexpectedly found, taking consent for an alternative vaginal approach may be a prudent precaution. In fact, this allows the surgeon to treat the vault prolapse safely and minimize risk of bowel injury. It is our practice to consent for sacrospinous fixation in case laparoscopy identifies adhesions or anatomical variation that would make a sacrocolpopexy more hazardous.

Vascular Injuries

Vascular injuries are rare but life-threatening conditions which may be encountered during different steps of any laparoscopic procedure: placement of the Veress needle, insertion of lateral trocars, and tissue dissection. Injury of major vessels is probably the main concern for surgeons who are learning the closed entry technique. The main risk factor is a low body mass index, with a reduced distance between major vessels and the overlying skin. As a matter of fact, in very thin women, the Royal College of Obstetricians and Gynaecologists recommends the open technique or entry at the Palmer's point [1]. Vascular injuries from an uncontrolled rapid entry of the Veress needle may also occur in women with a reduced resistance of the anterior abdominal wall, as a result of previous surgery, ageing, and multiparity. A

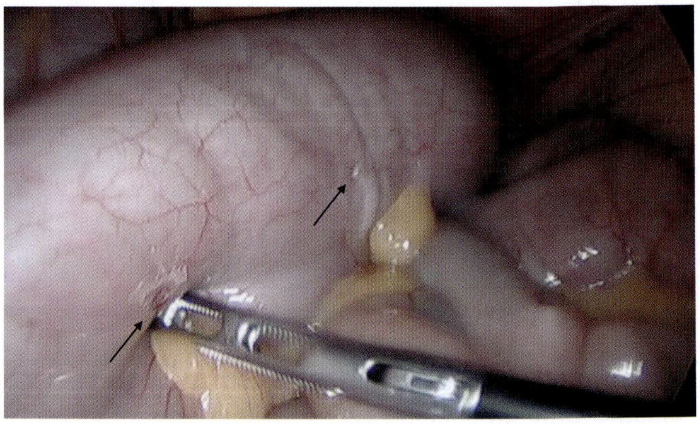

Figure 8.5 Bowel injury (see black arrows) caused by Veress needle. The on-call surgical team was asked to attend theatre. Conservative management was advised, and the recovery was uncomplicated.

vascular injury secondary to insertion of the Veress needle can be revealed through aspiration (Palmer's) test with syringe. If initially missed, concealed bleeding may cause a retroperitoneal haematoma or haemodynamic instability. Vascular surgeons should be promptly alerted. Treatment may involve immediate laparotomy, manual compression, fluid resuscitation with blood transfusion, and repair of the laceration, although in some cases fibrin sealant may suffice.

Insertion of the lateral trocars may cause transection of the inferior epigastric artery. This is a branch of the external iliac artery running cephalad between the rectus abdominis muscle and the posterior lamella of its sheath and it can often be visualized trans-peritoneally. Thus, lateral trocars should be introduced under direct vision. Prior to insertion, a straight needle can be used to inject local anaesthetic at the trocar site. This can also help to visualize the anatomical relationship between the entry site on the skin and the course of the inferior epigastric artery. If injury occurs, different strategies can be adopted to stop the bleeding. Firstly, a bipolar energy device may be used through the contralateral port to obtain coagulation. If haemostasis is not achieved, ligation can be attempted through the ipsilateral trocar site with an endoscopic fascial closure device. If this is not available, the skin incision can be extended in order to directly visualize, clamp, and ligate the bleeding vessel. Alternatively, mechanical compression can be applied with a 30-ml Foley catheter. This is inserted through the trocar site and secured externally with a clamp. Where available, interventional radiology and embolization of the bleeding vessel can be considered.

Vascular injuries can also complicate urogynaecological procedures. In order to safely perform a sacrocolpopexy, knowledge of the presacral space anatomy is vital. The iliac vessels and the aorta bifurcation represent its lateral and superior border, respectively. The left common iliac vein is the closest vessel to the sacral promontory, and also the most commonly injured. Due to the effect of the pneumoperitoneum compressing the left common iliac vein, its course is less obvious in laparoscopic surgery compared to open surgery and often looks like a blue pillow that feels soft when touched with a blunt probe. The middle sacral artery and vein are generally identified directly on the sacrum. The presacral venous plexus is formed by the anastomosis of the middle sacral with the lateral sacral veins [28]. Presacral vessels may be damaged while surgeons attempt to expose the sacral promontory. The bleeding may be brisk and potentially life-threatening. Also, anatomy slightly differs between patients, with the location of the inferior vena cava bifurcation potentially lower than expected in both thin and elderly women [29]. The senior author has abandoned one case of sacrocolpopexy when the bifurcation was identified directly over the promontory. If the presacral vessels are injured, haemostasis can be difficult as the presacral vessels tend to retract inside the bone. Electrocautery and placement of sutures or clips can be attempted if the vessel is identified. Alternative options are sterile thumbtacks and topical haemostatic agents, including bone wax, gelatin matrix (Gelfoam®), oxidized regenerated cellulose (Surgicel®, Fibrillar™), gelatin matrix combined with thrombin (FloSeal®), and microporous polysaccharide spheres (Arista®). If all other measures fail, pelvic packing up to 48 hours may represent the last resort [30].

Bleeding can also be encountered during a colposuspension, in particular while dissecting and exposing the paravaginal fascia. This originates more commonly from a plexus of vessels lateral to the bladder neck. The laparoscopic approach is associated with less blood loss than the open approach as it is easier to visualize blood vessels and coagulate [19,20]. If the dissection into the space of Retzius is carried out too laterally, damage to the obturator vessels can occur. Attention should also be paid in order to avoid vessels close to the anterior abdominal wall, such as the inferior epigastric artery and, more laterally, the external iliac artery. Injury to the aberrant or accessory obturator artery, alias corona mortis, has also been reported. This is an aberrant anastomotic branch (between the inferior epigastric and the obturator vessels) which lies on the superior pubic ramus, with a reported prevalence of 27.9% [31]. Bleeding from the paravaginal tissues often stops following electrocautery, placement of colposuspension sutures, and knot tying. If oozing persists, a drainage in the space of Retzius may be left for 24 hours. In the unlikely scenario of a major vessel injury, topical agents can be tried (see above). However, if these do not succeed, vascular surgeons should be alerted.

Mesh Complications

Long-term complications from insertion of a sacrocolpopexy mesh include vaginal exposure, infection, perforation of a hollow organ (bladder/bowel), and chronic pain. However, long-term data available in the literature are limited. In a recent survey with median follow-up of 6.4 years, 9 out of 166 patients (5.4%) reported a complication related to mesh exposure following a laparoscopic sacrocolpopexy [32]. Previously, an exposure rate of 10.5% was found at seven years follow-up from open sacrocolpopexy [33]. The use of different mesh materials may contribute to this drop observed over the years. In fact, macroporous and monofilament polypropylene meshes have been associated with a reduced risk of infection and exposure compared to other synthetic grafts, such as the microporous multifilament expanded Polytetrafluoroethylene (ePTFE) mesh [34]. Also, the use of delayed absorbable sutures to the vagina seem to cause less exposures when compared to permanent sutures. Concomitant hysterectomy and smoking have also been identified as risk factors for mesh exposure [35]. Patients may present with a history of painful intercourse, vaginal discharge, and bleeding. This can be many years after the mesh placement procedure. In our experience, magnetic resonance imaging is helpful when a sacrocolpopexy mesh complication is suspected [36]. In case of small erosions, options include a trial with local oestrogens (to promote growth of the vaginal mucosa over the exposed mesh), although this has a cure rate as low as 14% [37]. The next step is represented by vaginal excision under anaesthetic. A success rate of approximately 48% has been reported for the first attempt, while this significantly drops if repeat mesh trimming is required [38]. Thus, a concomitant vaginal and laparoscopic removal of the mesh may need to be considered in recurrent cases. Bowel involvement in sacrocolpopexy mesh complications is not uncommon, so the assistance of a colorectal surgeon is very helpful.

Bladder mesh perforation has been found in patients complaining of dysuria, bladder pain, and recurrent urinary tract infections. Persistent microscopic haematuria is also a possible sign. Bladder injury during index surgery has been argued to be a risk factor for developing bladder perforation (Figure 8.6). In this scenario, the current consensus is to insert the sacrocolpopexy mesh as long as this is placed away from the bladder repair. A cystoscopy is required to make a diagnosis of mesh perforation. Also, this will be able to inform the clinicians regarding the amount of bladder involved and the anatomical relationship with the ureters. Although urogynaecologists may have some expertise from previous cases with MUS, patients should be managed within a multi-disciplinary team including a urologist. Laparoscopic removal of the mesh must be offered with bladder reconstruction +/– ureteric reimplantation (in case of involvement of the ureteric orifices).

Bowel perforation is quite a rare long-term complication of sacrocolpopexy mesh. Surprisingly, patients may be asymptomatic [39]. Alternatively, red flag symptoms are rectal mucous discharge or bleeding. The underlying mechanism is not entirely understood. It is plausible that risk factors are conditions affecting blood supply and immunological response, such as diabetes and smoking [40]. Clinicians should have a low threshold to investigate anorectal symptoms if a mesh has been previously inserted. In exceptional cases, the bowel can grow around the mesh and a through-and-through perforation is found. In case a large bowel or a complicated small bowel injury (e.g. caused by diathermy) occurs intraoperatively, insertion of the mesh should be avoided as this can be associated with a high risk of sepsis and bowel perforation [24]. If a simple small bowel injury occurs, sacrocolpopexy mesh can be inserted as long as the mesh is not in contact with the repair. A mesh perforating the bowel (Figure 8.7) invariably needs a joint procedure with the colorectal surgeons. A complete mesh removal should be carried out with concomitant segmental bowel resection +/– temporary ileostomy or colostomy (according to the portion involved).

In the last few years, since mesh-related warnings from the Food and Drug Administration in 2008 and 2011, clinicians and patients have been more aware of the potential complications associated with synthetic material. An increasing number of women have sought medical attention, reporting new onset or worsening chronic pain and requesting mesh removal. Short-term data are available regarding complete removal of retropubic MUS in women with chronic pain. At 12-week follow-up, complete resolution of the symptoms was reported in 48% of cases, while no improvement was noted in a minority of cases (11%) [22]. However, there is a lack of data regarding removal of sacrocolpopexy mesh and outcomes. Moreover, despite mesh removal, there is a chance that pain symptoms may recur in the long-term. Given the uncertainties related to mesh removal and the associated risks, a thorough assessment of the symptoms from a pain clinician is recommended prior to embarking on complex surgery.

Other Complications

There is growing interest regarding patient positioning during laparoscopic surgery. Urogynaecological procedures are performed with the patient in Lloyd-Davies position in order to facilitate access to the pelvis. This is defined as a supine position of the body with hips flexed at 15 degrees and with a 30-degree head-down tilt. Legs are placed in support boots. Concerns have been raised as prolonged adoption of this position may compromise local blood flow to the calf muscle, leading to the development of compartment syndrome.

Incorrect patient positioning during laparoscopic surgery can cause nerve injuries defined as neurapraxia, with disruption of nerve conduction across a small part of the axon, which usually resolves within weeks to months. The brachial plexus is more commonly involved, with an incidence of 0.16%. This can derive from hyper-abduction of the arms (compression of the lower roots between the clavicle and the first rib) or a steep Trendelenburg position (head-down tilt ≥ 45 degrees) with two medial shoulder braces (overstretch of the upper roots). The former causes Erb's palsy, with the arm typically hanging by the side and medially rotated and the forearm extended and pronated, while the latter will result in Klumpke's palsy, with weakness of the distal forearm and hand. Thus, arms should be tucked and pronated or kept at less than 90 degrees from the body. Shoulder braces should not be used to support the Trendelenburg position and the head must be kept in the neutral position.

Improper tucking of the arm can also cause injury to the ulnar nerve through pressure on the medial aspect of the elbow

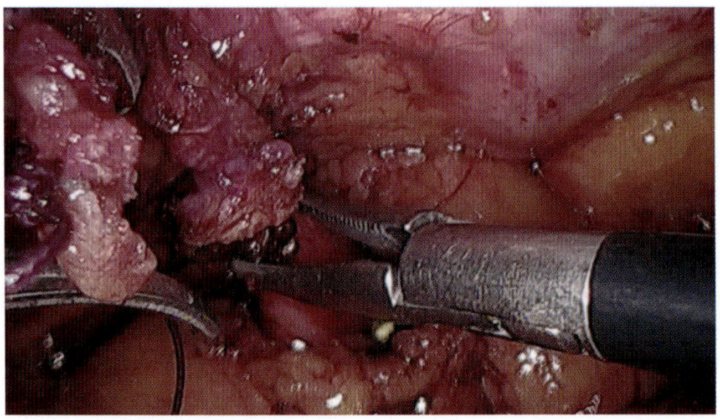

Figure 8.6 Long-term bladder perforation following retropubic tension-free vaginal tape. A complete removal of the tape was carried out through concomitant laparoscopic and vaginal approach. The bladder defect was closed and a Foley catheter was left in situ for two weeks postoperatively.

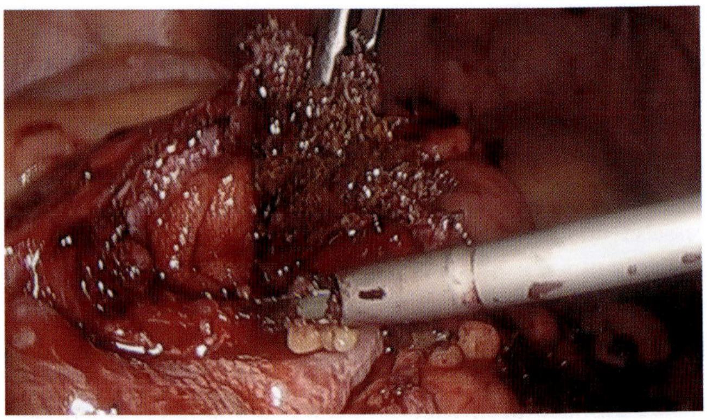

Figure 8.7 Sacrocolpopexy mesh perforating the small bowel. Complete laparoscopic removal of the mesh, segmental bowel resection, and side-to-side anastomosis was performed with colorectal surgeons.

(compression of the nerve in the cubital tunnel). This results in sensory loss in the tips of the small finger and medial aspect of the ring finger and in a 'claw hand' from muscle paralysis. The recommendation is to use a soft external padding at the level of the cubital tunnel to protect the nerve. Also, arms should be pronated if they are tucked and supinated if they are on arm boards.

In case of concomitant vaginal surgery, the patient's position will be changed from Lloyd-Davies to lithotomy, where legs are separated, flexed, and supported in raised stirrups. Surgeons must be mindful that thighs should be flexed no greater than 90 degrees and abducted no greater than 45 degrees. Hyperflexion and extreme abduction of the thighs with external rotation at the hip may result in the following neuropathies: femoral (kinking of the nerve under the inguinal ligament), obturator (compression against the obturator foramen), sciatic (overstretch), and common peroneal (compression by the head of the fibula) [41]. It is good practice to pause for at least 15 minutes in case of prolonged surgery and allow the legs to be dropped down to minimize the risk of peripheral nerve injury.

Placement of lateral trocars can cause injury to the iliohypogastric and ilioinguinal nerves, as they run in the abdominal wall approximately 2–3 cm medial and 1–3 cm inferior to the anterior superior iliac spine [42]. These nerves may be damaged through trocar insertion or nerve entrapment secondary to fascial closure, resulting in pain of the lower abdomen, upper thigh, and groin. Insertion of the trocars 2 cm above the anterior superior iliac spine or within 1 cm from the midline is deemed to minimize this risk.

Injury of the pelvic autonomic nervous system and de novo visceral dysfunction can occur following sacrocolpopexy. Currently, the recommended site for mesh fixation is at the sacral promontory, which is defined as the anterior surface of the S1 vertebra. This is in close proximity with the superior hypogastric plexus, a network of nerves situated in the presacral space predominantly below the aortic bifurcation and to the left of the midline [43]. The first sacral nerve branches out approximately 2–3 cm below the sacral promontory and 1–2 cm from the midline. Attention must be paid as this nerve is not visualized during the dissection as it runs outside the presacral space, just behind the fascia covering the piriformis muscle [44]. Moreover, the dissection of the peritoneum along the right utero-sacral ligament can cause interruption of nerve fibres arising from the inferior hypogastric plexus. Nerve-sparing techniques have been described to minimize postoperative sequelae [45]. However, their reproducibility is uncertain.

Injury to the obturator nerve may occur following laparoscopic colposuspension and removal of retropubic tapes. Lateral colposuspension sutures have been found 1–3 cm distant from the obturator nerve [46]. Thus, although injury has not been reported yet in the literature, surgeons should be aware of this anatomic relationship when dissecting the space of Retzius. Also, when a total removal of MUS is planned, the mesh may not be found where expected. In fact, transection of the transobturator nerve has been reported following incorrect insertion of a retropubic MUS [47] (Figure 8.8). This is a rare scenario, which has also been encountered in the authors' experience, where a complete laparoscopic removal carries a risk of complete interruption of the nerve fibres. We suggest abandoning the procedure and discussing with the patient the potential risks. Neurophysiology testing may be helpful. In case nerve reconstruction is anticipated, a joint procedure with plastic surgeons should be arranged.

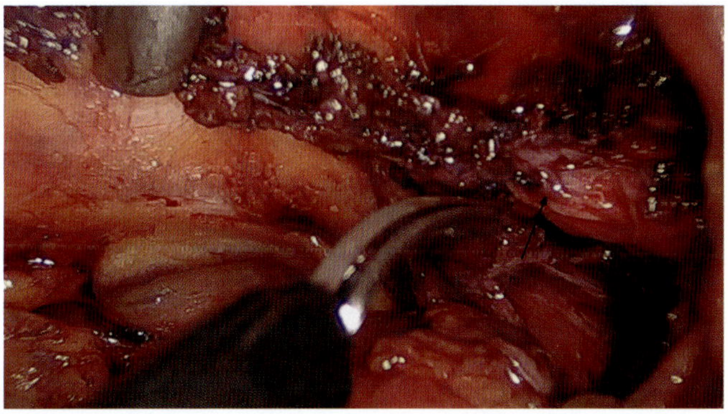

Figure 8.8 Right retropubic arm of tension-free vaginal tape transecting the right obturator nerve (see black arrow). The surgery was abandoned, and complete removal of the residual tape was arranged as an open procedure with plastic surgeons, who performed nerve reconstruction. Pictures from the Warrell Unit archive.

Finally, trocar site hernia can complicate laparoscopies, and this mainly occurs at the umbilical site. Fascial closure is recommended in trocar sites ≥ 10 mm, although this complication has also been reported with 5-mm trocar sites. Endoscopic suturing devices (Endo Close™) have been introduced to facilitate sheath closure. Alternatively, this can be accomplished by direct visualization, with a suture on a 'J' needle. Radially expanding trocars (VersaStep™) have been devised in order to cause less trauma to the rectus sheath. However, their routine use is supported by little evidence. Trocar site hernia can cause early onset small bowel obstruction. In these cases, prompt intervention is recommended as there is an increased risk of bowel necrosis secondary to an incarcerated hernia.

Conclusion

Proficiency in laparoscopic urogynaecology procedures is best obtained through structured training programmes. Outside of these, it is now becoming more common for surgeons to be formally proctored by colleagues with expertise in laparoscopy. Knowledge of the anatomy, diagnosis, and management of possible complications is an integral part of the required skills to provide safe care. Patient selection is critical to surgical success and clear operative documentation, including steps carried out to minimize complications, is prudent.

References

1. RCOG. Preventing entry-related gynaecological laparoscopic injuries. In: Green-top Guidelines. Green-top No. 49. Royal College of Obstetricians and Gynaecologists; 2008.
2. RANZCOG/AGES. Consensus statement of the Royal Australian & New Zealand College of Obstetricians & Gynaecologists (RANZCOG) and the Australasian Gynaecological Endoscopy and Surgery Society (AGES). Use of the Veress needle to obtain pneumoperitoneum prior to laparoscopy; 2017.
3. SAGES. Society of American Gastrointestinal and Endoscopic Surgeons. Guidelines for Diagnostic Laparoscopy; 2010.

4. Makai G, Isaacson K. Complications of gynecologic laparoscopy. Clin Obstet Gynecol 2009; 52(3): 401–11.
5. Ahmad G, Baker J, Finnerty J, Phillips K, Watson A. Laparoscopic entry techniques. Cochrane Database Syst Rev 2019; 1: CD006583.
6. Chapron CM, Pierre F, Lacroix S, Querleu D, Lansac J, Dubuisson JB. Major vascular injuries during gynecologic laparoscopy. J Am Coll Surg 1997; 185(5): 461–5.
7. Llarena NC, Shah AB, Milad MP. Bowel injury in gynecologic laparoscopy: a systematic review. Obstet Gynecol 2015; 125(6): 1407–17.
8. Epstein J, Arora A, Ellis H. Surface anatomy of the inferior epigastric artery in relation to laparoscopic injury. Clin Anat 2004; 17(5): 400–8.
9. Swank HA, Mulder IM, la Chapelle CF, Reitsma JB, Lange JF, Bemelman WA. Systematic review of trocar-site hernia. Br J Surg 2012; 99(3): 315–23.
10. Abboudi H, Ahmed K, Royle J, Khan MS, Dasgupta P, N'Dow J. Ureteric injury: a challenging condition to diagnose and manage. Nat Rev Urol 2013; 10(2): 108–15.
11. Wong JMK, Bortoletto P, Tolentino J, Jung MJ, Milad MP. Urinary tract injury in gynecologic laparoscopy for benign indication: a systematic review. Obstet Gynecol 2018; 131(1): 100–8.
12. Saidi MH, Sadler RK, Vancaillie TG, Akright BD, Farhart SA, White AJ. Diagnosis and management of serious urinary complications after major operative laparoscopy. Obstet Gynecol 1996; 87(2): 272–6.
13. Peacock LM, Young A, Rogers RG. Universal cystoscopy at the time of benign hysterectomy: a debate. Am J Obstet Gynecol 2018; 219(1): 75–7.
14. Zacche MM, Mukhopadhyay S, Giarenis I. Changing surgical trends for female stress urinary incontinence in England. Int Urogynecol J 2019; 30(2): 203–9.
15. Deprest J, Krofta L, Van der Aa F, Milani AL, Den Boon J, Claerhout F, Roovers JP. The challenge of implementing laparoscopic sacrocolpopexy. Int Urogynecol J 2014; 25(9): 1153–60.
16. Freites J, Stewart F, Omar MI, Mashayekhi A, Agur WI. Laparoscopic colposuspension for urinary incontinence in women. Cochrane Database Syst Rev 2019; 12: CD002239.
17. Vandendriessche D, Sussfeld J, Giraudet G, Lucot JP, Behal H, Cosson M. Complications and reoperations after laparoscopic sacrocolpopexy with a mean follow-up of 4 years. Int Urogynecol J 2017; 28(2): 231–9.
18. Sato H, Abe H, Ikeda A, Miyagawa T, Sato K. Complications and clinical outcomes of laparoscopic sacrocolpopexy for pelvic organ prolapse. J Obstet Gynaecol 2021; 41(1): 128–32.
19. Maher CF, Feiner B, DeCuyper EM, Nichlos CJ, Hickey KV, O'Rourke P. Laparoscopic sacral colpopexy versus total vaginal mesh for vaginal vault prolapse: a randomized trial. Am J Obstet Gynecol 2011; 204(4): 360 e1–7.
20. Coolen AWM, van Oudheusden AMJ, Mol BWJ, van Eijndhoven HWF, Roovers JWR, Bongers MY. Laparoscopic sacrocolpopexy compared with open abdominal sacrocolpopexy for vault prolapse repair: a randomised controlled trial. Int Urogynecol J 2017; 28(10): 1469–79.
21. Pacquee S, Nawapun K, Claerhout F, Werbrouck E, Veldman J, D'Hoore A, Wyndaele J, Verguts J, De Ridder D, Deprest J. Long-term assessment of a prospective cohort of patients undergoing laparoscopic sacrocolpopexy. Obstet Gynecol 2019; 134(2): 323–32.
22. Goodall EJ, Cartwright R, Stratta EC, Jackson SR, Price N. Outcomes after laparoscopic removal of retropubic midurethral slings for chronic pain. Int Urogynecol J 2019; 30(8): 1323–8.
23. Tanagho EA. Colpocystourethropexy: the way we do it. J Urol 1976; 116(6): 751–3.
24. Costantini E, Brubaker L, Cervigni M, Matthews CA, O'Reilly BA, Rizk D, Giannitsas K, Maher CF. Sacrocolpopexy for pelvic organ prolapse: evidence-based review and recommendations. Eur J Obstet Gynecol Reprod Biol 2016; 205: 60–5.
25. Clapp B, Klingsporn W, Lodeiro C, Wicker E, Christensen L, Jones R, Tyroch A. Small bowel obstructions following the use of barbed suture: a review of the literature and analysis of the MAUDE database. Surg Endosc 2020; 34(3): 1261–9.
26. Palmer R. Safety in laparoscopy. J Reprod Med 1974; 13(1): 1–5.
27. Hasson HM. A modified instrument and method for laparoscopy. Am J Obstet Gynecol 1971; 110(6): 886–7.
28. Wieslander CK, Rahn DD, McIntire DD, Marinis SI, Wai CY, Schaffer JI, Corton MM. Vascular anatomy of the presacral space in unembalmed female cadavers. Am J Obstet Gynecol 2006; 195(6): 1736–41.
29. Berger AA, Abramowitch S, Moalli PA. 3D vascular anatomy of the presacral space: impact of age and adiposity. Int Urogynecol J 2019; 30(3): 401–7.
30. Hokenstad ED, Occhino JA. Management of presacral bleeding. Int Urogynecol J 2020; 31(1): 215–17.
31. Duenas-Garcia OF, Kim Y, Leung K, Flynn MK. Vascular anatomical relationships of the retropubic space and the sacrospinous ligament, using three-dimensional imaging. Int Urogynecol J 2017; 28(8): 1177–82.
32. Thomas TN, Davidson ERW, Lampert EJ, Paraiso MFR, Ferrando CA. Long-term pelvic organ prolapse recurrence and mesh exposure following sacrocolpopexy. Int Urogynecol J 2020; 31(9): 1763–70.
33. Nygaard I, Brubaker L, Zyczynski HM, Cundiff G, Richter H, Gantz M, Fine P, Menefee S, Ridgeway B, Visco A, Warren LK, Zhang M, Meikle S. Long-term outcomes following abdominal sacrocolpopexy for pelvic organ prolapse. JAMA 2013; 309(19): 2016–24.
34. Kelly M, Macdougall K, Olabisi O, McGuire N. In vivo response to polypropylene following implantation in animal models: a review of biocompatibility. Int Urogynecol J 2017; 28(2): 171–80.
35. Cundiff GW, Varner E, Visco AG, Zyczynski HM, Nager CW, Norton PA, Schaffer J, Brown MB, Brubaker L, Pelvic Floor Disorders Network. Risk factors for mesh/suture erosion following sacral colpopexy. Am J Obstet Gynecol 2008; 199(6): 688e1–5.
36. Mahoney C, Hindle A, Rajashanker B, Kearney R. MR scan evaluation of pelvic organ prolapse mesh complications and agreement with intra-operative findings. Int Urogynecol J 2020; 31(8): 1559–66.
37. Deffieux X, Huel C, de Tayrac R, Bottero J, Porcher R, Gervaise A, Bonnet K, Frydman R, Fernandez H. Vaginal mesh extrusion after transvaginal repair of cystocele using a prosthetic mesh: treatment and functional outcomes. J Gynecol Obstet Biol Reprod (Paris) 2006; 35(7): 678–84.
38. Quiroz LH, Gutman RE, Fagan MJ, Cundiff GW. Partial colpocleisis for the treatment of sacrocolpopexy mesh erosions. Int Urogynecol J Pelvic Floor Dysfunct 2008; 19(2): 261–6.
39. Paine M, Harnsberger JR, Whiteside JL. Transrectal mesh erosion remote from sacrocolpopexy: management and comment. Am J Obstet Gynecol 2010; 203(2): e11–13.

40. Deng T, Liao B, Luo D, Shen H, Wang K. Risk factors for mesh erosion after female pelvic floor reconstructive surgery: a systematic review and meta-analysis. BJU Int 2016; 117(2): 323–43.
41. Deveneau NE, Forbis C, Lipetskaia L, Kinman CL, Agrawal A, Herring NR, Francis SL. The effect of lithotomy position on nerve stretch: a cadaveric study. Female Pelvic Med Reconstr Surg 2017; 23(6): 457–61.
42. Whiteside JL, Barber MD, Walters MD, Falcone T. Anatomy of ilioinguinal and iliohypogastric nerves in relation to trocar placement and low transverse incisions. Am J Obstet Gynecol 2003; 189(6): 1574–8; discussion 8.
43. Ripperda CM, Jackson LA, Phelan JN, Carrick KS, Corton MM. Anatomic relationships of the pelvic autonomic nervous system in female cadavers: clinical applications to pelvic surgery. Am J Obstet Gynecol 2017; 216(4): 388e1–e7.
44. Florian-Rodriguez ME, Hamner JJ, Corton MM. First sacral nerve and anterior longitudinal ligament anatomy: clinical applications during sacrocolpopexy. Am J Obstet Gynecol 2017; 217(5): 607e1–e4.
45. Sarlos D, Aigmueller T, Magg H, Schaer G. Laparoscopic sacrocolpopexy: demonstration of a nerve-sparing technique. Am J Obstet Gynecol 2015; 212(6): 824e1–3.
46. Kinman CL, Agrawal A, Deveneau NE, Meriwether KV, Herring NR, Francis SL. Anatomical relationships of Burch colposuspension sutures. Female Pelvic Med Reconstr Surg 2017; 23(2): 72–4.
47. Baines G, Jackson SR, Price N. Obturator nerve injury: a rare complication of retropubic tension-free vaginal sling. Int Urogynecol J 2016; 27(10): 1597–9.
48. Carey MP, Goh JT, Rosamilia A, Cornish A, Gordon I, Hawthorne G, Maher CF, Dwyer PL, Moran P, Gilmour DT. Laparoscopic versus open Burch colposuspension: a randomised controlled trial. BJOG 2006; 113(9): 999–1006.
49. Kitchener HC, Dunn G, Lawton V, Reid F, Nelson L, Smith AR, Group CS. Laparoscopic versus open colposuspension – results of a prospective randomised controlled trial. BJOG 2006; 113(9): 1007–13.

Chapter 9

Mesh: Types and Indications for Use for Laparoscopic Urogynaecology

Amy Park, Graham Chapman , Marie Fidela Paraiso

Introduction

Pelvic floor disorders are exceedingly common in women, with the reported incidence reaching as high as 23.6% [1]. It is estimated that one in five women will undergo surgery for pelvic organ prolapse (POP) or stress urinary incontinence prior to the age of 80 [2]. Surgical management of POP varies widely, including reconstructive versus obliterative procedures, vaginal versus abdominal techniques, and native tissue versus mesh-augmented repair. Similar to other reconstructive surgical fields, the rate of anatomical and symptomatic recurrence is of the utmost importance to both patients and surgeons when performing urogynecologic surgery. While much controversy exists as to the optimal approach, surgical augmentation with mesh or other grafting materials has long been suggested as a means to increase the durability of the repair and decrease the risk of recurrent POP or urinary incontinence [3–5].

However, prolapse repair with vaginal implantation of mesh has come under scrutiny in recent years, with significant restrictions placed on this practice by the US, UK, and others [6,7]. Abdominal placement of mesh has remained a mainstay treatment for POP, and is considered by many to be the gold standard procedure [8,9]. While this was traditionally performed via laparotomy, laparoscopic and robotic approaches have quickly become the primary modality for many surgeons. This chapter aims to review and describe the various types of mesh implants as well as the indications and uses for mesh in laparoscopic urogynaecology.

Historical Perspective

Implants have been utilized to reinforce reconstructive surgical repairs since the early 1900s. Hernia surgeons first used various synthetic materials at the end of the nineteenth century, and polypropylene mesh was introduced in 1954 [10,11]. Biologic grafts have been used in urogynaecology as early as 1917, when fascia lata was used to perform a pubovaginal sling for stress urinary incontinence [3]. While various graft materials were subsequently used for vaginal repair of POP throughout the twentieth century, the first reports of a graft-augmented abdominal approach to POP surgery occurred in 1958 and 1962, when a biologic graft was used to create a bridge between the top of the vagina to the anterior longitudinal ligament of the sacrum, thereby performing a sacrocolpopexy [12–14]. Today lightweight, macroporous, polypropylene mesh is the dominant material utilized, though innovation continues. The majority of the data regarding abdominal or laparoscopic placement of mesh lies in the sacrocolpopexy literature, though a number of other urogynaecologic applications exist including fistula repair, neovagina creation and repair, and vaginoplasty. Throughout the evolution of the use of various mesh and grafting materials in urogynaecologic surgery, a number of risks, benefits, and unique properties have been elucidated about a vast array of biologic and synthetic grafting materials.

Biologic Mesh

Biologic grafts are intended to augment reconstructive surgery by providing an extracellular scaffolding that will attract host stromal cells, stimulate angiogenesis, and promote the generation of strong, healthy tissue [15]. In urogynaecology, biologic grafts have consistently been shown to be efficacious when used to treat stress urinary incontinence via a retropubic or transobturator fascial sling [16–18]. Contrarily, when considering abdominal or laparoscopic surgery for POP, quality evidence exists that biologic graft materials provide lesser efficacy, with no improvement in the risk profile compared to more commonly performed native tissue or synthetic mesh procedures [19–21]. However, unique situations may render both native tissue and synthetic mesh not acceptable in a patient requiring laparoscopic urogynaecologic surgery. In this scenario, three biologic graft categories may be considered: autografts, allografts, and xenografts. Autografts are tissue that is harvested from the actual patient who is undergoing the procedure, allografts are harvested from cadaveric human donors, and xenografts are harvested from non-human sources. Each has important advantages and disadvantages that dictate their clinical utility.

Autografts

The most common examples of autografts in urogynaecology include rectus fascia and tensor fascia lata used for the pubovaginal sling or sacrocolpopexy. Other pertinent examples of autografting include buccal mucosal grafting for urethral or vaginal reconstruction. The primary advantage of autografting is the absence of risk for a negative host response such as graft rejection or mesh erosion. Given this factor, there is no need for processing to render the tissue non-immunogenic. Thus, this approach is more cost-effective than the other biologic grafting options. However, major drawbacks of autografting include notably increased surgical morbidity, limited tissue quantity, increased postoperative pain, and more extensive recovery. Walter et al studied harvest-site complications following fascia lata use in urogynaecologic surgery, and reported a 7% rate of cellulitis, 3% rate of seroma, and 1% rate of hematoma [22]. Additionally, two years after surgery, 13% of patients expressed dissatisfaction due to cosmesis or pain at the harvest site. Despite this risk associated with harvest-site morbidity, autografts have historically been the most commonly used biologic graft material in urogynaecology.

Allografts

Allografts utilized in urogynaecology most commonly include fascia lata and dermis obtained from cadaveric human donors. These products are harvested in a relatively standardized process, including donor screening for infectious diseases, and the use of aseptic surgical technique. After the tissue harvest, the graft is sterilized and preserved using a variety of techniques which can involve the use of various solvents, irradiation, and freezing or freeze-drying [23,24]. These efforts are primarily intended to eradicate the tissue of antigenicity to minimize the risk of a negative host response, while preserving the collagen scaffolding that provides strength and structure to the graft material. While the risk of disease transmission is greatly reduced by these sterilization techniques, antigenicity is unlikely to be completely eliminated. Studies of graft material after surgical removal have indicated that residual donor antigens and DNA exist even after a year of remaining in situ [23,25]. The clinical relevance of this is uncertain. While the risk of disease transmission is low, the presence of immunologic factors may increase the degradation of the material and decrease the efficacy of the graft, particularly in comparison to autografts or synthetic material. The major benefit of utilizing an allograft compared to an autograft is the lack of harvest site morbidity.

Xenografts

Xenografts have similar characteristics to allografts, although they are a more readily available resource compared to autografts or allografts. Given this, they are cheaper to manufacture, more well-studied, and used more commonly compared to allografts [15]. The donor source is typically either bovine or porcine, and the site of harvest may include small intestine, pericardium, or dermis. As with allografts, the processes involved in graft harvest includes standardized donor screening for infectious diseases and aseptic harvest, followed by various processing techniques to remove immunologic factors and generate an acellular scaffold [26]. Also similar to allografts, risks of using a xenograft include the theoretical possibility of infectious disease transmission and concern for graft breakdown and loss of strength due to a negative host response. Additionally, the processing required to produce xenograft and allograft materials renders them less economical than synthetic mesh or autografts.

Synthetic Mesh

Synthetic mesh is the most commonly used graft material in urogynaecology. While significant scrutiny exists regarding the vaginal placement of synthetic mesh to treat POP, abdominal placement is generally considered far more acceptable with a lower relative risk profile and evidence of superior anatomic durability when compared to native tissue repair. Compared to biologic mesh, advantages of synthetic mesh include a lack of risk for infectious disease transmission, lack of need for tissue harvest and the associated risks, lower cost, and higher tensile strength [27]. Synthetic mesh can be categorized as either absorbable or permanent, and the graft characteristics are described by the pore size, mesh weight, and classification.

Absorbable Synthetic Mesh

Absorbable synthetic mesh used in abdominal surgery includes polygalactin 910, which absorbs after approximately 30 days, and polyglycolic acid, which takes up to 90 days to absorb [27]. While absorbable mesh has been shown to be replaced by collagen-rich connective tissue after it degrades [28], this scar tissue does not retain its strength, thus is not useful in the abdominal repair of POP [29].

Non-Absorbable Synthetic Mesh

Non-absorbable synthetic mesh materials include polypropylene, polytetrafluoroethylene, and polyethylene, which provide longer lasting strength to augment reconstructive surgery. These materials each have distinct properties related to pore size, weight, and number of filaments. Pore size plays an important role in mesh flexibility and density, scar tissue formation, and risk of infection [30]. Macroporous mesh (pores >75 microns) provides a strong, flexible mesh that is less prone to infection due to the ability of host immune cells to access bacteria that may exist in the pore space. Microporous mesh (pores <10 microns) restricts host cell colonization to the periphery of the pores, resulting in encapsulation of scar tissue around the mesh. This decreases tissue integration within the mesh, diminishing the strength of the repair. Additionally the lack of access that host immune cells have to bacteria within the pore environment increases the risk of infection [27,31]. The mesh weight is dependent on the amount of synthetic material present (and thus the pore size). Thereby, macroporous meshes are of lighter weight. Light weight mesh has been shown to produce more flexible and elastic scar tissue and can reduce the risk of mesh-related complications [3,32,33]. Finally, synthetic mesh may be either monofilament or multifilament. In multifilament mesh, small (<10 micron) spaces exist between fibres of multifilament mesh, providing a nidus for bacterial growth without the ability of host immune cells to combat the growth, increasing the risk of bacterial colonization or infection in a similar fashion to microporous materials.

Synthetic Mesh Classification

Synthetic mesh is classified into four types, based on the abovementioned characteristics. Type I mesh is macroporous and is subdivided by heavy or light mesh weight. This includes the most commonly used mesh in urogynaecologic surgery, polypropylene. Type II mesh is microporous, and includes expanded polytetrafluoroethylene (Gore-Tex), which is commonly used as suture material in abdominal surgery for pelvic organ prolapse, though when used as a mesh graft has been associated with a significantly increased risk of erosion [21]. Type III mesh includes material that is macroporous with microporous components, or is multifilament, such as polyethylene. Type IV mesh is submicronic, with pore sizes less than 1 micron. Currently, the only synthetic mesh materials routinely used in urogynaecologic surgery are type I.

Indications, Risks, and Uses of Mesh in Urogynaecologic Surgery

In the planning and performance of surgery, the surgeon must weigh the risks and benefits of every move in order to maximize patient safety while optimizing the clinical outcome. In urogynaecologic surgery, this holds particularly true when determining which surgical approach is best: obliterative or reconstructive, abdominal or vaginal, native tissue or mesh-augmented. If a mesh-augmented repair is chosen, the ideal grafting material must be considered. While much research has been performed in an attempt to clarify these questions, it remains a complex issue that should be explored thoroughly to allow for shared decision-making between the patient and their surgeon. In order to understand the nuances of these decisions and convey them clearly to patients, the surgeon must have a deep understanding of the risks and benefits associated with the use of mesh.

Risks of Mesh Use

Mesh erosion

Erosion or exposure of mesh is the most notorious complication associated with mesh use in urogynaecologic surgery. Perforation of mesh into the vagina, bowel, or bladder can result in chronic pain, infectious complications, reoperation, and a number of other debilitating scenarios. While this risk is generally lower in abdominal placement of mesh as opposed to vaginal placement, true risk is still present. Most data regarding erosion after abdominal placement of mesh pertains to patients who underwent open abdominal sacrocolpopexy, as opposed to the laparoscopic approach. While baseline and surgical risk factors for erosion may differ in patients undergoing laparoscopic versus open surgery, it is presumed that the risks translate to a large degree. In a thorough review of the literature on laparoscopic or robotic sacrocolpopexy performed by van Zanten et al, the median mesh erosion rate was 1.9% with a range of 0–13% [34]. While some factors such as smoking are consistently accepted to increase the risk for mesh erosion, the risk conveyed by hysterectomy performance and type, as well as graft or suture materials used, differs between studies [21].

Mesh Erosion in Post-hysterectomy Patients

Mesh erosion after laparoscopic sacrocolpopexy for post-hysterectomy prolapse is relatively uncommon. In two randomized controlled trials of laparoscopic versus abdominal sacrocolpopexy for post-hysterectomy vault prolapse, no patients were found to have mesh erosion 12 months after surgery [35,36]. In a single randomized controlled trial of laparoscopic versus robotic sacrocolpopexy for post-hysterectomy prolapse, two patients (2.6%) out of 78 experienced a mesh erosion, both in the robotic group [3]. In a randomized controlled trial of laparoscopic sacrocolpopexy versus transvaginal mesh for post-hysterectomy prolapse, one patient (1.95%) out of 53 who underwent laparoscopic sacrocolpopexy experienced a mesh erosion at two years after surgery, compared to five (9.1%) out of 55 patients who had transvaginal mesh (p=0.11) [37]. These trials suggest a very low rate of mesh erosion in post-hysterectomy patients undergoing any form of abdominal sacrocolpopexy. It should be mentioned that the risk of mesh complications persists with time. A small prospective cohort study of laparoscopic sacrocolpopexy for post-hysterectomy prolapse suggested that the rate of erosion at five years after surgery is as high as 9.3% (four out of 43 participants) [38]. Although limited by sample size, this highlights the need for long-term follow-up and monitoring of these patients.

Mesh Erosion by Hysterectomy Type

The type of hysterectomy at the time of laparoscopic POP repair has been suggested to alter the risk profile for mesh erosion. While the risk of erosion may theoretically be increased when a total hysterectomy is performed, the data regarding this are inconclusive. In one retrospective cohort of patients who underwent laparoscopic sacrocolpopexy, the mesh erosion rate was significantly higher in those who underwent total vaginal hysterectomy (13/57, 22.8%) compared to laparoscopic supracervical hysterectomy (1/21, 4.8%) or no hysterectomy (5/110, 4.5%) [39]. Conversely, in a retrospective study of patients who underwent total versus supracervical robotic hysterectomy at the time of sacrocolpopexy, there was no difference in mesh erosion at one year after surgery (3/40, 7.5% versus 1/43, 2.3%, p=0.35) [40]. Similarly, in a retrospective study of patients who underwent hysterectomy at the time of laparoscopic sacrocolpopexy with follow up of 9–134 months, mesh erosion was found in 4/69 patients who had laparoscopic supracervical hysterectomy (6%), compared to 0/27 patients who underwent total laparoscopic or vaginal hysterectomy (p=0.22) [41]. Given the inconsistency in this data, the role that hysterectomy type plays in mesh exposure at the time of laparoscopic sacrocolpopexy is unclear, and performance of a total hysterectomy at the time of mesh placement may be considered. Long-term prospective studies are needed to address this issue.

Mesh Erosion with Synthetic versus Biologic Graft

The risk of mesh erosion when using synthetic versus biologic graft should also be considered. The risk of erosion of an allograft is extremely rare. Autografts and xenografts, however, do have a considerable risk of erosion, likely due to a negative host response. In a secondary analysis of the Colpopexy and Urinary Reduction Efforts prospective trial of open abdominal sacrocolpopexy using various mesh implants, Cundiff et al reported higher erosion rates when using expanded polytetrafluoroethylene (4/21, 19.0%, p=0.03) compared to 2/22 patients (9.1%) with porcine dermis, 10/134 patients (7.5%) with polyester, and 8/156 patients (5.1%) with polypropylene mesh. In a randomized controlled trial of polypropylene versus cadaveric fascia lata for abdominal sacrocolpopexy, Culligan et al reported no difference in mesh erosion at one year, with rates of 2/54 patients (3.7%) for polypropylene and 0/46 patients in the cadaveric fascia lata group [19]. In a retrospective study with mean follow-up of 13 months, Quiroz et al report higher erosion rates of porcine dermis (11/102, 10.8%) compared to synthetic mesh (4/134, 2.9%) or autologous fascia lata (1/23, 4.3%) (p=0.05) [42]. When considered together, this data suggests that there is no reduction in the risk of mesh erosion when using a biologic graft compared to a type I synthetic graft. It should be noted that innovation has improved the risk profile associated with type 1 mesh materials, as light-weight mesh is associated with significantly favourable biomechanical properties of the vagina compared to heavier type 1 mesh.

Mesh Infection

Whenever a foreign material is surgically implanted, the risk of infection must be considered. The incidence of reoperation for infected mesh after abdominal hernia repair is estimated to be around 1% [43]. When using mesh to augment POP repair, a unique risk factor for infection exists given the close proximity of the mesh material to the vagina and potentially direct exposure to vaginal flora. Perioperative administration of prophylactic antibiotics that target these bacteria is imperative when performing urogynaecologic surgery with mesh. The rate of mesh infection in vaginal POP surgery has been estimated to range from 0–8% [44,45]. Conversely, evidence of mesh infection after abdominal or laparoscopic POP surgery is limited to case reports. Thus, while the true incidence is unknown, it is assumed to be significantly lower in abdominal compared to vaginal surgery due to the fact that direct exposure to vaginal flora is significantly lower [46].

It should be noted that while clinical infection resulting in systemic symptoms and obvious need for mesh removal is rare, bacterial colonization of mesh is quite common, and occurs in the majority of patients undergoing vaginal mesh placement [47]. While it may not always be evident, it is hypothesized that subclinical infection may play a role in the host-response to mesh placement and lead to other mesh-related complications such as mesh erosion and chronic pain [48].

Chronic Pain and Sexual Dysfunction

Use of mesh in the surgical repair of pelvic floor disorders has been associated with the development of chronic pain, which can in turn develop into sexual dysfunction. Similar to the risk of infection, this is less likely with abdominal placement of mesh compared to vaginal placement. Geller et al reported on incidence of persistent pain one year after various POP surgeries augmented with synthetic mesh [49]. In this study, 10.3% of sacrocolpopexy patients had pain, compared to 17.6% of patients who underwent vaginal or rectal mesh placement for POP or a sling for urinary incontinence. In regards to dyspareunia as a specific cause of sexual dysfunction, a Cochrane review reported an increased risk with vaginal procedures for POP compared to sacrocolpopexy (RR 2.53, 95% CI 1.17 to 5.50) [50]. A separate systematic review and meta-analysis identified a similar trend of lower risk for dyspareunia in sacrocolpopexy patients compared to vaginal mesh patients (OR 0.44, 95% CI 0.23–0.88; P = 0.02) [51]. When comparing sacrocolpopexy to vaginal native tissue repairs over five comparative studies, Siddiqui et al report decreased risk of dyspareunia with sacrocolpopexy (OR 0.42, 95% CI 0.25–0.72), however this difference was no longer evident when including non-comparative data [52]. It is plausible that the risk of dyspareunia and chronic pain are less likely in laparoscopic or abdominal approaches due to limited contamination with vaginal bacterial flora, or it may simply be due to the increased distance between the mesh and vaginal epithelium and decreased risk of mesh erosion.

Bowel Dysfunction

Postoperative bowel dysfunction is a risk of laparoscopic urogynaecologic surgery, particularly with sacrocolpopexy [53]. Ganatra et al report an incidence of 9.8% of bowel dysfunction after sacrocolpopexy, including severe constipation and anal pain [46]. However, others, including Bradley et al, report an improvement in most bowel symptoms at one year after sacrocolpopexy [54]. Laparoscopic pectopexy has been suggested as an alternative abdominal approach to perform a mesh-augmented procedure for POP [55]. In this procedure, the mesh does not cross the rectum as it can in sacrocolpopexy, theoretically reducing the risk of de novo bowel symptoms. More prospective research thoroughly investigating the impact of various laparoscopic approaches to POP repair on bowel function is needed. In regards to short-term perioperative complications, abdominal prolapse surgery is associated with a significantly elevated risk of small bowel obstruction or ileus compared to vaginal surgery [52].

Bladder Symptoms

Surgery for POP is known to be a risk factor for the development of lower urinary tract symptoms and stress urinary incontinence [56]. In a review of nine studies of laparoscopic sacrocolpopexy, Ganatra et al report 17.8% incidence of postoperative stress urinary incontinence, urinary urgency, or urinary retention [46]. Maher et al report an increased risk of stress urinary incontinence after vaginal compared to abdominal POP surgery (RR 1.86, 95% CI 1.17–2.94), but no difference in rates of repeat surgery for stress urinary incontinence, de novo urge incontinence, or postoperative voiding dysfunction [50]. Siddiqui et al cite very low-quality evidence regarding functional bladder outcomes after mesh sacrocolpopexy versus native tissue vaginal prolapse repair, limiting the ability to make comparisons between procedures [52].

Weighing the Pros and Cons of Various Graft Materials

The risks and benefits of laparoscopic urogynaecologic surgery do vary depending on the mesh material that is used. In regards to the various types of synthetic mesh, the only widely accepted option is a type I, macroporous, light-weight polypropylene. Absorbable mesh has not shown the ability to convey the long-term strength to provide lasting results in abdominal prolapse surgery. Microporous mesh materials such as expanded polytrafluroethylene have been shown to be associated with a greater than four-fold increased risk of mesh erosion [21]. Polypopylene is associated with the best durability and lowest rate of complications amongst synthetic meshes. Additionally, newer lightweight polypropylene meshes convey even lower rates of mesh erosion with similar efficacy compared to heavier polypropylene materials [57].

When comparing synthetic mesh to biologic mesh, some data is conflicting. In regards to efficacy, the majority of studies support synthetic mesh to have lower rates of failure and reoperation for prolapse, with similar rates of mesh complications compared to biologic materials. A large retrospective review of over 14,000 prolapse surgeries with synthetic or biologic mesh reported higher rates of reoperation for recurrent POP with biologic mesh (3.6 versus 2.5%, p=0.01), but lower rates of reoperation for mesh-related complications (2.0% versus 3.0%, p=0.02), culminating in an equivalent overall risk of reoperation [58].

In regards to efficacy, multiple studies have reported significantly higher rates of prolapse recurrence after sacrocolpopexy with biologic graft materials, with the recurrence rates ranging from 21–38% for biologic grafts compared to 3–9% for synthetic mesh, with no significant differences in mesh-related complications [19,59–61]. In one prospective study of 22 patients with POP who were deemed to be high risk for graft-related complications, all were given biologic graft for sacrocolpopexy. Two years after surgery, 25% had experienced a graft-related complication and only 31% were considered to be anatomically cured [60]. Some studies have reported more optimistic outcomes following abdominal prolapse repair with biologic materials. For example, in a randomized controlled trial by Culligan et al, sacrocolpopexy with synthetic mesh compared to porcine dermis resulted in similar success rates (86.2% versus 80.7%, p=0.2), mesh complications, and rates of dyspareunia [33]. Similar results were seen in a study of synthetic mesh versus xenograft for sacrocolpopexy by Altman et al [62]. However, both of these studies had limited follow-up time of 12 months or shorter, potentially underestimating the risk of both mesh complication and prolapse recurrence.

Mesh-augmented Urogynaecologic Procedures

While the vast majority of data regarding mesh use in laparoscopic urogynaecologic surgery pertains to sacrocolpopexy as detailed extensively throughout this chapter, a number of other procedures should be mentioned. While procedural details are discussed thoroughly in other chapters, a brief review of these procedures follows below.

Sacrocolpoperineopexy

While a sacrocolpopexy traditionally involved attachment of mesh to the upper posterior vaginal wall, sacrocolpoperineopexy specifically involves attachment of the posterior arm distally to the perineal body, and thus is attached to the entire length of the posterior vaginal wall [63]. This technique has been proposed to be of benefit in patients with posterior compartment prolapse and those with symptoms of obstructed defaecation. Evidence regarding this procedure is limited. While it does improve posterior compartment prolapse, sacrocolpoperineopexy has not been shown to be beneficial in improving bowel symptoms [64,65]. Visco et al reported a 4.3% rate of mesh erosion following sacrocolpoperineopexy, compared to 3.2% with sacrocolpopexy [66].

Rectopexy

Vaginal prolapse often exists concomitantly with rectal prolapse, and combined surgical management is indicated. Just as surgical management of POP has multiple routes including vaginal, open, or laparoscopic, the surgical treatment of rectal prolapse can be perineal, open, or laparoscopic. A recent Cochrane review reported that evidence was insufficient to decipher a difference in efficacy between the perineal, abdominal, and laparoscopic approach to rectopexy [67]. However, multiple studies have shown the laparoscopic approach is associated with decreased complications, shorter recovery, and decreased cost compared to the analogous open procedure [67,68]. The laparoscopic approach entails mobilization of the rectum and securing it to the sacral promontory, typically either with suture material or mesh. When mesh is used, it is typically a lightweight, type I, macroporous mesh. In comparing mesh versus suture rectopexy, mesh rectopexy has been associated with better long-term functional outcomes, and a mesh-complication rate around 2% [69,70].

Sacrohysteropexy

Uterine preserving surgery for the treatment of apical pelvic organ prolapse is becoming increasingly common. Sacrohysteropexy represents an abdominal approach to hysteropexy with a potential increase in durability due to the utilization of mesh. In a systematic review of nine studies comparing mesh sacrohysteropexy versus hysterectomy and sacrocolpopexy, sacrohysteropexy was associated with lower blood loss, shorter operating time, less cost, and lower risk of mesh exposure (OR 0.16, 95% CI 0.03–0.97) [71]. There was no difference in resolution of prolapse symptoms (89% versus 88%, OR, 0.95; 95% CI, 0.86–1.03), or objective success, though data were heterogenous and limited for this outcome. Data regarding sacrohysteropexy versus vaginal native tissue repair is limited to two studies, one of which used a laparoscopic sacrohysteropexy technique and the other open. Sacrohysteropexy was superior in total vaginal length, C-point, blood loss, recovery time, and length of hospitalization. However, eight years after surgery, open sacrohysteropexy was associated with a similar rate of reoperation for POP 26% versus 14%, RR 1.83, 95% CI, 0.75–4.50, p=0.26) but worse symptoms related to mental health, health change, bodily pain, obstructive voiding, overactive bladder, and urinary pain [72]. In a recently completed randomized controlled trial of mesh sacrohysteropexy versus sacrospinous hysteropexy, there were no differences in success rates, while sacrohysteropexy was associated with more bothersome urinary and bowel symptoms, and sacrospinous hysteropexy was associated with higher rates of dyspareunia [73]. When all data is considered, long-term data is lacking, but hysteropexy offers a safe and efficacious surgical option for the treatment of POP, and laparoscopic sacrohysteropexy is a good option for any patient desiring a uterine-sparing, highly efficacious repair.

Pectopexy

Initially developed as a technique to treat POP in obese patients, pectopexy involves attaching two pieces of mesh between the vaginal apex and the bilateral pectineal ligaments [74]. In a randomized controlled trial between pectopexy versus sacrocolpopexy, pectopexy was associated with decreased de novo bowel symptoms, with similar anatomic results [75]. This procedure, while not universally adapted, is touted as a safe alternative to sacrocolpopexy when access to the sacral promontory is difficult, and eliminates the risks of presacral dissection including presacral haemorrhage or injury to the hypogastric plexus.

Lateral Suspension

The lateral suspension procedure provides another abdominal approach to repair apical or anterior pelvic organ prolapse with mesh. In this procedure, the vesicovaginal space is dissected, and mesh is attached between the anterior vaginal wall and an anchoring point on the anterior abdominal wall located posterior to the anterior superior iliac spine. This procedure may be performed after hysterectomy or as a uterine-sparing procedure. Prospective observation studies have identified this as another promising alternative to sacrocolpopexy as a mesh-augmented abdominal route to correct for anterior wall prolapse, with anatomic and subjective success rates greater than 80% and mesh erosion rates of less than 5% [76]. However, quality comparative trials comparing lateral suspension to alternative surgical techniques are lacking.

Colposuspension

Colposuspension is traditionally performed by using two to three non-absorbable stitches bilaterally to elevate the anterior vaginal wall at the level of the bladder neck to Coopers ligament as an anti-incontinence procedure. Alternatively, the procedure can be performed using two pieces of mesh with surgical staples. In a Cochrane review by Freites et al, colposuspension with mesh and staples did not differ compared to traditional suture technique in regards to subjective cure or rates of de novo detrusor overactivity, but may be associated with lower rates of perioperative complications [77].

Conclusion

In general, laparoscopic urogynaecologic surgery with mesh is safe, and may offer benefits when compared to native tissue repairs. Benefits in anatomical efficacy and symptom profiles must be weighed against potential risks associated with mesh use. Synthetic mesh likely provides a higher rate of long-term success in the repair of POP compared to the use of biologic grafting materials. Unlike transvaginal procedures, there does not seem to be a safety benefit to the use of biologic materials over type I synthetic mesh in laparoscopic urogynaecologic surgery when considering the outcomes of mesh erosion, infection, dyspareunia, or other potentially mesh-related complications. A light-weight, synthetic, type I mesh should be the first option in most cases of laparoscopic surgery for POP. However, the pros and cons of various mesh materials unique to the case at hand should be discussed and considered by the patient and their surgeon during a thorough, informed consent process.

References

1. Nygaard I, Barber MD, Burgio KL, et al. Prevalence of symptomatic pelvic floor disorders in US women. JAMA 2008; 300(11): 1311–16.
2. Wu JM, Matthews CA, Conover MM, et al. Lifetime risk of stress urinary incontinence or pelvic organ prolapse surgery. Obstet Gynecol 2014; 123(6): 1201–6.
3. Paraiso MF, Chen CCG. The use of biologic tissue and synthetic mesh in urogynecology and reconstructive pelvic surgery. In: MD Walters and M Karram (eds), *Urogynecology and Reconstructive Pelvic Surgery*. Saunders: 2014, pp. 411–27.
4. Maher C, Feiner B, Baessler K, et al. Transvaginal mesh or grafts compared with native tissue repair for vaginal prolapse. Cochrane Database Syst Rev 2016; 2(2): CD012079.
5. Lavelle ES, Giugale LE, Winger DG, et al. Prolapse recurrence following sacrocolpopexy vs uterosacral ligament suspension: a comparison stratified by Pelvic Organ Prolapse Quantification stage. Am J Obstet Gynecol 2018; 218(1): 116.e1–116.e5.
6. US Food and Drug Administration. Urogynecologic Surgical Mesh Implants. Available at: www.fda.gov/medical-devices/implants-and-prosthetics/urogynecologic-surgical-mesh-implants. Published 16 April 16, 2019.
7. National Institute for Health and Care Excellence. Transvaginal mesh repair of anterior or posterior vaginal wall prolapse. Interventional Procedures Guidance [IPG599]. Published 15 December, 2017.
8. Slopnick EA, Petrikovets A, Sheyn D, et al. Surgical trends and patient factors associated with the treatment of apical pelvic organ prolapse from a national sample. Int Urogynecol J 2019; 30(4): 603–9.
9. Serati M, Bogani G, Sorice P, et al. Robot-assisted sacrocolpopexy for pelvic organ prolapse: a systematic review and meta-analysis of comparative studies. Eur Urol 2014; 66(2): 303–18.
10. Stoppa R, Amid P, Bendavid R, et al. Hernia of the abdominal wall. In JP Chevrel (ed), *Hernias and Surgery of the Abdominal Wall*, 3rd edn. Springer-Verlag: 1998, pp 181–237.
11. Bendavid R. Foreword. In M Deysine (ed), *Hernia Infections*. Marcel Dekker; 2005, p iv. Taylor and Francis e-library.
12. Huguier J, Scali P. Posterior suspension of the genital axis on the lumbosacral disk in the treatment of uterine prolapse. Presse Med 1958; 66: 781–4.
13. Lane FE. Repair of posthysterectomy vaginal-vault prolapse. Obstet Gynecol 1962; 20: 72–7.
14. McDermott CD, Hale DS. Abdominal, laparoscopic, and robotic surgery for pelvic organ prolapse. Obstet Gynecol Clin North Am 2009; 36(3): 585–614.
15. Smart NJ, Bryan N, Hunt JA, Daniels IR. Porcine dermis implants in soft-tissue reconstruction: current status. Biologics 2014; 8: 83–90.
16. Paparella R, Marturano M, Pelino L, et al. Prospective randomized trial comparing synthetic vs. biological out-in transobturator tape: a mean 3-year follow-up study. Int Urogynecol J 2010; 21: 1327–36.
17. Arunkalaivanan AS, Barrington JW. Randomized trial of porcine dermal sling (Pelvicol implant) vs. tension-free vaginal tape (TVT) in the surgical treatment of stress incontinence: a questionnaire-based study. Int Urogynecol J 2003; 14: 17–23.
18. Amaro JL, Yamamoto H, Kawano PR, et al. Clinical and quality-of-life outcomes after autologous fascial sling and tension-free vaginal tape: a prospective randomized trial. International Braz J Urol 2009; 35: 60–7.
19. Culligan PJ, Blackwell L, Goldsmith LJ, et al. A randomized controlled trial comparing fascia lata and synthetic mesh for sacral colpopexy. Am J Obstet Gynecol 2005; 106: 29–37.
20. Deprest J, De Ridder D, Roovers JP, et al. Medium-term outcome of laparoscopic sacrocolpopexy with xenografts compared to synthetic grafts. J Urol 2009; 182: 2362–8.

21. Cundiff GW, Varner E, Visco A, et al. Risk factors of mesh/suture erosion following sacral colpopexy. Am J Obstet Gynecol 2008; 199: 688.e1–e5.
22. Walter AJ, Hentz JG, Magrina JF, Cornella JL. Harvesting autologous fascia lata for pelvic reconstructive surgery: techniques and morbidity. Am J Obstet Gynecol 2001; 185(6): 1354–459.
23. Fitzgerald MP, Mollenhauer J, Brubaker L. The antigenicity of fascia lata allografts. BJU Int 2000; 86(7): 826–8.
24. Dällenbach P. To mesh or not to mesh: a review of pelvic organ reconstructive surgery. Int J Womens Health 2015; 7: 331–43.
25. Choe JM, Bell T. Genetic material is present in cadaveric dermis and cadaveric fascia lata. J Urol 2001; 166(1): 122–4.
26. Cox A, Herschorn S. Evaluation of current biologic meshes in pelvic organ prolapse repair. Curr Urol Rep 2012; 13(3): 247–55.
27. Chen CC, Ridgeway B, Paraiso MF. Biologic grafts and synthetic meshes in pelvic reconstructive surgery. Clin Obstet Gynecol 2007; 50(2): 383–411.
28. Klinge U, Schumpelick V, Klosterhalfen B. Functional assessment and tissue response of short- and long-term absorbable surgical meshes. Biomaterials 2001; 22(11): 1415–24.
29. Barbolt TA. Biology of polypropylene/polyglactin 910 grafts. Int Urogynecol J Pelvic Floor Dysfunct 2006; 17(Suppl 1): S26–S30.
30. Falagas ME, Velakoulis S, Iavazzo C, Athanasiou S. Mesh-related infections after pelvic organ prolapse repair surgery. Eur J Obstet Gynecol Reprod Biol 2007; 134(2): 147.
31. Trabuco EC, Klingele CJ, Gebhart JB. Xenograft use in reconstructive pelvic surgery: a review of the literature. Int Urogynecol J Pelvic Floor Dysfunct 2007; 18(5): 555–63.
32. Cobb WS, Burns JM, Peindl RD, et al. Textile analysis of heavy weight, mid-weight, and light weight polypropylene mesh in a porcine ventral hernia model. J Surg Res 2006; 136(1): 1–7.
33. Culligan PJ, Salamon C, Priestley JL, Shariati A. Porcine dermis compared with polypropylene mesh for laparoscopic sacrocolpopexy: a randomized controlled trial. Obstet Gynecol 2013; 121(1): 143–51.
34. van Zanten F, van Iersel JJ, Paulides TJC, et al. Long-term mesh erosion rate following abdominal robotic reconstructive pelvic floor surgery: a prospective study and overview of the literature. Int Urogynecol J 2020; 31(7): 1423–33. https://doi.org/10.1007/s00192-019-03990-1
35. Coolen AWM, van Oudheusden AMJ, Mol BWJ, et al. Laparoscopic sacrocolpopexy compared with open abdominal sacrocolpopexy for vault prolapse repair: a randomised controlled trial. Int Urogynecol J 2017; 28(10): 1469–79.
36. Freeman RM, Pantazis K, Thomson A, et al. A randomised controlled trial of abdominal versus laparoscopic sacrocolpopexy for the treatment of post-hysterectomy vaginal vault prolapse: LAS study. Int Urogynecol J 2013; 24(3): 377–84.
37. Maher CF, Feiner B, DeCuyper EM, et al. Laparoscopic sacral colpopexy versus total vaginal mesh for vaginal vault prolapse: a randomized trial. Am J Obstet Gynecol 2011; 204(4): 360.e1–360.e3607.
38. Ross JW, Preston M. Laparoscopic sacrocolpopexy for severe vaginal vault prolapse: five-year outcome. J Minim Invasive Gynecol 2005; 12(3): 221–6.
39. Tan-Kim J, Menefee SA, Luber KM, et al. Prevalence and risk factors for mesh erosion after laparoscopic-assisted sacrocolpopexy. Int Urogynecol J 2011; 22(2): 205–12.
40. Myers EM, Siff L, Osmundsen B, et al. Differences in recurrent prolapse at 1 year after total vs supracervical hysterectomy and robotic sacrocolpopexy. Int Urogynecol J 2015; 26(4): 585–9.
41. Davidson ERW, Thomas TN, Lampert EJ, et al. Route of hysterectomy during minimally invasive sacrocolpopexy does not affect postoperative outcomes. Int Urogynecol J 2019; 30(4): 649–55.
42. Quiroz LH, Gutman RE, Shippey S, et al. Abdominal sacrocolpopexy: anatomic outcomes and complications with Pelvicol, autologous and synthetic graft materials. Am J Obstet Gynecol 2008; 198(5): 557.e1–557.e5575.
43. Kokotovic D, Bisgaard T, Helgstrand F. Long-term recurrence and complications associated with elective incisional hernia repair. JAMA 2016; 316(15): 1575–82.
44. Falagas ME, Velakoulis S, Iavazzo C, Athanasiou S. Mesh-related infections after pelvic organ prolapse repair surgery. Eur J Obstet Gynecol Reprod Biol 2007; 134(2): 147–56.
45. Glazener CM, Breeman S, Elders A, et al. Mesh, graft, or standard repair for women having primary transvaginal anterior or posterior compartment prolapse surgery: two parallel-group, multicentre, randomised, controlled trials (PROSPECT). Lancet 2017; 389(10067): 381–92.
46. Ganatra AM, Rozet F, Sanchez-Salas R, et al. The current status of laparoscopic sacrocolpopexy: a review. Eur Urol 2009; 55(5): 1089–103.
47. Vollebregt A, Troelstra A, van der Vaart CH. Bacterial colonisation of collagen-coated polypropylene vaginal mesh: are additional intraoperative sterility procedures useful? Int Urogynecol J Pelvic Floor Dysfunct 2009; 20(11): 1345–51.
48. Mangir N, Roman S, Chapple CR, MacNeil S. Complications related to use of mesh implants in surgical treatment of stress urinary incontinence and pelvic organ prolapse: infection or inflammation? World J Urol 2020; 38(1): 73–80. https://doi.org/10.1007/s00345-019-02679-w
49. Geller EJ, Babb E, Nackley AG, Zolnoun D. Incidence and risk factors for pelvic pain after mesh implant surgery for the treatment of pelvic floor disorders. J Minim Invasive Gynecol 2017; 24(1): 67–73.
50. Maher C, Feiner B, Baessler K, et al. Surgery for women with apical vaginal prolapse. Cochrane Database Syst Rev 2016; 10(10): CD012376.
51. Zhang CY, Sun ZJ, Yang J, et al. Sacrocolpopexy compared with transvaginal mesh surgery: a systematic review and meta-analysis. BJOG 2020; 10.1111/1471–0528.16324.
52. Siddiqui NY, Grimes CL, Casiano ER, et al. Mesh sacrocolpopexy compared with native tissue vaginal repair: a systematic review and meta-analysis. Obstet Gynecol 2015; 125(1): 44–55.
53. Antiphon P, Elard S, Benyoussef A, et al. Laparoscopic promontory sacral colpopexy: is the posterior, recto-vaginal, mesh mandatory? Eur Urol 2004; 45(5): 655–61.
54. Bradley CS, Nygaard IE, Brown MB, et al. Bowel symptoms in women 1 year after sacrocolpopexy. Am J Obstet Gynecol 2007; 197(6): 642.e1–642.e6428.
55. Biler A, Ertas IE, Tosun G, et al. Perioperative complications and short-term outcomes of abdominal sacrocolpopexy, laparoscopic sacrocolpopexy, and laparoscopic pectopexy for apical prolapse. Int Braz J Urol 2018; 44(5): 996–1004.
56. Brubaker L, Cundiff G, Fine P, et al. Pelvic Floor Disorders Network. A randomized trial of colpopexy and urinary reduction efforts (CARE): design and methods. Control Clin Trials. 2003; 24(5): 629–42.
57. Kenton K, Mueller ER, Tarney C, et al. One-year outcomes after minimally invasive sacrocolpopexy. Female Pelvic Med Reconstr Surg 2016; 22(5): 382–4.

58. Sohlberg EM, Dallas KB, Weeks BT, et al. Reoperation rates for pelvic organ prolapse repairs with biologic and synthetic grafts in a large population-based cohort. Int Urogynecol J 2020; 31(2): 291–301.
59. Deprest J, De Ridder D, Roovers JP, et al. Medium term outcome of laparoscopic sacrocolpopexy with xenografts compared to synthetic grafts. J Urol 2009; 182(5): 2362–8.
60. Claerhout F, De Ridder D, Van Beckevoort D, et al. Sacrocolpopexy using xenogenic acellular collagen in patients at increased risk for graft-related complications. Neurourol Urodyn 2010; 29(4): 563–7.
61. Tate SB, Blackwell L, Lorenz DJ, et al. Randomized trial of fascia lata and polypropylene mesh for abdominal sacrocolpopexy: 5-year follow-up. Int Urogynecol J 2011; 22(2): 137–43.
62. Altman D, Anzen B, Brismar S, Lopez A, Zetterström J. Long-term outcome of abdominal sacrocolpopexy using xenograft compared with synthetic mesh. Urology 2006; 67(4): 719–24.
63. Reddy J, Ridgeway B, Gurland B, Paraiso MF. Robotic sacrocolpoperineopexy with ventral rectopexy for the combined treatment of rectal and pelvic organ prolapse: initial report and technique. J Robot Surg 2011; 5(3): 167–73.
64. Ramanah R, Ballester M, Chereau E, et al. Anorectal symptoms before and after laparoscopic sacrocolpoperineopexy for pelvic organ prolapse. Int Urogynecol J 2012; 23(6): 779–83.
65. Grimes CL, Schimpf MO, Wieslander CK, et al. Surgical interventions for posterior compartment prolapse and obstructed defecation symptoms: a systematic review with clinical practice recommendations. Int Urogynecol J 2019; 30(9): 1433–54.
66. Visco AG, Weidner A, Barber MD, et al. Vaginal mesh erosion after abdominal sacral colpopexy. Am J Obstet Gynecol 2001; 194: 297.
67. Tou S, Brown SR, Nelson RL. Surgery for complete (full-thickness) rectal prolapse in adults. Cochrane Database Syst Rev 2015; 2015(11): CD001758.
68. Wallace SL, Syan R, Sokol ER. Surgery for apical vaginal prolapse after hysterectomy: transvaginal mesh-based repair. Urol Clin North Am 2019; 46(1): 103–11.
69. Hidaka J, Elfeki H, Duelund-Jakobsen J, et al. Functional outcome after laparoscopic posterior sutured rectopexy versus ventral mesh rectopexy for rectal prolapse: six-year follow-up of a double-blind, randomized single-center study. EClinicalMedicine 2019; 16: 18–22.
70. Evans C, Stevenson ARL, Sileri P, et al. A multicenter collaboration to assess the safety of laparoscopic ventral rectopexy. Dis Colon Rectum 2015; 58(8): 799–807.
71. Meriwether KV, Antosh DD, Olivera CK, et al. Uterine preservation vs hysterectomy in pelvic organ prolapse surgery: a systematic review with meta-analysis and clinical practice guidelines. Am J Obstet Gynecol 2018; 219(2): 129–46.e2.
72. Roovers JP, van der Vaart CH, van der Bom JG, et al. A randomised controlled trial comparing abdominal and vaginal prolapse surgery: effects on urogenital function. BJOG 2004; 111: 50–6.
73. van IJsselmuiden MN, van Oudheusden A, Veen J, et al. Hysteropexy in the treatment of uterine prolapse stage 2 or higher: laparoscopic sacrohysteropexy versus sacrospinous hysteropexy - a multicentre randomised controlled trial (LAVA trial). BJOG 2020 ;127(10): 1284–93.
74. Banerjee C, Noe KG. Laparoscopic pectopexy: a new technique of prolapse surgery for obese patients. Arch Gynecol Obstet 2011; 284: 631–5.
75. Noé KG, Schiermeier S, Alkatout I, Anapolski M. Laparoscopic pectopexy: a prospective, randomized, comparative clinical trial of standard laparoscopic sacral colpocervicopexy with the new laparoscopic pectopexy - postoperative results and intermediate-term follow-up in a pilot study. J Endourol 2015; 29(2): 210–15.
76. Veit-Rubin N, Dubuisson JB, Gayet-Ageron A, et al. Patient satisfaction after laparoscopic lateral suspension with mesh for pelvic organ prolapse: outcome report of a continuous series of 417 patients. Int Urogynecol J 2017; 28(11): 1685–93.
77. Freites J, Stewart F, Omar MI,. Laparoscopic colposuspension for urinary incontinence in women. Cochrane Database Syst Rev 2019; 12(12): CD002239.

Chapter

10

Medicolegal Issues in Laparoscopic Urogynaecology

Swati Jha

Introduction and Background

Medicine is an inaccurate science and errors leading to adverse events will occasionally occur. When patients come to harm due to avoidable errors which impacts on their life, adequate support through compensation pay-outs allows them to resume life at the standards to which they are accustomed. To bring a successful claim it must first be proven that there was a duty of care owed to the patient. In clinical negligence claims this is usually a given. It must then be proven that there has been a breach in that duty of care. And lastly it must be shown that there is a causality which means that the injury occurred as a result of the breach. There is usually a limitation period in bringing a claim. This is three years from the injury or three years from the date of recognition that an injury has ensued. The exceptions to the limitation period include negligence claims made by children and those with mental health conditions which affect capacity but is not relevant to thearea of practice being discussed here.

Litigation in urogynaecology has skyrocketed in the past decade. This is in keeping with litigation in other areas of obstetrics and gynaecology and has been further fuelled by the mesh controversy in recent years. In the UK in 2019–2020 there were 433 claims in gynaecology alone and a total payment in excess of £52 million for this period. Gynaecology claims [1] accounted for 7% of the total number of claims, and 3% of the pay-outs (see Figures 10.1 and 10.2). In the annual report from NHS Resolutions [1,2] for 2019/2020, it was noted that compared to 2018/2019 there was an overall increase of 404 reported incidents by Trusts in clinical negligence schemes for all specialties. Incidents reported in the gynaecology specialty accounted for 208 of the 404 incidents reported, an increase of 145% compared to 2018/2019. This increase is due to a large number of vaginal-mesh-related incidents being reported. These claims are related to tension-free vaginal tape, transobturator tape or vaginal mesh to treat symptoms of stress urinary incontinence or pelvic organ prolapse, and allegations tend to centre around (but not exclusively) failure to obtain adequate consent (e.g. failure to warn of risks of procedures or failure to offer alternative treatment) and/or substandard performance of surgery. In this same time period, the number of cases settled out of court was 71%, with 28.4% settled after commencement of court proceedings and only 0.6% reaching trial.

Lawsuits in the UK are increasingly becoming common. Two decades ago, this was viewed as more of a US problem, and the UK as a country from which lessons could be learnt. A big difference between the UK legal system compared to the US is that judges rather than juries decide medical malpractice suits including the pay-outs. Judges tend to be more objective, and it was believed this was one of the reasons why the size of the pay-outs were less. This trend appears to be changing quite dramatically.

Several factors are responsible for rising pay-outs in the NHS.

i) ***No win no fee***: Until 1998, the UK courts had a 'loser pays' policy which meant that the loser paid the legal costs of the winning party. The advantage was that baseless claims did not progress and frivolous lawsuits were avoided. However, with the introduction of the 'no win no fee' arrangements, given claimants only pay the attorney if they win the case, sometimes meritless lawsuits are initiated. It was found that up to 30% of outstanding claims against the NHS comprised such lawsuits. To protect attorneys, claimants are required to take out an insurance which covers

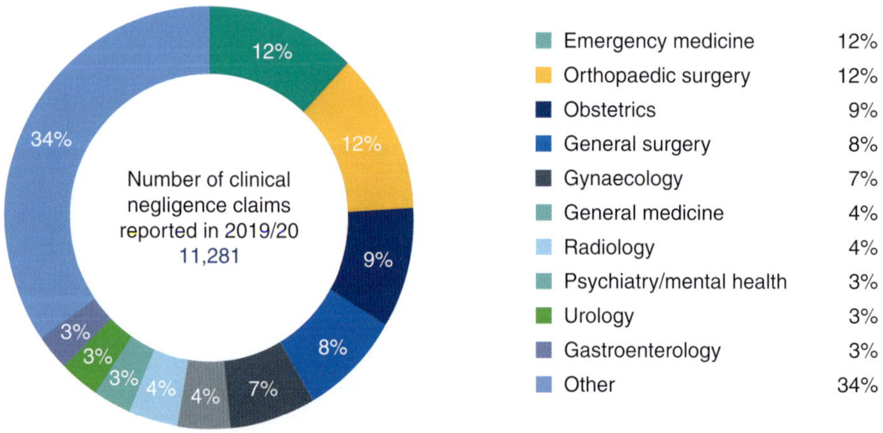

Figure 10.1 Number of claims reported in 2019/2020 by specialty from a total of 11,281.

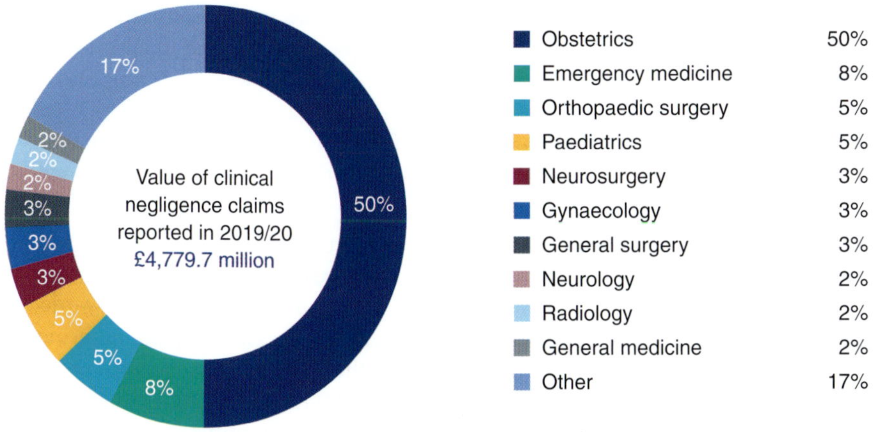

Figure 10.2 Value of claims by specialty across all clinical negligence schemes from a total of £4,779.7 million.

the legal fees should they lose. In many cases, however, the costs involved in going to trial are actually more than the actual pay-out would have been and for this reason, a vast majority of the cases are settled before going to court. For these reasons the 'no win, no fee' has actually encouraged solicitors to take on cases that were not a sure win.

ii) ***Maternity lawsuits***: Millions are paid out for cases involving babies who have suffered hypoxic ischaemic encephalopathy (HIE) due to mismanaged labour and delivery. Maternity pay-outs account for half of all NHS pay outs.

iii) ***Increasing cost of legal fees***: The amount paid to cover court costs and expert witnesses is gradually increasing.

iv) ***Reduction in the discount rate***: When claimants of serious harm are paid a lump sum, the actual amount they receive is adjusted according to the interest they are likely to receive if they invest the compensation given. The discount rate used to be 2.5%, but was reduced to minus 0.75% in 2017. This has resulted in compensation pay-outs increasing to the tune of £1.2 billion each year, with its obvious knock-on effect.

v) ***Unpredictable size of the pay-outs:*** There is a large degree of uncertainty about the size of an award, making it difficult to settle cases and resulting in extended disputes. It has been noted that the number of claims made remains constant, but due to increasing value of pay-outs, the total amount paid out is increasing year on year [3].

Broadly speaking, four main reasons for litigation have been identified and include:

- Concerns with standards of care and the desire to prevent similar problems occurring in future
- The need for an explanation to understand why a particular problem occurred
- Accountability and the need to hold someone responsible
- Desire for compensation for losses incurred as well as the pain and suffering that has ensued as a result of the injury arising from the treatment.

Litigation in the realm of laparoscopic urogynaecology is not unique and relates to the usual causes of litigation in urogynaecology practice, laparoscopic surgery, as well as the issues relating to the use of synthetic mesh.

Stages in Litigation

A claim goes through various stages before reaching court. Resolving claims is preferred to a trial as both claimants and defendants are spared the distress and cost of a trial, funders and insurers know their expenses for the case early in the process, pay-outs occur more promptly, and valuable court time is spared. Most cases are settled out of court without an acknowledgement of negligence for these reasons, with only 1–2% actually reaching the trial phase. If a case goes to trial for breach of duty, clinicians should have the satisfaction that there was significant dispute as to whether there was negligence, with a 50/50 chance of the case going either way. In some cases, breach of duty (liability) is admitted early, and the court case is simply to determine the value of the claim (quantum).

A claim goes through various stages before reaching trial but can be settled at any stage along this journey, including the pre-action stage. The various stages of a claim include the steps that lead to the trial (pre-trial) and the stages of the trial itself. These include the following:

Pre-trial

i) ***Letter before action:*** One early indicator that a patient is considering legal action is a complaint to the hospital where the injury occurred. However, this is not always the case and sometimes the first indicator that a claim is on its way is a letter from the patient's solicitors. This will usually give a summary of the allegations and be accompanied by a signed consent from the patient requesting all medical records relating to the patient. A response is usually required within four weeks.

ii) ***Letter of claim:*** It is usually many months after the initial letter that a letter of claim is actually sent. This is because the claimant's lawyers will sometimes feel there is no merit in the case. Many cases will proceed no further. If, however, the claimants solicitors feel there is a case to be made based on expert opinion obtained, they will send a letter of claim. The letter of claim will lay out the case summary, allegation, injury sustained as a result of the negligence, and the financial losses sustained as a result of the negligence. The receipt of the letter of claim has to be acknowledged within 14 days and a full response provided in four months.

iii) ***The response:*** Following receipt of the letter of claim, the response could be to deny the claim in its entirety, admit part or all of the claim, or make an offer to settle the claim. Clinicians are often keen to defend their stance but for the reasons alluded to earlier may be encouraged to settle to avoid costs from rising.

iv) ***Formal proceedings commence:*** If the claim cannot be resolved informally, then legal proceedings are initiated, and the court then serves a claim. The particulars of the claim, which includes a condition and prognosis report detailing the pain and suffering endured due to the injury, as well as past and future loss of earnings, accompanies the claim or follows within 14 days. Once the defense organization for the defendant is informed of the claim, a solicitor will be assigned the case to work on.

v) ***Track allocation:*** The case is allocated to one of three possible routes depending on its value and complexity, which include small claims, a fast-track, or a multi-track. Most clinical negligence cases are assigned to multi-track. Once allocated, the case has to stick to a strict schedule. The judge responsible for the case ensures the issues are narrowed down and looks at alternative ways of settling the case out of court.

vi) ***Witness statement:*** In response to the letter of claim, the clinician prepares a witness statement. This is prepared by the solicitors with detailed instruction from the defendant. A statement of truth forms part of this document.

vii) ***Exchange of witness statements:*** In preparing a report, an expert's duty is to the court, hence should be an unbiased opinion on the facts of the case. The reports of the experts for both the claimant and defendant are exchanged. Experts may also meet to narrow down the issues for discussion. Claimants may sometimes drop their case at this phase or settlements may be sought by defendants based on the expert statements.

Trial

It will usually be several years from the start of a claim to the point where it reaches court. The vast majority are settled before they reach trial.

i) ***The media:*** High profile cases will generate media attention. It is important to be able to interact with the media in a professional way. The patient's confidentiality must be maintained at all times.

ii) ***Court proceedings***: In a court proceeding, a claimant's account of a consultation will often carry more weight than a doctor's description of their usual practice, hence the importance of documenting clearly and comprehensively in the medical records. The claimant's barrister is heard first and will call witnesses for examination and ask questions based on their witness statement. This is followed by cross-examinations by the claimant's barrister. The same format is then followed by the defendant's barrister, with examination and cross-examination of witnesses. A closing statement is made by both barristers before the judge considers their decision.

iii) ***Judgement:*** This can take a week to six months to be issued, based on the complexity of the case. It takes into account whether the care provided was in keeping with what would be expected of a reasonable body of clinicians of similar standing; if the cause of the harm was actually the negligence alleged; and the claimant's condition and prognosis.

iv) ***Damages:*** The award of compensation is aimed at allowing the claimant to return to the state they would have been in had the negligence not occurred. Damages are awarded in two categories; general damages for the pain, suffering and loss of amenity, but the financial consequences of the injury is usually much higher and includes loss of earnings, pensions, cost of adaptations in the home and any equipment required.

The final sum awarded is through negotiation, and the losing party pays the cost of fees for both sides.

v) ***Appeals:*** To appeal a judgement requires the permission of the court. This is usually within 21 days of the judgement with a written request seeking permission from court.

Mediation

Mediation is used in all cases as a forum for resolution of claims. It provides patients who have been injured an opportunity to articulate concerns that may not otherwise be addressed in alternative dispute resolution. It allows patients and families to be given a face-to-face explanation and apology, while understanding and responding to patients concerns. A majority of cases that go to mediation are settled on the day or within 28 days [4]. Mediation allows patient concerns to be placed at the heart of the claim and shifts the focus away from compensation as the sole driver.

Causes for Litigation in Laparoscopic Urogynaecology

The reasons for litigation related to laparoscopic urogynaecology can be broadly grouped into the following:

Communication including Consent

When reviewing a patient with pelvic floor problems, a detailed assessment of all symptoms should be made. Quality-of-life questionnaires should be used. Asymptomatic prolapse identified during the course of an examination for other gynaecological problems does not warrant invasive treatments. Often simple reassurance that vaginal laxity is found in up to 50% [5,6] of women who have had vaginal deliveries will sufficiently allay anxieties. There are few specific investigations required for women with POP. Urodynamics is usually only advised if women have concurrent urinary incontinence [7] and this is their presenting, most bothersome complaint. In women with an enlarged uterus or adnexal masses, an ultrasound scan should be considered to assist in planning treatment and the options.

Conservative options should always be offered before considering surgery. Increasingly, a common cause for litigation centres around consent and failing to offer alternatives to surgery, including doing pelvic floor muscle training and the option of doing nothing. POP is rarely dangerous, particularly when it is stage 1 or 2, and therefore the mere diagnosis should not equate to treatment. Lifestyle advice including losing weight, avoidance of activities that worsen pelvic floor problems such as lifting weights, and advice regarding management of constipation should be given. Women with a high BMI may not be well suited to a laparoscopic urogynaecology procedure and as surgeons we will have a cut-off above which we will be uncomfortable performing a laparoscopic procedure.

In women who have not completed their families, surgery should be advised against and deferred till after childbearing is complete. Women wishing to proceed should be informed that further childbearing carries the risk of requiring a caesarean for delivery as well as recurrence of pelvic floor problems.

When a decision has been made to proceed to surgical correction, patient decision aids should be used in reaching a decision about the most appropriate type of surgery [8]. Most laparoscopic urogynaecology procedures have the option of vaginal or open procedures and these should be discussed in detail when offering a laparoscopic urogynaecology procedure and most mesh procedures have a non-mesh alternative.

Women should be assessed for suitability for a laparoscopic procedure, including suitability for general anaesthetic, pneumoperitoneum, and Trendelenburg position. Poor patient selection can result in a claim of negligence. For example, women with multiple laparotomies are high risk for laparoscopic procedures. The pros and cons of open versus laparoscopic procedures should be weighed and cases discussed at an MDT prior to proceeding with surgery.

In addition, all material risks of the procedure should be discussed. The material risk refers to risks a patient would attribute significance to rather than those a doctor perceives are significant. The RCOG provides guidance on how risk should be discussed in a healthcare setting [9]. In the context of laparoscopic urogynaecology, women should be informed of the risks and potential complications associated with laparoscopy. This includes a discussion of the entry technique used, specifically injury to the bowel, blood vessels, and urinary tract. Port site hernias can develop in later years. All patients should be informed of the risk of needing a laparotomy when any laparoscopic procedure is undertaken. There are increased risks of surgery in women who are overweight and who have had previous surgery or inflammatory bowel disease. It is important to bear in mind that these procedures are undertaken for conditions that impact on quality of life rather than as a lifesaving procedure, hence a woman's acceptance of risk may be different to a woman undergoing surgery for cancer/precancer.

The burden of proof in cases relating to consent is no longer the Bolam [10] test, which has been superseded by the Montgomery [11]. Further details of counselling and principles of consent are described in Chapter 2.

Treatment Complications

Claims arising from the surgical aspect of laparoscopic urogynaecology procedures may be related to a variety of different issues. It is important to be able to justify that the decision to perform a procedure laparoscopically was well considered and the surgeon had the appropriate skill sets to undertake this procedure. An allegation of the wrong choice of surgery can arise when a case is performed laparoscopically which would have been better performed as a laparotomy and complications arose as a result.

The commonest cause of litigation related to laparoscopic urogynaecology is internal injury or a delay in recognition of these complications. The initial laparoscopic entry into the peritoneal cavity is the major contributor to bowel injury and delayed recognition is a major factor in assessment of negligence. If the patient's medical records do not document that they have been closely monitored and deterioration in their condition managed in a timely and appropriate fashion, these cases can be difficult to defend. The need to proceed to a laparotomy, particularly a midline incision as opposed to a transverse incision to manage the bowel injury, also increases the risks of litigation. Whereas following a laparotomy, patients should be seen to improve on a daily basis, in laparoscopic surgery they should be improving on an hourly basis. Failure to see progressive improvement should raise concerns postoperatively.

There is no consensus on the safest entry technique. The closed technique using a Veress needle has been the preferred technique but increasingly direct entry using a Visiport is being used. The use of direct trocar entry reduces the risk of failed entry compared to the use of a Veress entry. The Hassan's technique, or the open technique, has been the method of choice by general surgeons. The advantage of the Hassan's technique over the Veress entry is that it is less likely to cause major blood vessel injury and when a bowel injury occurs it is more likely to be recognized. It does not however reduce the incidence of the bowel injury from occurring, and a meta-nalysis of the various techniques failed to show a superiority of any one technique in reducing the risk of injury [12]. Basic principles of any laparoscopic procedure should be adhered to including [13]:

- The primary umbilical incision should be vertical from the base of the umbilicus rather than below the umbilicus.
- The operating table should be horizontal at the start of the procedure.
- When using a Veress needle this should be tested to ensure the spring action is working. The needle should be inserted at right angles to the abdomen and two audible clicks heard during the entry as it penetrates the fascia and the peritoneum.
- An intra-abdominal pressure of 20–25 mm Hg should be achieved for insertion of the primary trocar. The primary trocar is inserted at a 90-degree angle and a 360-degree check performed once the laparoscope has been inserted to inspect for any bowel injury. All secondary trocars should be inserted under direct vision. If there is a concern regarding bowel injury, the umbilical port can be inspected using a 5 mm laparoscope down one of the secondary ports. Once the ports are inserted the pressure should be dropped to 12–15 mm Hg.
- Best possible vision should be maintained at all times.

- The use of sharp instruments should be avoided unless absolutely necessary.
- The use of diathermy, or ultrasonic devices, requires knowledge of their use and utmost care. The tip of the instrument may remain hot even if the power has been switched off.
- On completion of the procedure and when removing trocars, check all areas where possible injury to tissue or bleeding may have occurred.
- All trocar sites should be inspected after withdrawal by lightly placing a finger over the skin wound at the time so that any bleeding will run into the abdominal cavity and be identified.

The choice of sutures should be considered carefully. If using non-dissolvable sutures as for laparoscopic colposuspension or sacrohysteropexy, patients should be informed of this. Many surgeons will give patients the choice of dissolvable or non-dissolvable sutures when performing a laparoscopic colposuspension. The performance of all the laparoscopic urogynaecology procedures requires an understanding of the anatomy to ensure safe dissection.

When complications arise during surgery, involving other specialists is good practice.

Management of patient expectations helps ensure that they are satisfied with their care and there is early recognition of warning signs of complications post-surgery.

Patients should be given appropriate contact details and instructed to contact the hospital if problems occur postoperatively.

Medical Device Problems

Increasingly, litigation related to urogynaecology cases is centred on the use of meshes and related complications. Following the Class action against Johnson and Johnson vaginal mesh kits in the US, J and J publicly declared their decision to withdraw their vaginal meshes by the first quarter of 2013, and this was followed by a sharp decline in the use of vaginal meshes elsewhere, including the UK. These scares have made patients reluctant to have other procedures that involve the use of synthetic mesh, which has resulted in a decline in laparoscopic urogynaecology procedures that use a synthetic mesh. NICE recommend that when meshes and non-dissolvable stitches are used, patients should be given written information about these for their own records.

When a synthetic mesh is used in a procedure this should be a type 1, polypropylene macroporous mesh. Patients should be adequately counselled when using a mesh about the risks specific to a mesh, as this has been one of the principal reasons for litigation. Using a mesh carries the risk of mesh exposure and extrusion due to mesh migration, and this would inevitably result in the need for further surgery. Extrusion of mesh into adjacent viscera has the added risk of requiring major surgery in future, which is a risk inherent to the use of mesh. All procedures that involve the use of a mesh have alternatives that do not involve a mesh, and this should be discussed and patients given sufficient time to consider options before proceeding to a mesh procedure.

Failing to Meet Governance Requirements

NICE have issued guidance relating to the performance of several of these procedures [14,15] and this should be adhered to when offering these procedures. Clinicians undertaking laparoscopic urogynaecology procedures for the treatment of pelvic organ problems should familiarize themselves with NICE guidance on these procedures. Surgeons should be adequately trained and audit their outcomes. They should be familiar with the equipment, instrumentation, and energy devices being used and should have adequately trained assistants. They should have authorization to undertake this work by the hospital they are working at and patients should be managed within a multidisciplinary setting. All patients should be discussed at an MDT. Continuing professional development to maintain skills should be undertaken. There is a requirement to demonstrate through the annual appraisal process that adequate caseload is being maintained. In the UK, there is also a requirement to enter details of procedures that involve the use of a device on a national database or registry and to report all complications related to the device to the Medicines and Health Regulatory Authority (MHRA).

It would also be an expectation that women undergoing laparoscopic urogynaecology procedures have patient reported outcomes (PROMs) collected before and after surgery.

Avoidance of Litigation

The basic principles of avoiding litigation include:

a. ***Good documentation***: The old saying 'If it's not in the record, it didn't happen' still holds true. Good record keeping includes:
   - information provided by the patient that factored into the diagnoses or treatment decisions
   - the physical findings that guided decisions
   - the options discussed and the pros and cons of each
   - the patient information leaflets/PDA provided in reaching a decision
   - the treatment selected.

   Due to the restraints on time, sometimes making such detailed documentation can be difficult.
b. ***Good communication***: Good communication with the patient and valid informed consent is the cornerstone of all surgical treatment. Informed consent is a dialogue and should be viewed as a process which culminates in the signature on the consent form. It requires physicians to discuss:
   - risks of the treatment
   - benefits of the treatment
   - alternatives to the treatment, including doing nothing, as well as pros and cons of the individual treatment options. Any risks associated with serious long-term sequelae must be discussed, even if the probability of the risk occurring is remote, particularly if the patient is likely to attach significance to this risk.
c. ***Training and CPD***: It is imperative that clinicians undertake adequate training before performing procedures

independently. Laparoscopic urogynaecology procedures are inherently complex and require advanced surgical skills which can only be acquired with due diligence and training. Clinicians must not misrepresent their experience. A doctor's greatest asset is their advanced training and experience, but it is important to work and operate within the remit of their expertise. Newly appointed consultants can be particularly vulnerable and should be willing to call for assistance. It is also important to give patients realistic expectations about their outcomes and providing outcomes based on one's own performance can be helpful, which is only possible if this is collected as a matter of routine.

d. ***Discharge instructions:*** Increasingly, procedures are being performed as very short hospital stays and inpatient stay is relatively short. Discharge instructions should therefore address all areas of potential concern, including pain, wound care, and signs of infection. There should also be information regarding whom to contact if there is a change in condition or if there are any further questions.

e. ***Saying Sorry:*** Doctors are human and errors will sometimes happen. Acknowledging responsibility does not equate to accepting negligence but rather an acceptance that a complication has occurred [16]. It may be prudent to consider referral to a different clinician when a complication occurs as there can be a breakdown of trust. The vast majority of patients just want two things when things go wrong: an explanation and an apology.

   The Francis report, in keeping with the Duty of Candour, states 'Every healthcare organization and everyone working for them must be honest, open and truthful in all their dealings with patients and the public, and organizational and personal interests must never be allowed to outweigh the duty to be honest, open and truthful.'

f. ***Integrity:*** Physicians are expected to act with integrity and higher standards of conduct are placed on the medical profession. A physician should not allow their own interests to influence a patient's treatment. This is particularly true when cases are undertaken in the independent sector and practice in the private sector should mimic that in the public sector.

Ethical Issues

The effect of litigation on the healthcare professional is often underestimated. Studies have shown that a malpractice suit can have the same impact as a major illness, loss of a loved one, or a severe career setback [17]. In fact, the emotional impact involves the same stages as grief and have been described by Kubler-Ross. Facing a negligence claim can cause headache, insomnia, lack of concentration, irritability, depression insomnia, and even suicidal thoughts.

Increasingly, litigation in obstetrics and gynaecology impacts on junior doctors wanting to join the specialty with increasing reluctance, given rising costs of litigation [18,19]. It has also had an impact on practice, which results in clinicians practising defensive medicine [20]. Often unnecessary tests and investigations are performed which can sometimes be invasive and also drive up the cost of healthcare [21].

Medical Indemnity

Urogynaecologists' working on the NHS receive indemnity from NHS Resolution through the Clinical Negligence Scheme for Trusts (CNST). However, this does not cover cases reaching Coroners court or GMC proceedings, so all active clinicians should still have defence cover. Clinicians undertaking private work in the independent sector should have additional insurance through defence organizations such as the Medical Defence Union (MDU) or Medical Protection Society (MPS), though there are now a large number of other organizations that provide this cover. Clinicians undertaking mesh-related work on the public sector should have authorization to do so from their Hospital Executive board and in the private sector need to inform their insurers of this and ensure their medical indemnity covers this work, given the rising cost of litigation related to the nature of this work.

Conclusion

Increasing litigation costs in a publicly funded healthcare system means that funds which would otherwise be used to improve the health of the nation are diverted to paying compensation. In the UK this is fast reaching a point where pay-outs may well become unsustainable.

The fear of litigation also affects clinical practice, resulting in defensive medicine with unnecessary investigations being ordered, increasing secondary care referrals being made, and heightened levels of stress and anxiety. There has been no evidence to show that the quality of clinical care has changed or professional standards have altered and this makes it difficult to prevent. However, a better understanding of clinical negligence drivers and specific risks surrounding scenarios that result in large pay-outs, improving education of risk management, improving the culture and systems of dealing with concerns, and establishing realistic expectations of what the healthcare system can deliver, may go some way to reducing the spiralling costs of litigation.

References

1. NHS Resolution. Annual report and accounts 2019–20. Published 2020.
2. NHS Resolution. Annual report and accounts 2018–19. Published 2020.
3. Lacobucci G. Clinical negligence: NHS paid out £2.4bn last year. BMJ 2019; 366: 14688.
4. NHS Resolution. Mediation in healthcare claims: an evaluation. Published 2020.
5. Haya N, Feiner B, Baessler K, Christmann-Schmid C, Maher C. Perioperative interventions in pelvic organ prolapse surgery. Cochrane Database Syst Rev 2018; 8: CD013105.
6. Maher C, Feiner B, Baessler K, Schmid C. Surgical management of pelvic organ prolapse in women. Cochrane Database Syst Rev 2013; 4: CD004014.
7. National Institute for Health and Care Excellence. NICE Guideline NG123. Urinary incontinence and pelvic organ prolapse in women: management. Published 2019.
8. National Institute for Health and Care Excellence. NICE Clinical Guideline CG123. Urinary incontinence and pelvic organ prolapse in women: management. Published 2019.

9. Royal College of Obstetricians and Gynaecologists. Understanding how risk is discussed in healthcare. Published 2015.
10. Bolam v Friern Hospital Management Committee. 1957.
11. Montgomery v Lanarkshire Health Board. 2015.
12. Ahmad G, Baker J, Finnerty J, Phillips K, Watson A. Laparoscopic entry techniques. Cochrane Database Syst Rev 2019; 1: CD006583.
13. Royal College of Obstetricians and Gynaecologists. Preventing entry-related gynaecological laparoscopic injuries. Published 2020.
14. National Institute for Health and Care Excellence. NICE IPG583. Sacrocolpopexy using mesh to repair vaginal vault prolapse. Published 2017.
15. National Institute for Health and Care Excellence. NICE IPG584. Uterine suspension using mesh (including sacrohysteropexy) to repair uterine prolapse. Published 2017.
16. Robbennolt JK. Apologies and medical error. Clin Orthop Relat Res 2009; 467(2): 376–82.
17. Kerr CD. The personal cost of medical litigation. Med J Aust 2004; 181(7): 384–5.
18. Barber HR. The malpractice crisis in obstetrics and gynecology: is there a solution? Bull N Y Acad Med 1991; 67(2): 162–72.
19. MacLennan A, Nelson KB, Hankins G, Speer M. Who will deliver our grandchildren? Implications of cerebral palsy litigation. JAMA 2005; 294(13): 1688–90.
20. Medical Protection Society (MPS) (South Africa). 'On the defensive': case book series (January) 2011; 19(1).
21. Bishop TF, Federman AD, Keyhani S. Physicians' views on defensive medicine: a national survey. Arch Intern Med 2010; 170(12): 1081–3.

Chapter 11

Total and Supracervical Laparoscopic Hysterectomy at Sacrocolpopexy: Procedure Steps and Evidence

Tsung Mou, Kimberly Kenton

Introduction

Hysterectomy rates at the time of uterovaginal prolapse repair increased drastically in the latter part of the twentieth century when perioperative morbidity and mortality reduced significantly due to the improvement of surgical techniques and widespread use of prophylactic antibiotics. Currently, when uterovaginal prolapse repair is managed surgically, concomitant hysterectomy is commonly performed even when uterine pathology is not suspected [1]. In fact, out of the 430,000 hysterectomies performed annually in the US, approximately 74,000 of them were done with uterovaginal prolapse as the primary indication [2].

Concomitant hysterectomy with laparoscopic sacrocolpopexy is an effective treatment for uterovaginal prolapse and is often considered as the standard of care for primary repair [3,4]. As sacrocolpopexy continues to hold an important role in the wide repertoire of surgical treatments for uterovaginal prolapse, total and supracervical hysterectomies are two of the most commonly performed concomitant procedures with laparoscopic sacrocolpopexy.

When compared to abdominal hysterectomy, laparoscopic hysterectomy is clearly superior, as demonstrated in many randomized controlled trials and meta-analyses [5,6]. The advantages of laparoscopic hysterectomy over laparotomy include reduced blood loss, shorter recovery periods, and decreased postoperative pain. Many variations of laparoscopic hysterectomy exist; the three most common approaches are total laparoscopic hysterectomy (TLH), supracervical hysterectomy (SCH), and laparoscopic-assisted vaginal hysterectomy (LAVH). We will focus on the surgical steps and evidence for concomitant TLH and SCH at the time of laparoscopic sacrocolpopexy in this chapter.

Materials and Surgical Team Set-up

To set up for laparoscopic hysterectomy and sacrocolpopexy, we place four laparoscopic ports across the abdomen for both traditional and robotic-assisted laparoscopy. In this chapter, we will discuss the surgical steps of traditional laparoscopy without robotic assistance. For traditional laparoscopy, we first place a 5 mm port at the umbilicus followed by two additional 5 mm ports on the left lower abdomen and an 8 mm port on the right lower abdomen as seen in Figure 11.1.

The most medial 5 mm port in the left lower quadrant should be parallel to the umbilical port, and the other 5 mm port should be inferior and lateral above the anterior superior iliac spine (ASIS). It is important to visualize the hypogastric arteries bilaterally when placing the lateral ports, by tracing the round ligament cranially on the anterior abdominal wall. The primary surgeon is positioned at the patient's left using the two left lower quadrant ports. One of the two surgical assistants would be positioned at the patient's right using the umbilical port for the camera and the right lower abdomen port for intra-abdominal retraction and needle transfers. The second surgical assistant would be stationed at the pelvis between the patient's legs for vaginal manipulation and specimen retrieval in TLH.

Prior to starting the case, it is important to clear the pelvis from any adhesions and to restore anatomy. Moreover, it is imperative to retract small bowel from the pelvis. Steep Trendelenburg positioning is critical for this step, as is adequate adhesiolysis, allowing the bowels to fall out of the pelvis. The primary surgeon starts with a laparoscopic bipolar energy device in their dominant hand and a Maryland grasper in the other. The first assistant (standing on the patient's right) holds the camera with their left hand and a self-locking laparoscopic tenaculum to grasp at the uterine fundus with their right hand. The tenaculum allows the assistant to provide upward counter

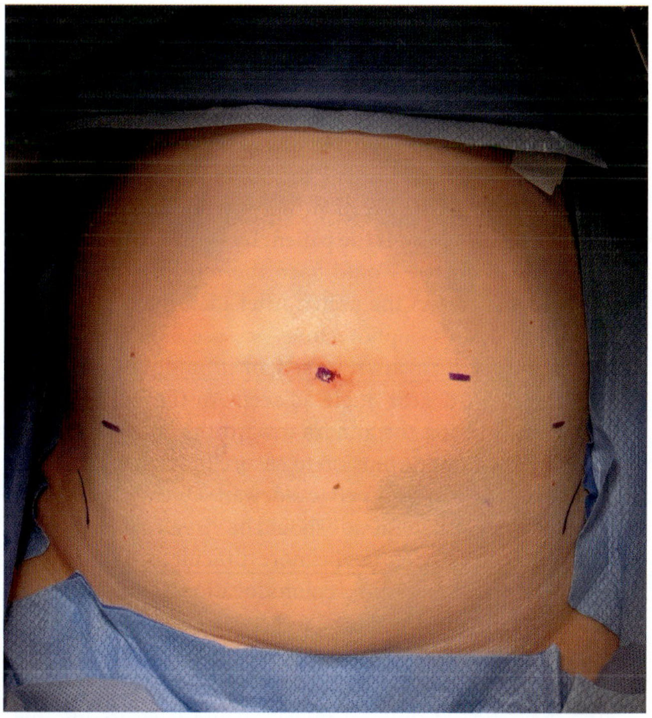

Figure 11.1 Laparoscopic ports placement marked in purple: 5 mm port at the umbilicus, two additional 5 mm ports on the left lower abdomen, and an 8 mm port on the right lower abdomen.

traction on the uterus, obviating the need for a uterine manipulator. The surgical assistant with the tenaculum can retract the uterus cranially and contralaterally from the side of dissection.

The second surgical assistant standing in between the patient's legs provides vaginal manipulation and retrieval of the specimen if a colpotomy was made. We use a Lucite vaginal stent placed in the vagina to facilitate making the colpotomy (Figure 11.2). The surgical assistant places the vaginal stent only when the primary surgeon is ready to make the colpotomy or when the surgeon needs additional retraction during anterior dissection. Alternatively, there are many uterine/vaginal manipulators available, with most placed vaginally with or without a transcervical anchoring device. Common uterine manipulators are limited by their restricted range of motion, difficulties in assembly of certain devices, challenges in manipulator placement through the cervix, and potential traumatic injuries to the patients [7]. Little evidence exists regarding the efficacy and safety of the available uterine manipulators, and there are no high-quality data to demonstrate that the uterine manipulator is effective in preventing ureteral injuries [8]. We prefer to retract the uterus intra-abdominally (similar to a total abdominal hysterectomy) with a self-locking tenaculum, as it provides optimal countertraction, full range of motion, and easy manipulation by the first assistant.

Surgical Steps

Please refer to our surgical videos here for reference (Video 11.1: 'Total laparoscopic hysterectomy and bilateral salpingo-oophorectomy'; Video 11.2: 'Laparoscopic supracervical hysterectomy and bilateral salpingectomy').

Treatment of the Adnexa and Fallopian Tubes

Prior to starting hysterectomy, we proceed with either risk-reducing salpingectomy or elective bilateral salpingo-oophorectomy (BSO). This choice is based on each patient's preferences, founded on shared decision-making after appropriate preoperative counselling. First, we identify the location of the ureter by transperitoneal visualization, starting at the pelvic brim. We do not routinely dissect and isolate the ureter by opening the pelvic side wall due to the excellent intraperitoneal visualization afforded by laparoscopy. If the patient has significant adhesions or altered anatomy, we would open the retroperitoneal space to visualize and retract the ureter. After identifying the ureter, if the patient desires oophorectomy, we use bipolar energy to seal and transect the ovarian vessels, or infundibulopelvic (IP) ligament, at a 90-degree angle adjacent to the ovary. This is done by gently lifting the adnexa toward the anterior abdominal wall without undue tension to ensure the furthest distance away from the ureter and pelvic sidewall. During these steps, the ureter on the ipsilateral side should be visualized at all times. The left ureter can sometimes be more difficult to visualize than the right ureter due to sigmoid colon's location. If this is the case, we advise clearing of any adhesion between the pelvic sidewall and sigmoid colon at the pelvic brim to facilitate the exposure of the left ureter in respect to the left IP ligament.

The incidence of ureteral injury during laparoscopic hysterectomy is between 0.05% to 0.5%, with risk factors being intraoperative haemorrhage, endometriosis, large pelvic mass, malignancy, and history of prior pelvic surgeries [9]. However, these risk factors are less common when hysterectomy is done at the time of sacrocolpopexy; therefore, ureteral dissection for a routine hysterectomy during sacrocolpopexy may not be necessary. Studies have shown that the ureter may still be injured during laparoscopic hysterectomy for benign conditions even with ureteral dissection and lateralization [10]. However, if there is anatomic distortion causing poor visualization or tenting of the ureter, lateralization of the ureter from the ovary and IP ligament is indicated.

The technique of opening the broad ligament to identify the ureter and drop it away from the operative field is the same laparoscopically as during laparotomy. We recommend sealing and transecting the round ligament followed by opening the anterior and posterior leaves of the broad ligament using monopolar energy. We then gently dissect the areolar tissue to identify the external iliac vessels and superiorly the bifurcation of the common iliac vessels at the level of pelvic brim. At the pelvic brim, the ureter should be identified on the medial leaf of the broad ligament anterior to the common iliac bifurcation. We then elevate the fallopian tube and ovary with an atraumatic grasper to create a window with laparoscopic scissors on the medial leaf of the peritoneum between the IP ligament and ureter. We subsequently lateralize the ureter by expanding the peritoneal window, which is achieved by bluntly pushing the ureter away from the IP ligament. Finally, the newly isolated IP ligament is sealed and transected adjacent to the ovary.

If the patient desires to preserve her ovaries, we would perform salpingectomy followed by transection of the utero-ovarian ligament. The fallopian tube is placed on tension anteriorly toward the abdominal wall then bipolar or monopolar energy is used to transect the mesosalpinx. This incision is extended from lateral to medial, originating from below the fimbriae towards the uterine cornua with fallopian tubes remaining attached to the uterus. It is important to remove all fimbriae tissue and avoid incision too close to the IP ligament when performing salpingectomy. After the fallopian tube is detached from the mesosalpinx, we turn our attention to transecting the utero-ovarian

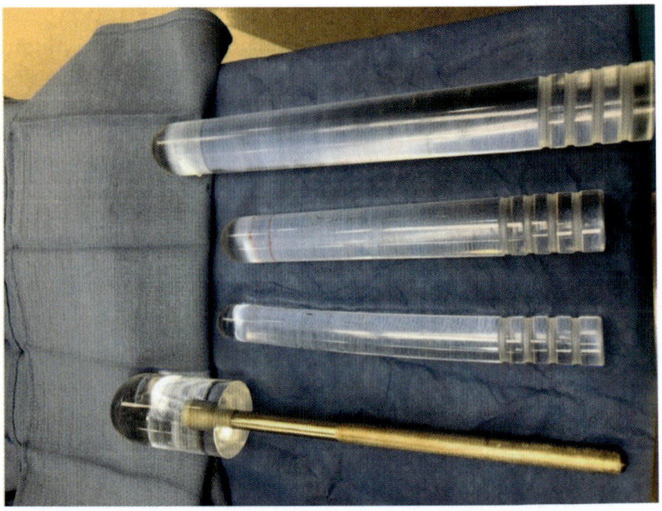

Figure 11.2 Lucite vaginal stent. From left to right: extra-large, small, medium, and large.

ligament. This is done by gently retracting the ovary and uterus away from each other. This puts countertraction in the utero-ovarian vessels and provides surgeons with a clear view to seal the middle segment of the vessels at a 90-degree angle to avoid thermal spread to the ipsilateral ovary.

Shared decision-making is important when surgeons discuss the risks and benefits of risk-reducing salpingectomy versus elective BSO at the time of sacrocolpopexy. The discussion in this section applies to only average-risk patients whose risk for developing ovarian cancer is estimated to be 1.4% [11]. We do not encourage routine preoperative ultrasound to evaluate the ovaries unless it is indicated clinically. For the general population, the decision of whether to proceed with BSO warrants a thorough discussion with the patients. The final decision should be guided by patients' personal goals as well as surgeons' clinical expertise. Women with age greater than 60–65 years, postmenopausal status, nulliparity, and family history of breast or ovarian cancer without a hereditary gene mutation would often be offered elective BSO at the time of sacrocolpopexy. However, if a woman is at low risk for developing ovarian malignancy, ovarian preservation may be favoured. BSO appears to increase long-term mortality and cardiovascular risk in women under age 59 years based on large cohort studies [12]. Additionally, emerging evidence demonstrates that ovaries retain functionality well after menopause [13]. This is echoed by a decision analysis that showed the risks and benefits of elective BSO approximate each other after age 65. As for the fallopian tubes, we recommend universal salpingectomy at the time of sacrocolpopexy due to growing evidence that malignancy may arise from the fallopian tubes [14]. In our practice, we see many women with an average risk of ovarian malignancy younger than 60 years who would prefer risk-reducing salpingectomy and ovarian preservation, whereas women older than 65 often choose concomitant elective BSO during sacrocolpopexy. As for women between age 60 and 65 years of age, patients and their surgeons would jointly decide whether to preserve the ovaries or not based on clinical counselling as well as patients' preferences and goals.

Development of the Vesico-uterine Space

After securing the ovarian vessels, we develop the vesico-uterine space. The round ligaments are transected close to the uterus and away from the pelvic sidewall. We then incise the anterior and posterior leaflets of the broad ligament with bipolar energy from the round ligament to the vesico-uterine junction without transecting the uterine arteries. The vesico-uterine junction can be identified by a fold of peritoneum that is firmly attached to the uterus. During this dissection, the first assistant is retracting the uterus cephalad and toward the contralateral side to provide maximum countertraction for the primary surgeon. Sometimes it may be helpful to re-grasp the uterus at the cornua or lower on the uterine body with a self-locking tenaculum to create optimal countertraction and avoid unnecessary thermal spread to the surrounding structures.

We do not routinely open the anterior and posterior folds of the broad ligament during the dissection prior to entering the vesico-uterine space. Our approach of using energy to transect the anterior and posterior leaflets of the broad ligament together has been previously described [15]. This technique is efficient, time saving, and prevents unnecessary dissection that may lead to blood loss. If the uterus is enlarged with or without fibroids, the surgeon may open the anterior and posterior leaflets of the broad ligament to skeletonize the ascending branches of the uterine artery. In this dissection, the anterior leaflet of the broad ligament will be incised toward the vesico-uterine junction. This is followed by the dissection of the posterior peritoneum towards the uterosacral ligaments. When the ureter is easily visible, there is no advantage to separating the leaflets of the broad ligament, especially when this dissection can cause unexpected bleeding. Excess bleeding can obscure the surgical planes and makes the upcoming sacrocolpopexy dissection more challenging.

To develop the vesico-uterine space, we use monopolar energy to make a small peritoneal incision in the midline just proximal to the bladder (at the vesico-uterine fold or reflection). Gently elevating the incised peritoneum allows carbon dioxide gas from the insufflation to enter the loose areolar tissue, therefore dissecting and separating the peritoneum from the bladder and uterus. Subsequently, it becomes easy to only incise a single layer of peritoneum in an inverted V shape, which outlines the bladder flap and also gives the surgeon easy access to begin the anterior sacrocolpopexy dissection later. In more difficult cases where there are adhesions or distortion of the vesico-uterine junction due to prior caesarean sections, we recommend accessing the vesico-uterine space slightly more laterally to avoid the scarred tissue. Excellent haemostasis is essential, as even small bleeding can obscure tissue planes needed for sacrcolpopexy. Again, during this dissection, the first assistant uses the laparoscopic tenaculum to retract the uterus cephalad and just slightly dorsal to provide adequate countertraction.

After scoring the bladder flap with monopolar energy, we sharply dissect the loose areolar tissue separating the bladder and uterus/cervix with laparoscopic scissors. The surgeon's non-dominant had should retract the anterior peritoneum toward the anterior abdominal wall to provide optimal countertraction. With the tips of the monopolar scissors pointing toward the uterus/cervix, the bladder is gently pushed toward the patient's feet using a snip and push technique. In this avascular plane, the tissue usually separates easily in this correct plane. If one encounters excess bleeding, the surgeon should re-evaluate the dissecting plane until avascular space is identified. The dissection principles here are to gently push the tissue distally against the cervix/vagina then cut the remaining thicker connective tissue projections that do not fall away during the snip and push dissection. During the bladder flap dissection, it is of utmost importance that the surgeon provides adequate countertraction by lifting the bladder peritoneum anteriorly towards the abdominal wall. The bladder peritoneum should be grasped judiciously to prevent traumatic vesical injury.

During the bladder dissection, we only use electrocautery to seal blood vessels when they are encountered. Thermal bladder injury may occur when there is an excessive use of electrocautery, which is one of the leading causes of cystotomy during laparoscopic hysterectomy [16]. It is important to note that fat belongs to the bladder and it is crucial to stay below fat to avoid cystotomy during dissection. If the dissection is bloody, the surgeon should re-evaluate to ensure he/she is in the correct plane, as bleeding is indicative of dissection into the cervix or detrusor muscle, especially if the surgeon is not near bladder trigone. We often carry out the anterior dissection as far caudally as possible behind the bladder foley balloon when sacrocolpopexy is planned.

The vesico-uterine space is an avascular plane, so this dissection does not typically yield significant bleeding. If the dissection is difficult, placing the Lucite stent in the vagina and aiming it cephalad often provides more countertraction and allows surgeons to delineate the vesico-uterine junction better. The Lucite stent can be used as a visual and tactile guide. The vagina under the Lucite stent is shiny and white. Likewise, irrigating the blood-stained tissues frequently helps with re-visualization of the distorted plane. It is common to adjust bladder peritoneum retraction periodically, especially when the anterior dissection is becoming more distal. Again, we normally carry down the dissection to the level of the trigone or just distal to the Foley catheter balloon.

Uterine Artery Ligation and Pedicle Lateralization

After developing the vesico-uterine space, we seal and transect the uterine arteries followed by lateralizing the uterine artery pedicles. The first assistant is still elevating the uterus with the tenaculum. If the vaginal stent was used during dissection, it is removed prior to sealing the uterine arteries, to prevent the possibility of the Lucite stent pushing the ureters cranially toward the surgical field. Having a retraction device against the vaginal fornix may also prohibit surgeons from transecting the uterine arteries close and parallel to the uterus. During this time, the first assistant is retracting the uterus cephalad and contralateral to the side of dissection with a tenaculum, to allow spontaneous separation of the uterine artery pedicle away from the uterine body after being sealed and transected. If the surgeon is using a uterine manipulator with a cup device positioned against the cervix and vaginal fornix, it is important that the surgical assistant pushes the manipulator cranially in addition to pointing the uterine axis away from the dissecting field, in order to create as much distance as possible from the ipsilateral ureter. Prior to sealing and transecting the uterine arteries, the ureter should be identified. An advantage of creating the bladder flap prior to this step is the bladder and ureters should have already been dropped away from the uterine artery. The uterine arteries are secured using bipolar energy either at the level of internal cervical os during a supracervical hysterectomy, or just proximal to the cervicovaginal junction during a total hysterectomy. The bipolar energy is first applied perpendicularly to the uterine vessel on the surgeon's side to ensure the most precise use of the thermal energy. After the uterine vessel is transected, the surgeon would turn the bipolar instrument parallel to the uterus and place it tightly against the cervix for supracervical hysterectomy, or cervicovaginal junction for total hysterectomy, to lateralize the uterine artery pedicle. Alternatively, one can take several small and perpendicular bites while moving caudally after each transection to lateralize the pedicle. It is especially important to take these lateralizing bites as close to the cervix/vagina as possible so bipolar device bounces off the cervix/vagina to minimize thermal spread to the lateral structures, particularly the ureters. Clinical judgement and surgical experience play a significant role in this important step to minimize blood loss.

After creation of the uterine artery pedicles during a TLH, the Lucite vaginal stent is placed in the vagina. The stent will expand the anterior vaginal fornix and delineate the white vaginal tissue from the cervix. For less experienced surgeons, tactile feedback by palpating the firm Lucite stent compared to the soft cervical tissue may be helpful. As for SCH at the time of sacrocolpopexy, the level of pedicle lateralization should be distal to the internal cervical os. Lateralization of the uterine artery pedicles is important to avoid inadvertent bleeding when performing colpotomy or uterine body amputation.

Colpotomy and Uterine Body Amputation

The main difference between TLH and SCH is whether the cervix is removed with the uterus or not. TLH is the removal of the uterus and cervix via a colpotomy. In contrast, SCH is the removal of the uterus by amputation of the uterine body at the internal os.

A Lucite stent or uterine manipulator is placed to perform the colpotomy during TLH. There is no evidence to support superiority of one device over the other, so the surgeon should choose the technique or device with which they are most familiar. To make the colpotomy, monopolar energy is applied circumferentially. It is important that the colpotomizer is placed firmly against the cervicovaginal junction to provide adequate countertraction. This countertraction is vital so the surgeon can use the least amount of energy possible to prevent accidental thermal spread to the surrounding tissue as well as to avoid excessive thermal injury which may impair proper healing. The first assistant continues to provide maximal traction cephalad and away from the colpotomy site. This counter traction will allow the vagina and cervix to separate easily and enable the surgeon to visualize the projection for the rest of the colpotomy. The surgical assistant may readjust the tenaculum by grasping more caudally toward the lower uterine body or cervix for optimal countertraction.

With a Lucite stent in the vagina, we start the colpotomy anteriorly at the 12 o'clock position and extend it away from the primary surgeon toward the 6 o'clock position (clockwise position when the surgeon is standing on the patient's left). This is why retracting the bowel out of the cul-de-sac with steep Trendelenburg at the beginning of the case is critical, as mentioned previously. It is important to visualize all surrounding organs and be constantly aware of the monopolar device's location. When the first half of the colpotomy is completed, the attention is returned back to the 12 o'clock position and the other half of the circumferential incision is made counterclockwise toward the 6 o'clock position.

When most of the colpotomy is made, the vaginal stent or manipulators without a transcervical anchoring device will no longer be able to provide adequate countertraction to expose the posterior vaginal wall. At this time, the first assistant should reposition the tenaculum on the posterior lip of the cervix while the primary surgeon places a coated laparoscopic instrument behind the posterior vaginal tissue serving as a counter-traction for the uterus and cervix to flip 180 degrees into the cul-de-sac. With this maneuver, the posterior vaginal wall is exposed on tension and the primary surgeon can apply monopolar energy over the vaginal epithelium to complete the posterior colpotomy. It is important that the primary surgeon is able to visualize the coated laparoscopic instrument on the contralateral side of the vaginal wall at all times to avoid inadvertent deviation of the colpotomy leading to injury of nearby pelvic structures.

With SCH, it is important to leave enough cervical stump in place without entering the vagina, while amputating the uterine body. The level of amputation should be slightly distal to the internal cervical os and proximal to the uterosacral ligaments. The first assistant will be retracting the uterus cephalad and laterally using the tenaculum. We recommend starting the amputation anteriorly and moving posteriorly. Again, it is important to provide adequate countertraction, so the cervical stroma naturally separates as the thermal energy moves through the plane. It is of the utmost importance to visualize the monopolar energy source at all times to prevent injury to surrounding organs. No uterine manipulation is needed for uterine body amputation. If there is a uterine manipulating device through the cervix, removal of this device at time of amputation may be needed. After the uterine body is amputated from the cervix, the remaining cervical stump should have a cut edge that appears flat and haemostatic. Some surgeons would choose to perform ablation of the endocervical canal to decrease the risk of postoperative cyclic bleeding. Reverse cervical conization has also been described. However, there is no definitive evidence that supports one method over the other [17,18].

Decision to Do Total Laparoscopic Hysterectomy or Supracervical Hysterectomy

The decision to do a TLH or SCH at the time of sacrocolpopexy is hotly debated. There are pros and cons of each technique, which surgeons should discuss with each patient to guide shared decision-making. Several studies showed higher mesh erosion rates when sacrocolpopexy was done at the time of total hysterectomy [19,20]. Cundiff et al reported a five-fold increase in sacrocolpopexy mesh erosions when a concomitant total hysterectomy was done; however, this study has limited generalizability to current procedures where ultralightweight polypropylene meshes are used. Over half of the meshes in the Cundiff study were braided polyester or extended polytetrafluoroethylene. Mesh exposure rates with newer ultralightweight polypropylene meshes are significantly lower, likely mitigating the magnitude of this difference. On the other hand, Myers et al found that women who had SCH were nearly three times more likely to have stage 2 or greater recurrent prolapse at one year compared to women who had TLH [21]. In addition, a larger umbilical incision or morcellation is necessary to remove the specimen during SCH.

Removal of the Specimen

After TLH, the specimen can usually be removed via colpotomy with a ring forceps without difficulty. In this section, we will discuss the surgical technique of laparoscopic suturing of the vaginal cuff after the TLH. As for SCH, we will discuss the abdominal approach to removal of the specimen by contained tissue extraction in a post-power morcellation era.

After the colpotomy is made, the first assistant needs to detach the tenaculum from the specimen, close the tenaculum, and remove the instrument under direct visualization. The other surgical assistant can easily remove the uterus through the vagina. After the specimen is removed, we usually insert a bulb from a large syringe to maintain pneumoperitoneum while closing the vaginal cuff. We always close the vaginal cuff laparoscopically with a series of figure-of-eight delayed absorbable sutures, which are tied extracorporeally. There is high-quality evidence demonstrating that vaginal closure of the cuff has increased risk for dehiscence and wound complications when compared to laparoscopic closure [22].

To close the vaginal cuff after TLH, the first assistant passes a loaded needle to the surgeon via the 8 mm port on the right as seen in Figure 11.3. This technique allows the surgeon to pick up the needle at a right angle and be ready to suture without repositioning the needle. This is especially helpful for learners or less experienced laparoscopic surgeons. The tail of the suture is placed through a closed knot pusher with a clamp at the end, allowing the assistant to efficiently tie after the vaginal cuff suture is placed. To place the suture, the surgeon and first assistant both hold the edge of the posterior vaginal cuff on tension to allow easy placement of the needle through the vaginal epithelium. The surgeon then regrasps the needle and anterior vaginal cuff, while the first assistant also grasps the anterior vagina and the suture is easily placed. The suture should be pulled all the way through to allow placement of a figure-of-eight suture. If the suture is not pulled all the way through, it can lock and make tying more difficult. After completing the figure-of-eight suture, the first assistant removes the needle and ties extracorporeally.

This same action is repeated until the whole vaginal cuff is closed. After the vaginal cuff is closed, we continue with anterior and posterior vaginal dissection portions of sacrocolpopexy. We typically do not routinely perform cystoscopy until after the sacrocolpopexy is completed, unless a different surgical team completed the hysterectomy, when we would perform cystoscopy prior to sacrocolpopexy.

To remove the specimen after SCH, we always perform contained tissue extraction through the umbilicus after the sacrocolpopexy is completed. Retrieving the specimen requires slight extension of the umbilical incision; therefore, the surgeon should complete all necessary procedures prior to removal of the specimen. In the modern, post-power morcellation era after the FDA's warning statement in 2014, we adapted a version of the extracorporeal tissue extraction technique [23]. We first extend the umbilical port incision and introduce a 15 mm endoscopic specimen retrieval bag to bring up the specimen. We then extend the umbilical port site to approximately 3 cm and secure the rolled-down edges of the retrieval bag with several Kelly clamps. We would finally 'core' the specimen with an 11-inch blade scalpel to extract the specimen, which is coined as the ExCiTE technique (Extracorporeal C-incision Tissue Extraction) [24]. It is important to not disrupt the containment bag during the extraction process with the scalpel by visualizing where the scalpel is at all times. After the extraction is completed and the specimen

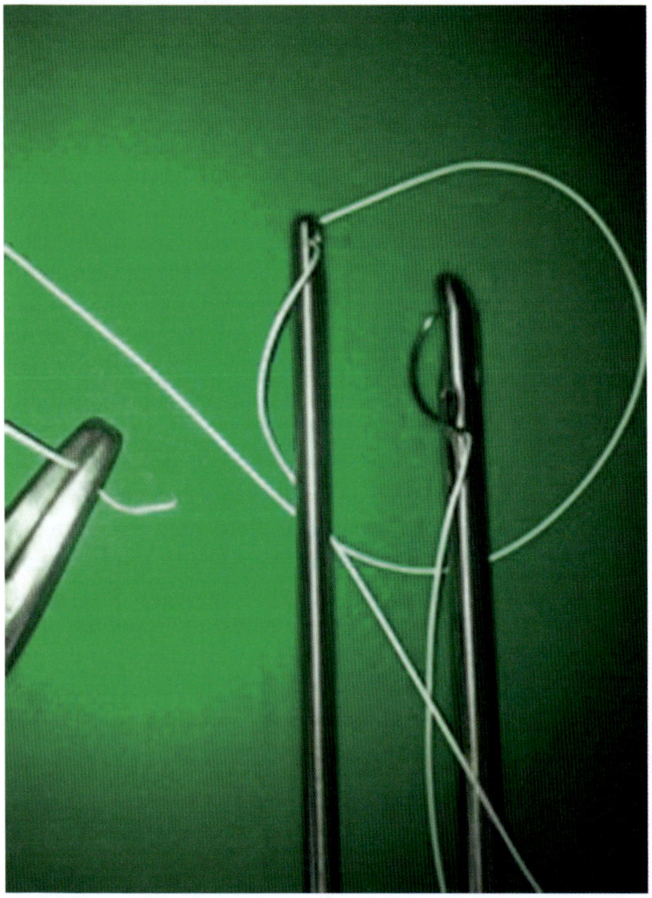

Figure 11.3 Laparoscopic needle holder and suture threaded with a closed knot pusher; end of the suture secured with a clamp.

as well as containment bag are completely removed, the fascia of the extended umbilical port site is closed with a 0-Vicryl suture. Of note, the ExCiTE technique might be needed in order to remove the specimen vaginally in TLHs if the uterine size is enlarged. The ExCiTE technique is an efficient way to remove the specimen in an efficient and controlled manner.

Conclusion

Hysterectomy is a commonly performed concomitant procedure at the time of sacrocolpopexy. Both total and supracervical hysterectomies require the surgeons' thorough understanding of the pelvic anatomy and surgical principles. Moreover, operating team members' contributions in anticipating surgical needs and providing seamless support during the surgery are vital to complete TLH and SCH both safely and efficiently. Laparoscopic surgery continues to demonstrate its proven benefits over laparotomy, and it is important for surgeons and their team members to develop a set of standardized techniques supported by evidence. However, there are many techniques and versions of performing hysterectomies, with no high-quality data supporting one way over the others. Nonetheless, as evidenced throughout many surgical specialties, the efforts to standardize surgical approaches within each practice will lead to consistent and favourable outcomes for all patients [25,26].

References

1. Ridgeway BM. Does prolapse equal hysterectomy? The role of uterine conservation in women with uterovaginal prolapse. Am J Obstet Gynecol 2015; 213(6): 802–9.
2. Wright JD, Herzog TJ, Tsui J, et al. Nationwide trends in the performance of inpatient hysterectomy in the United States. Obstet Gynecol 2013; 122(2): 233.
3. Nygaard I, Brubaker L, Zyczynski HM, et al. Long-term outcomes following abdominal sacrocolpopexy for pelvic organ prolapse. JAMA 2013; 309(19)): 2016–24.
4. Costantini E, Brubaker L, Cervigni M, et al.. Sacrocolpopexy for pelvic organ prolapse: evidence-based review and recommendations. Eur J Obstet Gynecol Reprod Biol 2016; 205: 60–5.
5. Aarts JWM, Nieboer TE, Johnson N, et al. Surgical approach to hysterectomy for benign gynaecological disease. Cochrane Database Syst Rev 2015; 8: CD003677. https://doi.org/10.1002/14651858.CD003677.pub5.
6. Nieboer TE, Hendriks JCM, Bongers MY, et al. Quality of life after laparoscopic and abdominal hysterectomy: a randomized controlled trial. Obstet Gynecol 2012; 119(1): 85–91.
7. Van den Haak L, Alleblas C, Nieboer TE, et al. Efficacy and safety of uterine manipulators in laparoscopic surgery: a review. Arch Gynecol Obstet 2015; 292(5): 1003–11.
8. Janssen PF, Brölmann HAM, Huirne JAF. Causes and prevention of laparoscopic ureter injuries: an analysis of 31 cases during laparoscopic hysterectomy in the Netherlands. Surg Endosc 2013; 27(3): 946–56.
9. Clarke-Pearson DL, Geller EJ. Complications of hysterectomy. Obstet Gynecol 2013; 121(3): 654–73.
10. Janssen PF, Brölmann HAM, Huirne JAF. Causes and prevention of laparoscopic ureter injuries: an analysis of 31 cases during laparoscopic hysterectomy in the Netherlands. Surg Endosc 2013; 27(3): 946–56.
11. ACOG Practice Bulletin No 89. American College of Obstetrics and Gynecologists. Elective and risk-reducing salpingo-oophorectomy. Obstet Gynecol 2008; 111: 231–41.
12. Manson JE, Aragaki AK, Bassuk SS, et al. Menopausal estrogen-alone therapy and health outcomes in women with and without bilateral oophorectomy: a randomized trial. Ann Intern Med 2019; 171(6)): 406–14.
13. Fogle RH, Stanczyk FZ, Zhang X et al. Ovarian androgen production in postmenopausal women. J Clin Endocrinol Metab 2007; 92(8): 3040–3.
14. Tone AA, Salvador S, Finlayson SJ, et al. The role of the fallopian tube in ovarian cancer. Clin Adv Hematol Oncol 2012; 10(5): 296–306.
15. Ghirardini G, Mohamed M, Bartolamasi A, et al. Minimally invasive vaginal hysterectomy using bipolar vessel sealing: preliminary experience with 500 cases. J Obstet Gynaecol 2013; 33(1): 79–81.
16. Ostrzenski A, Ostrzenska KM. Bladder injury during laparoscopic surgery. Obstet Gynecol Surv 1998; 53(3): 175–80.
17. Donnez J, Nisolle M, Smets M, et al. Laparoscopic supracervical (subtotal) hysterectomy: a first series of 500 cases. Gynaecol Endosc 1997; 6(2): 73–6.
18. Lyons TL. Laparoscopic supracervical hysterectomy. Obstet Gynecol Clin 2000; 27(2): 441–50.

19. Cundiff GW, Varner E, Visco AG, et al. Risk factors for mesh/suture erosion following sacral colpopexy. Am J Obstet Gynecol 2008; 199(6): 688–e1.
20. Bensinger G, Lind L, Lesser M, et al. Abdominal sacral suspensions: analysis of complications using permanent mesh. Am J Obstet Gynecol 2005; 193(6): 2094–8.
21. Myers EM, Siff L, Osmundsen B, et al. Differences in recurrent prolapse at 1 year after total vs supracervical hysterectomy and robotic sacrocolpopexy. Int Urogynecol J 2015; 26(4): 585–9.
22. Uccella S, Malzoni M, Cromi A, et al. Laparoscopic vs transvaginal cuff closure after total laparoscopic hysterectomy: a randomized trial by the Italian Society of Gynecologic Endoscopy. AJOG 2018; 218(5): 500.e1–13.
23. United States Food and Drug Administration. Laparoscopic uterine power morcellation in hysterectomy and myomectomy: FDA safety communication. Published 2014.
24. Truong MD, Advincula AP. The extracorporeal C-incision tissue extraction (ExCITE) technique. OBG Manag 2014; 26(11): 56.
25. Bertelsen CA, Bols B, Ingeholm P, et al. Can the quality of colonic surgery be improved by standardization of surgical technique with complete mesocolic excision? Colorect Dis 2011; 13(10): 1123–9.
26. Working Group of the European Society for Gynaecological Endoscopy. Surgical steps of total laparoscopic hysterectomy. Part 1: Benign disease by the European Society for Gynaecological Endoscopy (ESGE). Facts, Views & Vision in ObGyn 2019; 11(2): 103–10.

Chapter 12

Laparoscopic Sacrohysteropexy: Oxford Technique: Procedure Steps and Evidence

Matthew Izett-Kay, Rufus Cartwright, Natalia Price

Background

The International Urogynecological Association (IUGA) defines prolapse as 'The descent of one or more of the anterior vaginal wall, posterior vaginal wall, the uterus (cervix) or the apex of the vagina (vaginal vault or cuff scar after hysterectomy) [1]. Uterine prolapse specifically is found in at least 14% of postmenopausal women according to large population studies [2]. Symptoms from this are common, and 40% of women over the age of 45 report having had symptoms of prolapse [3]. The risk of surgical intervention for this condition is therefore quite high, reportedly between 11% and 19% in a woman's lifetime [4]. Laparoscopic mesh sacrohysteropexy (LSH) is one option that has emerged over the last decade as a solution for women with symptomatic uterine prolapse who have failed conservative measures. At our centre, this procedure is now offered routinely and we have published widely on outcomes generally, as well as in specific populations [5–10]. More recently, we have presented safety data in an attempt to address issues surrounding the use of mesh in pelvic floor surgery [11].

Before surgery is offered, it is essential that patients have considered, and where appropriate, engaged with non-surgical approaches to managing pelvic organ prolapse (POP). The latest guidance in the UK from the National Institute for Health and Care Excellence (NICE) outlines this, stating [12]:

> Discuss management options with women who have pelvic organ prolapse, including no treatment, non-surgical treatment and surgical options.

This forms part of the authors' routine practice, with support from clinical nurse specialists and women's health physiotherapists in ensuring that patients avoid the risks of surgery where possible. While success rates for conservative measures vary, large meta-analyses have shown that pelvic floor muscle therapy (PFMT) is associated with subjective improvement in prolapse symptoms, as well as objective improvements in severity of POP [13]. Up to 76% of patients require no further treatment following PFMT and over half of women report their symptoms to be better [14]. Vaginal support devices known as pessaries may also be used. While few randomized studies exist to support their use, large observational studies illustrate similar success rates of between 41% and 68% [15–17].

For those women who eventually undergo surgery for uterine prolapse, in the UK as in many other countries, vaginal hysterectomy (VH) with apical suspension is the most commonly performed procedure. Three-quarters of UK urogynaecologists offer this as first-line according to a survey undertaken in 2018 [18]. However, studies have shown the re-operation rate for prolapse following such procedures to be between 4.6% and 18% [19,20]. Re-operation rates after native tissue surgery more generally may be as high as 29% [21,22]. There is also an increasing trend to avoid hysterectomy at the time of prolapse surgery; indeed some studies suggest that the majority of women would prefer uterine preservation if given an equally efficacious alternative [23,24]. The Manchester-Fothergill repair would be one alternative to VH, with recent population data from Denmark suggesting this has a lower risk of re-operation as compared to VH [25]. Colpocleisis offers another surgical option, however it is generally reserved for the elderly, given it precludes the possibility of penetrative intercourse. Hysteropexy is therefore the principle uterine sparing alternative to VH for many clinicians and their patients, and can be undertaken with an abdominal or vaginal approach.

The anatomical advantage of an abdominal approach to prolapse repair is the surgical access to the entire pelvis, potentially allowing for higher suspension of the apex. As with any abdominal operation, a laparoscopic approach is the natural progression for twenty-first-century practice given the well-established advantages associated with the avoidance of laparotomy. Broadly, these advantages are better visualization of anatomy, reduced postoperative pain, and a return to normal activities [26]. While sutures may be used to suspend the uterus to either the sacrospinous ligament or the anterior longitudinal ligament over the sacral promontory, this is associated with a high rate of failure [27]. Mesh hysteropexy therefore provides a viable alternative to the use of suture suspension, with mesh materials offering more robust tissue support. A meta-analysis comparing sacrohysteropexy to VH reported advantages including higher suspension of pelvic organ prolapse quantification (POP-Q) point C, longer total vaginal length (TVL), blood loss, pain, and return to normal activity all favouring hysteropexy [28].

The consideration of mesh-augmented surgical techniques calls for examination of the controversies surrounding the use of non-absorbable mesh. For women with prolapse, the transvaginal placement of mesh has been recognized as having unreasonably high rates of mesh-associated complications [29]. In contrast, despite well-established efficacy and low complication rates in numerous high-quality studies, there also remain patient concerns around transvaginal mesh use for stress urinary incontinence (SUI) [30]. There have been multiple national and international reviews of the issue, and in some countries, pelvic mesh remains partially or completely restricted from use [31–35]. While mesh complications may be asymptomatic, they are often associated with chronic pain, leading to devastating impacts on quality of life [36]. Despite quality evidence refuting an association between systemic autoimmune disorders and mesh, some patients continue to worry about a possible link [37]. Regulators and reports into mesh have repeatedly identified a need for more high-quality, long-term data to support the use of mesh-augmented pelvic floor surgery [12,38]. As with any intervention, a change in practice must be justified by appropriate evidence for both safety and efficacy.

Finally, it is important that surgical approaches to LSH are considered each on their own merit and evidence base, particularly given that techniques continue to evolve. At our centre, we have developed an approach that avoids dissection and placement of mesh on the vagina. We would advocate therefore, that the Oxford Hysteropexy confers all of the benefits of hysteropexy and mesh augmentation, yet avoids the potential for vaginal mesh erosion, a theoretical advantage that appears substantiated by some of our more recent work [11]. This chapter aims to familiarize readers with the context for utilization of laparoscopic mesh sacrohysteropexy. We will discuss lessons learnt from the development of the surgical technique over the last decade, as well as presenting the data we have published to date in support of this surgical approach.

Preoperative Assessment and Considerations

Comprehensive history taking is essential when considering surgery for prolapse. Many patients present with coexisting bladder and bowel dysfunction, and it is important that patients are not subjected to surgical intervention to correct prolapse when their primary complaint is that of coexisting pelvic floor dysfunction that could be treated conservatively. History-taking may be supplemented by the use of patient reported outcome measures (PROMs). These are questionnaire-based tools that enable a more objective assessment of symptom status, among other measures [39]. With respect to the assessment of POP, the available PROMs have been appraised by the International Consultation on Incontinence (ICI) and a number are supported by Grade A evidence [40]. Not only do these quantify symptoms and symptom bother, they provide a medicolegal justification for surgical intervention as well as providing a benchmark when assessing postoperative resolution of symptoms.

Clinical examination remains fundamental to the assessment of POP. It can be done in the dorsal lithotomy or Sims' position with the use of Valsalva, or undertaken with the patient standing. For the Baden-Walker system, the hymen provides a landmark, with classification of prolapse within each of the three compartments from Stage 0–IV. The Pelvic Organ Prolapse Quantification (POPQ) system has been widely adopted and has been validated, showing good inter- and intra-observer reliability [41,42]. The POPQ allows a more meaningful, quantified, and objective assessment of not just the various vaginal compartments, but also the genital hiatus and perineal body as well as vaginal length. Using the hymen as a reference point, various landmarks are identified within the vagina, with their lowest position on Valsalva documented. Those above the hymen are demarcated by a '–' and those beyond the hymen with a '+'. The pelvic floor muscles should also be digitally assessed by vaginal examination to determine tone, as a marker of functional capacity as first described by Kegel in 1948 [43]. The strength can then be quantified using the Modified Oxford Grading System, although the reliability and reproducibility of this mode of assessment is debated [44,45].

For those diagnosed with uterine prolapse we generally offer the options of doing nothing, PFMT, a ring pessary, or surgery. In accordance with NICE guidance in the UK, for those at the stage of requesting surgery, we offer vaginal hysterectomy with apical suspension, hysteropexy (either vaginal approach with suture or laparoscopic approach with mesh), Manchester-Fothergill procedure, or colpocleisis [12]. Patients are routinely provided with either national or local patient information leaflets (PILs) outlining the procedure, risks and benefits, and expected safety and efficacy outcomes. Following counselling, patients are discussed at a multi-disciplinary meeting (MDT) which comprises of at the least: two consultant physicians with expertise in managing POP, a clinical nurse specialist, and a pelvic floor physiotherapist, in accordance with NICE [12].

Patient Selection: When to Offer Laparoscopic Mesh Sacrohysteropexy

Generally, LSH is offered in our unit to all women with symptomatic uterine prolapse who are requesting surgery. There are some specific contraindications to LSH which may shape the surgical options on offer. We do not offer the procedure to women with un-investigated abnormal uterine bleeding (including post-menopausal bleeding), known endometrial or cervical pathology, and large uterine fibroids (specifically that would preclude anatomical placement of mesh). It is available to those who desire further children, the outcome of which is discussed later in this chapter, as long as they understand the lack of safety data and the need for caesarean section as cervical dilatation is not possible with the circumferential placement of mesh that we undertake. We consider the procedure particularly suitable for those who wish for uterine preservation, those who have had previously failed uterine preserving prolapse procedures, failed primary anterior or posterior repair, younger women, and for those with a strong aversion to further prolapse surgery.

Counselling for Laparoscopic Mesh Sacrohysteropexy: What to Discuss

Framing the discussion for primary surgical correction for uterine prolapse will be shaped significantly by the patient desires and the surgeon's expertise. In the absence of contraindications to a specific intervention, our counselling generally covers the available evidence for the varying procedures and the relative safety and efficacy from the short- to longer-term. This is guided in UK practice by the NICE patient decision aids (PDA) which compare the various options [46]. It is made clear to our patients that VH with apical suspension is the standard and most common procedure undertaken, with the largest body of evidence to support its use. In accordance with NICE we quote that following this surgery patients can expect at one year an anatomical success rate of 90%, and a 65% symptomatic success rate [46]. We explain that despite a lack of high-quality evidence, a Manchester repair is likely to be associated with similar outcomes [25]. For those considering colpocleisis, the lack of comparative data is highlighted and a 90–100% success rate quoted, albeit highlighted to the patient that this is in unrepresentative patient populations, skewed towards the older woman [47]. The absence of mesh is highlighted as an advantage for all of these interventions and for all procedures we discuss the expected recovery along with possible changes in bladder and bowel dysfunction.

The evidence to support LSH is discussed in detail later in this chapter. Broadly, we highlight to patients the lack of high-quality comparative studies and the low quality of the available data. We explain the potential benefits, which we consider to be uterine preservation, higher apical suspension, maintenance of vaginal length, reduced blood loss and quick recovery, and a theoretical but as of yet unsubstantiated benefit of improved longevity due to the use of mesh. It must be explicit to patients that non-absorbable mesh is implanted and we discuss the application of mesh in pelvic floor surgery. It is important to distinguish the procedure from transvaginal mesh for prolapse, which is associated with at least an 8% risk of re-operation for mesh erosion [29,48]. In the UK, all mesh procedures are subject to 'high vigilance scrutiny' requiring the procedures to only be undertaken by those with appropriate training. As we outline here patients must be informed about the lack of evidence and controversies around use of mesh. Appropriate clinical governance structures must be documented including registration of each case in a national audit database such as that provided by the British Society of Urogynaecology (BSUG) [49]. This allows for national tracking of outcome data and complications.

Development of Surgical Technique

The evolution of LSH follows two paths, that of the development of mesh-augmented surgery and that of uterine sparing prolapse surgery. The term 'mesh' encompasses a range of materials and devices but is defined by IUGA and the International Continence Society (ICS) as 'a (prosthetic) network fabric or structure; open spaces or interstices between the strands of the net' [50]. Originally, surgical mesh was developed to augment the repair of abdominal herniae. A range of materials were used in the mid-twentiethcentury prior to the advent of plastics and ultimately polypropylene, which was first used clinically to repair inguinal hernias in the 1960s [51]. The initial use of mesh in pelvic floor surgery was for the treatment of stress urinary incontinence (SUI), in the form of a synthetic pubovaginal sling described by Zoedler and Boeminghaus in 1965 [52]. The first transvaginal mesh implant for SUI approved by the US Food and Drug Agency (FDA) was the ProteGen™ sling in 1996 [53]. Work by Petros and Ulmsten in the late 1980s led to the birth of the most popular such device, the tension free vaginal tape (TVT) [54]. This led to the propagation of mesh as both a customized inlay, and branded devices for the treatment of both SUI and POP.

The first sacrohysteropexy utilized suture material and was undertaken as an abdominal procedure, reported in 1956 by Arthure and Savage [55]. In 1979, SK Chaudhuri utilized autologous tissue as a sling to elevate the uterus, taking fascia from the external oblique and attaching it to the anterior aspect of the cervix [56]. A Goretex mesh was utilized by Farkas in 1993, and then polypropylene by Leron and Stanton in 2001 to undertake an open sacrohysteropexy [57,58]. Our technique builds on that reported by Cutner et al in 2007, who reported a laparoscopic sacrohysteropexy utilizing a merseline tape [59]. We reported our first series of 51 women in 2010, followed by a larger cohort with one to four years follow-up and a video of the surgical technique in 2014 (Video 12.1), and an initial randomised trial comparing with vaginal hysterectomy [8–10]. These studies were followed by a large cohort of over 500 women and 10 years of experience in 2017, and more recently, long-term four year follow-up looking at the safety of a cohort of 1,121 women, the data from which are presented within this chapter [5,11].

Principle Surgical Technique

Preoperative Preparation

All patients undergoing surgery will have been counselled, discussed at an MDT, and consented, as already outlined within this chapter. We routinely consent for conversion to vaginal hysterectomy should anatomical findings preclude hysteropexy, although such a need is rare. All patients are consented for concurrent colporrhaphy and perineorrhaphy. There are no international guidelines with respect to antimicrobial prophylaxis in the case of LSH, and guidance from the European Association of Urology does not reference the procedure [60]. In accordance with local recommendations, we use broad-spectrum antibiotics as antimicrobial prophylaxis immediately prior to operating, commonly co-amoxiclav, because LSH is considered a clean-contaminated procedure [61]. Patients are initially positioned supine without tilt, in lithotomy with 30-degress flexion at the hips. They then undergo skin cleaning with either chlorhexidine or betadine skin preparation and are draped. The uterus is instrumented with a disposable Spackman cannula and the bladder is emptied with an indwelling catheter.

Surgical Approach

Pneumoperitoneum is created with the use of a Veress needle in accordance with Royal College of Obstetrics and Gynaecology (RCOG) guidance [62]. Generally, we utilize four ports, one 10mm sub-umbilical, one 7mm suprapubic port, and two 5mm lateral ports. We undertake a full survey of the abdomen and pelvis to exclude incidental pathology and anatomical suitability, for example we have encountered aortic bifurcation at a level precluding the safe attachment of mesh to the sacral promontory. The peritoneum over the sacral promontory is incised with bipolar graspers and monopolar scissors (Figure 12.1). The ureters are identified bilaterally, and a peritoneal relaxing incision is made medial to the right ureter to retract it away from the operative site using a combination of blunt and sharp dissection. Each broad ligament at the level of the cervico-uterine junction is opened through an avascular area. Finally, the vesico-uterine peritoneum is incised and the bladder reflected caudally for 2–3 cm.

To suspend the uterus from the sacral promontory, a bifurcated polypropylene type 1 monofilament macroporous non-absorbable mesh (Atrium Medical Corporation, Hudson, NH, USA) is cut to the required bifurcated shape and used (Figure

12.2). The arms of the bifurcated mesh are then introduced bilaterally through windows created in the broad ligaments (Figure 12.3). The arms of the mesh are sutured to the anterior cervix with three non-dissolvable, non-absorbable polyester 2–0 sutures (Ethibond Excel™, Ethicon Inc., Somerville, NJ, USA) (Figure 12.4). More recently, for women with small post-menopausal uteri, we have adopted a 'cravat' technique. This involves the creation of an aperture at one end of a strip of polypropylene mesh. The strip is then passed through the broad ligament windows, and one end passed through the aperture. For both approaches, the mesh is then largely re-peritonealized before being tacked to the sacral promontory using 5-mm helical fasteners (Protack, United States Surgical, Tyco Healthcare, Norwalk, CT, USA) to elevate the uterus (Figure 12.5). The mesh is placed under moderate tension, aiming to reposition the cervix at the vaginal apex. The sacral promontory is then re-peritonealized to completely cover the mesh (Figure 12.6).

Closure

The surgical technique we use for laparoscopic hysteropexy has evolved over the last decade. Initially, the mesh was not completely re-peritonealized, as previous research suggested this was unnecessary [63]. However, when performing subsequent

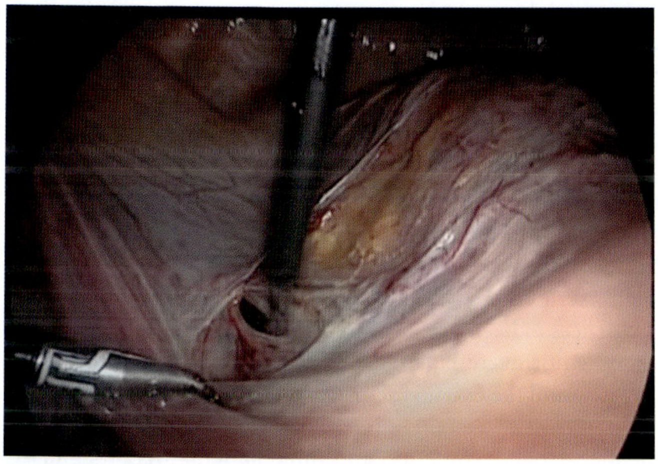

Figure 12.1 Peritoneum incised over sacral promontory.

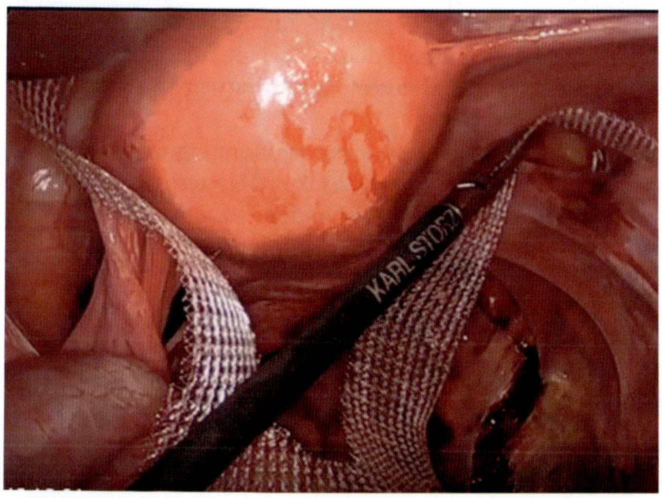

Figure 12.2 Custom-cut polypropylene mesh.

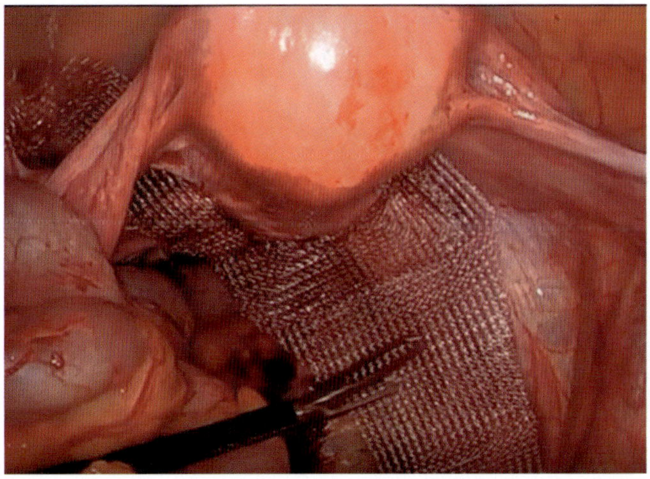

Figure 12.3 Mesh arms passed through broad ligament windows.

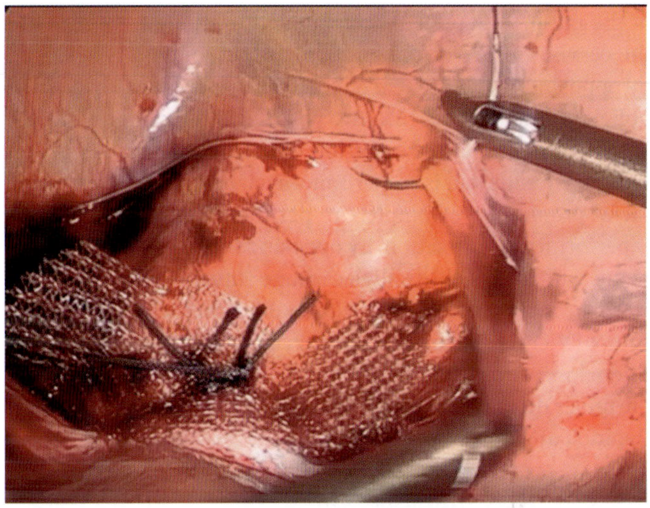

Figure 12.4 Mesh arms secured to anterior cervix.

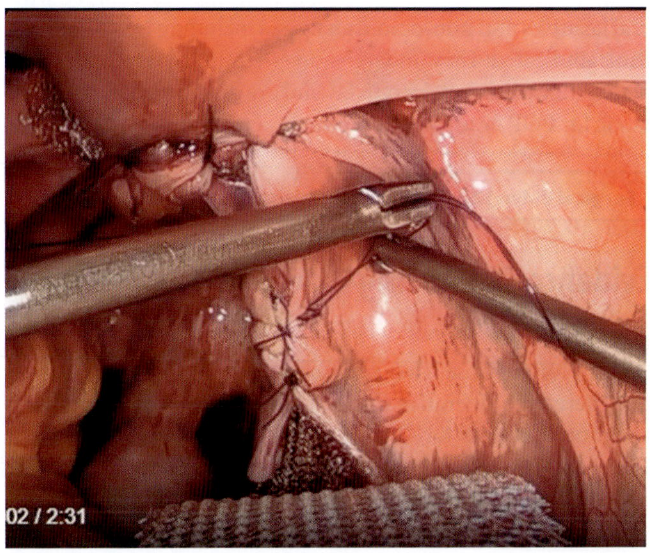

Figure 12.5 Fixation at sacral promontory with helical fasteners.

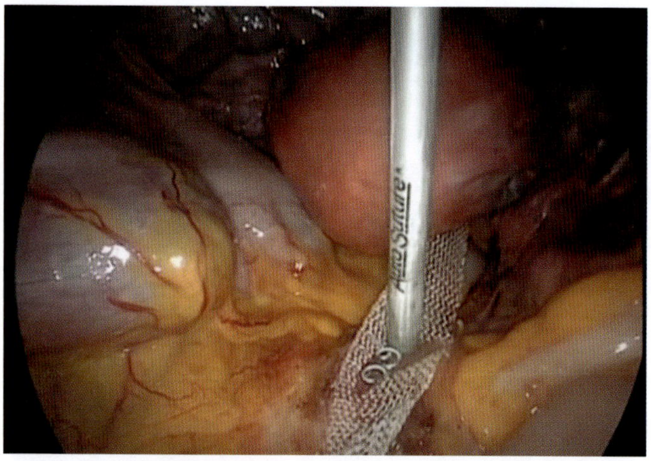

Figure 12.6 Complete re-peritonization of mesh.

laparoscopies on two of our patients, adhesions were noted between the mesh and loops of small bowel. Adaptation of the technique was undertaken to include full re-peritonealization of the mesh. Following placement and fixation of the mesh to the cervix, closure of the uterovesical peritoneum is achieved by opposing the peritoneal edges with two or three absorbable poliglecaprone sutures (Monocryl, Ethicon Inc., Somerville, NJ, USA). The mesh at the insertion of uterosacral ligaments and right pelvic sidewall is re-peritonealized prior to fixation to the sacral promontory. Complete re-peritonealization of the mesh is performed after fixation, by opposing the edges of the peritoneum with absorbable poliglecaprone sutures (Monocryl). We close the rectus sheath at the suprapubic port with 1 polyglactin suture (Vicryl, Ethicon Inc., Somerville, NJ, USA) passed on an Endoclose® device, and the umbilical port with 1 Vicryl a 'J' needle under direct vision. We use either 2/0 Monocryl®, 2/0 Vicryl Rapide®, or glue for the skin.

Postoperative Management

Patients are routinely discharged at postoperative day one, with criteria for mobilization and voiding only. A trial without catheter must be instituted, however we do not measure post void residual bladder volumes. Patients are routinely discharged with oral laxatives and non-opioid analgesia including NSAIDs if not contraindicated. They undergo nurse-led clinic visits at approximately 12 weeks postoperatively and are discharged if asymptomatic for POP or urinary symptoms.

Surgical Video 12.1 A video outlining our surgical approach.

Evidence Supporting Oxford Hysteropexy

Safety Data

Surgery for prolapse is a quality-of-life enhancing intervention. It is therefore imperative that any intervention we offer is safe, given our patients rarely face mortality should they be managed conservatively. Our first initial series included 51 women with a case note review and routine three-month follow-up [8]. There were no major intraoperative complications, however postoperatively two women developed abdominal pain and at laparoscopy were found to have bowel adhesions to exposed mesh. Adhesiolysis was undertaken for both and subsequently practice altered to include routine full re-peritonization of mesh. In our second, larger series we reported on 182 women, with follow-up of 140 women at a median of 2.1 years (range 1–4.4) [10]. Two women (1.1%) underwent subsequent hysterectomy, one for bowel symptoms and another for menstrual dysfunction. One woman (0.5%) had an intraoperative broad ligament vascular injury requiring laparotomy. Three women (2%) developed pain related to adhesions, which were laparoscopically divided, and one woman (0.5%) a pulmonary embolus. Other complications included infected perineal wounds (13 women, 9%), urinary retention (four women, 3%), urinary tract infection (four women, 3%), voiding dysfunction (five women, 4%), and constipation (18 women, 14%). There were no vaginal mesh erosions.

Subsequent to our first two cohort studies we undertook a pilot randomized controlled trial to compare LSH to the national gold standard of VH and apical suspension [9]. One-hundred-and-thirty-two patients were recruited and at one-year, data was available for 73 women (37 following LSH and 35 following VH), with a case note review for those that did not attend. There were no intraoperative complications in either group, but LSH was associated with significant lower blood loss, fewer nights in hospital, lower 24-hour postoperative pain scores and time to return to normal activity as shown in Table 12.1. There were no mesh-associated complications or serious adverse events at one year. Our largest single centre cohort was published in 2017, where we undertook a case note review of 507 women who had been operated on over a decade, most of whom had three-month routine follow-up [5]. It is worth noting that we are the only urogynaecology centre in our region and therefore the likelihood of patients having received care elsewhere is low. In this series there was one intraoperative bladder injury, three incidences of haemorrhage, and three instances of bowel adhesions requiring re-laparoscopy. There were no vaginal mesh erosions and the overall incidence of complications is shown in Table 12.2. Two patients underwent subsequent hysterectomy for menstrual dysfunction and three patients were diagnosed with gynaecological cancers (two with early endometrial cancer at 2 and 18 months postoperatively and a third with cervical cancer at two years postoperatively). Seventeen patients had their LSH abandoned due to deviant anatomy, with most undergoing vaginal hysterectomy for which they were consented preoperatively.

There are additional studies corroborating our findings in women that have undergone the Oxford Hysteropexy outside of our centre. University College London Hospitals (UCLH) offer the same surgical approach and have reported on data from 110 women at a mean follow-up of 2.6 years in a paper by Kupelian et al [64]. Authors reported that two women (1.8%) sustained adverse events, one a diathermy burn to the sigmoid colon that was over sewn and another a postoperative small bowel obstruction due to bowel tethering on to an exposed barbed suture. Both had longer inpatient stays but were discharged with no adverse morbidity. They reported no other visceral injuries, haemorrhages, thromboembolic events, or graft complications.

Table 12.1 Safety data favouring laparoscopic mesh sacrohysteropexy

	Laparoscopic hysteropexy (n=50)	Vaginal hysterectomy (n=50)	p value*
Mean duration of operation, min (range)	39.5 (25–60)	28.1 (15–50)	<0.001
Mean pain score 24 hours postoperatively, scale 1–10 (range)	3.6 (1–7)	4.6 (2–7)	0.002
Mean estimated blood loss, ml (SD)	19.6 (5–50)	82.1 (3–300)	<0.001
Mean number of nights in hospital (range)	2.1 (1–6)	2.5 (1–6)	0.005
Mean return to normal activity, weeks (range)	5.6 (3–16)	6.8 (2–16)	0.012

Table 12.2 Incidence of complications following laparoscopic mesh sacrohysteropexy

	n (%)
Major complications	
Pulmonary embolus	2 (0.4)
Bladder injury	1 (0.2)
Haemorrhage	3 (0.6)
Adhesions to mesh	3 (0.6)
Mesh extrusion	0 (0)
Minor complications	
Urinary tract infection	6 (1.2)
Perineal infection (concomitant posterior repair)	16 (3.2)
Voiding difficulty post-surgery	11 (2.2)

More recently, to address the concerns surrounding mesh-associated complications, we undertook a collaborative study between Oxford and UCLH [11]. This large cross-sectional study reported data from 1,121 women at a median of 46 months postoperatively, finding a re-operation rate for mesh-associated complications of 0.4% (four women). The incidence of chronic pain service use in the cohort was 1.78% and autoimmune disease rates were comparable to that reported in other studies.

It is worth noting that both the safety and efficacy data for the Oxford LSH appear favourable in comparison to other forms of native tissue and mesh-augmented prolapse surgery. From a safety perspective, a Cochrane review showed the risk of re-operation for mesh exposure following placement of transvaginal mesh for prolapse is 8%, and in the PROSPECT trial, the largest randomized trial of transvaginal mesh, 4% of women required re-operation for a mesh complication [29,48]. Following subtotal hysterectomy and cervicopexy, the reported mesh exposure rate is between 4.3% and 10.5% 65. Uterine preservation may confer the benefit of a lower risk of mesh erosion than that seen in other abdominal approaches to prolapse.

Other long-term cohort studies of alternative mesh hysteropexy techniques have reported mesh erosion rates of 4% following robotic-assisted sacrohysteropexy, and 5% following open sacrohysteropexy, with no details regarding the risk of re-operation [66,67].

Efficacy Data

The efficacy of surgical interventions for POP may be determined by objective measures such as POPQ score or re-operation rates, or alternatively subjective ones such as symptom relief or scores from validated PROMs. In our initial series we reported that 50 of the 51 patients (98%) had a Baden Walker classification of grade 1 or less for uterine POP or a POP-Q point C of less than -2 at 10 weeks and were therefore deemed a surgical success. Five women underwent a subsequent local anaesthetic anterior colporrhaphy giving an objective cure rate of 90%. It is worth noting that we undertook high rates of concurrent procedures in this series, predominantly posterior colpoperineorrhaphy which was undertaken in 71% of women. In the subsequent series, 17 women underwent re-operation for POP therefore the objective cure rate was 91%. Six women (4.3%) had recurrent uterine prolapse for which three underwent subsequent surgery (two with laparoscopic plication of mesh, one with cervical amputation). Two were asymptomatic of this and one declined further surgery. Ten women (7%) underwent re-operation for anterior wall prolapse, a further 35 (25%) had anterior wall prolapse beyond the hymen, of which 21 (15%) were symptomatic. Only two women reported no change in patient global impression of improvement (PGI-I) in prolapse symptoms at initial follow-up, and 89% reported them to be 'much better' or 'very much better'.

In our pilot randomized controlled trial, the objective cure rate was 90% at one-year on the basis of re-operation for POP [9]. There was no significant difference between this and the VH group. The risk of re-operation for apical prolapse however was lower in the LSH group (4% versus 8%). Our data did suggest that LSH was associated with a higher apical suspension of point C (-5.4 versus -4.3, p<0.001) and a longer TVL (8.35 versus 6.5, p<0.001). Eighty-two per cent of women rated their symptoms as 'much better' or 'very much better' after LSH, and there was no difference between the PGI-I and International Consultation on Incontinence Questionnaire– Vaginal symptoms (ICIQ-VS) between the two groups. In our large cohort, the objective cure rate based on re-operation for POP was 87.7% [5]. Fourteen women (2.8%) underwent subsequent apical surgery, for ten of whom this was simply a plication of the hysteropexy mesh to tighten it and increase elevation. Thirty-six women (7.1%) underwent colporrhaphy following LSH. There was a mean elevation of point C of 7.9 cm. With respect to PGI-I data, it was available for 404 patients, of whom 367 (93.8%) described their prolapse as 'much better' or 'very much better'. Considering the efficacy of alternatives, VH with apical suspension is associated with a high risk of recurrent vault prolapse; rates of re-operation for prolapse are between 4.6% and 18% [19,20].

With respect to the efficacy date from Kupelian et al, outcomes were reported at three months and then by telephone follow-up at variable timeframes with a median of 2.6 years [64]. The rate of concurrent vaginal repair in this cohort was 11% (12 women), which is significantly lower than the 54% (276 women) reported in our own paper by Jefferis et al [5]. At the three-month physical, the median point C was -7 and 98% of patients had an apical compartment prolapse stage 1 or less. There were however significant rates of anterior wall prolapse (41% stage 2 or higher) and posterior wall prolapse (25% stage 2 or higher). Overall, the objective cure rate based on re-operation for POP over the study period was 95%. Of the 81 women with telephone follow-up, 96% were satisfied with the surgery, reporting their prolapse as 'much better' or 'very much better' and 81% were asymptomatic for POP based on a screening question from the ICIQ-VS. The collaborative study with 1,121 participants at an average of four years found a re-operation rate of 13.56% (152 women) [11]. However, the majority of these were routine colporrhaphy and the apical re-operation rate was 3.7%. 81.4% of participants reported a PGI-I of 'very much better' or 'much better', and 82.2% of respondents would recommend the operation to a friend.

Outcomes in Specific Populations

Women Desiring Fertility Preservation

Our routine practice is to advise all patients to complete their family prior to undergoing surgery for POP. However, there are situations where this may not be possible due to severe POP that significantly impairs quality of life, or POP that is associated with morbidity such as recurrent UTI due to voiding dysfunction or more rarely ureteric obstruction. In this situation uterine conserving surgery is an option, however very careful counselling is mandated. Potential implications include a compromise of uterine blood supply and adverse outcomes for foetal growth, disruption of physiological uterine changes associated with pregnancy, and the risk of recurrence due to mesh stretching or detaching. We have reported a small series of six women who became pregnant following LSH [6]. All women were delivered by elective caesarean section, having had normal serial antenatal foetal growth scans, all giving birth to infants above the 10th centile, and none had apical prolapse at postpartum follow-up with a urogynaecologist at an average of nine weeks postpartum. Two women reported POP symptoms at this short-term follow-up but were found to have anterior wall prolapse. While these numbers are small and inadequate as to provide reassurance to women that post LSH pregnancy is safe, they are positive and suggest that for the most severe cases in women with future fertility desires, LSH is an option with appropriate counselling and recognition of the lack of data.

The Older Patient

The correlation between age and POP is well established and older patients, particularly in their eighth decade of life, require significantly more outpatient resources for care of the condition than younger women [68]. Associated with this are the concepts of frailty and biological age, which both correlate with an increased risk of morbidity and mortality [69]. Our centre has reported the outcomes of 55 women who underwent laparoscopic prolapse surgery over the age of 79 [7]. With a mean age of 93 (range 79–96), 26 underwent LSH and 30 underwent laparoscopic sacrocolpopexy. Most patients were ASA grade 2 or 3 (71.4% and 14.3% respectively). Prior to discharge, a high proportion of patients developed constipation (six women, 10.9%) and urinary tract infection and hypertension were also common (5% and 3.5% respectively). Constipation and UTI were common complaints at follow-up. There were no perioperative deaths or serious adverse events, and the average length of stay was 2.3 days; this did not correlate significantly with either age or ASA grade. Five women (9%) required further prolapse surgery, and the objective anatomical cure rate postoperatively was 80% at an average of 10 weeks. These efficacy outcomes mirror that reported in our large cohorts more generally.

Conclusion

Given the current climate surrounding the use of mesh in pelvic floor surgery, the evolving field of laparoscopic prolapse surgery is difficult to predict. Widespread adoption of LSH is limited by surgical training, access to laparoscopic equipment, and concerns around mesh use. The paucity of high-quality, prospective comparative data also creates a difficult case for more routine use. Despite these limitations, the procedure offers advantages including uterine preservation, a minimally invasive surgical approach, and the augmentation of repair with non-absorbable mesh which potentially enhances longevity. While further studies are required, systematic reviews do suggest a role for LSH and patients deserve the provision of the procedure as a choice where appropriate [28].

The Oxford hysteropexy appears to be safe and the avoidance of vaginal dissection and mesh placement is a likely reason for this. The outcome data available suggest at least equivalent efficacy in the medium term to alternative procedures. There is however a need for further prospective comparative studies of safety, efficacy, and cost efficiency, as well as data regarding long-term outcomes.

References

1. Haylen BT, Maher CF, Barber MD, et al. An International Urogynecological Association (IUGA)/International Continence Society (ICS) joint report on the terminology for female pelvic organ prolapse (POP). Int Urogynecol Journal 2016; 27(2): 165–94.
2. Hendrix SL, Clark A, Nygaard I, et al. Pelvic organ prolapse in the Women's Health Initiative: gravity and gravidity. Am J Obstet Gynecol 2002; 186(6): 1160–6.
3. Slieker-ten Hove MCP, Pool-Goudzwaard AL, Eijkemans MJ, et al. The prevalence of pelvic organ prolapse symptoms and signs and their relation with bladder and bowel disorders in a general female population. Int Urogynecol J 2009; 20(9): 1037–45.
4. Smith FJ, Holman CAJ, Moorin RE, Tsokos N. Lifetime risk of undergoing surgery for pelvic organ prolapse. ObstetGynecol 2010; 116(5): 1096–100.
5. Jefferis H, Price N, Jackson S. Laparoscopic hysteropexy: 10 years' experience. Int Urogynecol J 2017; 28(8): 1241–8.
6. Jefferis H, Price N, Jackson S. Pregnancy following laparoscopic hysteropexy—a case series. Gynecol Surg 2017; 14(1): 1–4.
7. King SW, Jefferis H, Jackson S, et al. Laparoscopic uterovaginal prolapse surgery in the elderly: feasibility and outcomes. Gynecol Surg 2017; 14(1): 2.

8. Price N, Slack A, Jackson S. Laparoscopic hysteropexy: the initial results of a uterine suspension procedure for uterovaginal prolapse. BJOG 2010; 117(1): 62–8.
9. Rahmanou P, Price N, Jackson SR. Laparoscopic hysteropexy versus vaginal hysterectomy for the treatment of uterovaginal prolapse: a prospective randomized pilot study. Int Urogynecol J 2015; 26(11): 1687–94.
10. Rahmanou P, White B, Price N, Jackson S. Laparoscopic hysteropexy: 1- to 4-year follow-up of women postoperatively. Int Urogynecol J 2014; 25(1): 131–8.
11. Izett-Kay ML, Aldabeeb D, Kupelian AS, et al. Long-term mesh complications and reoperation after laparoscopic mesh sacrohysteropexy: a cross-sectional study. Int Urogynecol J 2020: 31(12): 2595–602
12. National Institute for Health and Care Excellence. Urinary incontinence and pelvic organ prolapse in women: management [NG 123]. Published 2019.
13. Li C, Gong Y, Wang B. The efficacy of pelvic floor muscle training for pelvic organ prolapse: a systematic review and meta-analysis. Int Urogynecol J 2016; 27(7): 981–92.
14. Hagen S, Stark D, Glazener C, et al. Individualised pelvic floor muscle training in women with pelvic organ prolapse (POPPY): a multicentre randomised controlled trial. Lancet 2014; 383(9919): 796–806.
15. Brazell HD, Patel M, O'Sullivan DM, et al. The impact of pessary use on bowel symptoms: one-year outcomes. Female Pelvic Med Reconstr Surg 2014; 20(2): 95–8.
16. Jones K, Yang L, Lowder JL, et al. Effect of pessary use on genital hiatus measurements in women with pelvic organ prolapse. Obstet Gynecol 2008; 112(3): 630–6.
17. Abdool Z, Thakar R, Sultan AH, Oliver RS. Prospective evaluation of outcome of vaginal pessaries versus surgery in women with symptomatic pelvic organ prolapse. Int Urogynecol J 2011; 22(3): 273–8.
18. Jha S, Cutner A, Moran P. The UK national prolapse survey: 10 years on. Int Urogynecol J 2018; 29(6): 795–801.
19. Jelovsek JE, Barber MD, Brubaker L, et al. Effect of uterosacral ligament suspension vs sacrospinous ligament fixation with or without perioperative behavioral therapy for pelvic organ vaginal prolapse on surgical outcomes and prolapse symptoms at 5 years in the OPTIMAL randomized clinical trial. JAMA 2018; 319(15): 1554–65.
20. Edenfield AL, Amundsen CL, Weidner AC, et al. Vaginal prolapse recurrence after uterosacral ligament suspension in normal-weight compared with overweight and obese women. Obstet Gynecol 2013; 121(3): 554–9.
21. Aigmueller T, Dungl A, Hinterholzer S, et al. An estimation of the frequency of surgery for post hysterectomy vault prolapse. Int Urogynecol J 2010; 21(3): 299–302.
22. Olsen AL, Smith VJ, Bergstrom JO, et al. Epidemiology of surgically managed pelvic organ prolapse and urinary incontinence. Obstet Gynecol 1997; 89(4): 501–6.
23. Frick AC, Barber MD, Paraiso MFR, et al. Attitudes toward hysterectomy in women undergoing evaluation for uterovaginal prolapse. Female Pelvic Med Reconstr Surg 2013; 19(2): 103–9.
24. Zacche MM, Mukhopadhyay S, Giarenis I. Trends in prolapse surgery in England. Int Urogynecol J 2018; 29(11): 1689–95.
25. Husby KR, Larsen MD, Lose G, Klarskov N. Surgical treatment of primary uterine prolapse: a comparison of vaginal native tissue surgical techniques. Int Urogynecol J 2019; 11: 1887–93.
26. Cutner A, Rymer J. Patient recovery after laparoscopic colposuspension. Gynaecol Endosc 1998; 7(6): 307–8.
27. Nair R, Nikolopoulos K, Claydon L. Clinical outcomes in women undergoing laparoscopic hysteropexy: a systematic review. Eur J Obstet Gynecol Reprod Biol 2017; 208: 71–80.
28. Meriwether KV, Antosh DD, Olivera CK, et al. Uterine preservation versus hysterectomy in pelvic organ prolapse surgery: a systematic review with meta analysis and clinical practice guidelines. Am J Obstet Gynecol 2018; 219(2): 129–46.
29. Glazener CM, Breeman S, Elders A, et al. Mesh, graft, or standard repair for women having primary transvaginal anterior or posterior compartment prolapse surgery: two parallel-group, multicentre, randomised, controlled trials (PROSPECT). Lancet 2017; 389(10067): 381–92.
30. Gornall J. How mesh became a four-letter word. BMJ 2018; 363: k4137.
31. SCENIHR, European Commission. The safety of surgical meshes used in urogynaecological surgery. Available at: https://ec.europa.eu/health/scientific_committees/consultations/public_consultations/scenihr_consultation_27_en. Published 2015.
32. NHS England. Mesh Oversight Group Report. Available at:www.england.nhs.uk/publication/mesh-oversight-group-report/. Published 2017.
33. Therapeutic Goods Administration, Australian Department of Health. TGA undertakes regulatory actions after review into urogynaecological surgical mesh implants. Available at:www.tga.gov.au/alert/tga-actions-after-review-urogynaecological-surgical-mesh-implants. Published 2018.
34. Wise J. Surgical mesh for stress urinary incontinence to be halted immediately in England. BMJ 2018; 10; 362: k3035. https://doi.org/10.1136/bmj.k3035
35. Scottish Government. The Scottish independent review of the use, safety and efficacy of transvaginal mesh implants in the treatment of stress urinary incontinence and pelvic organ prolapse in women: final report. Available at: www.gov.scot/Publications/2017/03/3336/3. Published 2017.
36. Geller EJ, Babb E, Nackley AG, Zolnoun D. Incidence and risk factors for pelvic pain after mesh implant surgery for the treatment of pelvic floor disorders. J Minim Invasive Gynecol 2017; 24(1): 67–73.
37. Chughtai B, Sedrakyan A, Mao J, et al. Is vaginal mesh a stimulus of autoimmune disease? Am J Obstet Gynecol 2017; 216(5): 495. e491–495. e497.
38. Chapple CR, Cruz F, Deffieux X, et al. Consensus statement of the European Urology Association and the European Urogynaecological Association on the use of implanted materials for treating pelvic organ prolapse and stress urinary incontinence. Eur Urol 2017; 72(3): 424–31.
39. Nelson EC, Eftimovska E, Lind C, et al. Patient reported outcome measures in practice. BMJ 2015; 350: g7818.
40. Abrams P, Cardozo, L, Wagg, A, Wein, A. (eds). *Incontinence*, 6th edn. International Continence Society; 2017.
41. Athanasiou S, Hill S, Gleeson C, et al. Validation of the ICS proposed pelvic organ prolapse descriptive system. Neurourol 1995; 14: 4.
42. Hall AF, Theofrastous JP, Cundiff GW, et al. Interobserver and intraobserver reliability of the proposed International Continence Society, Society of Gynecologic Surgeons, and American Urogynecologic Society pelvic organ prolapse

classification system. Am J Obstet Gynecol 1996; 175(6): 1467–71.
43. Kegel AH. Progressive resistance exercise in the functional restoration of the perineal muscles. Am J Obstet Gynecol 1948; 56(2): 238–48.
44. Laycock J. Incontinence. Pelvic floor re-education. Nursing 1991; 4(39): 15–17.
45. Bø K, Finckenhagen HB. Vaginal palpation of pelvic floor muscle strength: inter-test reproducibility and comparison between palpation and vaginal squeeze pressure. Acta Obstet Gynecol Scandi 2001; 80(10): 883–7.
46. National Health Service. Excellence NIfHaC. Surgery for uterine prolapse. Patient decision aid. Available at: www.nice.org.uk/guidance/ng123/resources/patient-decision-aid-pdf-6725286112
47. FitzGerald MP, Richter HE, Siddique S, et al. Colpocleisis: a review. Int Urogynecol J 2006; 17(3): 261–71.
48. Maher C, Feiner B, Baessler K, et al. Transvaginal mesh or grafts compared with native tissue repair for vaginal prolapse. Cochrane Library 2016; 9(2): CD012079.
49. Moran P, Foon R, Assassa P. The BSUG national database: concept, design, implementation and beyond. Obstet Gynaecol 2013; 15(2): 120–7.
50. Haylen BT, Freeman RM, Swift SE, et al. An International Urogynecological Association (IUGA)/International Continence Society (ICS) joint terminology and classification of the complications related directly to the insertion of prostheses (meshes, implants, tapes) and grafts in female pelvic floor surgery. Neurourol 2011; 30(1): 2–12.
51. Usher F. Hernia repair with knitted polypropylene mesh. Surg Gynecol Obstet 1963; 117: 239–40.
52. Zoedler D, Boeminghaus H. On indication and technique of suspension plastic surgery. *Zeitschrift fur Urologie und Nephrologie* 1965; 58(7): 459.
53. Heneghan CJ, Goldacre B, Onakpoya I, et al. Trials of transvaginal mesh devices for pelvic organ prolapse: a systematic database review of the US FDA approval process. BMJ Open 2017; 7(12): e017125.
54. Petros PEP, Ulmsten UI. The combined intravaginal sling and tuck operation. An ambulatory procedure for cure of stress and urge incontinence. Acta Obstet Gynecol Scandi 1990; 69(S153): 53–9.
55. Arthure HG, Savage D. Uterine prolapse and prolapse of the vaginal vault treated by sacral hysteropexy. BJOG1957; 64(3): 355–60.
56. Chaudhuri S. The place of sling operations in treating genital prolapse in young women. Int J Gynecol Obstet 1979; 16(4): 314–20.
57. Farkas A, Shepherd J, Woodhouse C. Hysterosacropexy for uterine prolapse with associated urinary tract abnormalities. J Obstet Gynaecol 1993; 13(5): 358–60.
58. Leron E, Stanton SL. Sacrohysteropexy with synthetic mesh for the management of uterovaginal prolapse. BJOG 2001; 108(6): 629–33.
59. Cutner A, Kearney R, Vashisht A. Laparoscopic uterine sling suspension: a new technique of uterine suspension in women desiring surgical management of uterine prolapse with uterine conservation. BJOG 2007; 114(9): 1159–62.
60. Bonkat G, Pickard R, Bartoletti R, et al. EAU guidelines on urological infections. European Association of Urology; 2017, pp 22–6.
61. National Institute for Health and Care Excellence. Surgical site infections: prevention and treatment [NG125]. Published 2019.
62. Royal College of Obstetricians and Gynaecologists. Preventing entry-related gynaecological laparoscopic injuries. Published 2008.
63. Elneil S, Cutner AS, Remy M, et al. Abdominal sacrocolpopexy for vault prolapse without burial of mesh: a case series. BJOG 2005; 112(4): 486–9.
64. Kupelian AS, Vashisht A, Sambandan N, Cutner A. Laparoscopic wrap round mesh sacrohysteropexy for the management of apical prolapse. Int Urogynecol J 2016; 27(12): 1889–97.
65. Jia X, Glazener C, Mowatt G, et al. Systematic review of the efficacy and safety of using mesh in surgery for uterine or vaginal vault prolapse. Int Urogynecol J 2010; 21(11): 1413–31.
66. Grimminck K, Mourik S, Tjin-Asjoe F, et al. Long-term follow-up and quality of life after robot-assisted sacrohysteropexy. Eur J Obstet Gynecol Reprod Biol 2016; 206: 27–31.
67. Paek J, Lee M, Kim BW, Kwon Y. Robotic or laparoscopic sacrohysteropexy versus open sacrohysteropexy for uterus preservation in pelvic organ prolapse. Int Urogynecol J 2016; 27(4): 593–9.
68. Luber KM, Boero S, Choe JY. The demographics of pelvic floor disorders: current observations and future projections. Am J Obstet Gynecol 2001; 184(7): 1496–503.
69. Farhat JS, Velanovich V, Falvo AJ, et al. Are the frail destined to fail? Frailty index as predictor of surgical morbidity and mortality in the elderly. J Trauma Acute Care Surg 2012; 72(6): 1526–31.

Chapter 13

Laparoscopic Hysteropexy: Procedure Steps and Evidence

Yara Abdelkhalek, Nikolaus Veit-Rubin, Bruno Deval

Introduction

Pelvic organ prolapse is a condition that affects millions of women worldwide and has an enormous negative impact on their quality of life [1]. It is the downward displacement of the pelvic organs (uterus or vaginal vault, bladder and/or rectum) following a weakness in the pelvic floor support system (levator ani muscles, ligamentous and connective tissue and nerves) [2], and presents as a sensation of vaginal bulge associated with an impairment in urinary, bowel, and/or sexual functions. The apical prolapse consists of uterine prolapse, or vaginal vault prolapse in the case of hysterectomy. The uterus may herniate into or even beyond the hymeneal ring. When the prolapse is symptomatic, it usually affects multiple compartments (cystocele: anterior vaginal wall and/or rectocele: posterior vaginal wall) [3]. Thus, the correction of vaginal prolapse is a must to restore the woman's normal pelvic anatomy, treat urinary, bowel, and sexual dysfunctions, and improve their quality of life [4].

Historically, pelvic organ prolapse was cured by vaginal hysterectomy, but the uterus itself is not the cause of this disease, therefore removing it does not correct the defect in the pelvic floor support, which may lead to further recurrences and need for re-interventions hereafter [4,5].

Also, some studies have shown that hysterectomy is associated with damage to the nerve supply system, causing weakness to the pelvic floor, potentially increasing the risk of prolapse recurrence. Indeed, 11.6% of women treated with hysterectomy developed vaginal vault prolapse afterwards, with 6% to 8% of re-interventions [6]. In fact, the first-line therapy for pelvic organ prolapse is non-surgical conservative treatment (pelvic floor physical therapy, vaginal pessary) [3,7], but when surgical intervention is indicated, laparoscopic hysteropexy provides durable anatomic and physiologic restoration of the pelvic organs, with normal vaginal axis and thus good sexual satisfaction [5]. As well as its good anatomical and functional results, laparoscopic hysteropexy preserves the uterus, which allows further fertility if desired, along with better sexual well-being, self-esteem, and quality of life [4].

Epidemiology

Pelvic organ prolapse is a common condition and its incidence is increasing with the increase in life expectancy. In 1961, 3% of women reported a symptomatic vaginal bulge in one population-based study [8]. Nowadays, one woman in 12 reports symptoms of vaginal prolapse according to a study done in UK [9]. A loss of pelvic floor support is perceived in up to 30% to 76% of women during routine gynaecologic examination, with 3% to 6% of these prolapses protruding beyond the hymen [3]. A women's lifetime risk of any type of prolapse repair surgery is 11% to 19% [4,6,10]. After the procedure, there is a 30% risk of re-intervention for recurrence [4].

Pelvic organ prolapse represents the only indication in 15% to 18% of hysterectomies, and it is the most common cause for hysterectomy in postmenopausal women [11].

Clinical Presentation

Pelvic organ prolapse may be asymptomatic for years. With advanced stages of prolapse, symptoms vary from an isolated sensation of vaginal fullness to increased vaginal discharge, lower abdominal and back pain, and a vaginal bulge that can be in some cases seen [3,5].

Other symptoms may appear, such as urinary urgency (86%), stress incontinence (73%), difficulty to empty the bowel (31%) or rectal fullness, if cystocele or rectocele are associated [3,5]. In the case of severe prolapse (procidentia) (Figure 13.1), skin erosions of the vagina and cervix may develop, leading to vaginal bleeding and possible infections [3,5]. Other rare complications of untreated pelvic organ prolapse are obstruction at the level of the urethra, the bladder, or the ureters, with hydronephrosis and ultimately renal failure [2]. In addition to its physical limitations, pelvic organ prolapse is associated with major psychological and sexual discomfort; at this stage treatment is mandatory to improve women's quality of life.

Risk Factors

Many risk factors have been associated with pelvic organ prolapse; they can be classified into obstetric, medical, social, and family history factors.

Obstetric risk factors are:

- Multiple pregnancies. One observational study showed that compared to nulliparous women, those who had two deliveries have a relative risk of pelvic organ prolapse of 8.4, with this risk increasing to 10.9 with four or more deliveries [12].
- Vaginal childbirth, especially instrumental deliveries (Forceps). A study done in California with over 3,000 women concluded that vaginal birth increases the risk of prolapse by 46%, while caesarean delivery protects against pelvic organ prolapse [13].
- High infant birth weight (>4,500 g) [3].
- Prolonged second stage of labour [3].
- Maternal age <25 years at first delivery.

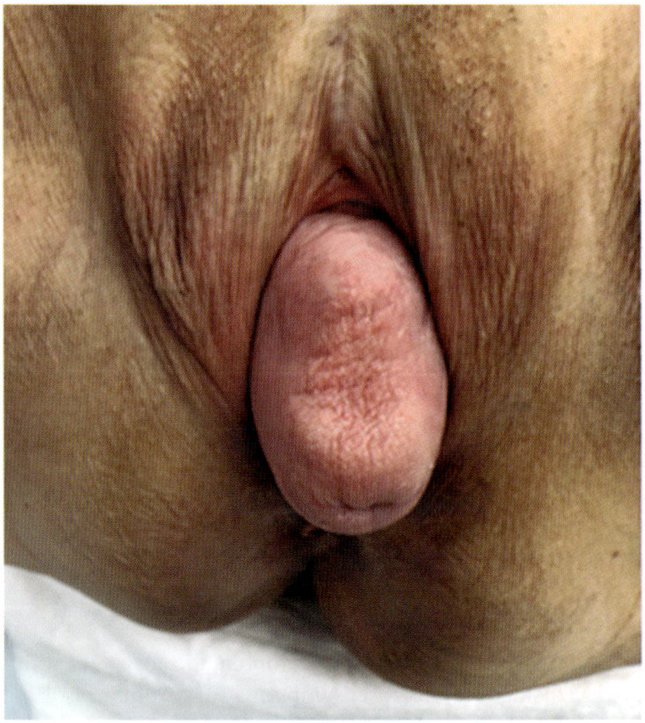

Figure 13.1 Genital prolapse.

Medical risk factors are:

- Advanced age. Studies show that the risk of prolapse increases by 40% after each decade of life, with the median age of surgical treatment 71 to 73 years [14].
- Increased body mass index [3].
- Prior hysterectomy [3].
- Connective tissue disorders, especially disease affecting the collagen type 1 gene COL1A1 [15].
- Chronic constipation [3].
- Shape and orientation of the pelvis [3].

Social risk factors:

- Occupational heavy lifting [3].

Family history risk factors:

- History of pelvic organ prolapse in close female relatives. A study showed that women are at significantly higher risk of prolapse if their mother or sister have had one [16].

Contra-indications

Laparoscopic hysteropexy is the first-line surgical treatment that should be offered to women presenting with grade 2 or more symptomatic pelvic organ prolapse, with whom conservative treatment no longer works.

Contra-indications to this procedure are few, they include [17]:

- Cervical dysplasia.
- Significant uterine abnormalities.
- Abnormal menstruation or post-menopausal bleeding.
- Current foreign body complications.
- Chronic pelvic pain.
- Prior prolapse repair with a synthetic mesh.

The presence of posterior wall fibroids is not a contra-indication for laparoscopic hysteropexy [5]. Myomectomy can be performed at the time of hysteropexy if its location is in the way of the correct placement of the mesh. Likewise, the desire of a future pregnancy may not necessarily defer the surgical treatment. Few cases of pregnancy have been reported after the procedure, as will be discussed later in this chapter.

Surgical Technique

Below we describe our technique in performing hysteropexy.

- Under general anaesthesia, the patient is placed in lithotomy position. Antibiotics are given according to individual hospital guidelines.
- Repeat clinical examination under general anaesthesia to recognize any weakness in the rectovaginal fascia, an indication to perform a combined anterior and posterior repair during the procedure.
- A bladder catheter is inserted along with a uterine manipulator to facilitate its mobilization.
- Pneumoperitoneum is created by using a Veress needle entry at Palmer's point.
- Four laparoscopic ports are needed: one umbilical 10 mm port and three 5 mm ports in the supra-pubic, right, and left iliac fossa.
- Before starting, perform an adequate evaluation of the abdominal cavity to rule out any pathology that may preclude hysteropexy.
- First the uterus is suspended to the anterior abdominal wall using a long straight needle to expose the uterosacral ligaments.
- If needed, the sigmoid colon is attached to the left lateral abdominal wall using the same technique to allow a better exposure of the posterior pouch of Douglas. Use this method with caution, especially when operating on the elderly or on patients with a known history of colonic diverticulosis.
- The sacral promontory is identified, as well as all the vital structures nearby (right common iliac vessels, right ureter).
- Start by opening the peritoneum at the level of the promontory. The pre-sacral space is an avascular space, so try to maintain the dissection as close to the midline to prevent any vascular damage. The dissection should not be excessive, and must be performed with extreme accuracy to preserve the superior hypogastric plexus below the promontory, thus protecting the autonomic innervation of the pelvic organs. The mean distance between the midsacral promontory and the right hypogastric nerve is 7 mm (0–17 mm) according to a vascular anatomy study conducted of female cadavers [18].
- A good haemostasis is a must to prevent any possible haemorrhagic complications afterwards. In our practice, we use a harmonic scalpel that allows precise dissection and adequate coagulation.

(a)

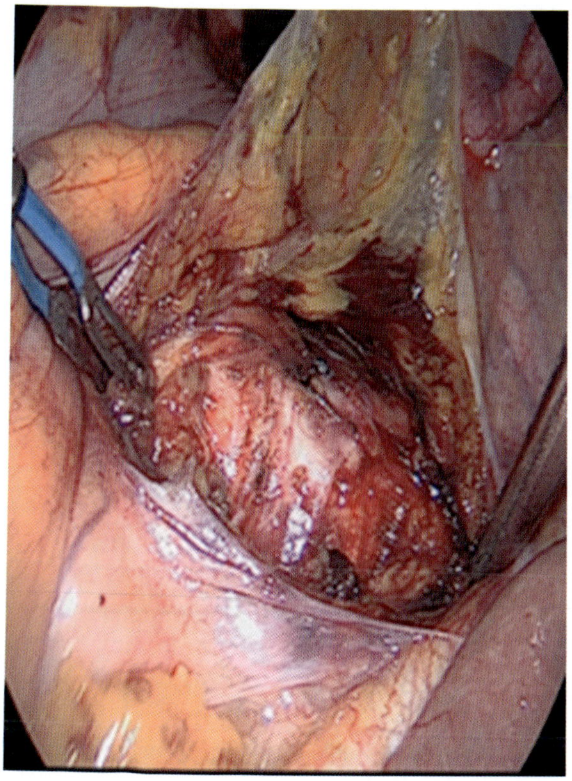

(b)

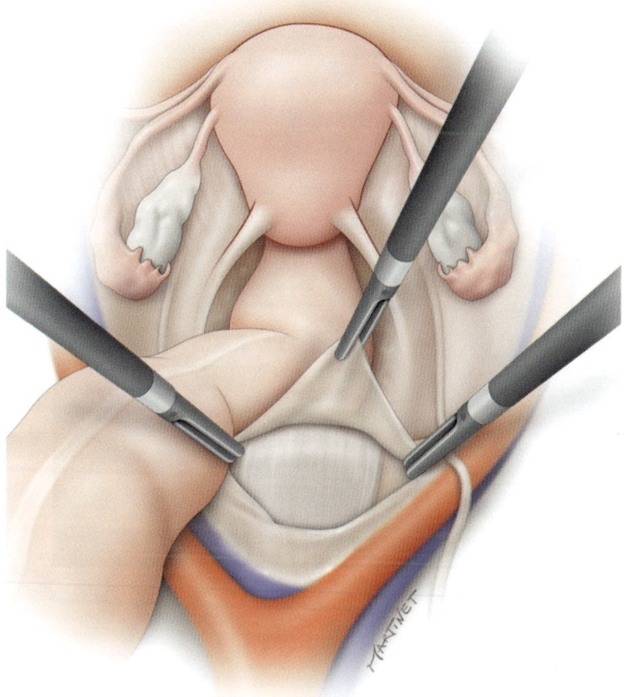

Figure 13.2 Promontory dissection and identification of the anterior longitudinal ligament.

- The anterior longitudinal ligament is identified; it consists of the solid support to which the uterus will be suspended (Figure 13.2).
- Initiate two stiches on the anterior longitudinal ligament using a non-absorbable Mersuture 2.0 to fix later on the meshes. Do not knot your threads at this point.
- Dissection of the peritoneum is continued towards the uterosacral ligaments.
- If a posterior mesh is needed, a malleable retractor is inserted in the posterior vaginal fornix to facilitate the dissection of the recto-vaginal space.
- Meticulous dissection following the posterior vaginal wall is done, to prevent any rectal bowel injury, which consists of a contra-indication to the use of the mesh afterwards. In our practice, we avoid dissection towards the levator ani because mesh fixation on these muscles may result in dyschezia and chronic pelvic pain.
- A single polypropylene 30 x 30 cm mesh is used to form the anterior and posterior mesh.
- The posterior mesh is first drawn and cut in a rectangular 4 x 15 cm shape.
- The mesh is introduced into the abdominal cavity and fixed to the posterior vaginal wall using at least six non-absorbable sutures of Mersuture 2.0.
- Attention is needed to avoid folding and wrinkling the mesh.
- Initiate the closure of the posterior peritoneum.
- The stich on the uterus is cut at this level, and the uterus is anteverted using the manipulator.
- Perform a dissection into the avascular space of the broad ligament at the level of the cervico-uterine junction bilaterally.
- The uterus is retroverted using the manipulator to proceed to the anterior repair.
- The vesico-uterine peritoneum is opened and the bladder is dissected distally 3 to 4 cm. The dissection is facilitated by using a malleable retractor inserted in the anterior vaginal fornix (Figure 13.3).
- Dissection should be maintained close to the anterior face of the vagina to prevent any bladder injury, especially if a previous caesarean section was performed. If opened, the bladder can be immediately sutured and the mesh can still be placed.
- A Y-shape, 15 cm mesh is drawn, cut, and introduced into the abdominal cavity.
- The mesh is fixed to the anterior vaginal wall using at least six non-absorbable sutures of Mersure 2.0.
- The arms of the anterior mesh are passed through windows created into the broad ligaments bilaterally, creating a loop around the cervix (Figure 13.4).
- Both meshes are well stretched towards the sacral promontory where they are anchored using ProTack, then sutured using the two knots initiated there before (Figure 13.5).
- Avoid excessive tension on the meshes, which may lead to urinary retention and constipation later on.
- Cut any extra portion of the meshes, then close the peritoneum to completely cover them.

(a)

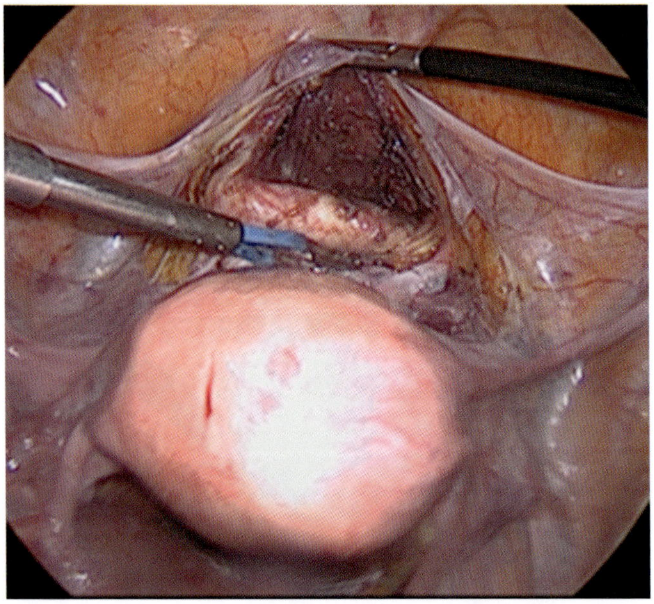

(b)

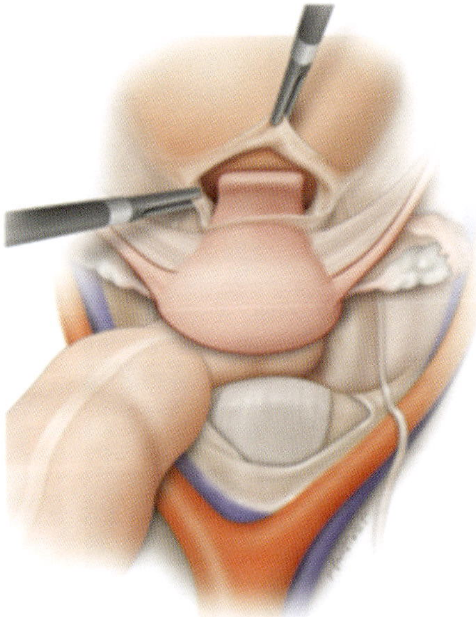

Figure 13.3 Vesico-uterine dissection.

(a)

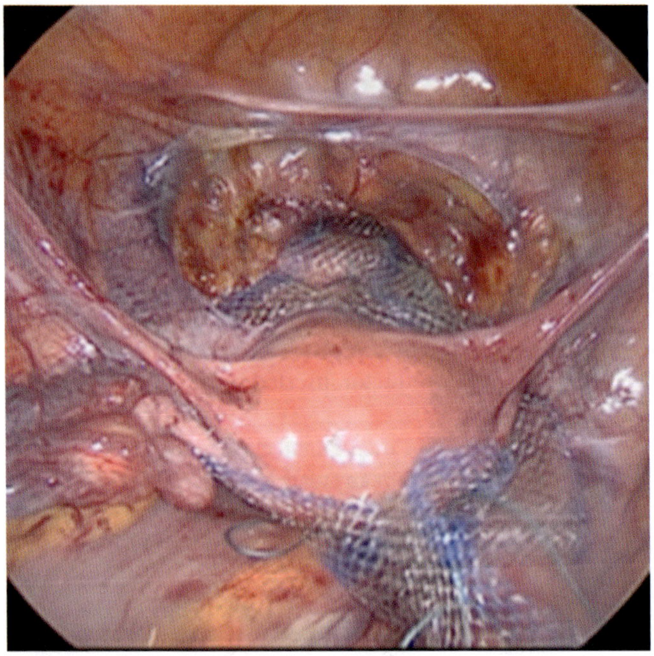

(b)

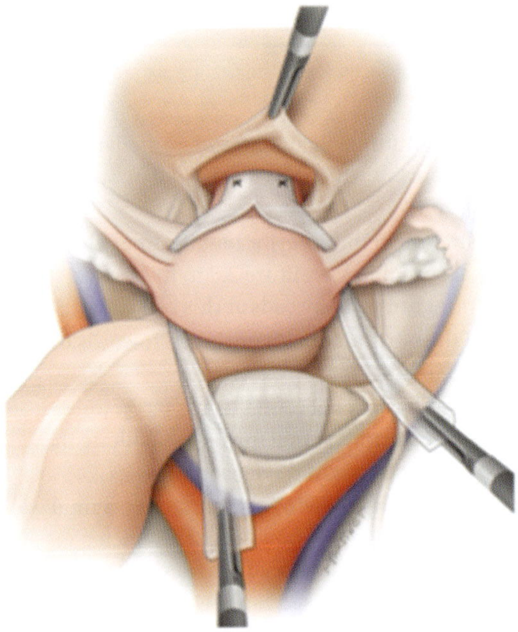

Figure 13.4 Mesh placement.

- No surgical drain is usually needed.
- Remove all laparoscopic ports and close the wounds.
- Vaginal examination is recommended to assess the degree of prolapse repair.
- We do not recommend any contemporary procedures such as tapes to treat stress urinary incontinence or posterior myorrhaphy.
- Mean operative time is 120 minutes, depending on the surgeon's experience. The learning curve for laparoscopic hysteropexy is over 60 procedures [7].
- Non-opioid analgesics usually provide adequate pain relief.
- Bladder catheter can be removed on day one after the surgery if no bladder injury occurred, and total hospital stay is around three days. In the case of bladder injury, keep catheterization for five days.
- We recommend abstinence from heavy physical activities for at least six weeks.

Postoperative Outcomes

Laparoscopic hysteropexy is considered the procedure of choice to restore the normal pelvic anatomy, with good apical support and normal vaginal axis. It is associated with a major

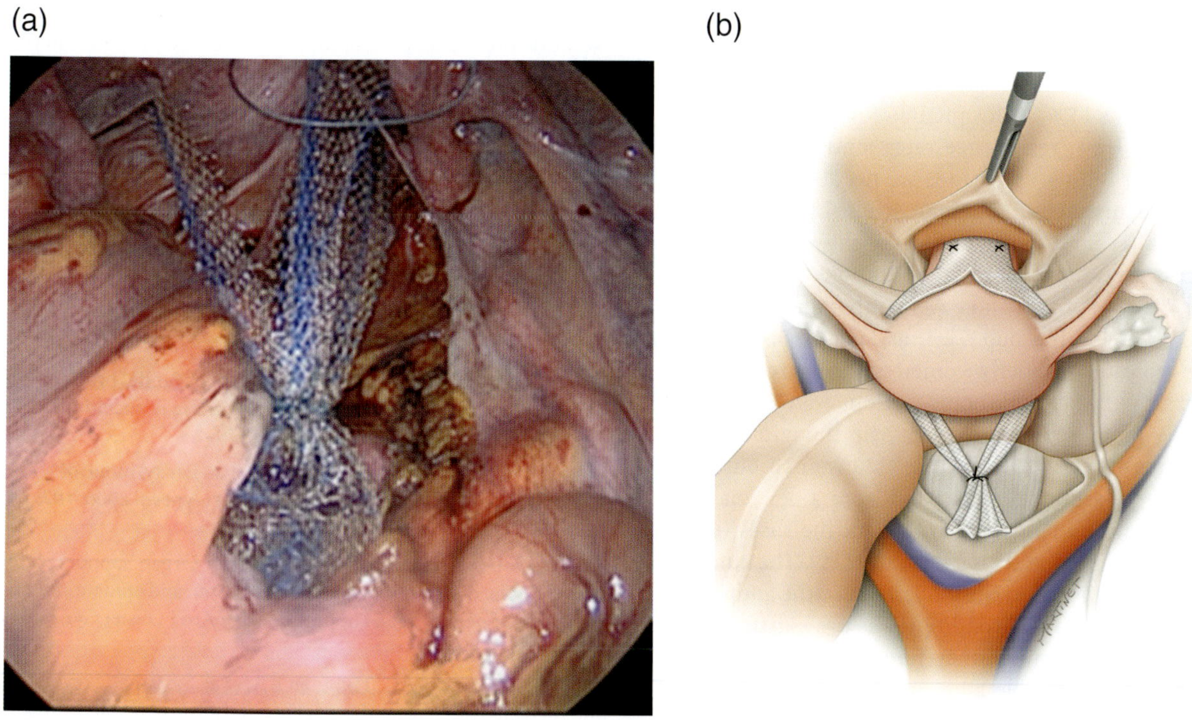

Figure 13.5 Mesh fixation on the promontory.

improvement in point C measurements on the POP-Q score [4]. Obviously, the correct mesh positioning is a major factor for its long-term success [5]. The good anatomical repair is associated with very high rates of patient satisfaction (84%) [4,6,19] and improved quality of life (94%) [20]. Overall satisfaction persists even at long-term follow-up (81.4% according to a recent cross-sectional study performed in the UK on 1,121 women over 46 months of follow-up) [19]. Sexual satisfaction appears better compared to vaginal hysterectomy and vaginal mesh hysteropexy. This may be related to a longer vaginal length after laparoscopic hysteropexy [17]. No increased risk of dyspareunia was noted [4], even in long-term follow-up studies, and women were able to resume their sexual activity faster (72% after laparoscopic hysteropexy versus 44% after vaginal mesh hysteropexy at one year) [17]. Furthermore, laparoscopic hysteropexy has all the potential advantages of any laparoscopic procedure. It is associated with quick post-operative recovery, less blood loss and adhesion formation, which may facilitate a desired pregnancy [4,5,17]. The laparoscopic approach reduces the risk of vaginal contamination of the synthetic mesh [3]. Ureteric injuries are rare compared to the vaginal approach (<0.1%), and other possible complications are spondylitis (0.3%), rectal injuries (0.4%), small and large bowel injuries, bladder injuries (2%), as well as retroperitoneal hematomas. The risk of a major complication after a laparoscopic hysteropexy is about 2% [4]. Other minor complications may occur in 13% of cases; they include: urinary infection or retention, constipation, port site infection, and umbilical hernia [4]. Long-term complications consist of two major complaints: vaginal mesh erosion and recurrence of the prolapse. They may require a re-intervention in some cases. A recent UK cross-sectional study showed a low rate of mesh complications requiring removal (0.4% after a follow-up of four years in 1,121 women treated with laparoscopic hysteropexy) [19]. Likewise, the investigators compared the risk of re intervention for mesh complications following the three most common gynaecological, mesh-related procedures, and concluded that there is no evidence of increased risk of mesh complications following a laparoscopic hysteropexy (5% versus 2.4% after synthetic mid-urethral sling and 4% to 8% after transvaginal mesh according to the Cochrane review by Maher et al [21] and the PROSPECT trial respectively [19, 22]. A systematic review regrouping 17 studies done between 2000 and 2016, among which eight studies used the laparoscopic mesh suspension of the uterus to the promontory, found only one case of erosion in only one of the studies (Rosenblatt et al, a retrospective 40 cases series report [4,23]. Other studies showed a risk of mesh erosion of 0% to 6% [24]. But when comparing hysteropexy to hysterectomy with sacral colpopexy, the risk of mesh erosion was five times lower [25]. Thus, the placement of the mesh on a healing vaginal suture appears to be a major risk for subsequent mesh erosion later on, while the conservation of the cervix and the presence of an intact vaginal wall in laparoscopic hysteropexy appear protective against erosion [4]. Many studies showed no recurrence of the prolapse or low recurrence rates over time. One shortcoming in the literature is that the majority of these studies had short follow-up periods [4]. In the same systemic review mentioned above, the prospective observational study on 140 cases of laparoscopic hysteropexy by Rahmanou et al had the longest follow-up period (48 months) [4]. In this series, the rate of recurrence requiring re-intervention was 9% [26]. Likewise, Kupelian et al showed a recurrence rate of vaginal wall prolapse of 5% after hysteropexy in their retrospective

110 cases cohort over a period of 3 months to 31 months of follow-up [4,27]. In parallel, the re-operation rates for prolapse recurrence in the cross-sectional study of 1,121 UK women mentioned was 11%, with a median follow-up period of 46 months [19]. Thus, recurrence rates tend to increase with time and longer follow-up periods are needed to clearly assess the risks of recurrence after a laparoscopic hysteropexy.

Furthermore, a recent comparative study showed no difference in success rates and risk of complications in women under or above 70 years of age. There were only more urinary symptoms seen in the elderly group [7]. Thus, laparoscopic hysteropexy can be indicated in elderly women suffering from pelvic organ prolapse. Other chronic complications were noticed in the literature. Women reported chronic pain thought to be attributed to the mesh in 1.8% of the cases (20 women out of 1,121 in the UK cross-sectional study) and from a new diagnosed systemic autoimmune disease in 5.8% of the cases (65 women out of 1,121 women in the same study) [19]. The autoimmune disorders were not an exclusion criteria so the authors were unable to determine if this condition was pre-existing or took place after mesh placement, therefore more studies are needed to establish any possible auto-immune mesh-related effects [19].

Pregnancy

Among the literature, multiple pregnancies were reported after pelvic organ prolapse repair surgeries, but only two pregnancies followed a laparoscopic hysteropexy [4]. In 2010, Busby et al were the first to describe a full-term pregnancy and a caesarean delivery [28], then Gaddoneix reported a similar uneventful birth in 2012 [29]. No adverse effects on the prolapse repair were noted after these deliveries, with no re-intervention needed [4].

References

1. Biler A, Ertas E, Tosun G, et al. Perioperative complications and short-term outcomes of abdominal sacrocolpopexy, laparoscopic sacrocolpopexy, and laparoscopic pectopexy for apical prolapse. Int Braz J Urol 2018; 44(5): 996–1004.
2. Dwyer L, Keamey R. Conservative management of pelvic organ prolapse. Obst Gynecol Reprod Med 2017; 28: 1.
3. Barber M. Pelvic organ prolapse. BMJ 2016; 354: 1–9.
4. Nair R, Nikolopoulos K, Claydon L. Clinical outcomes in women undergoing laparoscopic hysteropexy: a systematic review. Eur J Obstet Gynecol Reprod Biol 2017; 208: 71–80.
5. Faraj R, Broome J. Laparoscopic sacrohysteropexy and myomectomy for uterine prolapse: a case report and review of the literature. J Med Case Reports 2009; 3(99): 1–4.
6. Ijsselmuiden M, Coolen AL, Detollenaere R, et al. Hysteropexy in the treatment of uterine prolapse stage 2 or higher: a multicenter randomized controlled non-inferiority trial comparing laparoscopic sacrohysteropexy with vaginal sacrospinous hysteropexy (LAVA-trial, study protocol). BMC Women's Health 2014; 14: 112.
7. Boudy AS, Thubert T, Vinchant M. Outcomes of laparoscopic sacropexy in women over 70: a comparative study. Eur J Obst Gynecol Reprod Biol 2016; 207: 178–83.
8. Nygaard I, Barber MD, Burgio KL, et al. Pelvic Floor Disorders Network. Prevalence of symptomatic pelvic floor disorders in US women. JAMA 2008; 300: 1311–16.
9. Cooper J, Annappa M, Dracocardos D, et al. Prevalence of genital prolapse symptoms in primary care: a cross-sectional survey. Int Urogynecol J 2015; 26: 505–10.
10. Smith FJ, Holman CD, Moorin RE, Tsokos N. Lifetime risk of undergoing surgery for pelvic organ prolapse. Obstet Gynecol 2010; 116: 1096–100.
11. Whiteman MK, Hillis SD, Jamieson DJ, et al. Inpatient hysterectomy surveillance in the United States, 2000–2004. Am J Obstet Gynecol 2008; 198: 34.e1–7.
12. Mant J, Painter R, Vessey M. Epidemiology of genital prolapse: observations from the Oxford Family Planning Association Study. Br J Obstet Gynaecol 1997; 104: 579–85.
13. Lukacz ES, Lawrence JM, Contreras R, et al. Parity, mode of delivery, and pelvic floor disorders. Obstet Gynecol 2006; 107: 1253–60.
14. Swift S, Woodman P, O'Boyle A, et al. Pelvic Organ Support Study (POSST): the distribution, clinical definition, and epidemiologic condition of pelvic organ support defects. Am J Obstet Gynecol 2005; 192: 795–806.
15. Cartwright R, Kirby AC, Tikkinen KA, et al. Systematic review and metaanalysis of genetic association studies of urinary symptoms and prolapse in women. Am J Obstet Gynecol 2015; 212(199): e1–24.
16. Chiaffarino F, Chatenoud L, Dindelli M, et al. Reproductive factors, family history, occupation and risk of urogenital prolapse. Eur J Obstet Gynecol Reprod Biol 1999; 82: 63–7.
17. Gutman RE, Rardin CR, Sokol ER, et al. Vaginal and laparoscopic mesh hysteropexy for uterovaginal prolapse: a parallel cohort study. Am J Obstet Gynecol 2017; 216: 38.e1–11.
18. Wieslander CK, Rahn DD, McIntire DD, et al. Vascular anatomy of the presacral space in umembalmed female cadavers. Am J Obstet Gynecol 2006; 195: 1736.
19. Izett-Kay M, Aldabeeb D, Kupelian A, et al. Long-term mesh complications and reoperation after laparoscopic mesh sacrohysteropexy: a cross-sectional study. Int Urogynecol J. https://doi.org/10.1007/s00192-020-04396-0.
20. Grumeza D, Chira ID, Jinga V, et al. Results following laparoscopic lateral hysteropexy with mesh in anterior pelvic organ prolapse. Eur Urol Suppl 2019; 18(2): e2361.
21. Maher C, Feiner B, Baessler K, et al. Transvaginal mesh or grafts compared with native tissue repair for vaginal prolapse. Cochrane Database Syst Rev 2016; 2(2): CD012079.
22. Glazener CM, Breeman S, Elders A, et al. Mesh, graft, or standard repair for women having primary transvaginal anterior or posterior compartment prolapse surgery: two parallel-group, multicentre, randomised, controlled trials (PROSPECT). Lancet 2017; 389(10067): 381–92.
23. Rosenblatt P, Chelmow D, Ferzandi T. Laparoscopic sacrocervicopexy for the treatment of uterine prolapse: a retrospective case series report. J Minim Invasive Gynecol 2008; 15(3): 268–72.
24. Akl MN, Long JB, Giles DL, et al. Robotic-assisted sacrocolpopexy: technique and learning curve. Surg Endosc 2009; 23(10): 2390–4.
25. Gutman R, Maher C. Uterine-preserving POP surgery. Int Urogynecol J 2013; 24 (11): 1803–13.

26. Rahmanou P, White B, Price N, et al. Laparoscopic hysteropexy: 1- to 4-year follow-up of women postoperatively. Int Urogynecol J 2014; 25(1): 131–8.

27. Kupelian AS, Vashisht A, Sambandan N, et al. Laparoscopic wrap-round mesh sacrohysteropexy for the management of apical prolapse. Int Urogynecol J 2016; 27: 1889–97.

28. Busby G, Broome J. successful pregnancy outcome following laparoscopic sacrohysteropexy for second degree uterine prolapse. Gynecol Surg 2010; 7(3): 271–3.

29. Galdonneix P, Campagna G, Villet R. Pregnancy after laparoscopic sacral colpopexy: a case report. Int Urogynecol J 2012; 23(5): 651–3.

Chapter

14 Laparoscopic Sacrocolpopexy: Procedure Steps and Evidence

Christopher Maher, Zhuoran Chen

Introduction

Fredrick Lane in 1962 first described in detail the sacrocolpopexy procedure in four women with vault prolapse [1]. The dissertation is detailed, enlightening, and I would recommend reading to you all. He opens with the following statement: 'dissatisfied with accepted methods of vaginal plastic repair the author considered the practicability of correction without loss of function' and acknowledges viewing a 'motion picture' of a similar procedure at the April 1961 meeting of the American College of Obstetrics and Gynecology. This statement re-enforces the notion of very little change in vaginal native tissue repairs in the last 50 years and the value of visual learning. I suspect that Dr Lane would be surprised to learn that in 2010, sacrocolpopexy represented 11% of prolapse interventions performed in the US [2].

Significant variation exists in the rate, indication for and how the surgery is performed around the world. Haya et al described rates at which sacrocolpopexy was employed as apical suspending procedure, in OECD countries in 2012, and this ranged from nearly 66% in France to less than 5% in Denmark and Sweden [3]. These variations are difficult to understand and speak to a lack of consensus regarding the role of the procedure. This chapter will review the evidence surrounding sacrocolpopexy and the surgical technique.

Recent Data on Sacrocolpopexy

The 2016 Cochrane review identified six randomized trials comparing sacrocolpopexy to vaginal prolapse repair for vault prolapse, including three trials comparing abdominal sacrocolpopexy (ASC) to sacrospinous ligament suspension (SSLS) [4–6], one trial comparing ASC to uterosacral ligament suspension (ULS) [7], one trial comparing laparoscopic sacrocolpopexy (to transvaginal mesh repair) [8], and one comparing abdominal or laparoscopic sacrocolpopexy to ULS with mesh augmentation [9]. On meta-analysis, we concluded that, overall, sacrocolpopexy is associated with lower risk of awareness of prolapse, recurrent prolapse on examination, repeat surgery for prolapse, post-operative stress urinary incontinence (SUI) and dyspareunia when compared broadly with vaginal prolapse repairs with and without mesh augmentation.

In a more recent randomized controlled trial (RCT) not included in the above Cochrane review, Lucot et al reported the outcomes of a large French multi-centre RCT comparing laparoscopic sacrocolpopexy (LSC) (n=130) and transvaginal mesh (n=129) for those presenting with cystocele. They demonstrated no difference between the groups in symptoms of prolapse, re-operation for prolaps,e or validated satisfaction or quality-of-life outcomes. However, the LSC group had improved support at point C on examination, a longer total vaginal length (TVL), and lower risk of re-operation and dyspareunia as compared to the transvaginal mesh group [10].

A systematic review by the Society of Gynecologic Surgeons Systematic Review Group that included both randomized trials and cohort studies, comparing sacrocolpopexy with native tissue (non-mesh) vaginal repairs for both vault and uterine prolapse, found improved anatomic outcomes with sacrocolpopexy and no difference in re-operation rates or postoperative sexual function [11]. Adverse event data compiled from 79 studies (comparative and non-comparative) found sacrocolpopexy was associated with a higher rate of ileus or small bowel obstruction (2.7% versus 0.2%, p<.01), mesh or suture complications (4.2% versus 0.4%, p <.01) and thromboembolic disease (0.6% versus 0.1%, p=.03), but the authors acknowledged that adverse events were largely poorly reported. Two recently reported audits of nationwide databases exclusively designed to report on perioperative complications were unable to reproduce the increased perioperative adverse events associated with sacrocolpopexy reported above.

Kisby et al recently reported data from the American College of Surgeons National Surgical Quality Improvement Program database from 2005 to 2016, comparing adverse events in the first 30 days following minimally invasive sacrocolpopexy (MISC) (n-2753) and transvaginal mesh (n=3,149) in patients not undergoing concomitant hysterectomy. They found no difference in re-operation rates (1.6% versus 1.3% respectively) or in minor and major complications between the two groups, explicitly including no difference in thromboembolic events. Ileus or small bowel obstruction rates were not individually reported [12]. They did report that the MISC was associated with a lower rate of transfusion and urinary tract infections and a higher rate of requiring >2-day admission than the transvaginal mesh group.

Furthermore, Linder et al evaluated the same database from 2010 to 2016 for 30-day perioperative complications, comparing MISC (n=2,538) to non-mesh apical vaginal repair excluding those undergoing concomitant hysterectomy (n=3852). They demonstrated no difference between the groups on multivariate analysis for any complications, prolonged hospitalization, readmission, or re-operation [13].

In 2017, I lead a multinational group of leading Pelvic Organ Prolapse (POP) surgeons under the auspices of the International Collaboration on Incontinence (ICI) that prioritized data from all sources using the Oxford grading system for evidence. On rigorous evaluation of the data, we preferenced the sacrocolpopexy as the procedure of choice for the management of vault prolapse but not for uterine prolapse. When the group reconvenes in 2021 I suspect the findings preferencing sacrocolpopexy as the procedure of choice for vault prolapse will be unchanged.

Historical Data on Abdominal Sacrocolpopexy

Observational studies and clinical trials suggest that ASC is a highly effective procedure for apical prolapse. Barber et al reviewed the literature and the success rate of ASC, when defined as lack of apical prolapse, ranged from 78% to 100%. When success is defined as no recurrent prolapse in any segment, the published success rates are 56% to 100% [14]. Nygaard performed an early systematic review of ASC and reported a median re-operation rate for recurrent prolapse of 4.4% (range 0% to 18.2%), postoperative stress urinary incontinence (SUI) of 4.9% (range 1.2% to 30.9%), and a mesh erosion rate of 3.4% [15].

Long-term follow-up in the CARE trial (E-Care) suggested a substantial decline in anatomic and subjective outcomes and increase in mesh exposure. Subjects enrolled in the long-term follow-up (5–7 years) of the trial reported objective failure rates of 24% to 48% depending upon the definition of failure and a cumulative mesh erosion rate of 10.5% by seven years [16]. These results, demonstrating declining anatomic outcomes and escalating mesh erosion rate at 5–7 years, should be viewed with caution and may be explained by methodological issues with the trial. There was no standardization of sacrocolpopexy in the trial, with only 39% of cases having a type 1 monofilament polypropylene mesh that is recommended as the graft material of choice for sacrocolpopexy [17], with at least 50% receiving non monofilament polypropylene mesh, that is now not recommended due to high complication rates. One-third of participants also underwent concomitant hysterectomy which has been demonstrated to increase the mesh erosion rate fourfold when compared to ASC performed in post-hysterectomy prolapse [18]. Furthermore, non-absorbable sutures were utilized to fix the graft in over 50% of cases and their use is associated with a higher mesh erosion rate than absorbable sutures [19]. These three methodological realities would all contribute to a surprisingly high rate of mesh exposure reported in the E-CARE trial.

Recently, a Belgian group reported on a large cohort of 331 cases, with a mean seven-year review, and observed both a higher success rate and a lower rate of mesh erosion than in E-Care. The rate of improvement was 84%, mesh erosion was 7%, and re-operation rate for prolapse of 3.3% [20]. In this trial the authors changed to a monofilament polypropylene mesh and absorbable sutures after 200 cases and reported a significant reduction in the mesh exposure rate with these changes. Similarly, a Dutch group reported a 3% rate of mesh exposure three to six years following robotic sacrocolpopexy when employing both a type 1 monofilament polypropylene mesh and absorbable sutures from the outset of their trial [21]. Finally, an English group reported on over 600 LSC performed with a monofilament mesh and absorbable sutures with a four-year review that the mesh exposure rate was only 0.7% [22].

Route of Entry

Sacrocolpopexy, like most abdominal procedures, was traditionally performed via a laparotomy and then keyhole approach, and finally with robotic intervention. Trials comparing these three modes of accessing the abdomen have largely concentrated on perioperative outcomes rather than long-term success rates, with the assumption that the outcomes are dependent on the surgery rather than the access type.

In a 2013 Cochrane review of the surgical management of prolapse, including three RCTs comparing open sacrocolpopexy to vaginal sacrospinous colpopexy, we found level 1 evidence that there were no statistically significant differences in objective failure at any site (any POP RR 0.77, 95% CI 0.39–1.53), subjective failure (RR 0.53, 95%CI 0.25–1.09), re-operation for POP (RR 1.46, 95% CI 0.19–1.11) or patient satisfaction (RR 0.82, 95% CI 0.32–2.06) [23]. However, ASC was superior to SSLS for the following outcomes: prolapse ≤ Stage 2 (RR 0.29, 95% CI 0.09–0.97), recurrent vault prolapse (RR 0.23, 95% CI 0.07–0.77) postoperative SUI (RR 0.55, 95% CI 0.32–0.95), and less postoperative dyspareunia RR 0.39, 95% CI 0.18–0.86). In contrast, ASC was associated with a longer operating time (Weighted Mean Difference (WMD) 21 minutes, 95% CI 12–30), longer time to recover (WMD 8.3 days, 95% CI 3.9–12.7) and was more expensive (WMD US $1334, 95% CI 1027–1641) than SSLS [23].

Over the last decade, the laparoscopic approach has been popularized to minimize the postoperative admission and recovery time associated with open ASC. (Surgical instrumentation as per Table 14.1. Multiple prospective and retrospective case series demonstrate good short- to mid-term success rates with mean objective success rate of 91% (range 60–100%), subjective success rates of 79–98% [24–26], and mean re-operation rate of 5.9% [27] (ICI). Prospective studies demonstrate significant improvements in pelvic symptoms and quality of life after LSC [8,28,29]. Most RCTs observed that LSC is as effective as open abdominal procedure, with a reduced rate of intraoperative bleeding, hospitalization, and wound complications [30,31]. However, a recent RCT showed that LSC provides outcomes as good as those of open sacrocolpopexy for anatomical correction but not for anterior POP (Level 2 Evidence) [32].

Despite the clinical advantages of a laparoscopic approach, uptake of LSC has been relatively limited, probably because of the steep learning curve associated with attaining prerequisite dissection skills to open the various surgical planes and suturing skills to attach the mesh to the vagina and sacrum. Claerhout et al evaluated their learning curve in the first 206 cases performed by a single surgeon [33]. Operating times declined rapidly during the first 30 procedures in this series and reached steady state (175 minutes) after 90 cases. Using a cumulative sum (CUSUM) approach to evaluate operative time and failures (laparotomy, complication, or anatomic failures) they found that adequate learning occurred after 60 cases [33]. Complication rates remained unchanged throughout this series. Other studies have shown a decrease in operating time after 15–24 cases [34,35].

Many reviewers have evaluated the laparoscopic and robotic sacrocolpopexy jointly as minimally invasive sacrocolpopexy (MISC) (laparoscopic or robot-assisted) and concluded the MISC should be preferred over the open approach for sacral colpopexy. Indeed, similar anatomic/functional results have been observed, but mini-invasive approach is associated with a decrease in blood loss and shorter length of hospital stay in case control trials [36,37]. Linder et al, on data from the American College of Surgeons National Surgical Quality Improvement Program database from 2005 to 2016, comparing adverse events in the first 30 days following MISC (n=3183) and open ASC (n=1,179) reported that MISC was associated with lower rates of 30-day complications (p=0.001), deep vein thrombosis/pulmonary embolism (p=0.02), surgical site infections (p <0.0001), blood transfusions (p=0.01), and a shorter hospitalization (p <0.0001) [38]. Minimally invasive sacrocolpopexy was also associated with a lower 30-day readmission rate (2% versus 2.7%, p≤0.0001) and 30-day re-operation rate (1.1% versus 1.4%, p<0.0001).

The robot-assisted sacral colpopexy (RASC) was introduced in recognition of the advanced range of movements afforded to the clinician to attain the desired suturing and dissection skills. In two RCTs comparing the robotic and laparoscopic procedure, both had similar short-term anatomic cure rates and length of hospital stay [28, 39] (Level 2 Evidence). However, the robotic approach had longer operating time, greater postoperative pain, and higher costs than LSC [37] with the overall complication rates being similar in both laparoscopic and robotic approach. Separate to these, two trials have also recently analysed the RASC learning curve. In a US group, proficiency was demonstrated at 84 cases [13] and in a Dutch group, 75 cases were required prior to stabilization of intraoperative or postoperative complications [40]. This protracted learning curve is not dissimilar to that described for the LSC above and perhaps refutes the reduced learning curve as the one of the main advantages for robotic approach over LSC. On the basis of this data, the 2017 ICI pathway for the surgical management of vault prolapse preferences the laparoscopic approach above either open or RASC [27].

Changing Trends in Sacrocolpopexy

In recognition of increased perioperative morbidity with the open ASC, since 2009, MISC has overtaken open ASC as the commonest approach to all ASC [31] in the US, and in 2016 represented 82% of ASC procedures performed with CTP coding unable to differentiate between laparoscopic and robotic ASC in the national datasets [41].

The second change in sacralcolpopexy is the performance of concomitant surgery. Constantin et al reviewed data from RCTs that demonstrated superiority of ASC to vaginal interventions and found concomitant surgery at the time of ASC was the norm in these landmark trials [17]. Retropubic interventions (colposuspension or paravaginal repair) were performed in 87% of cases, and posterior repairs in 50%. As an observation, these interventions are currently not routinely performed by clinicians, with sacrocolpopexy frequently utilized as a stand-alone intervention. A recent large RCT of sacrocolpopexy and transvaginal mesh excluded retropubic surgery as an option at time of ASC [10]. This change may have occurred for a number of reasons including the rise in popularity of the mid-urethral slings as compared to colposuspensions as treatment for SUI and secondly, data from E-Care demonstrating that while urethropexy at sacrocolpopexy as compared to sacrocolpopexy alone had reduced SUI, no difference was seen in the overall rate of prolapse. However, no direct data from anterior vaginal wall was presented for evaluation to assess cystocele recurrence rate. Data from the E-Care trial needs to be reviewed with caution, as at least 20% in the no urethropexy group underwent paravaginal repairs, a methodological problem that serves to minimize the ability of the RCT to identify any real difference in prolapse outcomes between the sacrocolpopexy with and without urethropexy.

Trabuco et al randomly allocated women with occult or SUI undergoing sacrocolpopexy to mid-urethral retropubic sling or colposuspension and demonstrated, at two years, less postoperative SUI in the MUS group. However, the effects on symptomatic and anatomic prolapse are not able to be assessed from the results presented.

As discussed previously, Pacquee [20] recently reported 83% satisfaction with a seven-year follow-up of LSC, where the only regular concomitant surgery was MUS. While the anatomic failures at point C were low at 8.6%, anterior compartment (22%) and posterior compartment (28%) recurrences were much higher and suggest that the possible utilization of paravaginal and posterior compartment interventions in combination with LSC may be beneficial in improving long-term outcomes. The growing trend towards the ASC being viewed as a stand-alone intervention is not supported by the long-term data and is not consistent with the original RCTs that demonstrated anatomical and functional benefits of the sacrocolpopexy over vaginal-based interventions where the sacrocolpopexy was rarely performed in isolation.

The final trend to be discussed is the concept of 'nerve sparing' sacrocolpopexy. Recently Cosma et al [42] argued that some of the functional impairments after sacrocolpopexy, including bowel, sexual, and bladder dysfunction, may be secondary to interference with caudal superior hypogastric nerve damage during peritoneal dissection. They advocated a nerve-sparring technique with increased awareness of the course of the right hypogastric nerve during dissection on the sacral promontory and right pelvic sidewall. In their small series, they demonstrated improved bowel (Agachan-Wezner score) and sexual function (Prolapse and Incontinence Sexual Questionnaire; PISQ) in a group undergoing nerve preserving sacrocolpopexy compared to traditional sacrocolpopexy. Their literature review found 12.3% rate of bowel dysfunction (constipation, obstructed defaecation syndrome, or dyschezia) after LSC but did not quantify the extent of bowel dysfunction pre-intervention. While it may be difficult to demonstrate that the neve-sparring technique is absolutely beneficial to maximize functional outcomes following sacrocolpopexy, as Cosma argues, there appears to be little downside to incorporation of the change in technique that is required to minimize the risk of damage to the right hypogastric nerve during retroperitoneal dissection.

Why Sacrocolpopexy Fails

While we have ascertained above that sacrocolpopexy is an excellent procedure for the management of post-hysterectomy apical prolapse, recurrences do occur and Haya et al [43] reported on our experience with five such cases that underwent repeat sacrocolpopexy in 2012. In all cases at surgery the mesh was not attached to the anterior vaginal wall or vault and was intact on the sacrum as demonstrated in Video 14.1. Given these findings, we ensure a wide dissection of the bladder and bowel from the vaginal vault to ensure a large piece of mesh is secured to a wide area of the vaginal vault as demonstrated in Video 14.2.

Surgical Instruments Required for Laparoscopic Sacrocolpopexy

Table 14.1

Mesh	Lightweight monofilament partially absorbable macroporous polypropylene mesh ()
Trocars	3 x 5 mm trocars and 1 applied 5 mm balloon trocar (needle and mesh introduced via this trocar)
Sutures	3.0 polydioxanone (Ethicon)
Vaginal probe	Vaginal and rectal probe (Baynan Medical Rhode Island)
Camera	5 mm 0 degree
Scissors	Monopolar 5 mm diathermy scissors (Endopath Ethicon)
Tacker	5 mm titanium hernia tacker (Protack Medtronic)

Surgical Technique

Prior to surgery, the patient completes an exhaustive information transfer and consent process. Any medical comorbidities are optimized with the assistance of physicians in the pre- and perioperative periods. The initial set-up includes the patient positioned in low adjustable stirrups on a non-slip mattress in the Trendelenburg position with 25–27 degrees head down. The patient's buttocks should overhang the end of the bed by about 7 cm to ensure the vaginal and or rectal probes are able to be freely manipulated to maximize access to the rectovaginal space.

Trocar Placement

I classically utilize four trocars with a sub-umbilical primary optical access trocar (Video 14.3) and three secondary 5 mm trocars placed under direct vision. Two are placed low in the left and right iliac fossa approximately 3 cm medial and superior to the anterior superior iliac spine and lateral to the inferior epigastric vessels. The remaining trocar is placed also on the left side approximately 15 cm cranial to the left lower trocar and again lateral to the inferior epigastric vessels.

The steps of the procedure are:

1. Crafting the mesh: (Video 14.4) at the commencement of the surgery
2. Emptying the small bowel from the pelvis
3. Opening the retroperitoneal space from the sacrum to the vaginal vault
4. Creating the vesico-vaginal space
5. Creating the recto-vaginal space
6. Securing the mesh to the vaginal vault
7. Securing the mesh to the sacral promontory
8. Closing the retroperitoneal space
9. Completing middle vaginal compartment surgeries as planned, including colposuspension, paravaginal or posterior vaginal repairs, or mid-urethral slings
10. Cystoscopy

The first step is to clear the pelvis of the small bowel and adhesiolysis is frequently required to mobilize old adhesions and gain good access to the retroperitoneum which is opened on the sacrum. Once the retroperitoneal space is opened, the CO^2 rapidly enters the space and assists in dissection. Using traction and counter traction with the scissors in the left upper trocars, the retroperitoneal space is opened to the vaginal vault medial to the uterosacral ligament. During the dissection, the scissors blade provides upward traction on the peritoneum and frequently opens this space quite easily, minimizing any risk of traversing the right hypogastric nerves which classically run deep in the retroperitoneal space.

Once the dissection is at the vaginal vault, the insulated vaginal probe is introduced by the assistant and the peritoneum is opened over the vault. In large anterior wall prolapse the bladder should be manipulated anterior and distal along the probe to ensure the bladder is not inadvertently entered during the initial dissection. Again, using traction with the vaginal probe and countertraction with the non-toothed forceps, the bladder is mobilized from the anterior vagina wall with sharp dissection and monopolar diathermy to control small venous ooze. This dissection is continued distally until the bladder trigone is reached, which is identified when the bladder becomes firmly fixed to the vagina.

The posterior vaginal dissection is facilitated by the assistant maximally angulating the vaginal probe anteriorly. The posterior peritoneum is tented downward to facilitate countertraction for the dissection of the posterior vaginal wall which continues distally to the perineal body. Care is taken to minimize the use of inadvertent diathermy in this compartment to minimize any risk of thermal injury to the rectum.

Once the dissection is complete and haemostasis secured, the anterior and posterior spaces are revisited and self-styled Y-shaped mesh that was prepared initially is further crafted to fit the individual's needs. The aim is to ensure the mesh covers all the dissected vagina and lies flat on the vagina without folding or crimping. The anterior leaf of the Y-shaped mesh is secured to the vagina first using two to three 3.0 PDS sutures.

The sacral arm of the Y-mesh is then folded anteriorly and the vaginal probe angulated anteriorly to maximize posterior vaginal wall exposure. Again, the posterior leaf is secured to the posterior vagina with two to three PDS sutures, with the distal sutures placed first.

The sacral arm of the Y-shaped mesh is secured to the sacral promontory using three titanium tackers. Much is written about the importance of dissection of the sacrum to identify the anterior longitudinal ligament and middle sacral vessels. I classically do not identify the ligament or vessel and vision and tactile feedback from the tacker and left needle holder is utilized to ensure the mesh is on the sacrum. The tacker is placed between the open jaws of the needle holder to secure the mesh to the sacral promontory with three tacks. The retroperitoneal space is closed with a continuous 3.0 PDS suture as seen in Video 14.2.

Concomitant procedures are performed as required. A cystoscopy is always performed to confirm the bladder is intact and the ureters are functioning normally. The trocar sites are classically apposed with 3.0 vicryl rapide suture but most recently I am using Dermabond waterproof glue to which both the ward nursing staff and patients have responded positively.

In compliance with the National Health Medical Research Council perioperative recommendations, surgery is covered by a single dose of 2 g cephazolin and thrombo-embolic stockings for two weeks, 20 mg sub-cutaneous clexane for five days, and sequential compression devices overnight for the low-risk patient. The in-dwelling catheter is removed at 06:00 on the morning following surgery and a formal trial of void completed.

Conclusion

In summary, the findings and recommendations from this chapter are:

1. Sacrocolpopexy is preferenced as the procedure of choice for post-hysterectomy vault prolapse.
2. Concomitant surgery is performed commonly and is rarely undertaken as a stand-alone intervention and may serve to decrease the rate of middle compartment prolapse long-term.
3. Lightweight monofilament polypropylene mesh is the preferred graft.
4. Absorbable sutures are utilized to decrease the rate of mesh exposures.
5. Laparoscopic access is preferenced.
6. My surgical approach preferences minimalist dissection on the sacrum and pelvic side-wall with maximum dissection of the vagina.
7. Broad Y-mesh is applied to the vagina without folding.
8. The suspension arm of the mesh to the sacrum is applied with minimal tension.

References

1. Lane F. Repair of posthysterectomy vaginal-vault prolapse. Obstet Gynecol 1962; 20: 72–7.
2. Barber MD, Maher C. Epidemiology and outcome assessment of pelvic organ prolapse. Int Urogynecol J 2013; 24(11): 1783–90. https://doi.org/10.1007/s00192-013-2169-9
3. Haya N, Baessler K, Christmann-Schmid C, et al. Prolapse and continence surgery in countries of the Organization for Economic Cooperation and Development in 2012. Am J Obstet Gynecol 2015; 212(6): 755 e751–755 e727. https://doi.org/10.1016/j.ajog.2015.02.017
4. Benson JT, Lucente V, McClellan E. Vaginal versus abdominal reconstructive surgery for the treatment of pelvic support defects: a prospective randomized study with long-term outcome evaluation. Am J Obstet Gynecol 1996; 175(6): 1418–21.
5. Lo TS, Wang AC. Abdominal colposacropexy and sacrospinous ligament suspension for severe uterovaginal prolapse: a comparison. J Gynecol Surg 1998; 14: 59–64.
6. Maher CF, Qatawneh A, Dwyer P, et al. Abdominal sacral colpopexy or vaginal sacrospinous colpopexy for vaginal vault prolapse. A prospective randomized trial. Am J Obstet Gynecol 2004; 190: 20–6.
7. Rondini C, Braun H, Alvarez J, et al. High uterosacral vault suspension vs sacrocolpopexy for treating apical defects: a randomized controlled trial with twelve months follow-up. Int Urogynecol J 2015; 26(8): 1131–8. https://doi.org/10.1007/s00192-015-2666-0
8. Maher C, Feiner B, DeCuyper E, et al. Laparoscopic sacral colpopexy versus total vaginal mesh for vaginal vault prolapse: a randomized trial. Am J Obstet Gynecol 2011; 204(4): 360 e361–7. https://doi.org/10.1016/j.ajog.2010.11.016
9. Maher C, Feiner B, Baessler K, et al. Surgery for women with apical vaginal prolapse. Cochrane Database Syst Rev 2016; 10: CD012376. https://doi.org/10.1002/14651858.cd012376
10. Lucot JP, Cosson M, Bader G, et al. Safety of vaginal mesh surgery versus laparoscopic mesh sacropexy for cystocele repair: results of the prosthetic pelvic floor repair randomized controlled trial. Eur Urol 2018; 74(2): 167–76. https://doi.org/10.1016/j.eururo.2018.01.044
11. Siddiqui NY, Grimes CL, Casiano ER, et al. Mesh sacrocolpopexy compared with native tissue vaginal repair: a systematic review and meta-analysis. Obstet Gynecol 2015; 125(1): 44–55. https://doi.org/10.1097/aog.0000000000000570
12. Kisby CK, Occhino JA, Bews KA, et al. Perioperative complications in minimally invasive sacrocolpopexy versus transvaginal mesh in the management of pelvic organ prolapse: analysis of a national multi-institutional dataset. Female Pelvic Med Reconstr Surg 2019; 27(2): 72–7. https://doi.org/10.1097/spv.0000000000000738
13. Linder BJ, Chow GK, Elliott DS. Long-term quality of life outcomes and retreatment rates after robotic sacrocolpopexy. Int J Urol 2015; 22(12): 1155–8. https://doi.org/10.1111/iju.12900
14. Barber MD, Maher C. Apical prolapse. Int Urogynecol J 2013; 24(11): 1815–33. https://doi.org/10.1007/s00192-013-2172-1
15. Nygaard IE, McCreery R, Brubaker L, et al. Abdominal sacrocolpopexy: a comprehensive review. Obstet Gynecol 2004; 104(4): 805–23. https://doi.org/10.1097/01.aog.0000139514.90897.07
16. Nygaard I, Brubaker L, Zyczynski HM, et al. Long-term outcomes following abdominal sacrocolpopexy for pelvic organ prolapse. JAMA 2013; 309(19): 2016–24. https://doi.org/10.1001/jama.2013.4919
17. Costantini E, Brubaker L, Cervigni M, et al. Sacrocolpopexy for pelvic organ prolapse: evidence-based review and recommendations. Eur J Obstet Gynecol Reprod Biol 2016; 205: 60–5. https://doi.org/10.1016/j.ejogrb.2016.07.503
18. Gutman R, Maher C. Uterine-preserving prolapse surgery. Int Urogynecol J 2013; 24(11): 1803–13. https://doi.org/10.1007/s00192-013-2171-2
19. Shepherd JP, Higdon HL, 3rd, Stanford EJ, Mattox TF. Effect of suture selection on the rate of suture or mesh erosion and surgery failure in abdominal sacrocolpopexy. Female Pelvic Med Reconstr Surg 2010; 16(4): 229–33. https://doi.org/10.1097/SPV.0b013e3181d683a3
20. Pacquee S, Nawapun K, Claerhout F, et al. Long-term assessment of a prospective cohort of patients undergoing laparoscopic sacrocolpopexy. Obstet Gynecol 2019; 134(2): 323–32. https://doi.org/10.1097/aog.0000000000003380
21. van Zanten F, van Iersel JJ, Paulides TJC, et al. Long-term mesh erosion rate following abdominal robotic reconstructive pelvic floor surgery: a prospective study and overview of the literature. Int Urogynecol J 2020; 31(7): 1423–33.

22. Baines G, Price N, Jefferis H, et al. Mesh-related complications of laparoscopic sacrocolpopexy. Int Urogynecol J 2019; 30(9): 1475–81. https://doi.org/10.1007/s00192-019-03952-7
23. Maher C, Schmid C, Baessler K, Feiner B. Surgical management of pelvic organ prolapse in women. Cochrane Database Syst Rev (Online) 2013; (4): CD004014.
24. Higgs PJ, Chua HL, Smith AR (eds). Long-term review of laparoscopic sacrocolpopexy. BJOG 2005; 112: 1134–8.
25. Rivoire C, Botchorishvili R, Canis M, et al (eds). Complete laparoscopic treatment of genital prolapse with meshes including vaginal promontofixation and anterior repair: a series of 138 patients. J Minim Invasive Gynecol 2007; 14(6): 712–18. https://doi.org/10.1016/j.jmig.2007.06.017
26. Sarlos D, Brandner S, Kots L, et al. Laparoscopic sacrocolpopexy for uterine and post-hysterectomy prolapse: anatomical results, quality of life and perioperative outcome - a prospective study with 101 cases. Int Urogynecol J Pelvic Floor Dysfunc 2008; 19(10): 1415–22. https://doi.org/10.1007/s00192-008-0657-0
27. Maher C, Baessler KBM, Cheong C, et al. Surgical management of pelvic organ prolapse. In: P Abrahams, LWA Cardozo, and A Wein (eds). *International Consultation on Incontinence*, vol 2, 6th edn. ICUD ICS; 2017, pp 1855–992.
28. Paraiso M, Jelovsek J, Frick A, et al. Laparoscopic compared with robotic sacrocolpopexy for vaginal prolapse: a randomized controlled trial. Obstet Gynecol 2011; 118(5): 1005–13. https://doi.org/10.1097/AOG.0b013e318231537c
29. Sergent F, Resch B, Loisel C, et al. Mid-term outcome of laparoscopic sacrocolpopexy with anterior and posterior polyester mesh for treatment of genito-urinary prolapse. Eur J Obstet Gynecol Reprod Biol 2011; 156: 217–22. https://doi.org/10.1016/j.ejogrb.2011.01.022
30. Freeman R, Pantazis K, Thomson A, et al. A randomised controlled trial of abdominal versus laparoscopic sacrocolpopexy for the treatment of post-hysterectomy vaginal vault prolapse: LAS study. Int Urogynecol J 2013; 24: 377–84.
31. Tyson MD, Wolter CE. A comparison of 30-day surgical outcomes for minimally invasive and open sacrocolpopexy. Neurourol 2015; 34(2): 151–5. https://doi.org/10.1002/nau.22522
32. Costantini E, Mearini L, Lazzeri M. Laparoscopic versus abdominal sacrocolpopexy: a randomized, controlled trial. J Urol 2016; 196(1): 159–65. https://doi.org/10.1016/j.juro.2015.12.089
33. Claerhout F, Roovers JP, Lewi P, et al. Implementation of laparoscopic sacrocolpopexy – a single centre's experience. Int Urogynecol J Pelvic Floor Dysfunct 2009; 20(9): 1119–25. https://doi.org/10.1007/s00192-009-0914-x
34. Akladios CY, Dautun D, Saussine C, et al. Laparoscopic sacrocolpopexy for female genital organ prolapse: establishment of a learning curve. Eur J Obstet Gynecol Reprod Biol 2010; 149(2): 218–21. https://doi.org/10.1016/j.ejogrb.2009.12.012
35. Mustafa S, Amit A, Filmar S, et al. Implementation of laparoscopic sacrocolpopexy: establishment of a learning curve and short-term outcomes. Arch Gynecol Obstet 2012; 286(4): 983–8. https://doi.org/10.1007/s00404-012-2391-6
36. De Gouveia De Sa M, Claydon LS, Whitlow B, Dolcet Artahona MA. Laparoscopic versus open sacrocolpopexy for treatment of prolapse of the apical segment of the vagina: a systematic review and meta-analysis. Int Urogynecol J 2016; 27(1): 3–17. https://doi.org/10.1007/s00192-015-2765-y
37. De Gouveia De Sa M, Claydon LS, Whitlow B, Dolcet Artahona MA. Robotic versus laparoscopic sacrocolpopexy for treatment of prolapse of the apical segment of the vagina: a systematic review and meta-analysis. Int Urogynecol J 2016; 27(3): 355–66. https://doi.org/10.1007/s00192-015-2763-0
38. Linder BJ, Occhino JA, Habermann EB, et al. A national contemporary analysis of perioperative outcomes of open versus minimally invasive sacrocolpopexy. J Urol 2018; 200(4): 862–7. https://doi.org/10.1016/j.juro.2018.03.131
39. Anger J, Mueller E, Tarnay C, et al. Robotic compared with laparoscopic sacrocolpopexy: a randomized controlled trial. Obstet Gynecol 2014; 123(1): 5–12.
40. van Zanten F, Schraffordt Koops SE, Pasker-de Jong PCM, et al. Learning curve of robot-assisted laparoscopic sacrocolpo(recto) pexy: a cumulative sum analysis. Am J Obstet Gynecol 2019. https://doi.org/10.1016/j.ajog.2019.05.037
41. Linder BJ, Gershman B, Bews KA, et al. A national contemporary analysis of perioperative outcomes for vaginal vault prolapse: minimally invasive sacrocolpopexy versus nonmesh vaginal surgery. Female Pelvic Med Reconstr Surg 2019; 25(5): 342–6.
42. Cosma S, Petruzzelli P, Danese S, Benedetto C. Nerve preserving vs standard laparoscopic sacropexy: postoperative bowel function. World J Gastrointest Endosc 2017; 9(5): 211–19. https://doi.org/10.4253/wjge.v9.i5.211
43. Haya N, Maher M, Ballard E. Surgical management of recurrent upper vaginal prolapse following sacral colpopexy. Int Urogynecol J 2015; 26(8): 1243–5. https://doi.org/10.1007/s00192-015-2633-9

Chapter

15 Laparoscopic Native Tissue Repair: Procedure Steps and Evidence

Guenter K Noé

Introduction

The term native tissue repair describes surgical techniques mainly using fascia or other local tissue for the reconstruction of pelvic defects without the need for synthetic or biological grafts or mesh. The pelvic defects result due to distension or rupture/avulsion of fascia or ligamental structures. The main causes for these defects are pregnancy, childbirth, and being overweight. The pelvic fascia is subsequently exposed to increased risk of midline or lateral distension or rupture due to increased intrabdominal and pelvic pressure. A midline defect in the endopelvic fascia may cause a variety of symptoms including voiding difficulty (and in extreme cases urinary retention), urgency, pelvic pressure, and the feeling of a bulge in the vagina. In addition to midline defects in the endopelvic fascia, the vaginal epithelium can also be over-expanded to create a lateral defect. This can regularly be seen in prolapses of POPQ stage 2 or greater. The midline defect can be managed by classic midline repair (anterior/posterior colporrhaphy) and suturing the pelvic fascia between the vagina and the bladder rectum. However, suturing the mid-portion of the fascia may increase traction on the lateral attachments of the pelvic fascia. This may interfere with the lateral attachment of the pelvic fascia and increase a lateral defect.

In addition to fascial plication at anterior/posterior colporrhaphy, the vaginal epithelium is often also trimmed. Cutting vaginal epithelial tissue can cause subsequent narrowing of the vagina which has been described as far back as the nineteenth century [1]. Strategies such as cauterization, burning, or ligation with re-adaptation have also been developed and described. Breisky (1879), Savage (1868), and Fritsch (1881) developed and adopted new strategies as they developed greater knowledge of the anatomy of the pelvic floor [1]. Multiple vaginal approaches using local native tissue to support or just reduce the size and length of the tissue were described at the beginning of the twentieth century. These techniques were performed until the late 1990s; some of them are still in use [2–8].

In the last two decades the success rates achieved with native tissue have been considered to be low, therefore vaginal mesh surgery became increasingly popular. However, subsequent large trials have demonstrated similar efficacy and rates of recurrent prolapse when adopting vaginal mesh [17]. This may be due to lack of providing concomitant apical (level 1) support when repairing level 2 defects. The fact that the combination of vaginal native tissue repair and sufficient apical repair provides significantly better data was given little attention [9]. We have previously shown that excellent results can be achieved when combining a laparoscopic apical repair (sacropexy/pectopexy) with vaginal colporraphy and/or laparoscopic lateral repair [10–12]. For laparoscopic native tissue repair, many options are available and published. This chapter will focus on laparoscopic anterior and posterior midline (level 2 and 3) repair and a technique for lateral repair [12,13].

Laparoscopic Cystocele Repair

Vaginal Approach for (Native Tissue) Fascia Repair

Traditional access for the vaginal repair is to open the vaginal epithelium transversally and dissect the epithelium laterally to expose the pelvic fascia. The bulging overstretched or thinned tissue is duplicated by sutures similar to darts in textiles (see Figure 15.1). Frequently the dilated epithelium is shortened to avoid creating a midline fold. The vaginal approach has some advantages, including quick access, it can easily be learned, and long-standing clinical experience enables many surgeons to use this technique. The approach can be combined with vaginal and abdominal apex fixation as well.

Technique for Laparoscopic Anterior Midline Defect Repair

Why change a successful route? Combining laparoscopic apex-fixation (pectopexy or sacropexy) with laparoscopic fascia repair has some advantages. Both strategies can be performed in a single session respectively with no additional instruments needed for vaginal surgery, with only one sterile area being used. However, probably one of the most important factors is that the

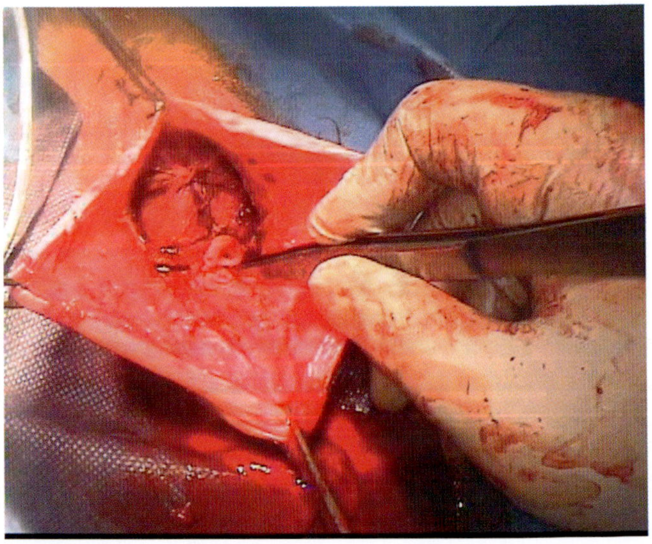

Figure 15.1 Vaginal anterior repair.

procedure preserves the integrity of the vaginal wall (no scar/no resection). This has greater emphasis in cases of recurrent prolapse where repeat surgery can cause significant scarring and shortening of the vagina.

At vaginal anterior colporrhaphy, after vaginal dissection the fascia is seen bulging in the direction of the surgeon. For the laparoscopic approach we use a retractor which is introduced into the vagina. (We favour the Breisky retractor). The retractor is plane and thin, permitting good traction of tissue in order to separate the layers. The retractor/vagina is pushed inside the abdomen in a cephaloid direction. First the bladder is dissected from the vagina or the pelvic fascia. This is similar to anterior preparation during laparoscopic sacral colpopexy (LSC) with a deep mesh fixation. The midline defect is dissected toward the urethra. The upper two-thirds of the anterior vaginal wall are regularly exposed (see Figures 15.2a, 15.3, and 15.4) depending on the size of the cystocele. The lower third should not be dissected as the ureter enters the bladder from the posterior aspect. The urethra itself should not be exposed.

Now the fascia is sutured with size 1 absorbable woven sutures (Figures 15.2b; 15.5). The fascia is penetrated five to six times (according to the size of the cystocele) (Figures 15.6–8). After placing three rows of sutures, the middle suture line is tied to compress the cystocele and enhance the thickness of the tissue (Figure 15.9). To avoid creating large vaginal folds, multiple stiches are crucial. The compression of tissue enables a thickening of the fascia as well as narrowing of the dilated vagina and enhances the firmness of the vaginal mucosa (Figure 15.2c. After tying the middle suture, both lateral sutures are tied additionally. To strengthen the whole tissue, a supplementary suture line is performed horizontal from left to right (Figure 15.10). The longitudinal suturing is easier if performed with the left hand from a lateral access port as the needle shows into the direction of the camera. The suture usually is performed with an absorbable suture. In case of relapse, we use a non-absorbable suture (PVDF).

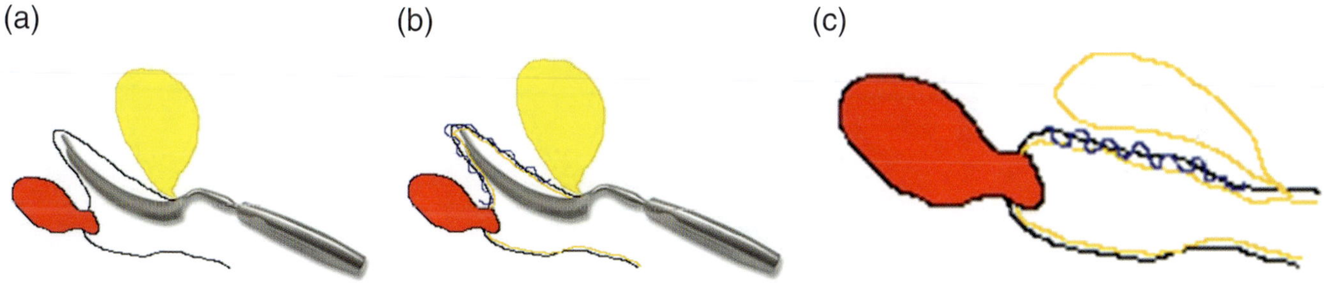

Figure 15.2 Exposure and suture placement for laparoscopic cystocele repair.

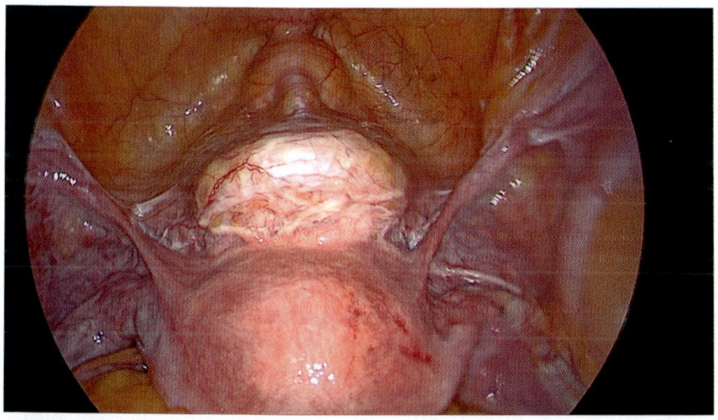

Figure 15.3 Dissection 1: Cystocele is pushed inside.

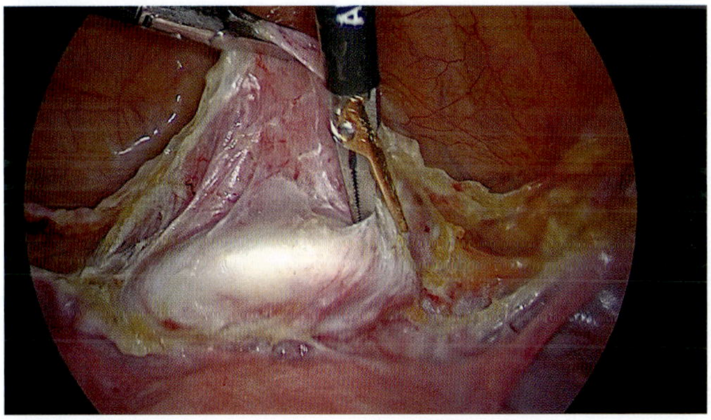

Figure 15.4 Dissection 2: Peritoneum is opened and fascia is exposed.

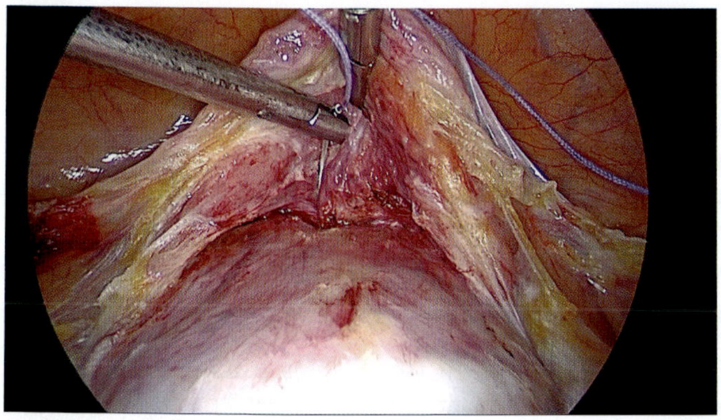

Figure 15.5 After complete exposure first suture is

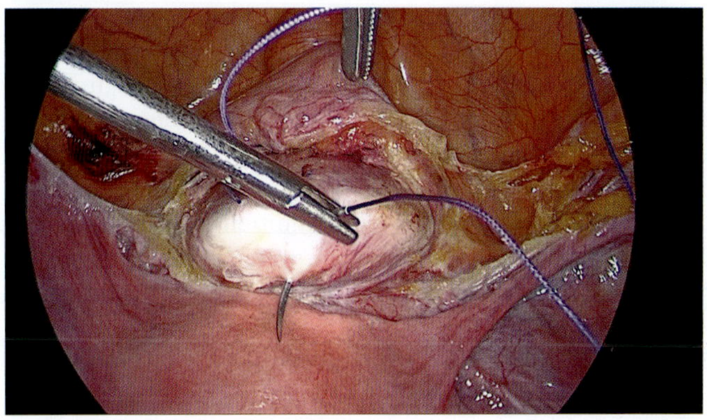

Figure 15.6 Five to seven stiches are performed, placed in the middle, beginning at the lowest point.

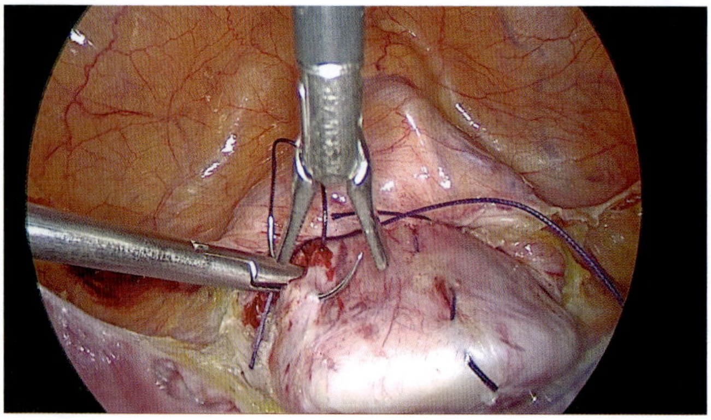

Figure 15.7 Lateral suture left.

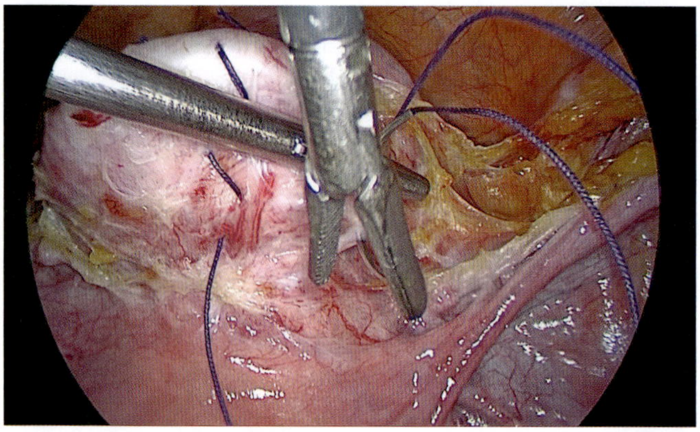

Figure 15.8 Lateral suture right.

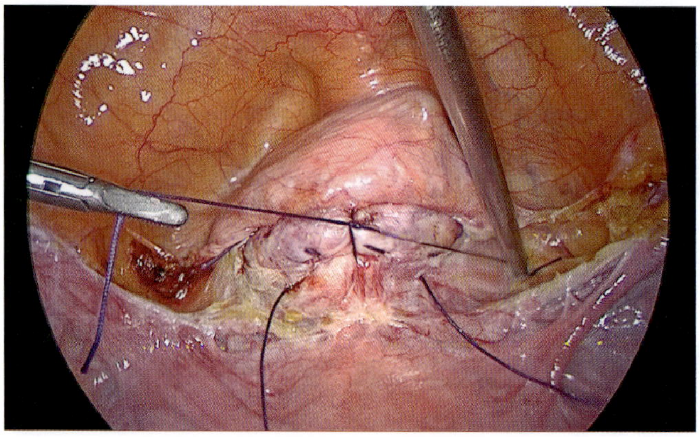

Figure 15.9 First the middle suture is closed, then the lateral sutures.

(a)

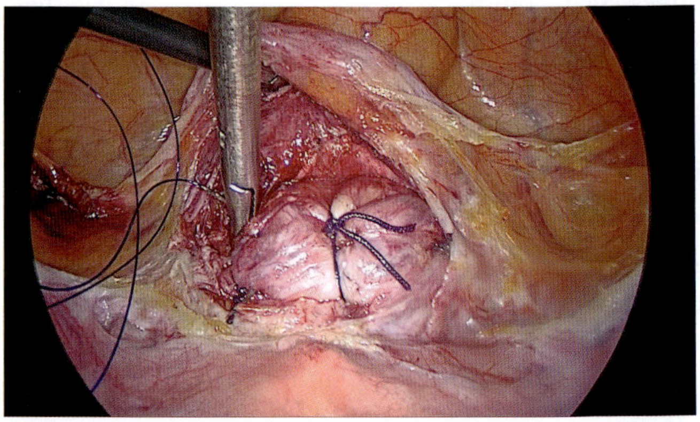

(b)

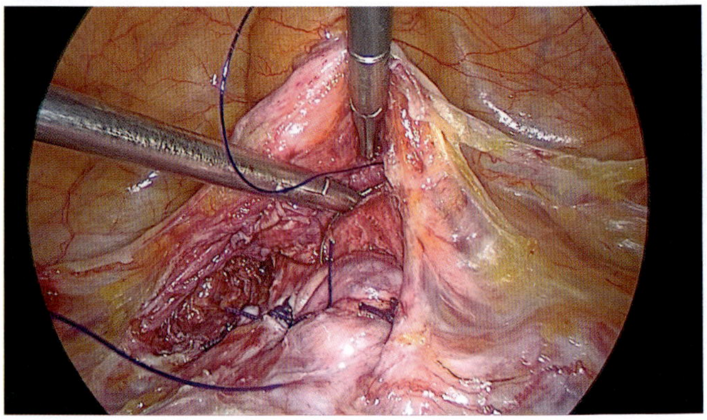

Figure 15.10 a /b Final horizontal suture with an absorbable or non-absorbable suture (PVDF).

Laparoscopic Posterior Defect Repair

The classic posterior repair is started by opening the vaginal epithelium. After pushing off the fatty tissue and the rectum, the lateral fascia is tied together to close the posterior defect. The cranial access is limited due to reduced view. Access to the deep utero sacral ligaments is difficult. In addition, the surgeon has to deal with the unclear position of the ureter and the deep pelvic nerve plexus. In many cases additional resection of the mucosa is performed to avoid big vaginal folds.

For the laparoscopic approach we also advise use of a retractor when dissecting the posterior vaginal wall as well. As the Breisky retractor is made of steel and available in different sizes, it is helpful to estimate the thickness of the tissue and find the lateral rim of the vagina. The procedure is started by opening the peritoneum in the pouch of Douglas. The borderline to the fatty tissue is used as the entering zone. Here we find the optimal area to enter the recto-vaginal septum to reach the non-vascular space. The vaginal wall should be exposed completely (Figure 15.11). The flat retractor provides good contact to the vaginal wall and optimal orientation. The area of the pre-anal canal is presented by blunt dissection. Lateral dissection requires the coagulation of small vessels. In the lower third, the levator muscles are exposed on both sides to visualize the lateral edge of the vaginal fascia. To avoid damage to the muscle this area should be exposed precisely (Figure 15.12).

To stimulate local scaring, we use a size 1 woven absorbable suture. Depending on the size of the defect, four to six sutures are placed. The sutures are placed in small steps and performed in a semicircular, horizontal way (Figures 15.13–15). As the cranial lower tissue is clearly exposed and the laparoscopic view provides direct access, additional suturing of the deep utero sacral ligaments is possible if required. The peritoneum is closed at the end of the procedure (Figure 15.16).

Lateral Defect Repair

The lateral defect repair (see Figures 15.17–22) can also be performed as part of native tissue repair. An extra-peritoneal approach can be performed to avoid scarring and suturing

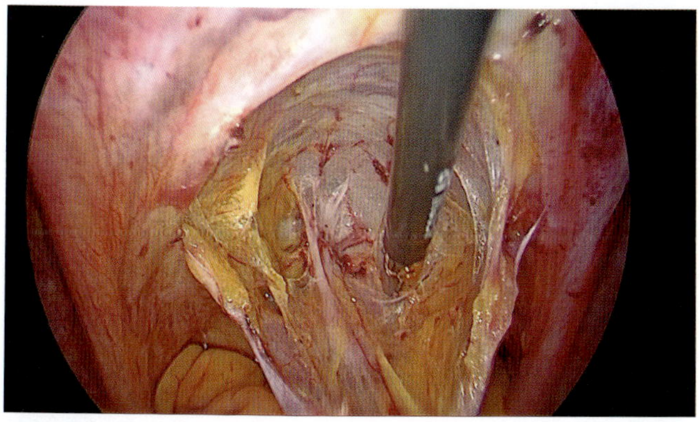

Figure 15.11 Fully entering the recto vaginal septum.

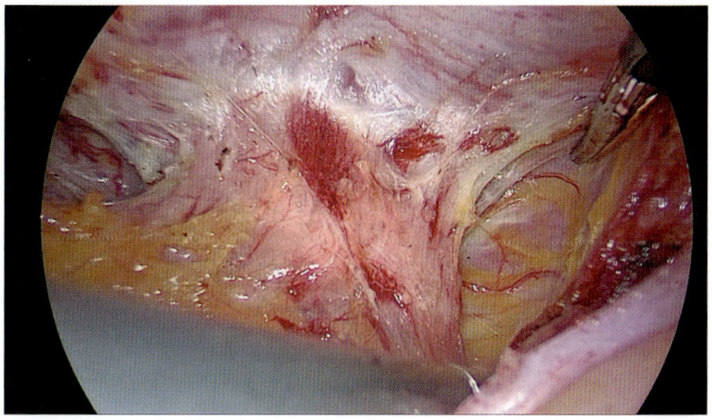

Figure 15.12 Deep rectum and levator muscles are exposed.

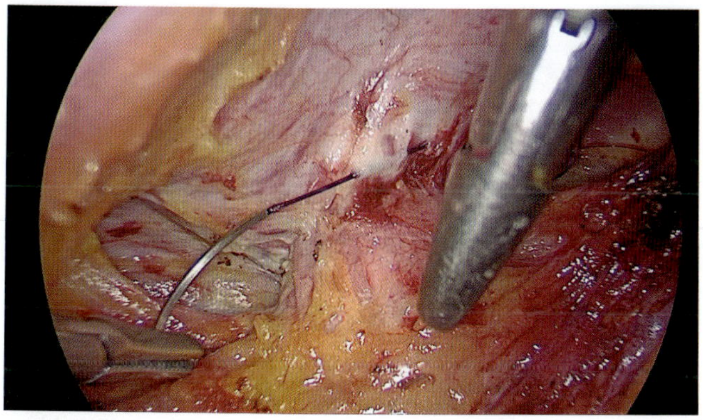

Figure 15.13 Multiple stiches are performed horizontal.

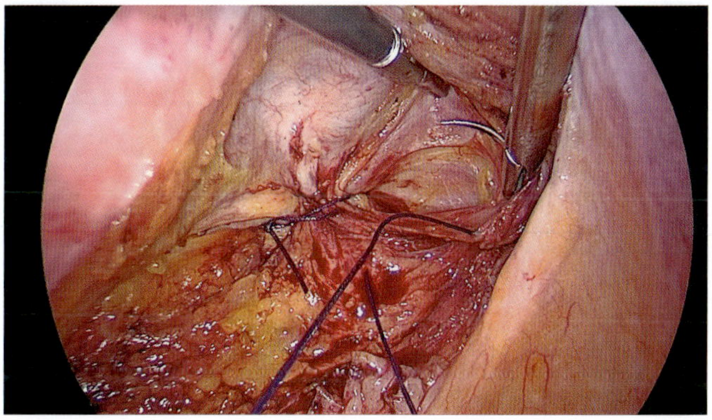

Figure 15.14 Second suture after closing the first suture.

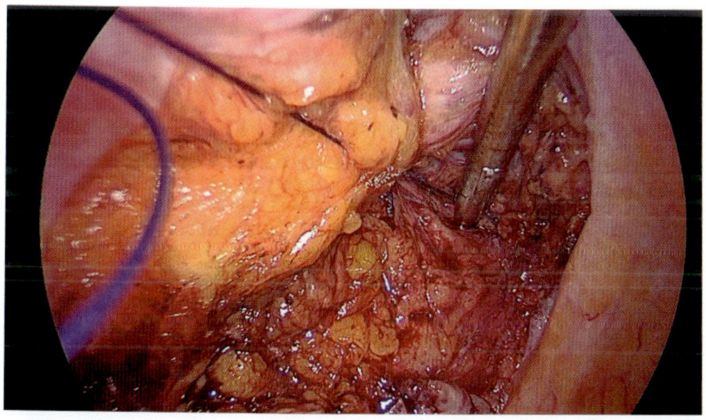

Figure 15.15 Closing the third suture.

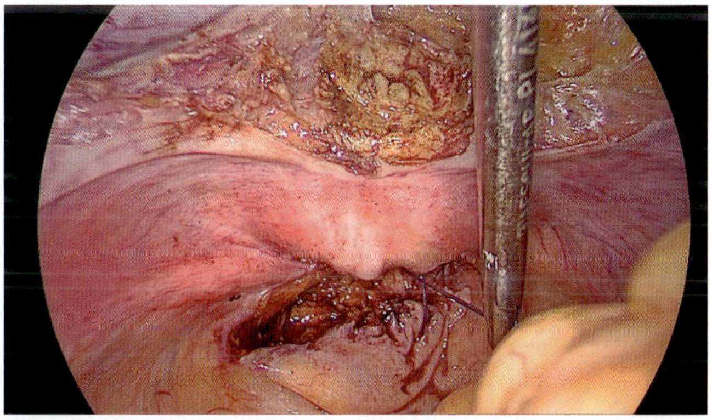

Figure 15.16 Last suture including utero sacral ligaments.

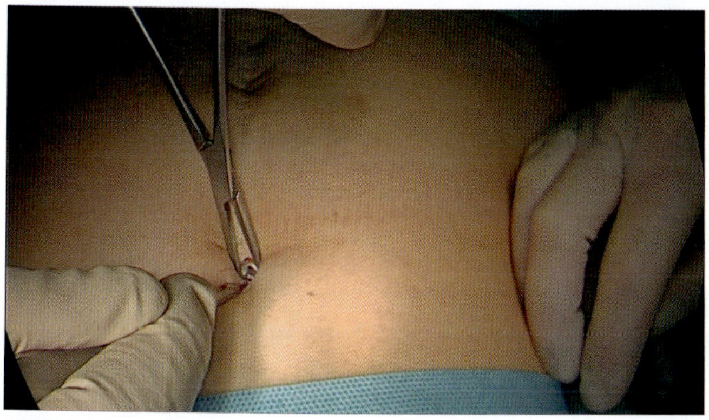

Figure 15.17 Fascial incision for extra-peritoneal approach.

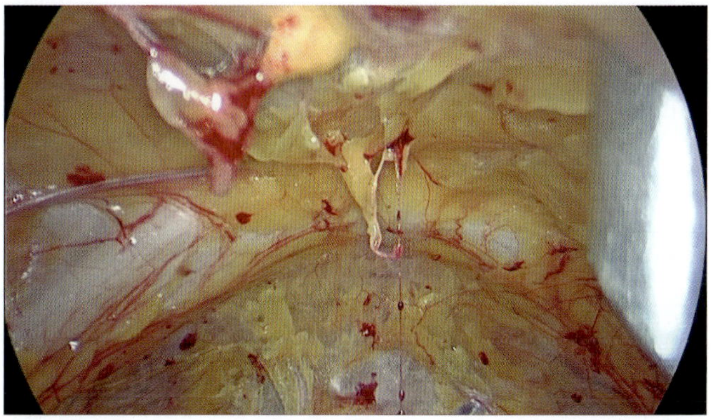

Figure 15.18 Blunt dissected space of Retzius by lenses and bipolar grasper introduces in the midline.

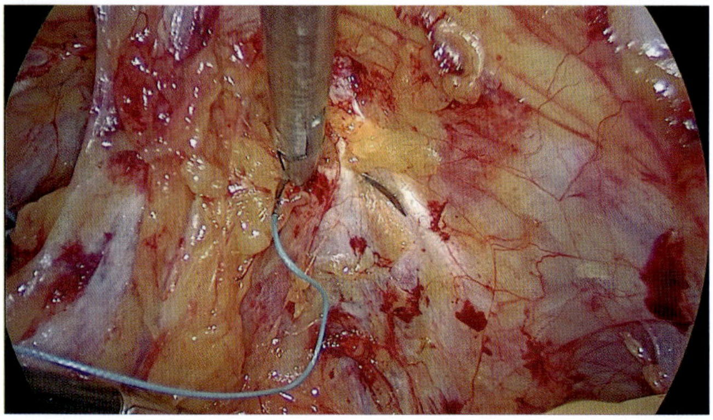

Figure 15.19 First stich close to the posterior lower rim of the pubic bone.

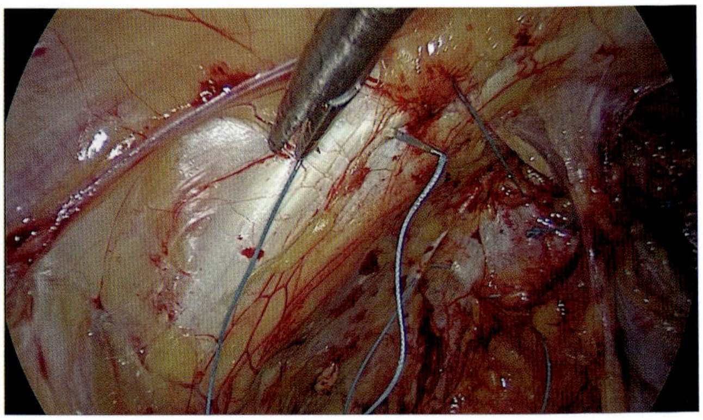

Figure 15.20 Puncturing the left pectineal ligament.

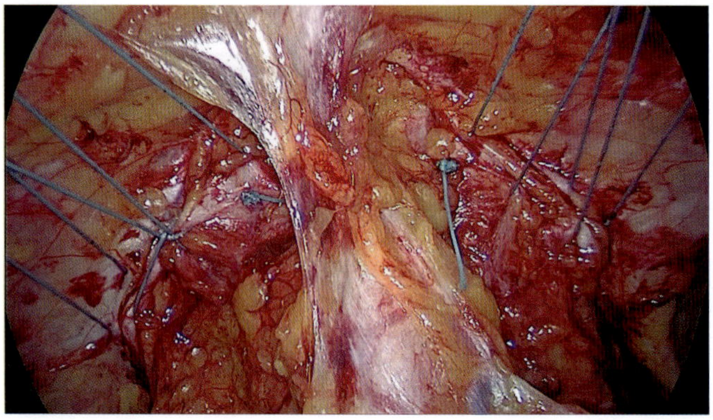

Figure 15.21 Lateral repair of two-thirds of the lateral fascia.

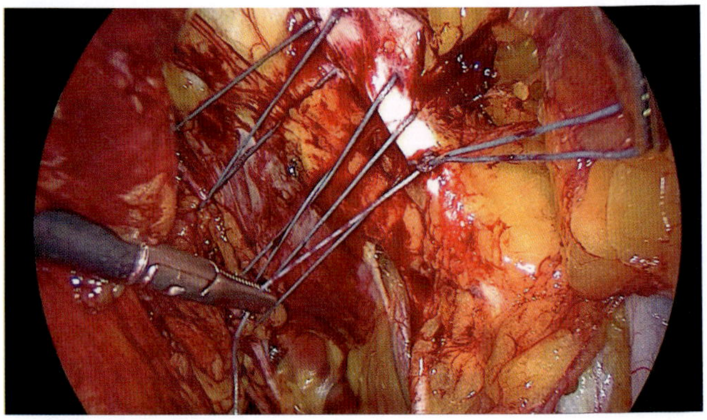

Figure 15.22 Lateral repair suspending the complete lateral fascia (transperitoneal lateral access).

of the peritoneum. A lateral repair combined with an apical suspension can compensate the missing lateral attachment in many cases. According to the author's experience, the simple lateral suturing of the pelvic fascia was less effective and so we changed in 2006 to a running suture suspending the lateral part of the pelvic fascia. If a simple lateral defect repair is planned without concomitant surgery, a pure extra-peritoneal access is used.

Evidence

Laparoscopic native tissue midline repair is still a relatively new technique and hence the evidence is limited but growing. The first follow-up for laparoscopic anterior and posterior fascia repair was published by our centre in 2019 [12]. We followed up 27 patients after 6 to 13 months with our standard quality assessment. The follow-up was performed by personal interview, a questionnaire (The German Version of the 'ICIQ Vaginal Symptoms Questionnaire' (German ICIQ-VS)) and a physical examination. All surgeries were performed concomitant to an apical support (pectopexy). The findings are listed below in Tables 15.1–15.3.

Table 15.1 Anatomical findings in the follow-up

Prior to surgery	13 cystoceles POPQ 2–4	23 recto-enterocele POPQ 2–3
After surgery	92.3% POPQ 0–1	98.7 % POPQ 0–1

Table 15.2 Clinical findings in the follow-up

De novo pain after surgery	De novo urgency	Satisfaction rate	Resumption of intercourse due to surgery	Voiding dysfunction	De novo Constipation
3.7%	3.7%	92.6%	2 patients	0%	0%

Table 15.3 Number of procedures followed up

Follow-up mean 15 months physically examined	Cystocele midline laparoscopic repair n=84; cystocele midline vaginal repair n=52
	Posterior defect laparoscopic repair n=53; posterior defect vaginal repair n=40
See also [18].	

This first quality study showed good anatomical results, a high satisfaction rate, and no new risks or disadvantage for the laparoscopic approach. Currently at the time of preparation of this chapter we have not published the results of a prospective multicentre trial delivered data to compare vaginal repair and laparoscopic repair.

Thus, as the data are not published yet we cannot go into detail in this chapter meanwhile published. In general, the anatomical findings for the vaginal approach were rated more favourably than the laparoscopic approach, however clinical findings and patient satisfaction rates were similar, and with no disadvantages for the laparoscopic approach.

During most vaginal surgeries the vaginal epithelium was shortened. This explains the different anatomical findings in the two groups. According to our experience this may induce a different outcome in the long-term due to future shrinkage or scaring which can occur later when patients stop using oestrogen. We feel, as there is no clinical difference but the risk for developing a tethered vagina is very low, the laparoscopic approach may also have a benefit in the longer term.

According to our first published data [10] the outcome for native tissue repair is satisfactory when combining with a sufficient apical support. These findings are supported by various publications [14,15]. Moreover, there is now a greater emphasis to focus on clinical outcomes and patient satisfaction more than anatomical findings based on POPQ [16], supporting the use of native tissue prior to mesh use. We have found, as experienced laparoscopic surgeons, that the combination of sufficient apical support with repair of accompanying defects in the same setting is a good option.

References

1. Kaltenbach H. *Die operative Gynäkologie*. Ferdinand Enke; 1886.
2. Küstner O. Abdominale totalexstirpation des uterus, ventrifixur des scheidengewölbes, kolporrhaphien; verfahren bei grossen prolapsen. Monatsschrift für Geburtshilfe und Gynäkologie 1910; 32(1):1–3.
3. Fothergill WE. The end results of vaginal operations for genital prolapse. BJOG 1921; 28(2):251–5.
4. Amreich J. *Ätiologie und Operation des Scheidenstumpfprolapses*. Wien Klin Wochensch 1951; 63: 74–7.
5. Ulfelder H. *Prolapse of the Vagina Following Hysterectomy. Progress in Gynecology*, vol 4. Grune & Stratton; 1963, p 676.
6. Ober KG. *Allgemeine und spezielle chirurgische Operationslehre: Gynäkologische Operationen* 1964; 2: 638.
7. Richardson AC, Lyon JB, Williams NL. A new look at pelvic relaxation. Am J Obstet Gynecol 1976; 126(5): 568–73.
8. Käser O., Hirsch HA. *Atlas der gynäkologischen Operationen*, vol 4. Thieme; 1983.
9. Rooney K, et al. Advanced anterior vaginal wall prolapse is highly correlated with apical prolapse. Am J Obstet Gynecol 2006; 195(6): 1837–40.
10. Banerjee C, et al. Komplikationen, Reprolapsraten und funktionelle Ergebnisse nach laparoskopischer Sakropexie: eine Kohortenstudie. Geburtshilfe Frauenheilkd 2010; 70(5): 379–84.
11. Noé KG, et al. Laparoscopic pectopexy: a prospective, randomized, comparative clinical trial of standard laparoscopic sacral colpocervicopexy with the new laparoscopic pectopexy-postoperative results and intermediate-term follow-up in a pilot study. J Endourol 2015; 29(2): 210–15.
12. Noé GK, et al. Laparoscopic anterior and posterior native tissue repair: a new pelvic floor approach. Minim Invasive Ther Allied Technol 2019; 28(4): 241–6.
13. Banerjee C, Noé GK. Endoscopic cystocele surgery: lateral repair with combined suture/mesh technique. J Endourol 2010; 24(10): 1565–9.
14. Chen L, et al. Interaction among apical support, levator ani impairment, and anterior vaginal wall prolapse. Obstet Gynecol 2006; 108(2): 324–32.
15. Maher CM, et al. Surgical management of pelvic organ prolapse in women: the updated summary version Cochrane review. Int Urogynecol J 2011; 22(11):1445–57.
16. Kowalski JT, et al. Systematic review of definitions for success in pelvic organ prolapse surgery. Int Urogynecol J 2018; 29(11): 1697–704.
17. Glazener CMA, et al. Mesh, graft, or standard repair for women having primary transvaginal anterior or posterior compartment prolapse surgery: two parallel-group, multicentre, randomised, controlled trials (PROSPECT). *Lancet* 2017; 389(10067): 381–92.
18. Noé GK, Barnard A, Spüntrup C, et al. Laparoscopic versus vaginal native tissue repair in combination with pectopexy. Subanalysis from an international, prospective, and multi-centre study: short term results. Minim Invasive Ther Allied Technol 2021. https://doi.org/10.1080/13645706.2021.1941118

Chapter 16

Laparoscopic Pectopexy: Procedure Steps and Evidence

Igor But, Tamara Serdinšek

Introduction

Vaginal surgical techniques have a long and respected tradition in surgical treatment of pelvic organ prolapse (POP). However, it is important to emphasize that traditional vaginal POP surgery is characterized by a substantially high recurrence rate and up to 30% re-operation rate [1–4]. Two major events happened in the last decades that have changed the way we address POP management: the introduction of vaginal mesh procedures, which have now almost entirely disappeared from the clinical practice in several countries, and the evolution of endoscopic surgery in urogynaecology [5].

Today, several different laparoscopic procedures are available for POP treatment, both uterine-sparing and for vaginal vault prolapse, and there seems to be an increasing trend towards their use [6,7]. One of the most common uterine-sparing laparoscopic procedures performed for POP is laparoscopic sacrohysteropexy, which is very effective and capable of restoring the physiologic axis of the uterus in the long term with very low re-operation rate [8,9]. For patients with vaginal vault prolapse, laparoscopic sacrocolpopexy can be utilized. The efficacy of sacrocolpopexy is very high and the 2004 Cochrane systematic review concluded that it is the procedure of choice for women with apical prolapse [8].

Despite very good outcomes, neither of these laparoscopic procedures are without drawbacks. During the dissection of the pararectal space, the risk of right ureteral and bowel injury is increased. Moreover, possible injury of the left common iliac vein during dissection of the anterior longitudinal ligament can lead to serious bleeding. Fixation of mesh to the promontory can damage the adjacent sympathetic fibres and lead to the occurrence of defaecatory symptoms such as constipation in up to 19.5% of patients [10,11]. Since laparoscopic suspension to the promontory may be difficult to perform in obese patients or in cases of some other anatomic obstacles or severe adhesions, new laparoscopic POP procedures have been developed to overcome these limitations. One of them is laparoscopic mesh pectopexy, which was introduced by Banerjee and Noé in 2010 [10,11]. The procedure avoids mesh placement to the promontory and the mesh is fixed to the pectineal ligament instead. The aim of the present chapter is to describe the key steps of this procedure and to provide the evidence behind it.

Anatomy of the Pectineal Ligament

The pectineal ligament (lat. *ligamentum (ilio)pectineum*) was first described in 1804 by Sir Astley Cooper [12] and starts in the vicinity of the lacunar ligament [13]. Throughout history, several different definitions of this structure have been proposed. While some authors defined it as the extension of the inguinal ligament, others described it as (i) an element of the attachment of the aponeurosis of the external oblique muscle, (ii) fascial thickening of the posterior wall of the inguinal canal, or as (iii) a thickening of the origin of the pectineus muscle fascia [14]. Histologically, it consists of a dense longitudinally and transversally arranged collagenous network with some fibrocartilaginous areas. This regular arrangement of fibres is thought to account for its strength [12]. The ligament itself is in the shape of a crescent, located along the posterior side of the pectineal line, and adheres to the periosteum of the superior pubic ramus [12,15]. Its medial insertion is to the pubic spine [12], after which it spreads dorsolaterally, passes over the superior pubic ramus, and merges with the iliopubic ramus laterally. On its dorsolateral side, it blends with the muscle fibres of the internal obturator muscle [15]. It extends to the medial border of the external iliac vein and marks the upper limit of the inguinal region [16] (Figure 16.1). According to anatomical studies, its mean length is 53 mm (range 26–65 mm) and it was found to be thicker in two regions: at its medial insertion and between the external iliac vessels and the pubic spine [12]. The ligament itself

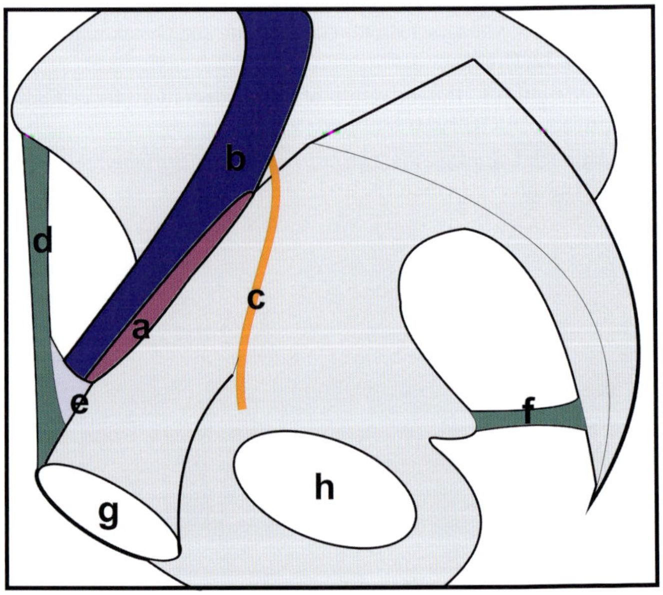

Figure 16.1 Anatomy of the pectineal ligament. The pectineal ligament is located along the posterior side of the pectineal line. It adheres to the periosteum of the superior pubic ramus and extends to the medial border of the external iliac vein. Legend: (a) pectineal ligament; (b) external iliac vein; (c) obturator nerve; (d) inguinal ligament; (e) lacunar ligament; (f) sacrospinous ligament; (g) pubic symphysis; (h) obturator foramen.

has several fascial connections. In its medial part, is it connected to the inguinal ligament via the lacunar ligament. Moreover, it has a connection with the (i) cranial extension of fascia lata (the iliopectineal fascia), (ii) with the tendinous origin of the rectus abdominis muscle, and (iii) with the iliopubic tract [15].

There are several clinically important structures in the vicinity of the pectineal ligament. The aberrant obturator vessel, which connects the external (external iliac or inferior epigastric) and internal iliac (obturator) vascular system, can cross the pectineal ligament and comprise the so-called circle of death [17,18] (Figure 16.2). Its name – circle of death or crown of death (lat. *corona mortis*) – implies the importance of this vascular connection, as profound haemorrhage might occur if accidentally cut [19]. Importantly, this anastomosis can be arterial, venous, or both. Anatomical studies have shown that it is present in up to 84% of cases. There are several different types of corona mortis and the distance between it and the pubic symphysis is variable, to as much as 96 mm [18,19]. Cases of corona mortis injury during different types of urogynaecological procedures such as Burch colposuspension, midurethral slings, pubovaginal slings, and paravaginal defect repairs have been described [18,20,21]. As mentioned previously, the pectineal ligament extends to the external iliac vein [16], which covers its lateral side, so that any dissection in this part must be approached with caution. Moreover, the pectineal ligament is supplied by the branches of the obturator nerve, which can be found along the back side of the ischiopubic ramus as it runs to the obturator canal, and represents another important structure in this area [15].

The value of pectineal ligament in surgery is well established. In 1898, Austrian surgeon Georg Lotheissen was the first to perform inguinal hernia repair by suturing the internal oblique and transversus abdominis muscle to the pectineal ligament [22]. After that, several modifications of hernia procedures utilizing the pectineal ligament have been developed. In orthopaedic and trauma surgery, the pectineal ligament represents an important landmark for dissection towards the iliac fossa and for occlusion or preparation of corona mortis or bleeding control [15]. In urogynaecology, Burch has demonstrated the usefulness of the pectineal ligament in stress urinary incontinence (SUI) treatment in 1961 [23]. Moreover, the pectineal ligament can serve as an anchor point in cases of uterovaginal prolapse [24,25] or neovaginal prolapse after reconstruction procedures in women with Mayer-Rokitansky-Kuester-Hauser syndrome [26].

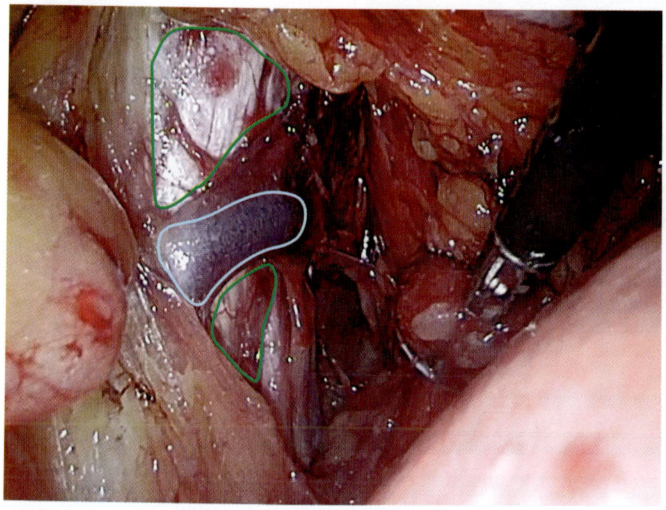

Figure 16.2 Corona mortis. Aberrant vessel (blue line) is seen crossing over the pectineal ligament (green line).

Procedure Steps

The key component of laparoscopic pectopexy is that the mesh for suspension of the uterus or the vaginal vault is fixed to the pectineal ligament. Although different modifications of this procedure have been described in the literature [27,28], we will mainly adhere to the description of the procedure as originally described by its authors [10].

Laparoscopic pectopexy is performed under general anaesthesia and can be divided in six steps, with step one being patient preparation. The patient lies in a dorsal lithotomy position; both arms are tucked by her side. A Foley catheter is inserted into the bladder and attached to a continuous drainage system [10].

In the second step of surgery, a 12 mm optic trocar is inserted through the paraumbilical incision and the abdomen is insufflated with CO_2 up to 12 mm Hg intra-abdominal pressure, which is followed by insertion of three access ports. Two 5 mm access ports are placed 2–4 cm medial and inferior of the anterior superior iliac spine bilaterally, while one 5 mm access port is placed 2–3 cm cranially to the pubic symphysis [10] (Figure 16.3).

The third step comprises the preparation of the pectineal ligament on both sides. After intra-abdominal survey, attention is turned to the round ligament of the uterus, which serves as a landmark for exposure of an area sized approximately 4 cm^2. This area includes the lateral part of the pectineal ligament and is bordered by the external iliac

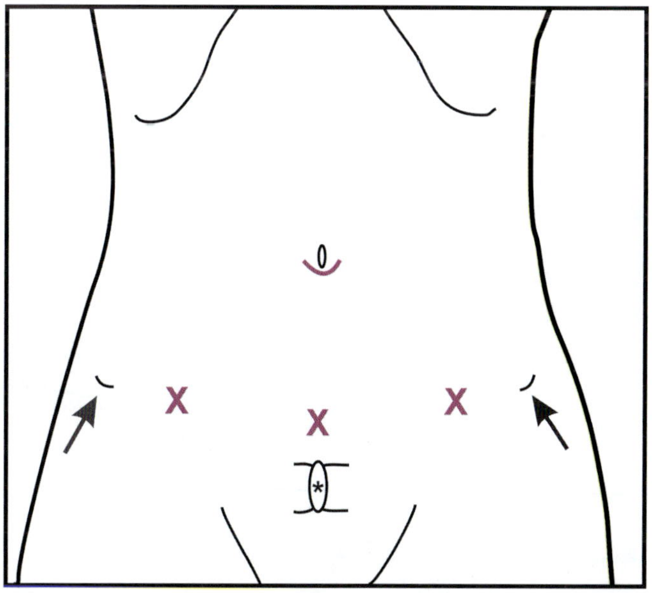

Figure 16.3 Trocar placement. For laparoscopic pectopexy, a 12 mm optic trocar is inserted through the paraumbilical incision (purple semicircle). Then, three 5 mm access ports (purple X) are placed. One access port is inserted 2–3 cm cranially to the pubic symphysis (grey asterisk) and one 2–4 cm medial and inferior of the anterior superior iliac spine (grey arrow) bilaterally.

vessels cranio-ventrally and the obturator nerve dorso-caudally. For the preparation, peritoneum next to the round ligament is superficially incised and the soft tissue of the pelvic sidewall is bluntly prepared until the pectineal ligament is reached. External iliac vessels are also prepared. Preparation of the pectineal ligament is performed up to the region of the obturator nerves, which allows enough space for mesh fixation [10] (Figure 16.4). During this step of the procedure, the

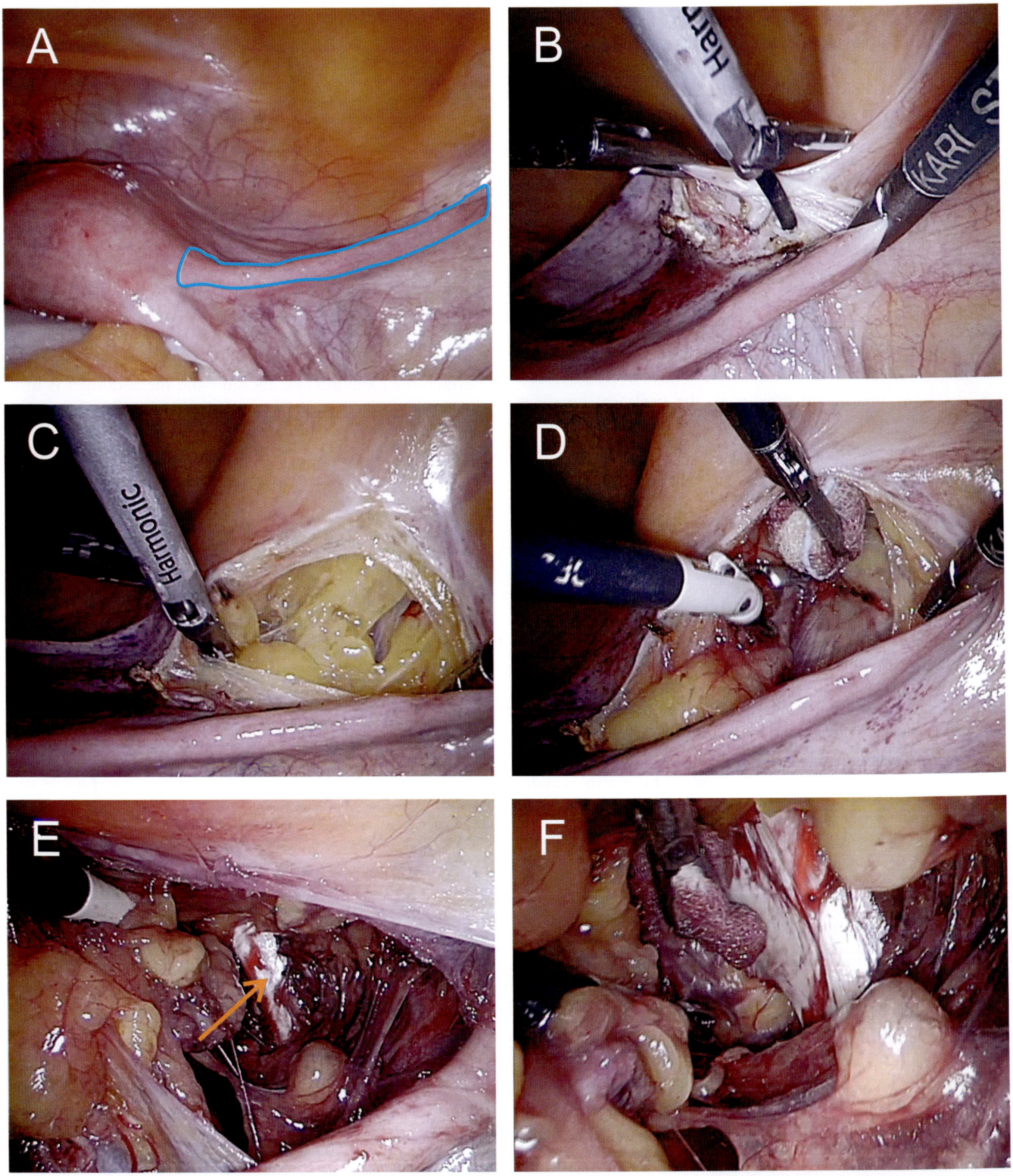

Figure 16.4 Preparation of the pectineal ligament for mesh placement. (A) The round ligament of the uterus (blue line) serves as a landmark for the ligament exposure. (B) Peritoneum at the lateral side of the round ligament is incised. (C–D) Soft tissue of the pelvic sidewall is bluntly prepared. Cotton swab can be very useful for this step of the procedure. (E) Preparation is performed until the pectineal ligament (orange arrow) is reached. (F) Appropriately sized area for mesh placement is prepared.

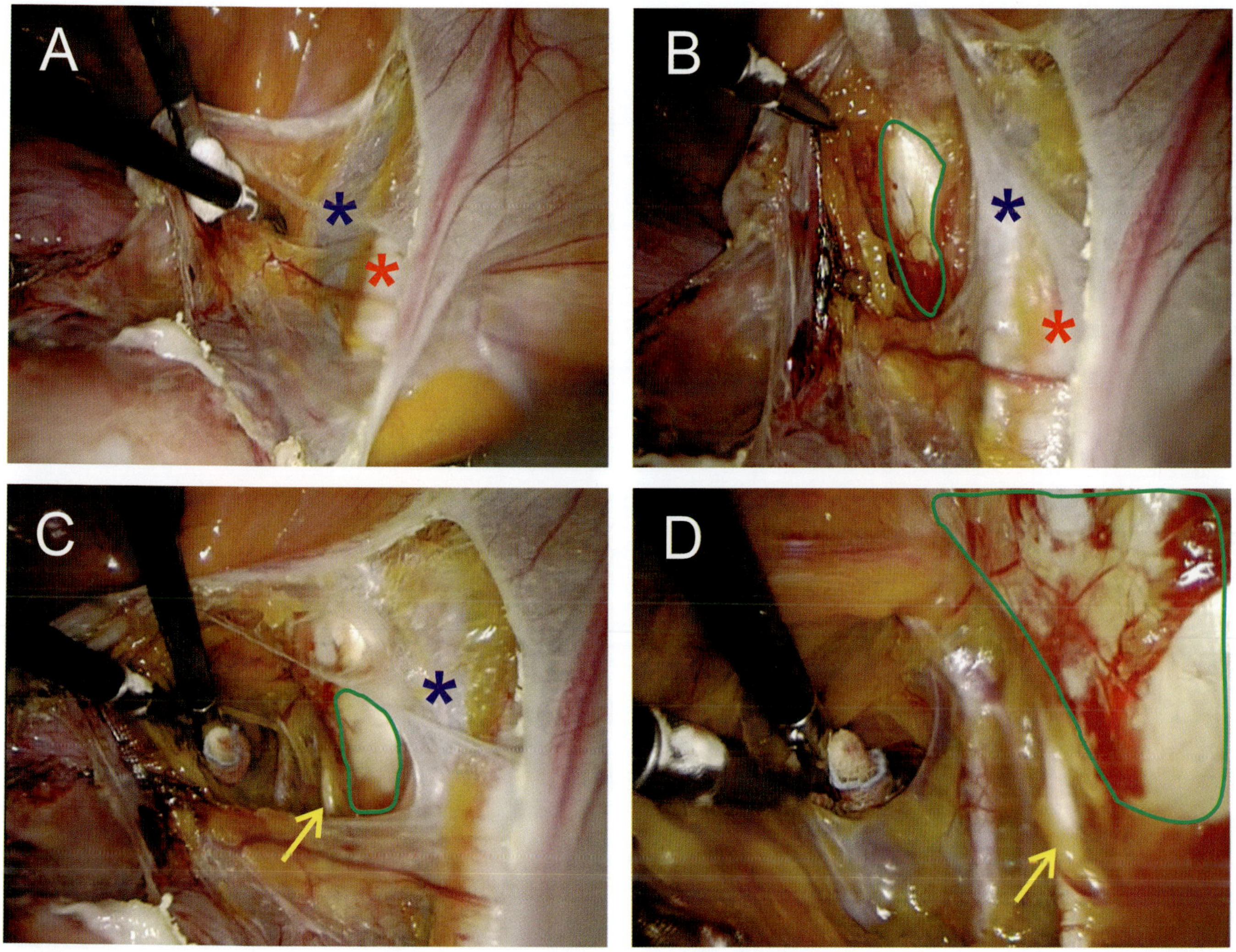

Figure 16.5 Important anatomical structures to be visualized during pectineal ligament preparation. (A–B) Upon opening of the peritoneum, external iliac vein (blue asterisk) and artery (red asterisk) can be seen and further prepared during the exposure of the ligament (green line). (C–D) During further dissection of the ligament (green line), obturator nerve (yellow arrow) and vessels can be seen. The obturator nerve can be found along the back side of the ischiopubic ramus as it runs to the obturator canal.

external iliac veins and obturator nerve need to be visualized and protected (Figure 16.5).

Step four differs whether we are performing suspension of the uterus or suspension of the vaginal apex/cervical stump. In both cases, we start by superficially enlarging the peritoneal incisions on both sides by a blunt dissection in an imaginative line between the physiological axis of the pectineal line and the cervical stump, vaginal apex, or the uterus, respectively. This preparation is performed using a blunt forceps and a bipolar clamp [10] or a harmonic scalpel [29]. We should aim to be as superficial as possible, as this reduces the danger of the accidental injury of nerves and vessels. Then, the lower insertion area is prepared. Its location depends on the existent structures. In case of fixation on the cervical stump, for example after previous or concomitant subtotal hysterectomy, the anterior and posterior brim of the cervical stump provide a good tissue for a stable fixation. If we have to perform a fixation directly to the vaginal vault, then the peritoneum has to be dissected and anterior and posterior parts of vaginal apex prepared as in laparoscopic sacrocolpopexy [10]. While the authors of this method prefer to perform a laparoscopic subtotal hysterectomy and then subsequent fixation of the cervical stump [10,30], uterus-sparing procedure is also possible. In this case, the anterior peritoneum of the uterus is dissected and lower uterine segment prepared for the mesh fixation [29] (Figure 16.6). At the end of this step, the lower insertion area should correspond to superficial peritoneal incisions [10].

Mesh fixation is performed in step five. Both use of polyvinylidene fluoride (PVDF) monofilament mesh [10] and use of polypropylene monofilament mesh [31] have been described. Mesh and a non-absorbable suture with attached needle are inserted via the large port. One end of the mesh is attached to the left pectineal ligament with two simple interrupted stiches, and the same is repeated on the right side [10]. Use of both non-absorbable tacks and absorbable mesh fixation devices instead of sutures for this step of the procedure has also been described in the literature [28,32] (Figure 16.7). If necessary, the mesh is shortened before fixation at the right

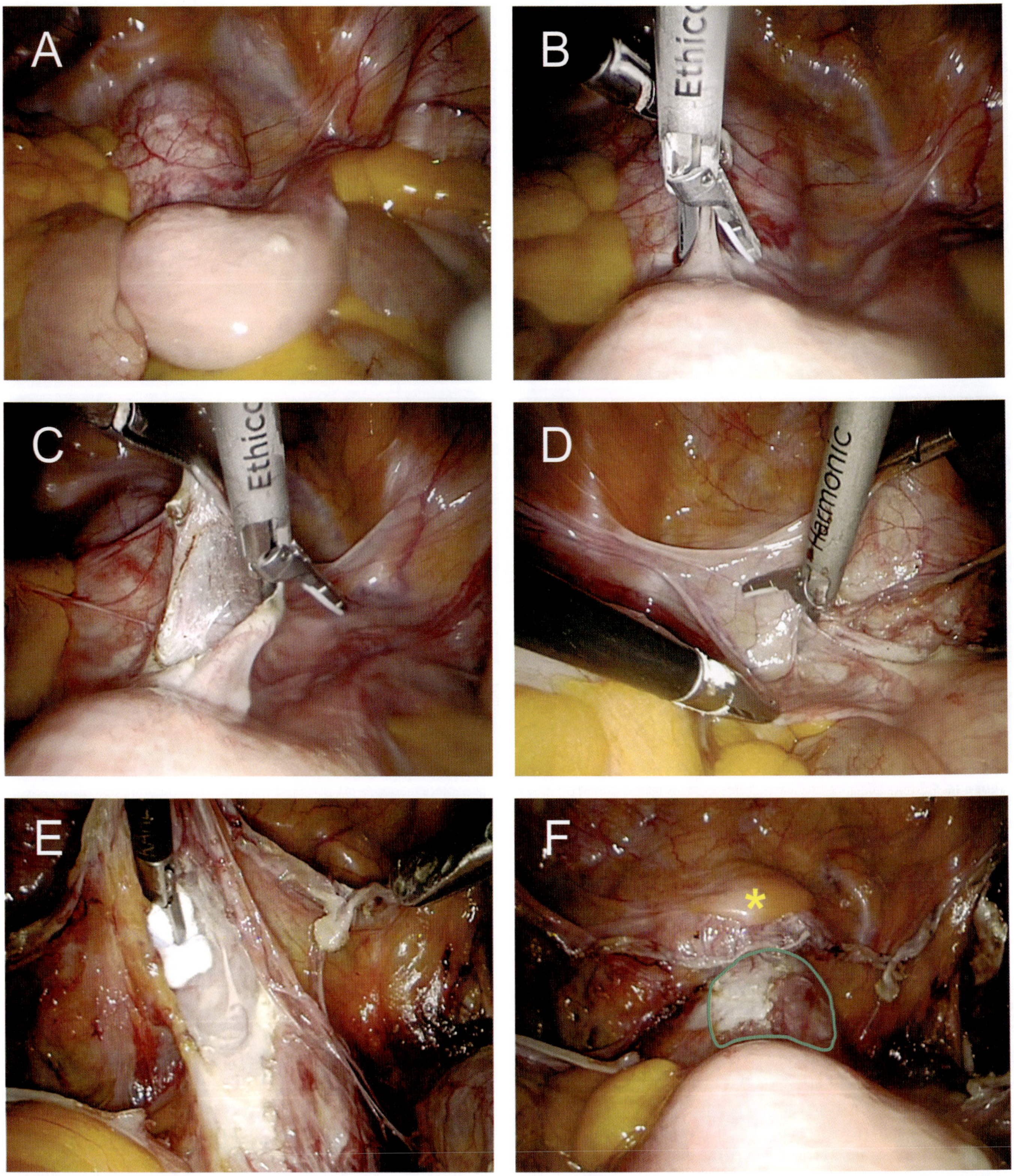

Figure 16.6 Preparation of the lower uterine segment for mesh fixation. (A–C) Peritoneum of the lower uterine segment is lifted and incised. (D) The incisions are then extended laterally towards pelvic sidewalls. (E) Using blunt dissection technique, the bladder is pushed distally. (F) In the end, area for mesh fixation (green line) is exposed and bladder (yellow asterisk) is safely deflected.

side. The needle is then removed and another non-absorbable suture is introduced. In case of vaginal apex fixation, the authors of the method suggest the use of polydioxanone (PDS) suture, while in case of cervical stump fixation, they opt for a non-absorbable suture. Vaginal apex or the cervical stump, respectively, is elevated to the intended position and fixed with 2–4 simple interrupted or continuous sutures to the middle of the mesh. It is important to emphasize that the elevation of the vaginal apex/cervical stump needs to be tension-free [10]. If uterus is present, the mesh is attached to the anterior

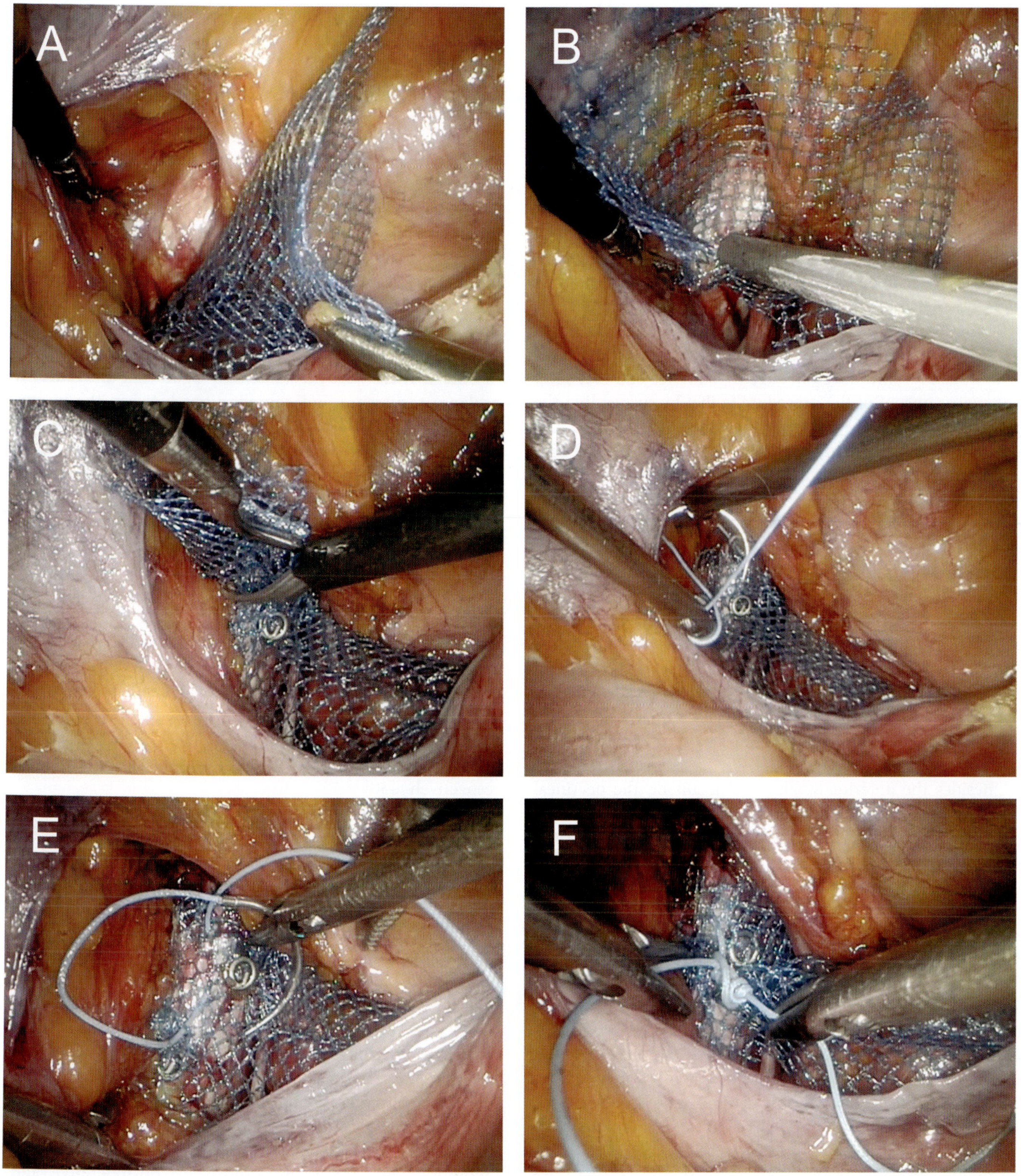

Figure 16.7 Mesh fixation to the pectineal ligament using tacks and non-absorbable suture. (A) One end of the mesh is positioned to the pectineal ligament. (B) Mesh is fixated using non-absorbable tacks. (C) If necessary, the mesh is shortened using scissors. (D–F) Mesh is attached to the pectineal ligament using non-absorbable suture.

side of the lower uterine segment [29]. At our centre, we aim to achieve a sufficient level 1 support of the uterus, which is why we introduce the mesh through the openings that we create in the avascular parts of the broad ligaments and attach it above the levels of the sacrouterine ligaments. Which one of these two approaches provides better clinical results is currently unknown.

In step six, which is a final step of the procedure, closure of the peritoneum is performed using a continuous absorbable suture of 35 cm length with an attached needle. Then, the ports and the Foley catheter are removed and CO_2 is evacuated from the abdominal cavity [10].

Evidence Regarding Laparoscopic Pectopexy

The idea of suspending the uterus or vaginal vault to the pectineal ligament is not entirely new. In 1993, Joshi published the results of his technique of uterine suspension to the pectineal ligaments through a Cherney incision. He used a mersilene tape for uterus suspension [25]. In 2013, he and seven other authors published the results of vaginal vault suspension to pectineal ligament by either open or laparoscopic route using a polyester tape. They included 119 women with a mean follow-up of 5.5 years. Only two women had prolapse recurrence and an additional two had an asymptomatic tape erosion [24].

However, laparoscopic mesh pectopexy as we perform it today, was first introduced in 2010 by Banerjee and Noé [10]. The main concept of the procedure is that by suspending the prolapsed organ to the pectineal ligaments, we follow the natural course of the round ligaments without crossing the ureters, hypogastric trunk, or the bowel, and without causing the restriction of the presacral space [11,33,34]. According to the authors, one of the main advantages of the method compared to anterior fixation methods is the reduction of the *de novo* rectocele formation and bowel obstruction occurrence due to more physiologic lateral fixation [10]. The segment of the pectineal ligament, to which the mesh is attached, corresponds to the level of the second sacral vertebra, which is supposed to be the optimal level for restoration of the physiological axis of vagina [29,30]. Moreover, the method was developed to be used in patients with difficult access to lesser pelvis or anterior longitudinal ligament due to adhesions, obesity, or other anatomical obstacles [10].

Besides the anterior longitudinal ligament, the pectineal ligament itself is one of the strongest ligaments used in female pelvic surgery. As shown in a cadaver study by Cosson et al, the pectineal ligament is statistically stronger than the arcus tendinous of pelvic fascia and the sacrospinous ligament. Although there is great variability between individuals and between the same ligaments on the opposite sides in the same person, the pectineal ligament can obtain a maximal tearing value up to 120 N with the average value of 81±37 N on the right side and 74±34 N on the left side. There was no statistically significant difference between the right and the left side [35]. Our experience with soft-embalmed cadavers showed that the extraction forces of a non-absorbable suture and a non-absorbable tack, embedded in the pectineal ligament, are 3.3±2.0 kg and 3.3±0.7, respectively [36]. In this view, the pectineal ligament provides a suitable mesh fixation point. Despite slight variations in the technique compared to the original description [10] and use of different suturing or anchoring materials for mesh fixation, there is currently no evidence that these factors affect the efficacy of the procedure. A biomechanical analysis by Sauerwald et al discovered that a single suture to the pectineal ligament is as sufficient as a continuous suture and would support loads up to 85 N [37]. Moreover, a small retrospective study suggested that there is no statistically significant differences in short-term outcomes when comparing laparoscopic pectopexy using sutures or absorbable mesh fixation tacks except for the shorter operation time [32].

Several short and intermediate follow-up studies that evaluate the outcomes of laparoscopic pectopexy are available. A six-month follow-up after laparoscopic pectopexy discovered significant changes in all postoperative Pelvic Organ Prolapse Quantification (POP-Q) system values compared to preoperative values. There was no subjective recurrences and a significant improvement in Female Sexual Function (FSFI) and Prolapse Quality of Life (P-QOL) scores [27]. Another six-month follow-up study by Biler et al that compared abdominal sacrocolpopexy, laparoscopic sacrocolpopexy, and laparoscopic pectopexy concluded that the mean operating time was significantly shorter in the laparoscopic pectopexy group than in others. There were no statistically significant differences in prolapse recurrence and complications between the groups. Subjective satisfaction rate in all three groups was over 95% [38]. Intermediate results of laparoscopic pectopexy versus vaginal sacrospinous fixation (SSF) found no significant differences in apical descensus relapse rate between both groups (11.1% versus 14%, respectively). However, there was more *de novo* cystoceles in patients after SSF with no differences in number of rectoceles. Patients' satisfaction rates were very high in both groups and exceeded 90% [31]. Another intermediate follow-up study compared laparoscopic pectopexy to laparoscopic sacrocolpopexy and the results showed no differences in apical descensus relapse rates between groups (2.3% for pectopexy and 9.8% for sacrocolpopexy group). The rates of *de novo* SUI and rectoceles were similar in both groups. However, the incidence of *de novo* defaecation disorders and *de novo* lateral defect cystoceles was significantly higher in the sacrocolpopexy group (0% versus 19.5%, respectively) [30].

As mentioned previously, laparoscopic sacrocolpopexy is considered as a gold standard for apical prolapse correction and reconstitution of physiological vaginal axis. However, the possibility of presacral haemorrhage and pelvic space reduction need to be taken into account. Especially the latter can lead to chronic pelvic pain, defaecation disorders, and hypogastric nerve damage, particularly in obese population. On the other hand, sacrospinous fixation can be associated with complications such as haemorrhage, cystocele formation, bladder, rectum or small bowel injury, ischiorectal abscess, perineal hernia, or even necrotizing infection [34]. In this view, the laparoscopic pectopexy appears as a compelling option, especially in obese patients or in patients with difficult access to the promontory [38]. Nevertheless, it is not entirely without complications, although they do not seem more prevalent than in other surgical methods for POP treatment. A short-term postoperative randomized comparison of laparoscopic sacrocolpopexy with laparoscopic pectopexy of the cervix or vaginal vault found no major complications and no *de novo* defaecation problems or incontinence in either group. Although the average operating time and blood loss were significantly lower in the pectopexy group, they were also quite low in the sacrocolpopexy group (43.1 versus 52.1 minutes and 4.6 versus 15.3 ml, respectively) [11]. Another small six-month follow-up series described no intraoperative or postoperative complications of the procedure and no conversion to laparotomy was required [29], while another series had 4.5% conversions to laparotomy, 4.5% of women had exacerbation of cystocele, 9.0% of rectoceles, there was 4.5% of *de novo* SUI, and 4.5% of *de novo* urgent urinary incontinence [27]. Astepe et al observed 2.8% of intraoperative bladder injuries, 2.8% of mesh erosions [31], while in a study by Biler et al overall complication rate of laparoscopic pectopexies was 3.6% [38].

To date, the largest prospective international multicentre pectopexy trial with the longest follow-up period was published by Noé et al in 2020. They included 501 surgical procedures, performed at 11 different clinics. All surgeries were performed following the same principle and using the same type of pre-manufactured mesh. Although the study did not address the apical descensus recurrence rate, it did provide the information regarding the operation time and complication rate. The mean operation time was 135±46 minutes and surgery was completed in less than 60 minutes in less than 79% of cases. Severe complications such as organ damage or larger bleeding occurred in 1%, but the authors emphasized that the organ damage was never related to pectopexy, but to concomitant approaches or the management of adhesions [39]. Overall, it seems that laparoscopic pectopexy is associated with a very low complication rate if performed with caution. During preparations of the ligament for mesh fixation, important anatomical structures such as external iliac vessels and obturator nerve need to be protected. On the other hand, preparation of structures such as hypogastric vessels or ureter is not necessary [10].

Laparoscopic pectopexy can be combined with different concomitant procedures such as anterior or posterior colporrhaphy, perineoplasty, vaginal paravaginal repair, hysterectomy, laparoscopic Burch procedure, or different tape procedures for SUI treatment [11,28,30,31,38]. Moreover, it can be combined with laparoscopic anterior and/or posterior native tissue repair or paravaginal repair. As the procedure can be performed in a single session, it requires no additional instruments or separate sterile area for vaginal surgery, and it enables the preservation of the integrity of the vaginal wall [40,41]. Different types of synthetic mesh can be used for the procedure, but a few reports of using hamstring autograft as a mesh alternative for different laparoscopic POP procedures have been described and could be worth investigating in the future [42]. If hamstring autografts were to be recognized as equally effective, they could represent a possible alternative to synthetic mesh, which is especially important in this transvaginal mesh ban era, when we are searching for new efficient native tissue reconstruction options.

In conclusion, laparoscopic pectopexy seems an efficient alternative to sacrocolpopexy/sacrohysteropexy with very low complication rate and relatively short operation time, especially in obese patients. However, there is scarcity of data regarding its long-term outcomes. The current view of The National Institute for Health and Care Excellence (NICE) from 2018 on the position of laparoscopic mesh pectopexy for apical prolapse is that the evidence on its safety and efficacy is insufficient and that it should only be used in the context of research [43]. Before including the procedure into clinical guidelines and everyday clinical practice, appropriate long-term randomized controlled studies need to be conducted.

References

1. Vergeldt TFM, Weemhoff M, IntHout J, Kluivers KB. Risk factors for pelvic organ prolapse and its recurrence: a systematic review. Int Urogynecol J 2015; 26(11): 1559–73.
2. Whiteside JL, Weber AM, Meyn LA, Walters MD. Risk factors for prolapse recurrence after vaginal repair. Am J Obstet Gynecol 2004; 191(5): 1533–8.
3. Bohlin KS, Ankardal M, Nüssler E, Lindkvist H, Milsom I. Factors influencing the outcome of surgery for pelvic organ prolapse. Int Urogynecol J 2018; 29(1): 81–9.
4. Bump RC, Norton PA. Epidemiology and natural history of pelvic floor dysfunction. Obstet Gynecol Clin North Am 1998; 25(4): 723–46.
5. Downing KT. Uterine Prolapse: From Antiquity to Today [Internet]. Obstetrics and Gynecology International. Published 2012. Available from: www.hindawi.com/journals/ogi/2012/649459/
6. Miller BJ, Seman EI, O'Shea RT, Hakendorf PH, Nguyen TTT. Recent trends in the management of pelvic organ prolapse in Australia and New Zealand. Aust N Z J Obstet Gynaecol 2019; 59(1): 117–22.
7. Zacche MM, Mukhopadhyay S, Giarenis I. Trends in prolapse surgery in England. Int Urogynecol J 2018; 29(11): 1689–95.
8. Gutman R, Maher C. Uterine-preserving POP surgery. Int Urogynecol J 2013; 24(11): 1803–13.
9. Jefferis H, Price N, Jackson S. Laparoscopic hysteropexy: 10 years' experience. Int Urogynecol J 2017; 28(8): 1241–8.
10. Banerjee C, Noé KG. Laparoscopic pectopexy: a new technique of prolapse surgery for obese patients. Arch Gynecol Obstet 2011; 284(3): 631–5.
11. Noé KG, Spüntrup C, Anapolski M. Laparoscopic pectopexy: a randomised comparative clinical trial of standard laparoscopic sacral colpo-cervicopexy to the new laparoscopic pectopexy. Short-term postoperative results. Arch Gynecol Obstet 2013; 287(2): 275–80.
12. Faure J-P, Hauet Th, Scepi M, et al. The pectineal ligament anatomical study and surgical applications. Surg Radiol Anat 2001; 23(4): 237–42.
13. Lytle WJ. The inguinal and lacunar ligaments. J Anat 1974; 118(Pt 2): 241–51.
14. Skandalakis JE, Gray SW, Skandalakis LJ, Colborn GL, Pemberton LB. Surgical anatomy of the inguinal area. World J Surg 1989; 13(5): 490–8.
15. Steinke H, Wiersbicki D, Völker A, et al. The fascial connections of the pectineal ligament. Clin Anat 2019; 32(7): 961–9.
16. Lytle WJ. Inguinal anatomy. J Anat 1979; 128(Pt 3): 581–94.
17. Avisse C, Delattre J-F, Flament J-B. The inguinofemoral area from a laparoscopic standpoint: history, anatomy, and surgical applications. Surg Clin North Am 2000; 80(1): 35–48.
18. Drewes PG, Marinis SI, Schaffer JI, Boreham MK, Corton MM. Vascular anatomy over the superior pubic rami in female cadavers. Am J Obstet Gynecol 2005; 193(6): 2165–8.

19. Rusu MC, Cergan R, Motoc AGM, Folescu R, Pop E. Anatomical considerations on the corona mortis. Surg Radiol Anat 2010; 32(1): 17–24.
20. Gobrecht U, Kuhn A, Fellman B. Injury of the corona mortis during vaginal tape insertion (TVT-Secur™ using the U-Approach). Int Urogynecol J 2011; 22(4): 443–5.
21. Hubka P, Svabik K, Martan A, Masata J. A serious bleeding complication with injury of the corona mortis with the TVT-Secur procedure: two cases of contact of TVT-S with the corona mortis during cadaver study. Int Urogynecol J 2010; 21(9): 1179–80.
22. Sachs M, Damm M, Encke A. Historical evolution of inguinal hernia repair. World J Surg 1997; 21(2): 218–23.
23. Burch JC. Urethrovaginal fixation to Cooper's ligament for correction of stress incontinence, cystocele, and prolapse. Am J Obstet Gynecol 1961; 81: 281–90.
24. Joshi VM, Otiv SR, Dagade VB, et al. Pectineal ligament suspension of prolapsed vaginal vault. Int J Gynecol Obstet 2013; 123(1): 29–32.
25. Joshi V. A new technique of uterine suspension to pectineal ligaments in the management of uterovaginal prolapse. Obstet Gynecol 1993; 81(5(Pt 1)): 790–3.
26. Freundt I, Toolenaar TA, Jeekel H, Drogendijk AC, Huikeshoven FJ. Prolapse of the sigmoid neovagina: report of three cases. Obstet Gynecol 1994; 83(5 Pt 2): 876–9.
27. Tahaoglu AE, Bakir MS, Peker N, Bagli İ, Tayyar AT. Modified laparoscopic pectopexy: short-term follow-up and its effects on sexual function and quality of life. Int Urogynecol J 2018; 29(8): 1155–60.
28. Pirtea L, Balint O, Secoşan C, Grigoraş D, Ilina R. Laparoscopic pectopexy with Burch colposuspension for pelvic prolapse associated with stress urinary incontinence. J Minim Invasive Gynecol 2019; 27(5): 1023–4.
29. Kale A, Biler A, Terzi H, Usta T, Kale E. Laparoscopic pectopexy: initial experience of single center with a new technique for apical prolapse surgery. Int Braz J Urol 2017; 43(5): 903–9.
30. Noé K-G, Schiermeier S, Alkatout I, Anapolski M. Laparoscopic pectopexy: a prospective, randomized, comparative clinical trial of standard laparoscopic sacral colpocervicopexy with the new laparoscopic pectopexy-postoperative results and intermediate-term follow-up in a pilot study. J Endourol 2015; 29(2): 210–15.
31. Astepe BS, Karsli A, Köleli I, et al. Intermediate-term outcomes of laparoscopic pectopexy and vaginal sacrospinous fixation: a comparative study. Int Braz J Urol 2019; 45(5): 999–1007.
32. Basol G, Kale A, Aytuluk HG, Kale E, Pence H, Sapmaz T. Polypropylene suture versus absorbable tack mesh fixation in laparoscopic pectopexy: a retrospective study. Int J Med Rev Case Reports 2019; 3(8): 521–7.
33. Cezarino BN. Editorial Comment: Laparoscopic pectopexy: initial experience of single center with a new technique for apical prolapse surgery. Int Braz J Urol 2017; 43(5): 910.
34. Bhattarai A, Staat M. A computational study of organ relocation after laparoscopic pectopexy to repair posthysterectomy vaginal vault prolapse. Biomech Biomed Eng Imaging Vis 2019; 8(3): 1–10.
35. Cosson M, Boukerrou M, Lacaze S et al. A study of pelvic ligament strength. Eur J Obstet Gynecol Reprod Biol 2003; 109: 80–7.
36. Serdinšek T, Zemljič M, Kocbek L, Pejkovic B, But I. 'Comparison of extraction forces of non-absorbable suture and different anchoring systems used in pelvic organ prolapse surgery using soft-embalmed female cadavers.' Conference presentation at 10th EUGA Meeting, Barcelona, Spain, 2017.
37. Sauerwald A, Niggl M, Puppe J, et al. Laparoscopic pectopexy: a biomechanical analysis. PLoS ONE 2016; 11(2): e0144143.
38. Biler A, Ertas IE, Tosun G, et al. Perioperative complications and short-term outcomes of abdominal sacrocolpopexy, laparoscopic sacrocolpopexy, and laparoscopic pectopexy for apical prolapse. Int Braz J Urol 2018; 44(5): 996–1004.
39. Noé GK, Schiermeier S, Papathemelis T, et al. Prospective international multicenter pectopexy trial: interim results and findings post surgery. Eur J Obstet Gynecol Reprod Biol 2020; 244: 81–6.
40. Noé GK, Alkatout I, Schiermeier S, Soltécz S, Anapolski M. Laparoscopic anterior and posterior native tissue repair: a new pelvic floor approach. Minim Invasive Ther Allied Technol 2019; 28(4): 241–6.
41. Bakir MS, Bagli I, Cavus Y, Tahaoglu AE. Laparoscopic pectopexy and paravaginal repair after failed recurrent pelvic organ prolapse surgery. Gynecol Minim Invasive Ther 2020; 9(1): 42–4.
42. Hornemann A, Hoch B, Germann G, Franz W, Sütterlin M. Hamstring autograft as a mesh alternative for pelvic organ prolapse. J Minim Invasive Gynecol 2020; 27(1): 17–18.
43. National Institute for Health and Care Excellence. Laparoscopic mesh pectopexy for apical prolapse of the uterus or vagina [Internet]. Published 2018. Available from: www.nice.org.uk/guidance/ipg608

Chapter

17

Laparoscopic Colposuspension: Procedure Steps and Evidence

Matthew Izett-Kay, Alfred Cutner, Arvind Vashisht

Background

Stress urinary incontinence (SUI) is defined by the International Urogynecological Association (IUGA) and International Continence Society (ICS) as the complaint of involuntary loss of urine on effort or physical exertion, or on sneezing or coughing [1]. Large population studies have shown the incidence is between 9% and 29%, with large variation between different countries and increasing incidence with age [2,3]. Approximately 6% of women report being regularly bothered by such symptoms, leading to a life-time risk of surgery for urinary incontinence of 3.6% and a risk of subsequent re-operation for recurrent incontinence of 8.8% [4,5].

The aetiology of SUI is multifactorial with age, parity, BMI, and medical comorbidity all having been implicated [6,7]. Broadly, continence is maintained in women by a striated muscle sphincter with intact pudendal innervation, the presence of a well vascularized urothelium and sub-mucosa, intact and functioning intrinsic urethral smooth muscle, and intact vaginal wall support [8]. The interplay of these structures and the resulting pelvic floor dysfunction associated with their disruption is well described in what is referred to as the integral theory [9]. Age is likely to be associated with vascular, hormonal, and degenerative changes in these structures. Childbirth may lead to pudendal nerve injury, disruption of fascia supporting the anterior vaginal wall and urethra, and disruption or detachment of the levator ani, all of which compromise the integrity of women's continence mechanisms [10–12].

First-line management of SUI consists of conservative therapies such as pelvic floor muscle therapy (PFMT) and employing a stepwise approach to intervention has been advocated by much of the latest guidance [13]. A Cochrane review has reported that the use of PFMT can result in a cure rate of 56% and cure or improvement as high as 74% [14]. For those patients failing initial conservative treatment there are a range of surgical interventions. For many years, open Burch colposuspension was the operative method favoured by most gynaecologists and it became the mainstay of surgery. Following the advent of the tension-free vaginal tape (TVT) in 1996, the synthetic mid-urethral sling (MUS) became widely recognized as the gold standard treatment for SUI [15]. However, concerns surrounding mesh-associated complications following mesh augmented gynaecological surgery have led to a resurgence of other techniques and a fall in synthetic MUS procedures shown in Figure 17.1 (copyright pending). With the use of mesh for SUI banned or subject to restricted use in many countries, there is a need for clinicians to offer definitive alternatives [16,17]. This poses difficulties for a generation of gynaecologists who largely relied on the synthetic MUS.

In the UK, current National Institute for Health and Care Excellence (NICE) guidance recommends the following surgical options for the initial surgical management [13]:

- colposuspension (open or laparoscopic)
- autologous rectus fascial sling
- retropubic mid-urethral mesh sling

There is also a recommendation to consider the use of intramural bulking agents if alternative surgical procedures are not suitable for or acceptable to the woman.

This chapter aims to equip readers with the necessary perioperative knowledge and surgical steps in order to undertake laparoscopic colposuspension for the treatment of SUI.

Preoperative Assessment and Considerations

Office Assessment

An initial history will help distinguish between those with isolated SUI and patients with other subtypes of urinary incontinence. For those with overactive bladder (OAB) syndrome, as well as for those with mixed urinary incontinence, initial conservative and medical therapy should be instituted [13]. Modifiable risk factors such as obesity, diabetes, and other endocrine disorders should be identified as these can be the target of conservative management and this has been shown to improve symptoms [19,20]. Clinicians may choose to use patient reported outcome measures (PROMs): these are questionnaires offering a standardized method of measuring the presence of symptoms, symptom severity, general health, and health-related quality of life. The International Consultation on Incontinence Questionnaire for Urinary Incontinence (ICIQ-UI) short form version is one such PROM and has been shown to correlate with pad testing to quantify the severity of SUI [21].

International guidelines recommend routine use of a bladder diary to facilitate the distinction of incontinence subtypes and aid conservative therapies, as well as urinalysis to exclude active urinary tract infection or renal tract malignancy as a contributing pathology to the patient's presentation [8]. In those with SUI and symptoms of voiding dysfunction, uroflowmetry and measurement of the post void residual will identify women with voiding difficulties who may require intermittent self-catheterization to facilitate bladder emptying either following treatment or instead of surgery for SUI. Pad usage and a one-hour pad test will objectively quantify the extent of the problem. A clinical examination will determine the presence of

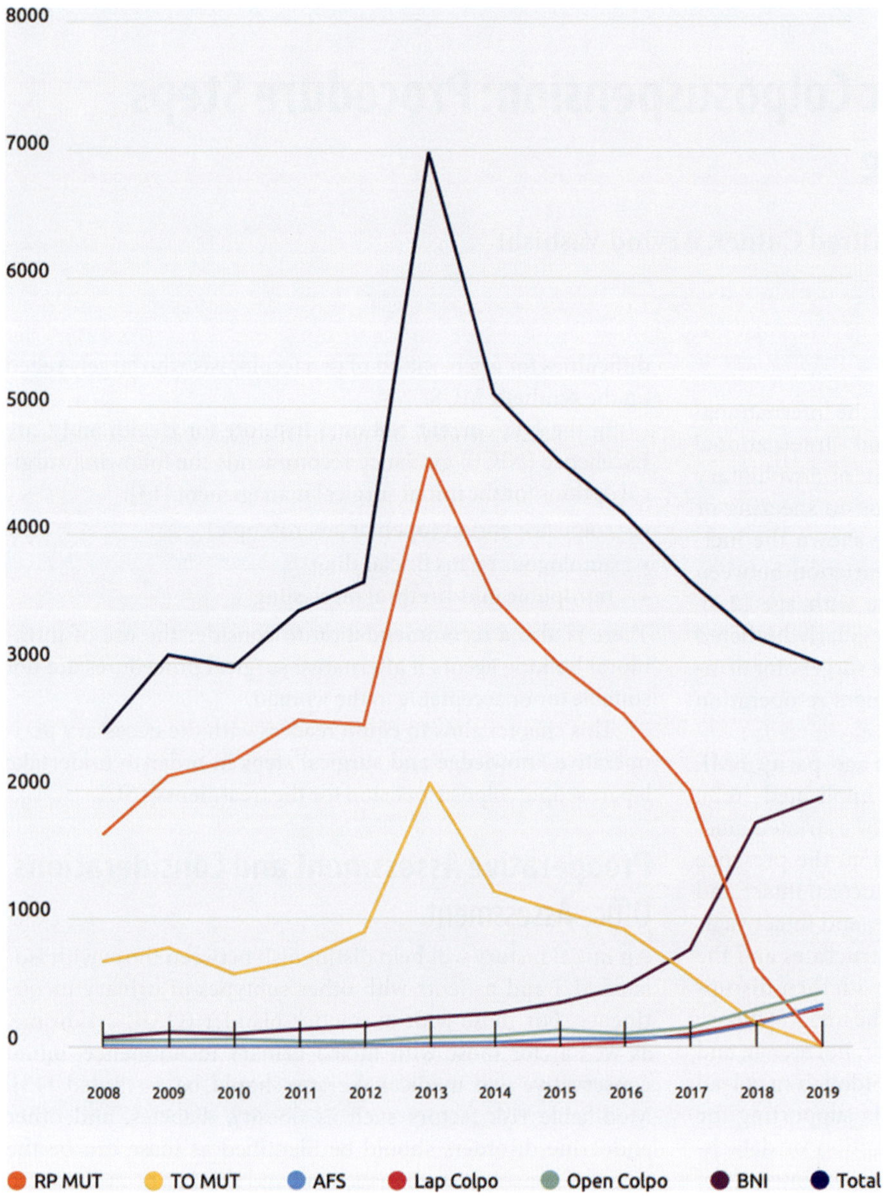

Figure 17.1 Number of procedures for SUI on BSUG database 2008—2019 [90].

concurrent pelvic organ prolapse or urethral pathology as well as allowing the clinician to undertake an office incontinence test. This is the most reliable clinical assessment for diagnosing SUI and involves the patient coughing or performing a Valsalva manoeuvre with a comfortably full bladder [8]. Urethral hypermobility should also be assessed, having been shown to be associated with a higher chance of surgical success in patients undergoing a colposuspension [22].

The Role of Urodynamic Studies

The role of urodynamic studies (UDS) prior to surgery for SUI is not clearly defined by the available literature and therefore its use remains controversial. Randomized studies in the US and UK have not shown any inferiority in the use of an office evaluation in place of invasive UDS [23,24]. Additionally, cost-effectiveness analyses do not seem to support one approach in favour of the other [25]. This has led to the general guidance that in women with isolated symptoms of SUI who have undergone office assessment as outlined above, including the presence of demonstrable SUI in clinic, that invasive UDS are not strictly necessary [8,13], although many urogynaecologists argue that the test gives invaluable baseline information, may identify additional diagnoses, and allows more detailed patient-specific counselling. The IUGA guidance concludes that UDS does not predict surgical failure rates, nor the chance of voiding dysfunction, however it is noteworthy that their guidance recommends counselling patients with concurrent detrusor overactivity (DO) that the success rates of surgery for SUI are lower than for those with isolated urodynamic stress incontinence (USI). Video cystourethrography allows for classification of USI on the basis of bladder neck descent, however routine use is not supported by current guidance [8,26].

Concurrent Procedures

Many patients present with a multitude of pelvic floor symptoms and pathology. Controversies persist as to whether to treat only the predominant presenting complaint, or alternatively to treat coexisting pathology. Access to the abdominal cavity allowing for concurrent procedures is a theoretical advantage of an intra-abdominal approach. Attempts to prevent postoperative SUI, a recognized feature of undertaking prolapse surgery, through the use of concurrent continence procedures has been studied [27–30]. The CARE trial, which is the largest and longest study using a concomitant colposuspension at the time of treatment of vault prolapse showed that continence is maintained in the long-term, with lower rates of SUI at seven years as compared to those who undergo an isolated vault procedure [28]. The study did not find a difference in rates of voiding dysfunction.

Patient Selection: When to Use Laparoscopic Colposuspension

Controversies surrounding the use of synthetic mesh have resulted in a renewed interest in Burch colposuspension for surgeons undertaking continence procedures. Evolutions in endoscopic surgery have cemented advantages over open approach predecessors including better visualization of anatomy, reduced postoperative pain, and a return to normal activities [31]. Technological advances in visualization together with advances in theatre design have further enabled more complex laparoscopic surgery to become mainstream [32]. Therefore, in the opinion of the authors, if similar clinical efficacy can be demonstrated, it should be the preferred route. Particular patient-specific characteristics lending themselves to a (laparoscopic) colposuspension include women who have significant anterior vaginal wall or bladder neck mobility, those undergoing concurrent abdominal procedures, and those with previous failure or removal of an MUS. There is evidence from retrospective cohort data to suggest that for those women who have recurrent SUI following a synthetic MUS, subjective cure rates of laparoscopic colposuspension at two years are as high as 93% [33]. A recent Cochrane review however, found insufficient high-quality evidence to support any particular surgical approach for women with recurrent SUI [34].

Development of Surgical Techniques

The surgical technique described within this chapter and referred to as laparoscopic colposuspension is a modified laparoscopic Burch colposuspension. Open Burch colposuspension has stood the test of time and the laparoscopic variants should be regarded as equivalent at least in the short term, by findings of a Cochrane meta-analysis [35]. The modified Burch technique utilizes a transperitoneal approach, opening the cave of Retzius, the use of absorbable sutures tied extra-corporeally, with elevation of the peri-urethral tissues to Copper's ligament. The first laparoscopic bladder neck suspension published within the literature was a variant of the Marshall-Marchetti-Kranz technique, undertaken in 1991 by Vancaille and Schuessler [36,37]. However, the term colposuspension is generally synonymous with the Burch colposuspension procedure, first described in 1961, and the Tanagho modification of this technique is now the standard method [38,39]. The first laparoscopic Burch colposuspension, using absorbable sutures and fixation of the peri-urethral sutures to Cooper's ligaments, as routinely undertaken, was described by Liu and Paek in 1993 [40].

As seen with any surgical procedure, multiple variants of laparoscopic colposuspension have been described with changes to approach, port size and site, dissection technique, suture placement and the number of sutures used, as well as choice of fixation material including the use of mesh, staples, clips and bone anchors being used to attach the suture to Cooper's ligament, or alternatively the pubic rami [41–44]. While we utilize a transperitoneal approach, some surgeons do advocate an extraperitoneal approach that offers the potential advantages of reduced risk of injury to intra-abdominal organs, reduced risk of conversion to open surgery, and a quicker dissection time. Data from a single study by Wallwiener et al comparing the approaches did not support these theoretical advantages [45]. Disadvantages include the fact that intraperitoneal abdominal and pelvic organs are not visualized, and it is not possible to undertake additional abdominal procedures such as prolapse surgery. It also requires close port placement and limited access for suturing. We would caution on the use of techniques that differ from the modified Burch colposuspension as there are no data to support equivalent efficacy.

Principle Surgical Technique

Preoperative Preparation

First-line conservative management in conjunction with relevant counselling and provision of appropriate decision-making tools and information resources follows initial assessment. Women needing surgery for SUI in our unit are generally offered laparoscopic Burch colposuspension, a mid-urethral sling (autologous or synthetic, although synthetic slings are currently unavailable in UK practice) or peri-urethral bulking (being made aware this is currently second-line treatment as declared by NICE). Having considered their surgical options, patients return to undertake surgical consent as well as inclusion within a national urogynaecology database, which is an NHS England requirement and considered best practice globally. Women are consented for the possibility of requiring concomitant apical suspension.

There are no international guidelines with respect to antimicrobial prophylaxis in the case of colposuspension, and guidance from the European Association of Urology does not reference the procedure [46]. In accordance with local recommendations we use broad-spectrum antibiotics, commonly gentamicin (and augmentin), as antimicrobial prophylaxis immediately prior to operating as a colposuspension is considered a clean-contaminate procedure [47]. Patients are initially positioned supine without tilt, in lithotomy with 30-degree flexion at the hips. They then undergo skin cleaning with either chlorhexidine or betadine skin preparation and are draped. A catheter is required that will allow free drainage, particularly in the event of bladder injury and haematuria, but that is comfortable for the majority of patients who have uncomplicated surgery. We use a size 14Ch Foley urethral catheter left on free drainage.

While uncommon, ureteric injury at the time of colposuspension has been well described within the literature [48]. The incidence after laparoscopy generally is estimated to be approximately 1% [49]. Both identification and repair of ureteric injuries is improved by the use of ureteric stenting. Our unit undertakes large volumes of complex laparoscopic surgery with close multi-disciplinary working, training, and input from colleagues in endourology. Therefore, prophylactic ureteric stenting with Pollack catheters is fairly routine and undertaken with minimal effect on overall operating time. We therefore routinely perform prophylactic ureteric catheterization prior to laparoscopic colposuspension, based on our preference and not guided by evidence within the literature.

Approach and Dissection

Initial port insertion is based on surgeon preference and patient comorbidity. Our routine practice is in accordance with the UK's Royal College of Obstetricians and Gynaecologists (RCOG) guidance [50]. We undertake a transperitoneal approach and for enhanced ergonomics we tend to place our lateral ports at least 8 cm from the midline at the level of the umbilicus. Two 5 mm ports are inserted and following dissection of the cave of Retzius, an 11 mm suprapubic port is placed to allow for passage of sutures into the abdominal cavity. The 11 mm suprapubic port is closed at the level of the rectus sheath and we avoid large lateral ports. These require closure to prevent incisional herniae, and in our experience this tends to be associated with increased postoperative pain [51].

Any concurrent pelvic procedures are performed prior to commencing the colposuspension. The exception to this rule is the sacral fixation of any apical prolapse procedures, as this reduces vaginal mobility and therefore makes adequate elevation of peri-urethral tissues difficult. We fill the bladder with 200 ml of normal saline and this can be mixed with methylene blue, to aid identification of the edge of the bladder dome. The obliterated median umbilical ligaments are identified and used as landmarks for entry into the cave of Retzius. They are incised between 2–4 cm cephalad from the bladder dome. The bladder is then emptied, allowing better access to the paravaginal tissues and dissection commenced. We utilize an ultrasonic scalpel with bipolar (Thunderbeat™) to allow bloodless tissue dissection. Alternative energy sources are used in other units. Careful attention at dissection is made for the urethra, the dorsal vein of the clitoris in the midline, and the obturator neurovascular bundle and external iliac vessels laterally. At completion, the pubic symphysis should be exposed, with the bladder neck in the midline and finally Cooper's ligament and the arcus tendinous fascia, both located laterally as shown in Figure 17.2.

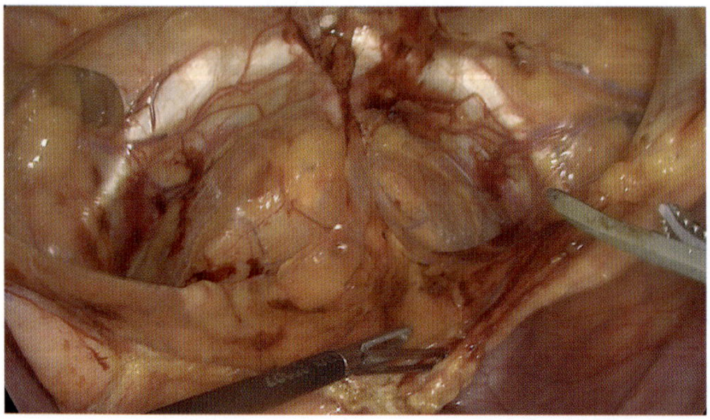

Figure 17.2 Following dissection into cave of Retzius. Cooper's ligament and arcus tendinous fascia exposed.

Suture Placement

To allow for suture placement and colposuspension, the bladder must be retracted medially. A pledget (either on a grasper with a marker thread, or disposable pledget on a stick) is used for blunt dissection to facilitate this. This process may be augmented by the placement of a finger vaginally to demarcate tissue planes. The use of a rectal probe or large Hagar is advocated to replace the finger at the time of suture placement to avoid inadvertent sharps injuries. There is no evidence to guide the choice of suture material and traditionally the non-absorbable suture No. 0 Ethibond® is used. There are case reports of late presenting complications associated with misplacement or erosion of non-absorbable sutures [52,53]. Some surgeons therefore opt to use slow-dissolving sutures as an alternative, part of wider moves to avoid surgical applications of non-absorbable materials. It is worth noting that the efficacy of the procedures is theorized to derive from fibrosis rather than the strength of the suture itself. The first two sutures are placed bilaterally, shown in Figures 17.3 and 17.4, either side of the bladder neck, and a second pair then placed slightly more cephalad. Each suture

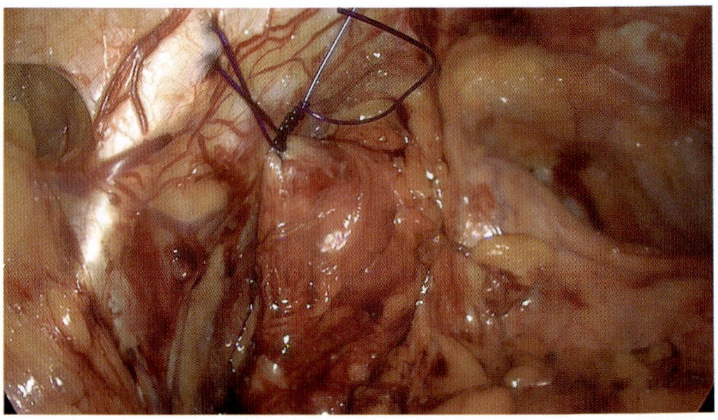

Figure 17.3 First suture.

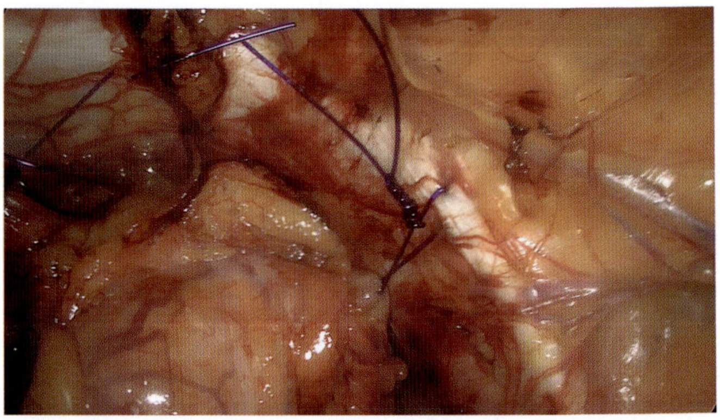

Figure 17.4 Second suture.

involves a double bite of the paravaginal tissues, with care not to transect through to the vaginal skin. The sutures are fixated on the ipsilateral Cooper's ligament, with each individual suture tied after insertion using limited tension and an extracorporeal knot, shown in Figure 17.5.

There is no published evidence exploring the optimal amount of tension to apply to these sutures. In our experience, approximately 15 mm distance is left between the paravaginal fascia and the ligament, allowing for sufficient elevation to facilitate continence, but avoiding postoperative voiding dysfunction. This however depends on vaginal wall mobility. We would always advocate the placement of at least two sutures either side of the urethra. This is supported by a study from Persson et al that reported higher objective and subjective perception of cure in women receiving two sutures versus those that received only one (89% and 65% respectively, relative risk (RR) 1.37, 95% confidence interval (CI) 1.14 to 1.64), with no increase in adverse events [54].

Closure

Peritoneal closure of the cave of Retzius has some merits in that it prevents the formation of bowel adhesions that could make future surgery difficult. This is therefore our usual routine practice, with the use of either a continuous or interrupted dissolvable suture as shown in Figures 17.6 and 17.7, acknowledging the theoretical risk of haematoma formation or collection. Placement of a drain within the cave is dependent on the course of each surgical case. A check cystoscopy is undertaken with a 120-degree cystoscope to ensure that no sutures have been placed in the bladder and to ensure ureteric patency by observation of urine jets from the ureteric orifice. Sutures in the bladder require immediate removal and replacement. Obstructive uropathy secondary to laparoscopic Burch colposuspension has been reported, and while rare, we would consider it good practice to ensure patency at the time of surgery [55]. We close the rectus sheath at the suprapubic port with 1 Vicryl an Endoclose® device and the umbilical port with a 'J' needle under direct vision. We use either 2/0 Monocryl®, 2/0 Vicryl Rapide®, or glue for the skin.

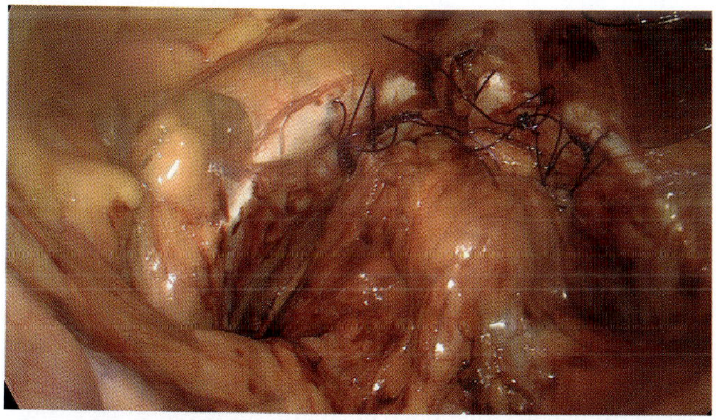

Figure 17.5 Completed suture.

Postoperative Management

Patients may be discharged at postoperative day one. The indwelling urethral catheter is left in-situ at our unit until day three, and variation in practice may be removal anywhere from day one to day ten. A strict trial without catheter must be instituted, and we measure the post void residual using a transabdominal bladder scan after the second void. Suprapubic catheters are no longer required with easily accessible bladder scanners, avoiding the restricted mobility, pain, and poor cosmesis associated with their use.

Surgical Video 17.1

For a step-by-step guide with reference to relevant anatomy, please consult the narrated Video 17.1 included within the digital version of this publication.

Evidence in Support of Laparoscopic Colposuspension

Efficacy and Long-term Outcomes

As with any surgical procedure, determining the safety and efficacy of an operation is greatly influenced by the chosen outcome measure. There is significant heterogeneity between reported subjective and objective definitions of cure or success within the literature for women following laparoscopic colposuspension. A 2017 Cochrane meta-analysis has reported subjective short-term success rates of between 62% and 100% [35]. The ICS sixth consultation on incontinence, published in 2017, collated data from the available level 1 and 2 evidence, and most studies report success rates for laparoscopic colposuspension in excess of 80%

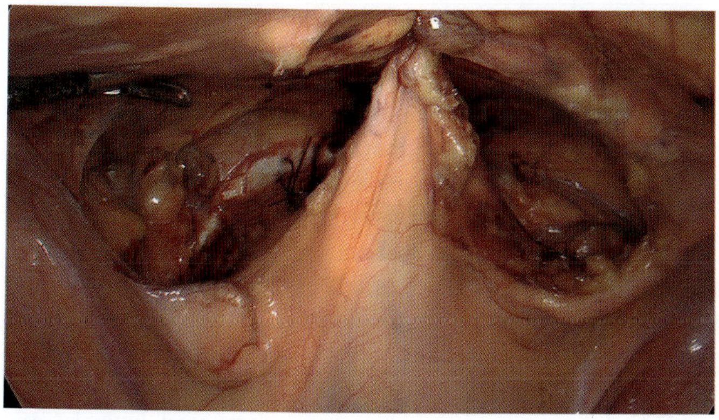

Figure 17.6 Reperitonealization commenced.

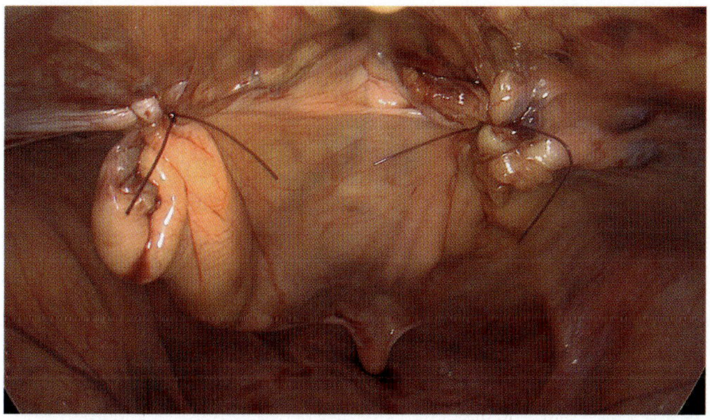

Figure 17.7 Completed reperitonealization of cave of Retzius.

[8]. In the UK, NICE have appraised the evidence more recently and reported a one- to five-year success rate for both open and laparoscopic colposuspension of 70% [56]. In the largest randomized study, Kitchener et al reported two-year outcome data for 123 women randomized to laparoscopic colposuspension, with an objective cure rate of 80% [57]. In this study, a subjective cure rate of 55% was reported and defined as being 'perfectly happy/pleased', as well as having patient-reported continence of 'never leaking/leaking <1/month'.

With respect to long-term outcomes, both the Cochrane analysis as well as the ICS guidance have noted the predominance of short-term prospective outcome data, generally limited to two years. Carey et al used non-validated telephone follow-up for 76 women at an average of 3.7 years postoperatively, who had been randomized to laparoscopic colposuspension [58]. While they did not report specific data, they commented that subjective cure rates were equivalent to the available data at 24 months, where 66% of those in follow-up reported being continent. This dropped to 50% if those lost to follow-up were considered to have ongoing incontinence. Most long-term follow-up data come from large cohort studies. Barr et al showed a subjective cure rate of 52% ten years after laparoscopic colposuspension in 96 women [59]. Describing an extraperitoneal approach, Hong et al report an objective cure rate of 72% at an average of 52 months; they noted a diminished cure rate over time [60]. A reasonable summary of the available evidence is that high rates of cure in excess of 80% are found in the two-year medium term therefore supporting the use of laparoscopic colposuspension, but that further data, while reassuring, are not able to provide definitive long-term success rates.

Efficacy Data: Laparoscopic versus Open Colposuspension

The 2017 Cochrane meta-analysis by Dean et al compared the laparoscopic and open approaches to colposuspension, using 10 studies shown in Table 17.1 [35]. They reported subjective cure rates at up to 18 months follow-up ranging from 58% to 96% in the open group, and 62% to 100% in the laparoscopic group. Two studies were excluded from the analysis of subjective cure; Su et al due to inconsistencies with surgical approach and randomization, and the trial by Burton et al due to the presentation of their data [61,62]. Within the 18-month follow-up period, the Cochrane review found a non-significant 5% lower relative subjective cure rate for laparoscopic colposuspension compared to an open technique (RR 0.95, 95% CI 0.90–1.00). One of the studies by Akardal et al utilized mesh implants rather than sutures to undertake the urethropexy, although a re-run of the analysis with this study excluded did not alter these findings [63]. With respect to objective measures of cure, included studies used either urodynamic testing or a negative pad test, the meta-analysis favoured open colposuspension in the short term at up to 18 months (RR 0.91, 95% CI 0.86–0.96). However, with longer term follow-up of up to five years, there was no significant difference between the two approaches (RR 1.01, 95% CI 0.88–1.16). Significant heterogeneity in the reporting of quality-of-life scores in the included studies meant that meaningful analysis of this data was not possible.

The largest study included in the Cochrane analysis included the randomized study by Kitchener et al, the Medical Research Council (MRC) funded COLPO (COlposuspension; is Laparoscopic Preferable to Open?) which recruited 291 women in six UK centres [57]. A non-absorbable suture (Ethibond) was used for both the open and laparoscopic approach. Of the 147 women allocated to open surgery, one had laparoscopic surgery and three had no operation. Of the 144 women allocated to laparoscopic surgery, 11 received open surgery and two had no operation. At two years on an intention-to-treat analysis, using an objective outcome (one-hour pad test) showed 80% of women were cured in the laparoscopic group (85.4% data available) and 70% cured in the open group (79.6% data available). The subjective cure rate was 55% in both groups. There was no difference in quality of life when assessed using a number of validated generic and symptom-specific scores. This study provides the highest quality dataset used within the analysis and findings from this study demonstrate that in the hands of surgeons experienced with laparoscopic surgery, an endoscopic approach does not produce an inferior cure rate as compared to open colposuspension.

Included within the Cochrane analysis was a randomized study by Cheon et al which enrolled 90 women to compare open and laparoscopic colposuspension, reporting similar objective cure rates at one year (86% versus 85%) [64]. Fatthy et al also reported similar success rate for open and laparoscopic approaches [65]. A randomized study not included within the meta-analysis of subjective cure due to methodological flaws with randomization and concurrent surgery, was that undertaken by Su et al [61]. In the majority of their cases, only one suture was placed in the laparoscopic group as compared to two or three sutures in the open group. They reported similar operating times, but lower blood loss in the laparoscopic group and lower success rate at one year compared to open (80.4% versus 95.6%). The complication rate in the open group was higher than in the laparoscopic group (17.4% versus 10.8%). An analysis in a systematic review by Moehrer et al also excluded this paper and found no statistically significant difference in objective cure when comparing both approaches [66].

The other study that was excluded from the Cochrane analysis of subjective cure was that by Burton et al, which randomized 60 women to either open or laparoscopic colposuspension, using two absorbable sutures on either side of the urethra for both techniques [62]. Data has only been published as a conference abstract and therefore not subject to formal peer review, making evaluation of the findings difficult. At three-year follow-up, women who underwent laparoscopic colposuspension were more likely to have objective stress incontinence than those who underwent an open procedure (60% versus 93%, p = <0.05).

Another meta-analysis published by Tan et al in 2007 identified 16 studies, published between 1995 and 2006, comparing the results of laparoscopic and open colposuspension [67]. Analysis was undertaken in 1,807 patients, with 861 (47.6%) undergoing laparoscopic and 946 (52.4%) undergoing open colposuspension. This study concluded that the approaches are associated with similar subjective and objective cure rates. Two published retrospective studies have compared laparoscopic

Table 17.1 Randomized controlled trials comparing synthetic open versus laparoscopic colposuspension [58,61-65,71,72,87,88]

Open colposuspension versus laparoscopic colposuspension								
Number	**Study**	**Type**	**Comparators**	**N (numbers at follow-up)**	**Follow-up**	**Cure (objective or subjective)**	**Level of evidence**	**Comments**
1	Ankardal et al [63]	RCT	OC vs LMC	OC = 120: LMC= 120 (97:105)	1y	Obj: OC 92% vs LMC 74% Subj: OC 89% vs LMC 62%	2	Randomization process not clear. Crossover of participants with other RCT. Not analysed on ITT.
2	Ankardal et al [87]	RCT	OC vs LSC vs LMC	OC = 79: LSC = 53: LMC = 79 (63:49:72)	1y	Subj: OC 92% vs LSC 90% vs LMC 63%, p<0.05 open vs.mesh	2	Randomization process not clear. Crossover of participants with other RCT. Not analysed on
3	Burton et al [62]	RCT	OC vs LSC	OC = 60: LSC= 60 (24:23)	1y 3y 5y	Obj: OC 97 % vs LSC 73%, p<0.05 Obj: OC 93 % vs LSC 60%, p<0.05 Obj: OC 90% vs LSC 57%, p<0.05	2	Abstract data only. VAS for subjective assessment making analysis difficult.
4	Carey et al [58]	RCT	OC vs LSC	OC = 104: LSC = 96 (88:76)	3–5y	Subj 72% vs 78%; p=0.22 (at 6m) 70% vs 63%; p= 0.38(at 2y)	2	Only 24 months data reported, 3–5-year data noted to be similar to findings at 24 months but not reported.
5	Cheon et al [64]	RCT	OC vs LSC	OC = 43: LSC = 47 (not reported)	1Y	Subj: OC 86% vs LSC 81% Obj: OC 86% vs LSC 85%	2	Both extra- and intraperitoneal approaches used. No significant difference in cure rates or satisfaction between groups.
6	Fatthy et al [65]	RCT	OC vs LSC	OC = 34: LSC = 40 (not reported)	6m and 18m	Subj: OC 88% vs LSC 85% (at 18m)	2	
7	Kitchenr et al [72]	RCT	OC vs LSC	OC = 147: LSC = 144 (128:128)	2y	Subj: OC 53% vs LSC 55% Obj: OC 70% vs LSC 80%	1	Following randomization – 12 women changed operation and five had no operation. Analysis undertaken on ITT. Objective data on 83% of particpants
8	Morris et al [71]	RCT	Manuscript unavailable					
9	Su et al [61]	RCT	OC vs LSC	OC = 46: LSC = 46	6m	Obj: OC 95% vs LSC 80% p= 0.044	2	Large proportion of LSC patients underwent subsequent open procedure (n=14). Prestated sample size calculation required 152 participants pants.
10	Summitt et al [88]	RCT	OC vs LSC	OC = ?: LSC = ? (34:28)	1y	Obj: OC 93% vs LSC 88%	2	No significant difference in objective outcomes between groups. Three laparoscopies converted to open.

LMC = laparoscopic mesh colposuspension; LSC = laparoscopic suture colposuspension; OC = open colposuspension.

and open routes and have shown similar success rates at one year [68,69]. Surgeons used non-absorbable sutures in both studies and reported lower use of analgesia, shorter hospital stay, and earlier return to work in the laparoscopic groups. A third study comparing the anatomic result of the two procedures by assessing the bladder neck position with postoperative ultrasound found no difference in urethral mobility, or resting and straining bladder neck positions at one year postoperatively [70].

Limited longer-term comparative data looking at efficacy are available. Carey et al found no difference in self-reported stress incontinence between the two operative routes, three to five years following surgery [58]. Although only available as data from an abstract, Morris et al concluded that the laparoscopic approach gave a significantly higher objective cure rate after a median follow-up of six years [71]. Barr et al performed structured interviews at least 10 years following surgery, and the authors reported a deterioration in subjective cure rates (defined as no urinary leakage in the last six months) from 71% and 67% at six months to 48% and 32% at 10 years, for the laparoscopic and open procedures respectively [59]. Again, no statistical difference was noted between the two surgical approaches.

Safety Data: Laparoscopic versus Open Colposuspension

With respect to surgical safety, findings from the 2017 Cochrane study favour a laparoscopic approach [35]. There were significantly fewer perioperative complications following laparoscopic colposuspension (RR 0.74, 95% CI 0.58–0.96), with the exception of bladder injuries which occurred in 4% (21/521) of patients versus 2% (10/507) of those undergoing open colposuspension (RR 1.88, 95% CI 0.93–3.83). Operative time favoured an open approach, while length of hospital stay favoured a laparoscopic technique [35]. Although not analysing such data with quantitative analysis, authors did conclude that women who underwent a laparoscopic colposuspension appeared to have less pain and lower postoperative analgesia requirements. There was no statistically significant difference in rates of detrusor overactivity in the short or long term nor in the rates of voiding dysfunction between the groups.

The meta-analysis by Tan et al reported similar findings in that a laparoscopic approach was associated with a lower operative blood loss, earlier postoperative recovery, and an earlier return to work [67]. Carey et al reported a shorter operative time for the open technique (44 versus 85 minutes) [58]. In contrast, Su et al reported shorter operative time with the laparoscopic approach, although less suturing was undertaken [61]. The laparoscopic approach took 17 minutes longer in the trial undertaken by Fatthy et al (in keeping with findings from the MRC trial), with nearly 200 ml less blood loss, 40 hours shorter hospital stay, and return to light work 23 days earlier [65,72]. Fatthy et al and Su et al both reported a longer hospital stay after an open approach. There was no significant difference in length of hospital stay in the studies by Cheon et al and Carey et al [58,64]. The latter group did however report a significantly quicker return to normal activities in the laparoscopic arm of patients. Of note, in the MRC study all patients had a suprapubic catheter which may have resulted in a longer hospital stay.

Efficacy Data: Laparoscopic Colposuspension versus Synthetic Mid-urethral Sling

With the available evidence suggesting comparable efficacy between a laparoscopic and open approach to colposuspension, and from the perspective of safety and recovery clear advantages to laparoscopy, comparison must then be made with what has been the gold standard approach to SUI, the synthetic MUS. Eight studies were used within the Cochrane analysis to compare laparoscopic colposuspension with vaginal synthetic MUS procedures, and these are shown in Table 17.2 [35]. It should be noted that both the TVT and the SPARC® system were analysed, as well as both suture and mesh colposuspension. Three of the studies used were only published as abstracts.

At 18 months follow-up, analysis revealed no significant difference in rates of subjective cure between the two approaches (RR 0.91, 95% CI 0.80–1.02), and in a study with four- to eight-year follow-up by Jelovsek et al, this continued to be the case [73]. Objective cure was determined by the various trials as either a negative pad test, negative clinical stress test, negative urodynamic test, or the absence of leaks recorded on a bladder diary, and was reported by all studies with the exception of that by Mirosh et al [74]. This analysis favoured the TVT procedure over laparoscopic suture colposuspension for objective cure rates at 18 months (RR 0.92, 95% CI 0.85–0.99). A re-run of this analysis of short-term data was undertaken excluding the study by Adile et al, due to uncertainty of the length of follow-up, and yielded similar findings, however the result was no longer statistically significant (RR 0.92 95% CI 0.93–1.02). Overall, the Cochrane review reported that laparoscopic colposuspension procedures have statistically significant lower objective cure rates (RR 0.88, 95% CI 0.81–0.95). Although heterogenous quality-of-life outcomes were used making comparison difficult, the 2017 Cochrane analysis noted that in all studies both groups had significant improvements in measures, with no significant difference between the two groups. In the longest follow-up study by Jelovsek et al that included 72 patients, 88% of subjects in the laparoscopic Burch group reported that if they had to do it all over again, they would choose the same treatment as compared to 79% in the TVT group [73].

Safety Data: Laparoscopic Colposuspension versus Synthetic Mid-urethral Sling

Concerning morbidity, seven studies reported perioperative complications and there were no statistically significant differences in the perioperative complication rates between laparoscopic colposuspension and vaginal sling procedures (RR 0.99, 95% CI 0.60–1.64). Laparoscopic surgery took significantly longer than MUS surgery by an average of 20 minutes [35]. An MUS procedure was associated with a lower average length of inpatient stay by one day (mean difference 1.10, 95% CI 0.79–1.41), as well as a shorter time to return to normal activities [35]. Two studies in the review looked at postoperative pain relief. In the study by Paraiso et al, authors reported similar length of use for patient-controlled analgesia in both groups, while Valpas et al found lower rates of analgesia use following TVT [75,76].

Table 17.2 Randomized controlled trials comparing synthetic mid-urethral sling versus laparoscopic suture colposuspension [73–80,84,89]

Synthetic mid-urethral sling versus laparoscopic colposuspension								
Number	**Study**	**Type**	**Comparators**	**N (numbers at follow-up)**	**Follow-up**	**Cure (objective or subjective)**	**Level of Evidence**	**Comments**
1	Adeileet al [78]	RCT	TVT vs LSC	TVT = 57: LSC = 56 (57:56)	6–24 m	Sub: TVT 89% vs LSC 45%		Abstract data only. Subjective cure rates reported were satisfaction only.
2	Foote et al [77]	RCT	SPARC device vs LSC	MUS = 49: LSC = 48 (44:43)	2y	Subj: MUS 77.4% vs LSC 81.4%	2	SPARC device used as MUS. Cure/ improvement defined as no leaks/week and VAS<2, or 50% improvement in leaks/ week and VAS.
3	Mirosh et al [74]	RCT	TVT vs LSC	TVT = 16: LSC = 14 (16:14)	12 m	Not reported		Abstract only. No difference in QoL scores.
4	Maher et al [80]	RCT	TVT vs LSC	TVT = 40: LSC = 42 (31:42)	18 m	Subj: TVT 85% vs LSC 81% (p=0.77) Obj: TVT 85% vs LSC 78% (p=0.56)	2	Abstract data only. No difference in symptom or QoL scores.
5	Paraiso et al [75]	RCT	TVT vs LSC	TVT = 33: LSC = 33 (not reported)	12–43 m (median 18m)	Obj: TVT 81% vs LSC 97% (18m)	1	Objective cure was no evidence of leakage on urodynamic studies.
	Jelowsek et al [73]			TVT = 36: LSC = 36(25:28)	12–88 m (median 65m)	Subj: TVT 52% vs LSC 43% (65 m)	2	Subjective cure defined as reporting to be leak free.
6	Persson et al [84]	RCT	TVT vs LSC	TVT = 38: LSC = 33 (37:31)	12 m	Subj: TVT 57% vs LSC 52% Obj: TVT 89% vs LSC 87%	1	No details on method of determining subjective cure. Objective cure was a negative postoperative pad test.
7	Ustun et al [79]	RCT	TVT vs LSC	TVT = 23: LSC = 23 (not reported)	3 m	Obj: TVT 83% vs LSC 83%	2	
8	Valpas et al [76]	RCT	TVT vs LMC	TVT = 70: LMC = 51 (not reported)	6w	Obj: TVT 93% vs LMC 88% (p=ns)	2	Objective cure was negative stress test (coughing) with 300ml bladder capacity.
	Valpas et al [89]	RCT			1y	Obj: TVT 8% vs LMC 57% (diff 95% a 12.7–43.9, p=0.000)	2	Stress test as above. Sample size calculation required.

LMC = laparoscopic mesh colposuspension; LSC = laparoscopic suture colposuspension; MUS = mid-urethral sling; TVT = tension free vaginal tape.

Regarding postoperative bladder function, the various studies seem to report conflicting outcomes with respect to OAB symptoms. Two studies showed urgency was more common after a sling procedure and a further three studies found higher rates of overactivity [75–79]. However, Maher et al reported the opposite, so overall meta-analysis found no difference in *de novo* detrusor overactivity at 18 months (RR 0.80, 95% CI 0.34–1.88) [80]. The numbers of women with voiding dysfunction following the two procedures were too small to allow for an adequate analysis, although there appeared to be no difference in the groups.

Comparison of the MUS to laparoscopic colposuspension suggests potential advantages to a sling procedure in terms of short-term subjective and objective cure as well as reduced morbidity. However, the landscape of incontinence surgery has change. Studies using large datasets have highlighted that the use of a synthetic MUS may be associated with mesh-associated complications requiring re-operation in 2% of women following the procedure, a complication avoided in suture colposuspension [81]. Pain has been recognized as a potential sequela of mesh-augmented surgery and none of the studies outlined have utilized validated pain scores when comparing the synthetic MUS to laparoscopic colposuspension. As laparoscopic colposuspension re-emerges as a more commonly performed procedure for SUI, there will be a need for further high-quality prospective studies assessing this approach.

Cost Effectiveness

As outlined, the laparoscopic approach is generally reported to require longer operating time than the open colposuspension or MUS procedures. The cost of disposable equipment is often cited as a negative factor regarding the laparoscopic approach. As part of the COLPO study group, Dumville et al undertook a cost-effective analysis comparing laparoscopic colposuspension versus open colposuspension [82]. While short-term costs favoured an open approach, those who underwent laparoscopic surgery had higher quality-adjusted life years (QALYs) when compared with those who underwent open surgery. They had shorter inpatient stays and fewer postoperative visits. At 24 months, the authors concluded 'the laparoscopic approach might be a cost-effective alternative in the medium term, provided that there are no major cost implications from treatment failure compared with the open group'. Given that there is little evidence to suggest that failure rates of the two procedures are particularly divergent after two years, the laparoscopic colposuspension could be assumed to be cost-effective at this time interval.

A retrospective two-year cost analysis of laparoscopic suture colposuspension compared with open colposuspension has been undertaken by Kohli et al [83]. They found that the laparoscopic approach was more expensive, costing $4,960 versus $4,079, although the postoperative care costs were lower than in the open group ($1,068 versus $1,561). Persson et al reported that a laparoscopic colposuspension is cheaper than a TVT (€1,273.4 versus €1,342.8), despite the TVT procedure being performed in less time [84]. In contrast, a more recent Swedish study reported that the TVT procedure generated a lower direct cost than colposuspension, either by the open or laparoscopic approach [85]. Cody et al have undertaken an analysis of cost effectiveness comparing TVT with three alternatives, open Burch colposuspension, laparoscopic colposuspension, and bladder neck injectables [86]. Utilizing data from a systematic review, they modelled ten-year follow-up based on experience and data from the UK's NHS and reported a cost, as of 2001, of £1,058 per woman for TVT, compared to £1,317 for laparoscopic colposuspension. Improved laparoscopic skills and therefore reduced operating times, as well as lower cost instruments, means more contemporaneous cost efficiency analysis is needed.

Limitations of Laparoscopic Colposuspension

There are two principal aspects of laparoscopic colposuspension that limit its more widespread adoption; a lack of quality long-term data and the provision of surgical training. Following the publication of persuasive studies supporting the efficacy of the synthetic MUS in the 1990s, there was limited interest in colposuspension. Two decades of literature investigating surgery for SUI focussed to a large extent on the TVT and its various progeny. Following the global re-appraisal of the role of mesh in pelvic floor surgery, patients, clinicians, and regulators find themselves in need of more high-quality prospective medium- and long-term data for other options.

The second limitation is surgeon training. Many practising gynaecologists were trained in the era of the synthetic MUS, with limited exposure to colposuspension. More senior clinicians abandoned the procedure in favour of devices such as the TVT. There is a steep learning curve in laparoscopic surgery, and this is likely to further account for the poor uptake of laparoscopic colposuspension. Clinicians in established practice are increasingly working with colleagues who have maintained the skills to undertake laparoscopic colposuspension, and formal mentorship programmes are being developed, such as that offered in the UK by the British Society of Urogynaecology (BSUG). Laparoscopic urogynaecology is now considered an essential component of training for urogynaecologists in training, and most generalists would now be trained in laparoscopic surgery. With clear advantages in terms of morbidity and cost effectiveness, not just for colposuspension but for abdominopelvic surgery generally, healthcare facilities in most developed countries are now providing infrastructure to support endoscopic surgery.

Conclusion

Given the current climate surrounding the use of mesh in pelvic floor surgery, the ever-evolving field of anti-incontinence surgery is likely to see laparoscopic colposuspension emerge as the gold-standard surgical treatment. This will require widespread training in the procedure as well as investment in healthcare infrastructure.

The procedure offers both the advantage of utilizing native tissue repair in combination with a minimally invasive surgical approach. With evidence of equivalence to open colposuspension, it provides an effective intervention for SUI and at the same time avoids the risks, perceived or otherwise, of the use of a synthetic MUS.

While differences remain in the exact techniques employed, the laparoscopic modified Burch colposuspension with the use of two sutures remains that most supported by the evidence. Subjective short- to medium-term cure rates appear to exceed 80%. There is however a need for further prospective comparative studies of safety, efficacy, and cost efficiency, as well as data regarding long-term outcomes.

References

1. Haylen BT, et al. An International Urogynecological Association (IUGA)/International Continence Society (ICS) joint report on the terminology for female pelvic floor dysfunction. Neurourol Urodyn 2010; 29(1): 4–20.
2. Coyne KS, et al. The prevalence of lower urinary tract symptoms (LUTS) in the USA, the UK and Sweden: results from the Epidemiology of LUTS (EpiLUTS) study. BJU Int 2009; 104(3): 352–60.
3. Hunskaar S, et al. The prevalence of urinary incontinence in women in four European countries. BJU Int 2004; 93(3): 324–30.
4. Abdel-Fattah M, et al. Primary and repeat surgical treatment for female pelvic organ prolapse and incontinence in parous women in the UK: a register linkage study. BMJ Open 2011; 1(2): e000206.
5. Perry S, et al. An epidemiological study to establish the prevalence of urinary symptoms and felt need in the community: the Leicestershire MRC Incontinence Study. J Public Health 2000; 22(3): 427–34.

6. Coyne KS, et al. Risk factors and comorbid conditions associated with lower urinary tract symptoms: EpiLUTS. BJU Int 2009; 103: 24–32.
7. Gyhagen M, et al. A comparison of the long-term consequences of vaginal delivery versus caesarean section on the prevalence, *severity and bothersomeness of urinary incontinence subtypes: a national cohort study in primiparous women*. BJOG 2013; 120(12): 1548–55.
8. Abrams P, Cardozo L, Wagg A, Wein A (eds). *Incontinence*, 6th edn. International Continence Society; 2017.
9. Petros P. The integral system. Cent European J Urology 2011; 64(3): 110.
10. Margulies RU et al. Origin and insertion points involved in levator ani muscle defects. Am J Obstet Gynecol 2007; 196(3): 251. e1–251. e5.
11. Martan A, et al. Ultrasonic evaluation of paravaginal defects before and after surgical treatment in women with urinary stress incontinence. Ceska gynekologie 2000; 65(3): 152–6.
12. Sajadi KP, et al. Neurogenic aspects of stress urinary incontinence. Curr Opin Obstet Gynecol 2010; 22(5): 425.
13. National Institute for Health and Care Excellence. Urinary incontinence and pelvic organ prolapse in women: management [NG 123]. Published 2019.
14. Dumoulin C, et al. Pelvic floor muscle training versus no treatment, or inactive control treatments, for urinary incontinence in women. Cochrane Database Syst Rev 2018; 10(10): CD005654. https://doi.org/10.1002/14651858.CD005654.pub4
15. Petros P. Creating a gold standard surgical device: scientific discoveries leading to TVT and beyond. Int Urogynecol J 2015; 26(4): 471–6.
16. Therapeutic Goods Administration, Australian Department of Health. TGA undertakes regulatory actions after review into urogynaecological surgical mesh implants. Published 2018. Available from: www.tga.gov.au/alert/tga-actions-after-review-urogynaecological-surgical-mesh-implants
17. Gornall J. How mesh became a four letter word. BMJ 2018; 363: k4137.
18. British Society of Urogynaecology (BSUG). Stress urinary incontinence surgery in the UK 2008–2017. First National Report. Published 2018.
19. Lenherr SM, et al. Glycaemic control and risk of incident urinary incontinence in women with type 1 diabetes: results from the Diabetes Control and Complications Trial and Epidemiology of Diabetes Interventions and Complications (DCCT/EDIC) study. Diabetic Med 2016; 33(11): 1528–35.
20. Vissers D, et al. The effect of non-surgical weight loss interventions on urinary incontinence in overweight women: a systematic review and meta-analysis. Obesity Rev 2014; 15(7): 610–17.
21. Franco AVM, et al. Is there an alternative to pad tests? Correlation of subjective variables of severity of urinary loss to the 1-h pad test in women with stress urinary incontinence. BJU Int 2008; 102(5): 586–90.
22. Viereck V, et al. Urethral hypermobility after anti-incontinence surgery: a prognostic indicator? Int Urogynecol J 2006; 17(6): 586–92.
23. Hilton P, et al. A mixed methods study to assess the feasibility of a randomised controlled trial of invasive urodynamic testing versus clinical assessment and non-invasive tests prior to surgery for stress urinary incontinence in women: the INVESTIGATE-I study. Trials 2015; 16(1): 400.
24. Nager CW, et al. A randomized trial of urodynamic testing before stress-incontinence surgery. New Engl J Med 2012; 366(21): 1987–97.
25. Homer T, et al. Invasive urodynamic testing prior to surgical treatment for stress urinary incontinence in women: cost-effectiveness and value of information analyses in the context of a mixed methods feasibility study. Pilot Feasibility Stud 2018; 4(1): 67.
26. Blaivas JG, Olsson CA. Stress incontinence: classification and surgical approach. J Urol 1988; 139(4): 727–31.
27. Brubaker L, et al. Abdominal sacrocolpopexy with Burch colposuspension to reduce urinary stress incontinence. New Engl J Med 2006; 354(15): 1557–66.
28. Nygaard I, et al. Long-term outcomes following abdominal sacrocolpopexy for pelvic organ prolapse. JAMA 2013; 309(19): 2016–24.
29. Van der Ploeg J, et al. Prolapse surgery with or without stress incontinence surgery for pelvic organ prolapse: a systematic review and meta-analysis of randomised trials. BJOG 2014; 121(5): 537–47.
30. Costantini E, et al. Pelvic organ prolapse repair with and without concomitant Burch colposuspension in incontinent women: a randomised controlled trial with at least 5-year follow-up. Obstet Gynecol Int 2012: 967923. https://doi.org/10.1155/2012/967923
31. Cutner A, Rymer J. Patient recovery after laparoscopic colposuspension. Gynaecol Endosc 1998; 7(6): 307–8.
32. Holland TK, et al. Gynaecologists' and general surgeons' preference for the features of integrated theatres: a discrete choice experiment. BMC Women's Health 2018; 18(1): 112.
33. De Cuyper EM, et al. Laparoscopic Burch colposuspension after failed sub-urethral tape procedures: a retrospective audit. Int Urogynecol J 2008; 19(5): 681–5.
34. Bakali E, et al. Interventions for treating recurrent stress urinary incontinence after failed minimally invasive synthetic midurethral tape surgery in women. Cochrane Database Syst Rev 2019; 9(9): CD009407. https://doi.org/10.1002/14651858.CD009407.pub3
35. Dean N., et al. Laparoscopic colposuspension for urinary incontinence in women. Cochrane Database Syst Rev 2017; 7(7): CD002239. https://doi.org/10.1002/14651858.CD002239.pub3
36. Vancaillie TG, Schuessler W. Laparoscopic bladderneck suspension. J Laparoendosc Surg 1991; 1(3): 169–73.
37. Marshall VF. The correction of stress incontinence by simple vesico-urethral suspension. Surg Gynecol Obstet 1949; 88: 509–15.
38. Je B. Urethrovaginal fixation to Cooper's ligament for correction of stress incontinence, cystocele and prolapse. Am J Obstet Gynecol 1961; 81: 281–90.
39. Tanagho EA. Colpocystourethropexy: the way we do it. J Urol 1976; 116(6): 751–3.
40. Liu C, Paek W. Laparoscopic retropubic colposuspension (Burch procedure). J Am Assoc Gynecol Laparosc 1993; 1(1): 31–5.
41. McDougall EM. Laparoscopic management of female urinary incontinence. Urol Clin North Am 2001; 28(1): 145–9, x.
42. Henley C. The Henley staple-suture technique for laparoscopic Burch colposuspension. J Am Assoc Gynecol Laparosc 1995; 2(4): 441–4.

43. Das S. Comparative outcome analysis of laparoscopic colposuspension, abdominal colposuspension and vaginal needle suspension for female urinary incontinence. J Urol 1998; 160(2): 368–71.
44. Ou, C-S, et al. Laparoscopic bladder neck suspension using hernia mesh and surgical staples. J Laparoendosc Surg 1993; 3(6): 563–6.
45. Wallwiener D, et al. Endoscopic retropubic colposuspension: 'Retziusscopy' versus laparoscopy – a reasonable enlargement of the operative spectrum in the management of recurrent stress incontinence? Endosc Surg Allied Technol 1995; 3(2–3): 115–18.
46. Bonkat G, et al. EAU guidelines on urological infections. European Association of Urology; 2017, 22–6.
47. National Institute for Health and Care Excellence (NICE). Surgical site infections: prevention and treatment [NG125]. Published 2019.
48. Rosen DM, et al. Ureteric injury at Burch colposuspension 4 case reports and literature review. Aust N Z J Obstet Gynaecol 1996; 36(3): 354–8.
49. Härkki-Siren P, et al. Major complications of laparoscopy: a follow-up Finnish study. Obstet Gynecol 1999; 94(1): 94–8.
50. Royal College of Obstetricians and Gynaecologists (RCOG). Preventing entry-related gynaecological laparoscopic injuries. Published 2008.
51. Coda A, et al. Incisional hernia and fascial defect following laparoscopic surgery. Surg Laparosc Endosc Percutan Tech 2000; 10(1): 34–8.
52. Dwyer P, et al. Suture injury to the urinary tract in urethral suspension procedures for stress incontinence. Int Urogynecol J 1999; 10(1): 15–21.
53. Shapiro R, et al. Delayed presentation of suture erosion following Burch colposuspension. Case Rep ObstetGynecol 2017; 2017: 8178361. https://doi.org/10.1155/2017/8178361
54. Persson J, Wølner-Hanssen P. Laparoscopic Burch colposuspension for stress urinary incontinence: a randomized comparison of one or two sutures on each side of the urethra. Obstet Gynecol 2000; 95(1): 151–5.
55. Asian P, Woo HH. Ureteric injury following laparoscopic colposuspension. BJOG 1997; 104(2): 266–8.
56. National Institute for Health and Care Excellence (NICE). Surgery for stress urinary incontinence – Patient decision aid. Published 2019.
57. Kitchener HC, et al. Laparoscopic versus open colposuspension – results of a prospective randomized controlled trial. Obstet Gynecol Surv 2007; 62(1): 24–5.
58. Carey M, et al. Laparoscopic versus open Burch colposuspension: a randomised controlled trial. BJOG2006; 113(9): 9991006.
59. Barr S, et al. The long-term outcome of laparoscopic colposuspension: a 10-year cohort study. In Urogynecol J 2009; 20(4): 443–5.
60. Hong JH, et al. Long-term results of laparoscopic Burch colposuspension for stress urinary incontinence in women. J Korean Med Sci 2009; 24(6): 1182–6.
61. Su TH, et al. Prospective comparison of laparoscopic and traditional colposuspensions in the treatment of genuine stress incontinence. Acta Obstet Gynecol Scandi 1997; 76(6): 576–82.
62. Burton B. A three-year prospective randomized urodynamic study comparing open and laparoscopic colposuspension. Neurourol Urodyn 1997; 16: 353–7.
63. Ankardal M, et al. A randomised trial comparing open Burch colposuspension using sutures with laparoscopic colposuspension using mesh and staples in women with stress urinary incontinence. BJOG 2004; 111(9): 974–81.
64. Cheon W. Prospective randomised controlled trial comparing laparoscopic and open colposuspension. Hong Kong Med J 2003; 9(1): 10–14.
65. Fatthy H, et al. Modified Burch colposuspension: laparoscopy versus laparotomy. J Am Assoc Gynecol Laparosc 2001; 8(1): 99–106.
66. Moehrer B, et al. Laparoscopic colposuspension: a systematic review. BJOG2003; 110(3): 230–5.
67. Tan E, et al. Laparoscopic versus open colposuspension for urodynamic stress incontinence. Neurourol Urodyn 2007; 26(2): 158–69.
68. Miannay E, et al. Comparison of open retropubic and laparoscopic colposuspension for treatment of stress urinary incontinence. Eur J Obstet Gynecol Reprod Biol 1998; 79(2): 159–66.
69. Saidi MH, et al. Extraperitoneal laparoscopic colposuspension: short-term cure rate, complications, and duration of hospital stay in comparison with Burch colposuspension. Obstet Gynecol 1998; 92(4): 619–21.
70. Huang W-C, Yang J-M. Anatomic comparison between laparoscopic and open Burch colposuspension for primary stress urinary incontinence. Urology 2004; 63(4): 676–81.
71. Morris A, et al. 5–7 year follow-up of a randomised trial comparing laparoscopic colposuspension (LC) and open colposuspension (OC) in the treatment of genuine stress incontinence. Intl Urogynecol J Pelvic Floor Dysfunct 2001; 12(Suppl 3): S6.
72. Kitchener H, et al. Laparoscopic versus open colposuspension—results of a prospective randomised controlled trial. BJOG 2006; 113(9): 1007–13.
73. Jelovsek J, et al. Randomised trial of laparoscopic Burch colposuspension versus tension-free vaginal tape: long-term follow up. BJOG 2008; 115(2): 219–25.
74. Mirosh M, Epp A. TVT vs laparoscopic Burch colposuspension for the treatment of stress urinary incontinence. In *Proceedings of the International Continence Society (ICS), 35th Annual Meeting.* Montreal, QC, Canada. 2005.
75. Paraiso MFR, et al. Laparoscopic Burch colposuspension versus tension-free vaginal tape: a randomized trial. Obstet Gynecol 2004; 104(6): 1249–58.
76. Valpas A, et al. Tension-free vaginal tape and laparoscopic mesh colposuspension for stress urinary incontinence. Obstet Gynecol 2004; 104(1): 42–9.
77. Foote AJ, et al. Laparoscopic colposuspension versus vaginal suburethral slingplasty: a randomised prospective trial. Aust N Z J Obstet Gynaecol 2006; 46(6): 517–20.
78. Adile B, et al. A prospective randomised study of Burch laparoscopy versus tension-free vaginal tape: 2-year follow-up. Urogynaecol Int J 2001; 15(1 Suppl): 121–2.
79. Üstün Y, et al. Tension-free vaginal tape compared with laparoscopic Burch urethropexy. J Am Assoc Gynecol Laparosc 2003; 10(3): 386–9.
80. Maher C, et al. Laparoscopic colposuspension or tension-free vaginal tape for recurrent stress urinary incontinence and/or intrinsic sphincter deficiency: a randomised controlled trial. Neurourol Urodyn 2004; 23(5–6): 433–4.

81. Keltie K, et al. Complications following vaginal mesh procedures for stress urinary incontinence: an 8-year study of 92,246 women. Sci Rep 2017; 7(1): 12015.
82. Dumville J, et al. Cost-effectiveness analysis of open colposuspension versus laparoscopic colposuspension in the treatment of urodynamic stress incontinence. BJOG 2006; 113(9): 1014–22.
83. Kohli N, et al. Open compared with laparoscopic approach to Burch colposuspension: a cost analysis. Obstet Gynecol 1997; 90(3): 411–15.
84. Persson J, et al. Cost-analyzes based on a prospective, randomized study comparing laparoscopic colposuspension with a tension-free vaginal tape procedure. Acta Obstet Gynecol Scandi 2002; 81(11): 1066–73.
85. Ankardal M, et al. Comparison of health care costs for open Burch colposuspension, laparoscopic colposuspension and tension-free vaginal tape in the treatment of female urinary incontinence. Neurourol Urodyn 2007; 26(6): 761–6.
86. Cody J, et al. Systematic review of the clinical effectiveness and cost-effectiveness of tension-free vaginal tape for treatment of urinary stress incontinence, in *NIHR Health Technology Assessment programme: Executive Summaries*. NIHR Journals Library; 2003.
87. Ankardal M, et al. A three-armed randomized trial comparing open Burch colposuspension using sutures with laparoscopic colposuspension using sutures and laparoscopic colposuspension using mesh and staples in women with stress urinary incontinence. Acta Obstet Gynecol Scandi 2005; 84(8): 773–9.
88. Summitt Jr RL, et al. Randomized comparison of laparoscopic and transabdominal Burch urethropexy for the treatment of genuine stress incontinence. Obstet Gynecol 2000; 95(4): S2.
89. Valpas A, et al. TVT versus laparoscopic mesh colposuspension: 5-year follow-up results of a randomized clinical trial. Int Urogynecol J 2015; 26(1): 57–63.
90. Jha S, Hillard T, Monga A, Duckett J. National BSUG audit of stress urinary incontinence surgery in England. Int Urogynecol J 2019; 30(8): 1337–41.

Chapter

18 Laparoscopic Paravaginal Repair: Procedure Steps and Evidence

Bobby Garcia, John R Miklos, Robert D Moore

Paravaginal defects, which may be seen in patients with anterior vaginal wall prolapse, are due to a loss of support or detachment of the pubocervical fascia from the arcus tendinous fascia pelvis (ATFP), at or near its lateral attachment. Originally described by White in 1909 as a vaginal procedure [1], an abdominal technique was then reported in 1976 [2] and then modified to a laparoscopic approach with reported efficacy of 60–89%. This minimally invasive approach affords numerous advantages, including a reduced risk of vaginal shortening and obviating the need for a vaginal incision. This operative space is easily accessible when performing other laparoscopic procedures such as a hysterectomy, sacrocolpopexy, and/or Burch urethropexy.

Introduction

Pelvic organ prolapse (POP) is a condition that negatively affects the quality of life of millions of women, with an 11% lifetime risk of women needing to undergo surgical correction [3]. Constituents of anterior vaginal wall support include the levator ani muscle, arcus tendinous fascia pelvis (ATFP), pubocervical fascia, and the uterosacral-cardinal ligament complex [4]. The rate of any anterior wall defect (cystocele) is estimated to be between 32–34% [5]. A break in support of this compartment can come at any point along the anterior wall but is largely attributed to either a midline or lateral wall defect and is diagnosed either during preoperative physical exam or during surgery. Treatment for the former, a midline defect, is addressed with a traditional anterior colporrhaphy while a lateral wall defect may require a paravaginal repair to restore anatomical support.

Diagnosis

During a new patient consultation, a thorough history of present illness is gathered, and a physical examination is performed to assess for POP. On initial speculum examination if an anterior vaginal wall defect is noted, a distinction must be drawn between a central and paravaginal defect. The presence of rugae on the anterior vaginal wall is suggestive of a paravaginal defect [6]. Loss of rugae on the other hand could be associated with a midline defect, however this could also be attributed to atrophy of the vaginal wall from a hypoestrogenic state [4].

A diagnostic technique was first described by Richardson using two tongue blades [7] and then by Shull using a sponge (ring) forceps. The forceps are opened and placed vaginally with the ends pointing toward the ischial spines and the patient is asked to Valsalva. If there is improvement in the anterior vaginal wall support, this suggests that she has a paravaginal defect, as the forceps are functioning to simulate or recreate lateral anatomic support along the arcus tendinous fascia pelvis. On the other hand, if the bulge persists, despite the forceps providing lateral support, it would suggest that she has a midline defect [8]. Additionally, the examiner can palpate the lateral attachment to the arcus tendinous fascia pelvis through the vaginal wall by feeling for any breaks in support where the finger enters the retropubic space. While these techniques can be helpful, preoperative diagnosis does not always correlate with intraoperative findings, particularly in women with a prior Burch colposuspension or Marshall-Marchetti-Krantz procedure [9]. Imaging modalities such as ultrasound and MRI have been employed to assist in the diagnosis of paravaginal defects. While they have demonstrated visual changes, these can be attributed to either levator ani or paravaginal support loss and more research is needed [4]. Ultimately, direct visualization of the retropubic space via an abdominal approach is the gold standard in the diagnosis of paravaginal defects. Nonetheless, identification of small or partial tears can be challenging.

Shull [10] described three variations of paravaginal defects:

1. The pubocervical fascia tears from the ATFP
2. The ATFP breaks away from the pelvic sidewall
3. A portion of the ATFP tears with a segment attached to the pubocervical fascia with the remnant staying connected to the pelvic sidewall

Along with other forms of pelvic organ prolapse, the aetiology of paravaginal defects is thought to be multifactorial including genetics, trauma (childbirth), obesity, and age. In addition to these mechanisms, it is also postulated that as the vaginal vault prolapses, the lateral attachments on the anterior wall tear away leading to a paravaginal defect. Irrespective of the variation, the operative technique remains unchanged. Originally described by White in 1909 as a vaginal procedure [1], an abdominal variant was then reported in 1976 [2] and subsequently minimally invasive options including laparoscopic and robotic adaptations have evolved. Here we will discuss the laparoscopic paravaginal repair (LPVR) technique and the evidence supporting its use.

Preoperative Considerations

Based on the patient's chief complaint and physical exam, a presumptive diagnosis is made and a series of conservative and surgical options are provided. This includes providing risk stratification and explaining the anticipated benefits for each procedure in our hands. Once the patient has selected the best therapeutic option for her, informed consent is signed and all questions are answered. Preoperative bowel preparation is recommended for our patients as it helps to decompress the bowel and improves intraoperative visualization. We suggest a full liquid diet two days before surgery, clear liquids 24 hours prior to, and 8 oz of magnesium citrate the evening before surgery. The authors acknowledge published data which questions the utility of preoperative bowel preparation, however we have found that it improves visualization and facilitates operative exposure and efficiency.

Surgical Technique

Prophylactic intravenous antibiotics are given 30 minutes prior to incision and the patient is placed under general anesthesia and positioned in the dorsal lithotomy position with the arms tucked bilaterally. Sequential compression devices are applied for DVT prophylaxis and a 16 French foley catheter is placed, with the balloon only insufflated with 5 cc to maximize visualization. A 10-mm access port is placed at the inferior aspect of the umbilicus and the abdomen is inflated with CO_2 gas to a total pressure of 15 mm Hg. In order to maintain heated insufflation and smoke evacuation, the Surgiquest Airseal® (SurgiQuest Company, Connecticut) is utilized. A zero-degree laparoscope is then inserted, and a survey performed. Three additional ports are placed under direct visualization – one in each lower quadrant and one suprapubic. At least one of these is a 12 mm port but this may vary depending on planned concomitant surgery. A typical urogynaecology procedure port placement is shown in Figure 18.1. If a hysterectomy or sacrocolpopexy is planned, it is performed prior to the paravaginal repair. If a laparoscopic Burch procedure is planned, this should be done after completion of the paravaginal repair since the anterior vaginal wall will then be at its normal anatomic position.

Prior to port placement, the bladder is backfilled with 300 cc of normal saline, which facilitates intra-abdominal identification of the superior aspect of the bladder. The retropubic space is entered with the aid of a Harmonic scalpel via a transverse incision, 3 cm cranial to the bladder reflection and medial to the obliterated umbilical ligaments, thereby avoiding the inferior epigastric vessels which run laterally. Immediately, the appearance of loose areolar tissue confirms entry into the appropriate space. Further dissection of the Space of Retzius reveals the following landmarks: pubic rami, Cooper's ligament, arcus tendinous fascia pelvis (ATFP)/white line, bladder, bladder neck, and obturator neurovascular bundle. The anterior vaginal wall originates at the pubic symphysis and inserts at the ischial spine. In patients with a paravaginal defect, a 'break' in the pubocervical fascia will be noted at the level of the ATFP (Figure 18.2). A laparoscopic kitner facilitates dissection of the bladder medially off the pubocervical fascia and improves visualization. These defects can be either unilateral or bilateral.

The surgeon's nondominant hand is inserted into the vagina to lift the anterior vaginal wall, temporarily reapproximating the lateral edge to the ATFP. A series of interrupted 2–0 non-absorbable sutures are then placed through the ATFP (incorporating the fascia of the levator ani and the obturator

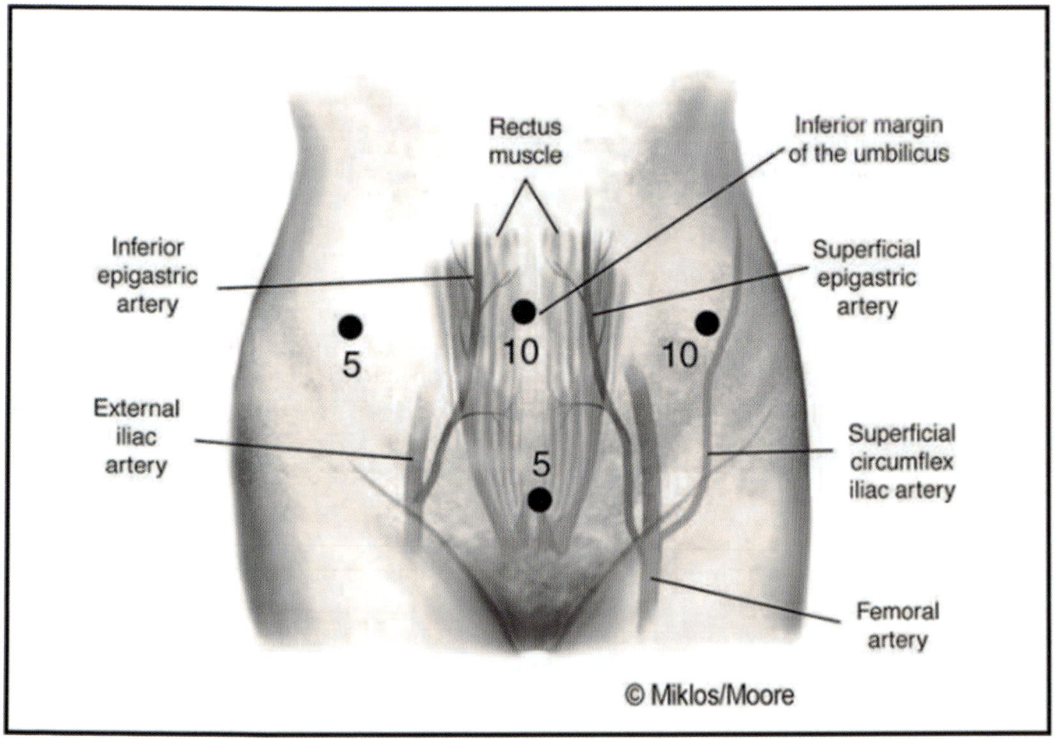

Figure 18.1 Laparoscopic port placement.

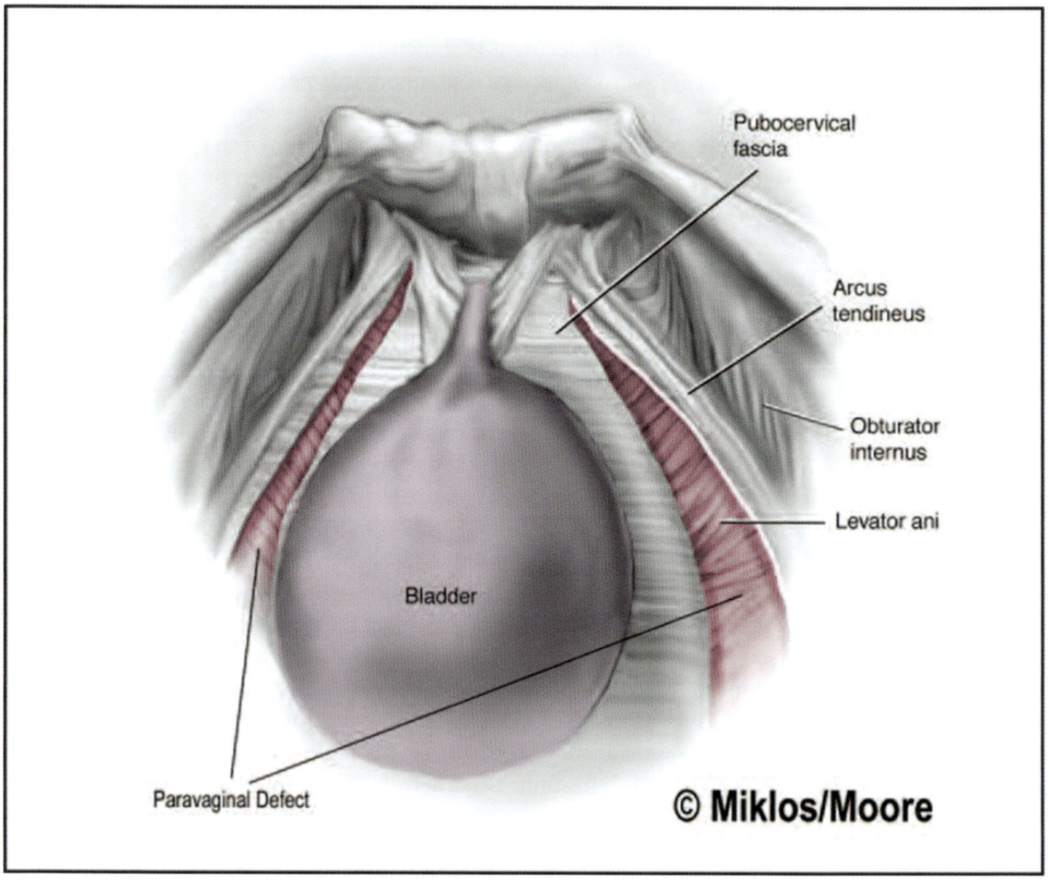

Figure 18.2a Paravaginal defect illustration.

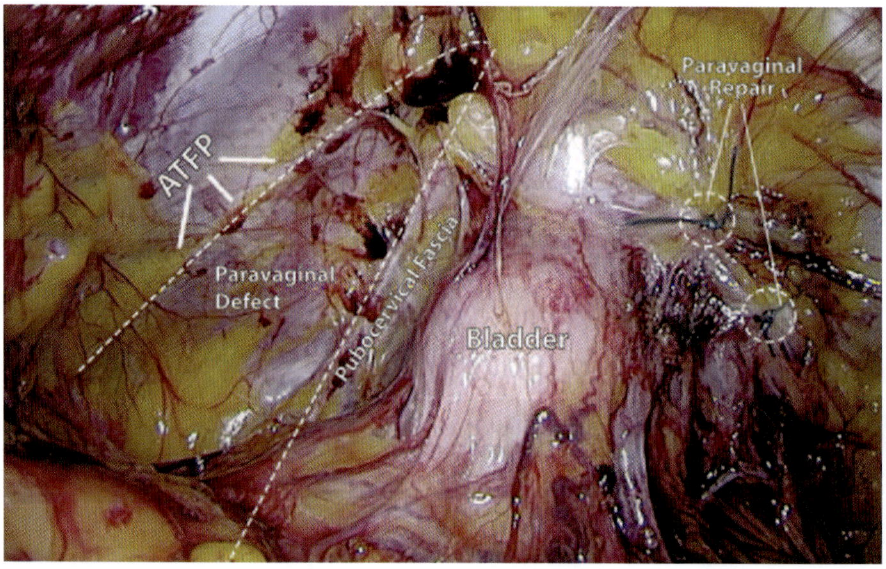

Figure 18.2b Paravaginal defect anatomy during laparoscopy.

internus) and the pubocervical fascia of the vagina, equally spaced between the ischial spine and the pubic symphysis. Typically, this will take about four to five sutures (Figure 18.3). In order to maximize efficiency, the assistant directs the camera and provides retraction. The surgeon passes the suture through the 10 mm port and performs all needlework and suturing. We use an extracorporeal knot-tying technique, ensuring direct apposition of the tissues without any suture bridging.

If the patient needs an anti-incontinence procedure, such as a Burch urethropexy or mid-urethral sling, the paravaginal repair should be completed first to facilitate determination of appropriate urethral correction. The peritoneum is then reapproximated with 2–0 monofilament suture closing the retropubic

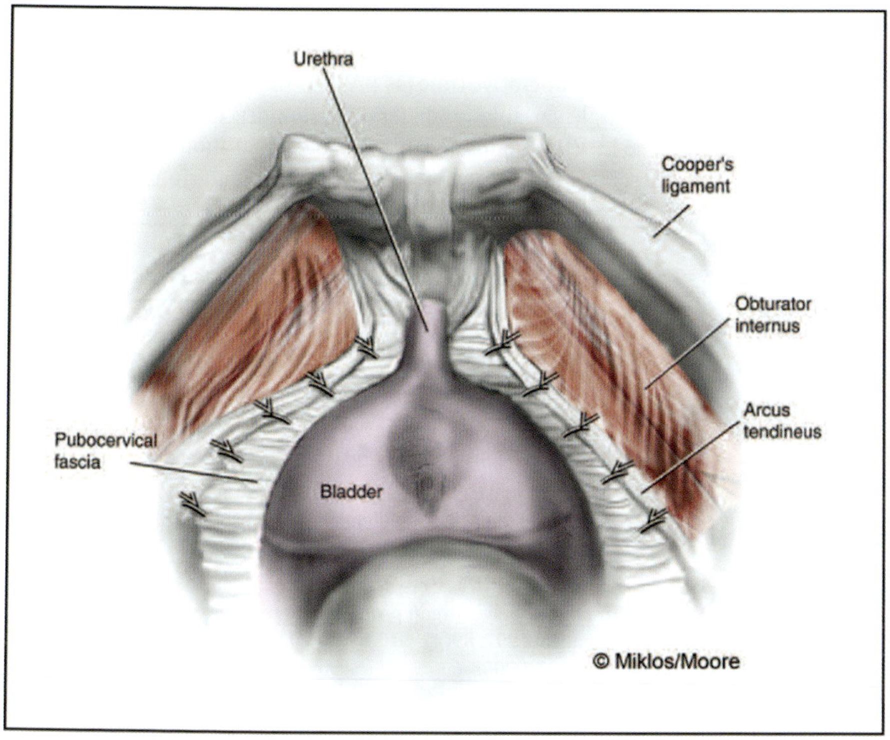

Figure 18.3 Paravaginal defect repair.

space. The abdomen is then desufflated of CO_2 gas, monitoring for any occult bleeding. The fascia of any incision greater than 10 mm is reapproximated and the trocar sites are closed. Even in the absence of an anti-incontinence procedure, a voiding trial (active or passive) is performed postoperatively, given the bladder manipulation and to confirm adequate emptying.

Complications

Overall, the adverse event rate is low and similar to other laparoscopic procedures. In a series of 212 LPVR procedures, the reported major complication rate was 4.2%, which included seven inadvertent cystotomies (3.3%), blood loss >1,000 ml (0.9%), and one bowel injury (0.5%). A 28.8% incidence of minor complications included prolonged urinary retention (10.4%) and urinary tract infection (8.5%) [11]. Author JM has previously reported a urinary tract injury rate of less than 3% in his series of 171 subjects [12].

Although dissection is performed under direct visualization, with the bladder backfilled, cystoscopic evaluation for injury at the conclusion of the procedure is prudent. While ureteral injury is unlikely, we routinely assess for efflux in any operation which involves manipulation or dissection around the bladder. This can be aided with the use of indigo carmine, furosemide, backfilling with a 50% glucose solution or 200 mg of pyridium taken orally prior to the start of the procedure.

Although the space of Retzius is classified as an avascular space, occasionally bleeding can be encountered. This will usually resolve with bipolar electrocautery but persistent oozing can be treated with the application of haemostatic agents such as Flowseal or Arista. Care should be taken to avoid the obturator neurovascular bundles bilaterally, the urethra and dorsal vein of the clitoris centrally. Identification of these structures upon entering the retropubic space is prudent to decrease the potential for injury.

Evidence

Authors JM and RM previously published a literature review of laparoscopic paravaginal repairs to determine objective anatomical success, defined as anterior compartment prolapse POP-Q point Ba <-1 or Baden Walker Grade 0–1 [6]. Of 111 citations reviewed, 28 studies met the inclusion criteria and described an overall paravaginal success rate of 54% to 95.8% for all approaches (abdominal, vaginal, and laparoscopic), with a laparoscopic success rate of 60% to 89%.

Behnia-Willison performed a longitudinal study of 212 women treated with a LPVR for anterior compartment prolapse, with a cure rate of 76% and an average follow up of 14.2 months [11].

Patients were categorized as having either only a paravaginal defect (absent sulci with intact rugae) or both paravaginal and central defects (absent sulci and rugae). The investigators decided not to combine LPVR with anterior colporrhaphy as the plication from the latter may result in undue tension on the paravaginal repair. Subjects with both central and lateral defects were counselled that they may need a secondary procedure in the future. This study showed that subsequent treatment of residual central defects with graft augmented anterior colporrhaphy increased the overall cure rate by 10%.

A comparative trial with abdominal paravaginal (APVR), vaginal paravaginal (VPVR), and laparoscopic paravaginal (LPVR) repair arms was described reporting lower efficacy for the laparoscopic approach relative to the other modalities

(60% versus 90%+) over a 12-month follow-up. However, this was not randomized and there were only five subjects in the laparoscopic group and 20 subjects in the other arms [13].

A few variants of the traditional LPVR have been described. Rivoire reported on the treatment of 138 women who underwent laparoscopic promontofixation, using mesh, of whom 40 were also treated with LPVR. Of those receiving LPVR, 16 subjects underwent a suture suspension as described above, while the remaining 24 had a paravaginal repair with mesh placement. The recurrence rate when using suture suspension was reported as 18.8% versus 0% with mesh over a follow-up period of 33 months [14]. Another mesh-based LPVR technique was published by Washington. A prolene graft was stapled to Cooper's ligament with a helical tacker. Subjective and objective improvement was noted in 91% and 82% respectively, over a follow-up period of 5–25 months [15]. Another group included a suture throw through the iliopectineal ligament, described as a 'key suture' for additional support [16].

Robotic paravaginal repairs have been described in the literature, but the main challenge is the loss of tactile sensation and the inability for the surgeon to elevate the vagina with his/her hand during suspension. While this procedure can be accomplished with the aid of a knowledgeable assistant, the laparoscopic approach circumvents these drawbacks.

As described above, accurate diagnosis of the anterior vaginal wall defect is of utmost importance. If a patient presents with a true paravaginal defect and is treated with an anterior colporrhaphy, the dissection and subsequent midline plication of the fibromuscularis would only further exacerbate the tear injury along the ATFP and potentially result in recurrent prolapse. In a similar scenario, if a patient elects to proceed with a sacrocolpopexy for treatment of her POP, a paravaginal repair should still be done if she is found to have a paravaginal defect. The apical attachment and anterior mesh arm may place traction and reduce the defect, but it is not the same as restoring anatomy via a reattachment of the pubocervical fascia to the ATFP.

Conclusion

In assessing anterior vaginal wall defects, it is crucial to determine if a paravaginal defect is the responsible aetiology. While these repairs have been described using vaginal, abdominal, and robotic techniques, a laparoscopic approach is beneficial, affording a minimally invasive approach with concomitant decrease in recovery time, excellent visualization, and tactile sensation. Additionally, this is a mesh-free option that can be performed at the same time as other POP or stress urinary incontinence procedures.

If a patient has significant POP, it is very likely that a paravaginal defect is present, and in order to optimize outcome all compartments must be addressed. This, in many instances, requires both a sacrocolpopexy and paravaginal repair. While it is possible to compensate for an uncorrected paravaginal defect with overzealous tension on the anterior sacrocolpopexy mesh, this is not the most anatomic repair and can increase the risk of postoperative pain or dyspareunia. In an article describing sacrocolpopexy efficiency, authors JM and RM performed concomitant LPVR 72% of the time without significantly adding to the total operative time [17]. While outcomes are dependent on multiple variables, the literature supports excellent results, and the LPVR remains a viable approach that should be considered a staple in the urogynaecologist's armamentarium.

Video 18.1
Laparoscopic paravaginal repair and Burch colposuspension.

References

1. White GR. Cystocele – A radical cure by suturing lateral sulci of the vagina to the white line of pelvic fascia. Int Urogynecol J 1997; 8(5): 288–92. https://doi.org/10.1007/BF02765486
2. Richardson AC, Lyon JB, Williams NL. A new look at pelvic relaxation. Am J Obstet Gynecol 1976; 126(5): 568–71. https://doi.org/10.1016/0002-9378(76)90751-1
3. Olsen A, Smith V, Bergstrom J, et al. Epidemiology of surgically managed pelvic organ prolapse and urinary incontinence. Obstet Gynecol 1997; 89(4): 501–6. https://doi.org/10.1016/S0029-7844(97)00058-6
4. Arenholt LTS, Pedersen BG, Glavind K, et al. Paravaginal defect: anatomy, clinical findings, and imaging. Int Urogynecol J 2017; 28(5): 661–73. https://doi.org/10.1007/s00192-016-3096-3
5. Hendrix SL, Clark A, Nygaard I, et al. Pelvic organ prolapse in the Women's Health Initiative: gravity and gravidity. Am J Obstet Gynecol 2002; 186(6): 1160–6. https://doi.org/10.1067/mob.2002.123819
6. Orawee C, Miklos JR, Moore RD. Laparoscopic paravaginal defect repair: surgical technique and a literature review. Surg Technol Int 2015; 27: 173–83.
7. Richardson AC, Lyon JB, Williams NL. A new look at pelvic relaxation. Am J Obstet Gynecol 1976; 126(5): 568–73. Available at: www.ncbi.nlm.nih.gov/pubmed/984127 [last accessed 31 October 2021].
8. Shull BL. Clinical evaluation of women with pelvic support defects. Clin Obstet Gynecol 1993; 36(4):9 39–51.
9. Barber MD, Cundiff GW, Weidner AC, et al. Accuracy of clinical assessment of paravaginal defects in women with anterior vaginal wall prolapse. Am J Obstet Gynecol 1999; 181(1): 87–90. https://doi.org/10.1016/S0002-9378(99)70440-0
10. Shull BL. How I do the abdominal paravaginal repair. J Pelvic Surg 1995; 1(1): 43–6.
11. Behnia-Willison F, Seman EI, Cook JR, et al. Laparoscopic paravaginal repair of anterior compartment prolapse. J Minim Invasive Gynecol 2007; 14(4): 475–80. https://doi.org/10.1016/j.jmig.2006.12.002
12. Miklos JR, Kohli N. Laparoscopic paravaginal repair plus Burch colposuspension: review and descriptive technique. Urology 2000; 56(6 Suppl 1): 64–9. https://doi.org/10.1016/s0090-4295(00)00510-0
13. Hosni MM, El-Feky AEH, Agur WI, et al. Evaluation of three different surgical approaches in repairing paravaginal support defects: a comparative trial. Arch Gynecol Obstet 2013; 288(6): 1341–8. https://doi.org/10.1007/s00404-013-2927-4
14. Rivoire C, Botchorishvili R, Canis M, et al. Complete laparoscopic treatment of genital prolapse with meshes including

vaginal promontofixation and anterior repair: a series of 138 patients.J Minim Invasive Gynecol 2007; 14(6): 712–18. https://doi.org/10.1016/j.jmig.2007.06.017
15. Washington JL, Somers KO. Laparoscopic paravaginal repair: a new technique using mesh and staples. JSLS 2003; 7(4): 301–3.
16. Seman EI, Cook JR, O'Shea RT. Two-year experience with laparoscopic pelvic floor repair. J Am Assoc Gynecol Laparosc 2003; 10(1): 38–45. https://doi.org/10.1016/S1074-3804(05)60232-0
17. Moore R, Moriarty C, Chinthakanan O, et al. Laparoscopic sacrocolpopexy: operative times and efficiency in a high-volume female pelvic medicine and laparoscopic surgery practice. Int Urogynecol J 2017; 28(6): 887–92. https://doi.org/10.1007/s00192-016-3179-1

Chapter 19

Choice of Sacrocolpopexy Route Including Vaginal Mesh Attachment

Emily Davidson, Karl Jallad

Introduction

While sacrocolpopexy is considered the gold standard procedure for pelvic organ prolapse repair, individual surgeons' techniques vary greatly [1,2]. Surgeons must choose which graft they use (see Chapter 9) as well as the materials and tools they use to affix this graft to the vagina and the sacral promontory (see Chapter 5). However, surgeons must also choose the route by which they will perform the surgery. While the original sacrocolpopexy was completed entirely abdominally through a laparotomy incision, the procedure has now been performed laparoscopically, with robotic-assistance, and most recently completely transvaginally. Additionally, surgeons can choose combinations of these techniques, hybridizing these procedures based on the two main steps: vaginal attachment of the graft and sacral fixation.

In this chapter, we will review minimally invasive routes of sacrocolpopexy and recommendations for how surgeons choose their preferred techniques. We will also discuss concurrent hysterectomy at the time of sacrocolpopexy. Additionally, we describe the surgical technique for a transvaginal attachment of the vaginal portion of the sacrocolpopexy graft. Finally, we briefly review the emerging topic of the vaginal sacrocolpopexy.

Route of Sacrocolpopexy

Laparoscopic Sacrocolpopexy versus Abdominal Sacrocolpopexy

The original abdominal sacrocolpopexy (ASC) was described prior to the advent of advanced laparoscopic technologies. As technologies and surgeons' skills have developed, the procedure has been modified to be performed laparoscopically [3-8]. Studies have compared ASC and laparoscopic sacrocolpopexy (LSC) and the findings are similar to what has been found with other gynaecologic procedures: minimally invasive procedures are associated with decreased patient morbidity, duration of hospital stay, blood loss, and postoperative bowel complications like ileus and obstruction but with the trade-off of increased operative time [9].

Laparoscopic versus Robotic-assisted Laparoscopic Sacrocolpopexy

With the advent of LSC, surgeons looked to find ways to facilitate the procedure. With the development of the robotic platform, surgeons could experience improved visualization with three-dimensional optics as well as increased ease of suturing with wristed instruments when performing a robotic-assisted laparoscopic sacrocolpopexy (RSC).

Several studies have compared the RSC and the LSC [10,11]. After multiple systematic reviews, there appears to be no difference in significant patient outcomes other than increased pain after RSC [12,13]. LSC requires less operative time than RSC. However, the learning curve is shorter with robotic assistance, with a decrease in OR time of 25% (60 minutes) after 10 cases [14]. In comparison, it took approximately twice that number of cases to reach a turning point in surgeon's operative time for LSC [15].

With the rising cost of healthcare, cost is an important consideration when comparing route of surgery, especially without demonstrated benefit to the patient. There is clear evidence that RSC is more expensive that LSC [10,11,16,17]. However, Anger et al found that this difference is primarily related to the initial purchase of the robotic platform, not related to day-of operating costs or hospital-related costs up to six weeks after surgery. However, one potential benefit of robotic assistance is the decreased incidence of surgeons' work-related injuries related to surgery [18]. Increased work-related injuries could potentially lead to an overall increase in the cost of healthcare, with the training of new surgeons if early retirement were to be needed.

Hysterectomy with Sacrocolpopexy

Concurrent hysterectomy may be performed with sacrocolpopexy. Multiple studies have investigated the impact on perioperative complications, prolapse recurrence, and mesh exposure. Regardless of route, concurrent hysterectomy does not impact perioperative complications or morbidity [19,20]. In a systematic review on LSC, no consensus could be reached on the preferred type of hysterectomy [21].

Prolapse Outcomes

If the patient has a uterus, a hysterectomy is typically performed during sacrocolpopexy. When deciding between a supracervical hysterectomy (SCH) and total hysterectomy, there is not enough data in a recent systematic review to reach a consensus [21]. However, two studies suggest a decreased risk of recurrent prolapse with complete hysterectomy. Myers et al reported increased recurrent stage 2 or greater prolapse one year after RSC in women with concurrent SCH compared to total hysterectomy; however, composite success outcomes and prolapse at or past the hymen were not different between groups [22]. Davidson et al compared vaginal and SCH with concurrent RSC or LSC and found that patients who underwent a complete hysterectomy with either RSC or LSC had less recurrent prolapse (stage 2 or greater and/or retreatment with surgery or a pessary) although this trend was not statistically significant [20].

Mesh Exposure

Supracervical hysterectomy with sacrocolpopexy is often performed instead of total hysterectomy with sacrocolpopexy with the idea that this may avoid future mesh erosion. Deng et al's systematic review of 7,084 patients included concurrent hysterectomy as a risk factor for mesh exposure, but the majority of studies included slings and transvaginal mesh [23]. Warner et al found an increased risk with either total laparoscopic hysterectomy (TLH) or vaginal hysterectomy compared to SCH [24], and Osmundsen showed increased risk of mesh exposure with TLH compared to SCH [25]. Tan-Kim et al also found an increased risk of mesh exposure with vaginal hysterectomy; however, their mesh exposure incidence of 23% is significantly higher than other published data.

Many other studies, however, have shown no increased risk of mesh exposure [20,26,27]. This mixed data exists for hysterectomy with ASC as well as minimally invasive sacrocolpopexy [28-32]. Potential mechanisms for the differences seen in these studies may be the use of electrosurgery, especially during TLH. Excessive electrosurgery at the vaginal cuff may compromise vascularity to the cuff, decrease wound healing, and increase the risk of mesh exposure. In addition, serial improvement in surgical technique may be a factor. The majority of studies showing increased mesh exposure are older studies, and there is a huge variation in the incidence of mesh exposure between authors (ranging from 2% [26] to 23% [33]).

Conclusions regarding Concurrent Hysterectomy

Given the mixed data on concurrent hysterectomy, surgeons may choose to perform concurrent hysterectomy or not. Factors that may come into play are risk for future cervical pathology, cervical size, potential need to morcellate the uterine specimen, and patient preference. Surgeons performing hysterectomy with RSC or LSC should track and assess their own outcomes.

Vaginal Mesh Attachment

Surgical efficiency is an important strategy for successful sacrocolpopexy. Suturing the mesh onto the vagina is a step during minimally invasive sacrocolpopexy where multiple variations have attempted to increase the efficiency. Robotic-wristed instruments led to increased ease of knot-tying. Use of both barbed suture and running locked sutures have been shown to decrease operative time during vaginal mesh attachment [34,35]. Surgical glue has even been shown to be a feasible alternative to suturing [36,37]. However, attachment of the mesh transvaginally is one option that may decrease operative time by up to one hour [26]. This may be especially of interest when the vaginal cuff is open as after TLH or VH. Multiple authors have described this technique [26,38]. This technique could also be used after opening the vaginal cuff in a vaginal vault prolapse as described by Park et al [39]. Various studies have demonstrated the safety of vaginal mesh attachment [20,40]. In this section we present our technique for transvaginal mesh attachment. The authors wish to thank Drs. Robert Gutman, Patrick Nosti, Andrew Sokol, Danielle Marshall, and Cheryl Iglesia for the images in Figures 19.1–19.9.

For this procedure, there are several key steps:

1. Vaginal dissection
2. Vaginal mesh attachment
3. Cuff closure
4. Attachment of the sacral aspect of the mesh

Considerations during Hysterectomy

When planning to attach the mesh transvaginally, we recommend that as much vaginal length is preserved as possible during a hysterectomy. Doing so will allow use of 1–2 cm of the cuff without mesh attached for performing a double layer closure. We can also preserve length for postoperative sexual function. Additionally, we recommend using as little electrosurgery at the cuff as possible. In this way, we can preserve vascularity at the cuff which we feel is important to minimize future mesh complications.

Vaginal Dissection

Posterior Vaginal Dissection

After the hysterectomy (or after entry into the peritoneal cul de sac in a post-hysterectomy prolapse) the vaginal cuff is open. Multiple Allis clamps are placed on the edges of the cuff for stabilization during dissection and mesh placement.

In preparation for mesh attachment, it is our practice to perform hydrodissection. We use a dilute mixture of local anaesthetic with a vasoconstrictor such as 0.5% lidocaine with 1:100,000 epinephrine. This can be further diluted with a 1:1 solution of normal saline if necessary, based on the use of local anaesthetic throughout the rest of the procedure. Alternatively, injectable saline alone can be used.

After hydrodissection, we perform the vaginal dissection. We prefer to start with the posterior dissection. The vaginal cuff is inverted with the surgeon's first two fingers against the vaginal epithelium. The surgical assistant grasps the rectovaginal tissue with forceps. We use a Mayo scissors to create the full thickness vaginal dissection (see Figure 19.1). We start approximately 2 cm from the edge of the cuff for preservation of full thickness tissue for vaginal cuff closure.

We recommend dissection to a length of at least 5 cm in the rectovaginal space or longer based on total vaginal length (see Figure 19.2). Other surgeons have performed the dissection all the way to the hymen which may require a transperineal incision [41].

Anterior Vaginal Dissection

After completion of the posterior dissection, we then proceed with the anterior dissection. The anterior cuff is inverted against the surgeon's fingers (see Figure 19.3). Again, it is important to preserve 2 cm of full thickness vaginal cuff away from the vaginal dissection.

During this portion of the dissection, the urethral catheter may be drawn toward the cuff edge to confirm proper dissection location (see Figure 19.4).

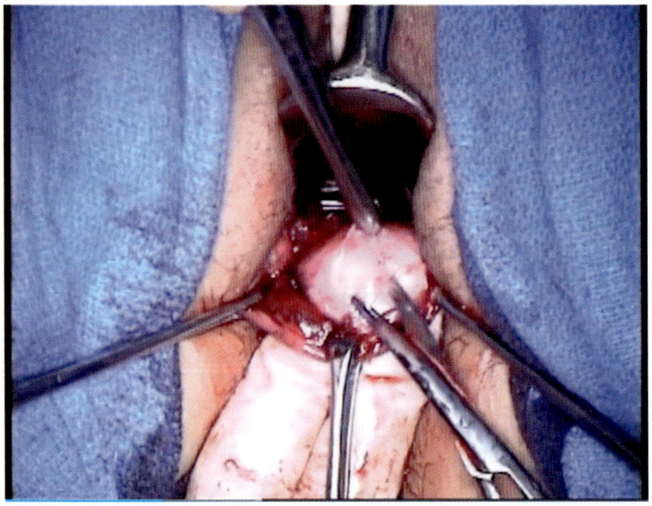

Figure 19.1 Initiation of rectovaginal dissection.

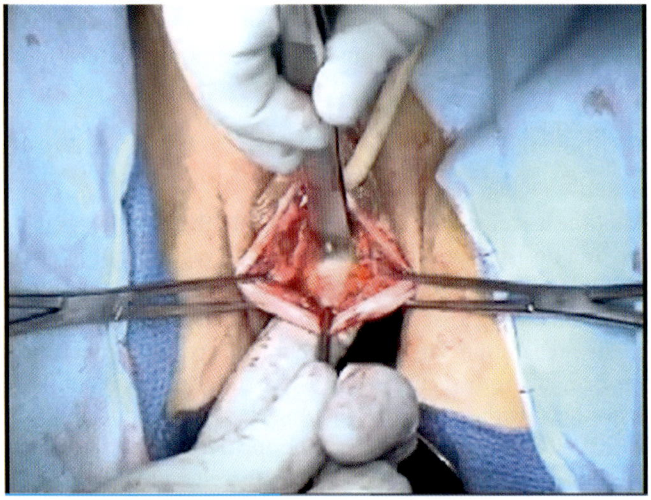

Figure 19.2 Completion of rectovaginal dissection.

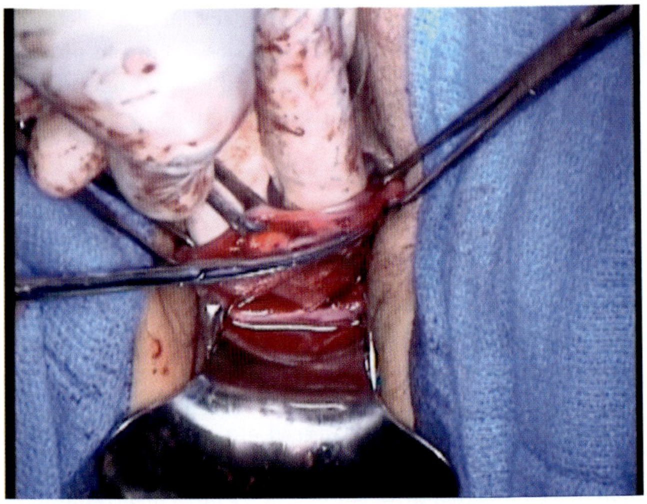

Figure 19.3 Anterior dissection.

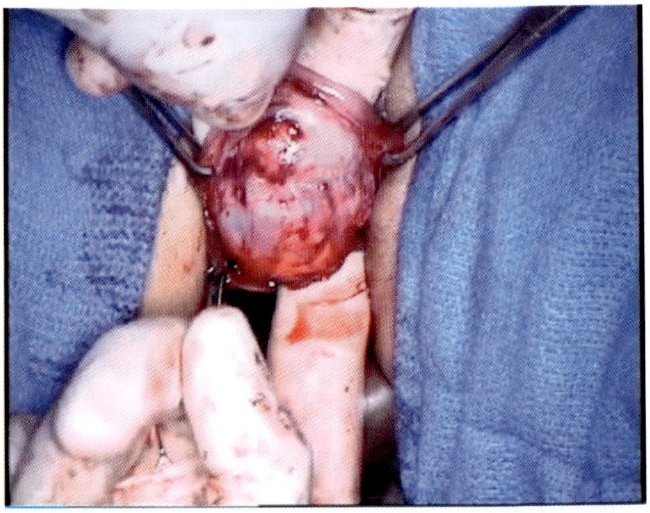

Figure 19.4 Urethral catheter balloon at the cuff edge.

We continue the anterior dissection to the level of the level of the bladder neck where one can feel the balloon of the urethral catheter (see Figure 19.5).

Graft Choice

We prefer to use large-pore, light-weight polypropylene mesh with dual anterior and posterior arms [42]. We use a full-length graft knowing we will need to shorten the graft abdominally. Alternatively, the graft can be trimmed prior to attachment based on an assessment of the predicted length of the distance from the vaginal cuff to the sacral promontory.

Vaginal Attachment

Proper orientation of the mesh is essential. During the posterior mesh attachment, the sacral portion should hang out of the vagina toward the surgical team. During replacement of the vaginal cuff, this will be displaced cephalad. We recommend ensuring this is protected with sterile towels from contamination around the anus. During anterior mesh attachment, the mesh also hangs out of the vagina but can rest on the mons pubis to improve visualization.

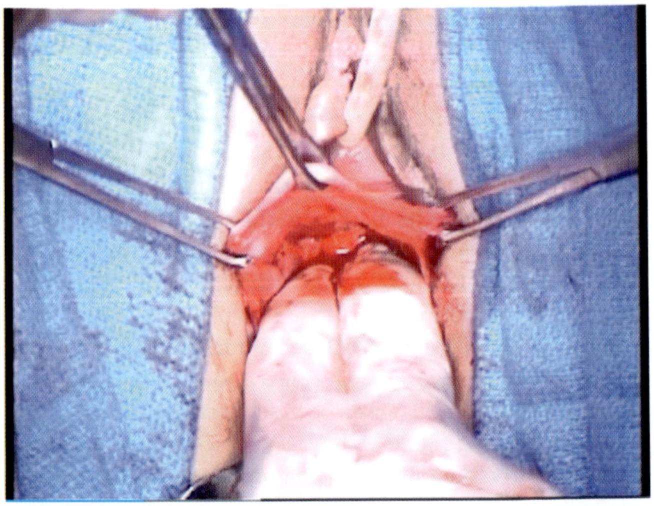

Figure 19.5 Completion of anterior dissection.

During vaginal mesh attachment, we utilize an end-to-end anastomosis (EEA) sizer to suture against the inverted cuff. Alternatively, a Breisky-Navratil retractor can be used. The sizer is placed in the distal vagina with the cuff pulled against the metal using Allis clamps. In this way, we flatten the vagina and increase visualization and a flat surface on which to suture. While a surgeon's fingers could also be used as during the dissection, the use of the EEA sizer minimizes the potential for a needlestick injury.

When suturing the mesh, the most distal sutures (farthest from the cuff) should be at one end of the graft (see Figure 19.6). We use multiple interrupted sutures of 2-0 delayed absorbable suture such as polydioxanone. Prior work has demonstrated no difference in outcomes between permanent and delayed absorbable sutures, and this eliminates the risk of permanent suture exposure in the future [43]. We typically perform six to eight total sutures on each mesh arm. The sutures should be approximately 1–2 cm apart. It is important that approximately 2 cm of the vagina at the cuff are free from mesh (see Figure 19.7).

After both meshes are sutured in place, we then grasp the two sacral ends of the mesh with a ring forceps, and after copious irrigation using dilute bacitracin antibiotic solution, we gently place the mesh into the peritoneal cavity (see Figure 19.8).

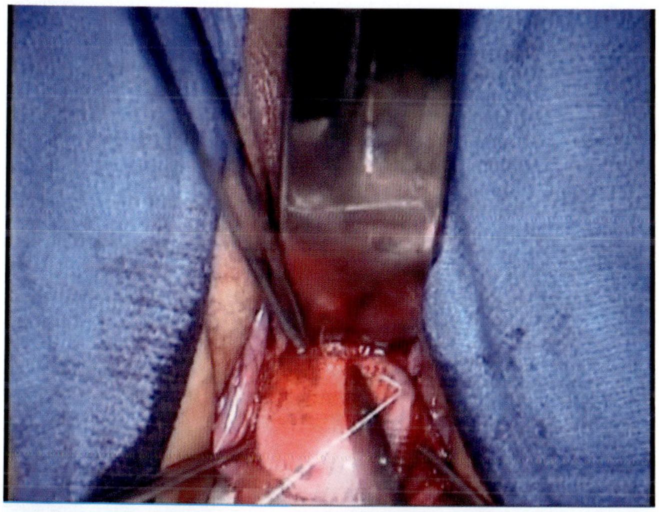

Figure 19.6 Distal attachment of posterior mesh.

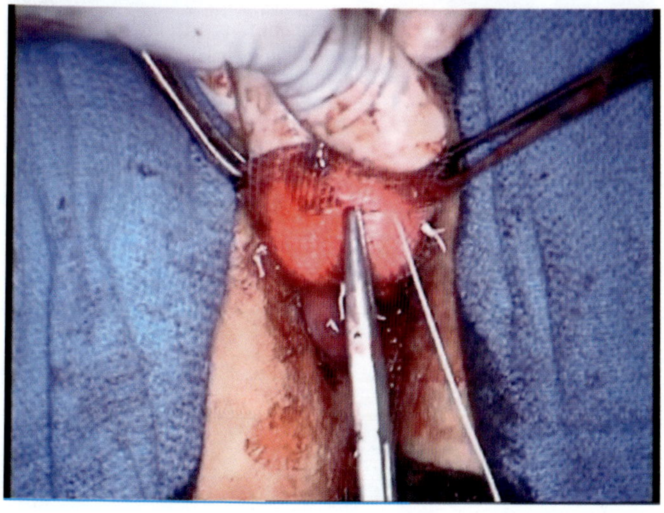

Figure 19.7 Proximal attachment of anterior mesh.

Closure of the Vaginal Cuff

After the two sacral arms of the mesh are placed into the abdomen, the vaginal cuff is closed. We prefer to close the vagina in a transverse fashion in two layers. Using a running suture of 2-0 absorbable suture such as polyglactin, we close the muscularis of the vaginal cuff. Finally, we suture the epithelium of the vaginal cuff with 2-0 absorbable suture in either a running locked suture or with multiple figures of eight. If a posterior colporrhaphy is planned, this can be performed at this time. However, we recommend avoiding performing a mid-urethral sling until after fixation of the sacral arm of the mesh establishing the final apical support, if an anti-incontinence surgery is planned.

Minimally Invasive Fixation of the Sacral Arm of the Graft

We then turn to the abdominal portion of the procedure, the sacral fixation. It is our practice to utilize traditional laparoscopic instruments for the sacral attachment when performing transvaginal attachment of the sacrocolpopexy mesh. We do not feel that robotic assistance is necessary given the minimal suturing and dissection required after vaginal mesh attachment. This portion of the procedure is no different to that which has been described in previous chapters (Chapters 11–14).

Prior to tensioning and sacral promontory attachment, it is necessary to straighten the sacral mesh arms. If these are difficult to straighten, we have found that irrigation of the arms is helpful to assist in the arms' release from each other and the vaginal cuff. Copious irrigation is also important given the mesh's transfer through the vagina. After attachment of the mesh at the sacral promontory and reperitonealization if performed, cystourethroscopy is performed to assess ureteral patency and integrity of the bladder.

Conclusions regarding Transvaginal Attachment of Sacrocolpopexy Mesh

Transvaginal attachment of the vaginal mesh arms during a minimally invasive sacrocolpopexy is one way to improve

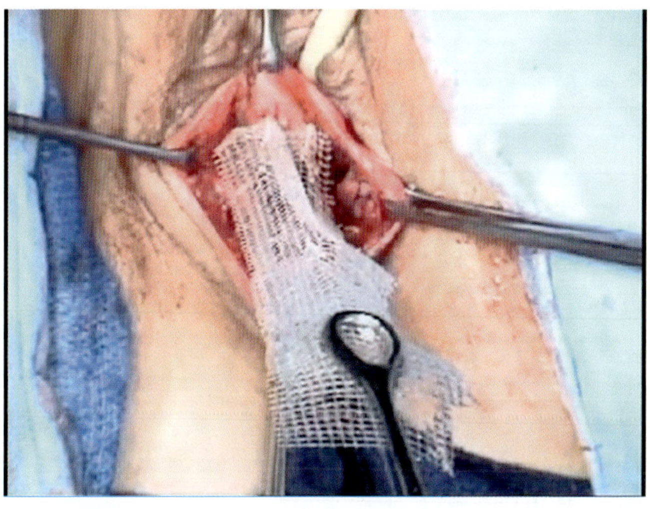

Figure 19.8 Placement of mesh into peritoneal cavity.

surgical efficiency. However, there remain some concerns about the risk of future mesh exposure as discussed previously. Surgeons who wish to perform this procedure need to be aware that the available data is not enough to reach consensus. Because of this, it is essential to be aware of one's own outcomes, as discussed with concurrent hysterectomy. Those who want to start performing this technique should be comfortable with this type of full thickness vaginal dissection which is less commonly performed with the decreasing availability of transvaginal mesh procedures.

Vaginal Sacrocolpopexy/Vaginal NOTES Sacrocolpopexy

Minimally invasive surgery technologies and techniques grow and evolve. In fields such as colorectal surgery and gastroenterology, there have been increasing numbers of Natural Orifice Translumenal Endoscopic Surgeries (NOTES). These procedures utilize natural anatomic orifices such as the stomach, anus, and vagina to access other organs resulting in an incisionless surgery. Well-described NOTES procedures in the surgery literature include cholecystectomy, transanal total mesorectal excision, and thyroidectomies [44].

Transvaginal approaches have also been described in gynaecology. Vaginal NOTES procedures that have been described in the literature include hysterectomy, adnexal surgery including treatment of ectopic pregnancy, uterosacral ligament suspension, and even pelvic lymphadenectomy for endometrial cancer [45-49]. Skilled gynaecologists adopting vaginal NOTES procedures have been shown to rapidly improve operative efficiency after only 10 cases [50].

Sacrocolpopexy is one such procedure that has been modified for a NOTES technique. Noblett et al published the feasibility of a vaginal sacrocolpopexy using cadavers in 2012 [51]. Since that time, multiple authors have published their techniques for the procedure [41,52,53]. While long-term data is not yet available, a case series of 26 patients who underwent vaginal NOTES sacrocolpopexy demonstrated good outcomes in terms of safety and short-term efficacy [53].

Surgeons performing vaginal NOTES procedures typically enter the peritoneal cavity after a hysterectomy is completed or by a technique similar to that described by Park et al [39]. Anatomic measurements are made of the vagina and the mesh trimmed appropriately. The vaginal arms of the mesh are secured to the vagina similar to the technique described above.

Pneumoperitoneum is then achieved by using a vaginal single-port device. This can be purchased as a prefabricated single-port or can be created using a surgical glove, circular wound retractor, and laparoscopic trocars (see Figures 19.9–19.11, previously published by Jallad and Walters [54] and reproduced with permission). The sacral dissection is performed using rigid instruments through this port. Based on surgeon preference, retroperitoneal dissection or tunnelling can be performed. Tensioning of the mesh is usually accomplished using measurement of the distance from the sacral promontory to the level of the cuff or hymen for the specific patient. The sacral arms (or

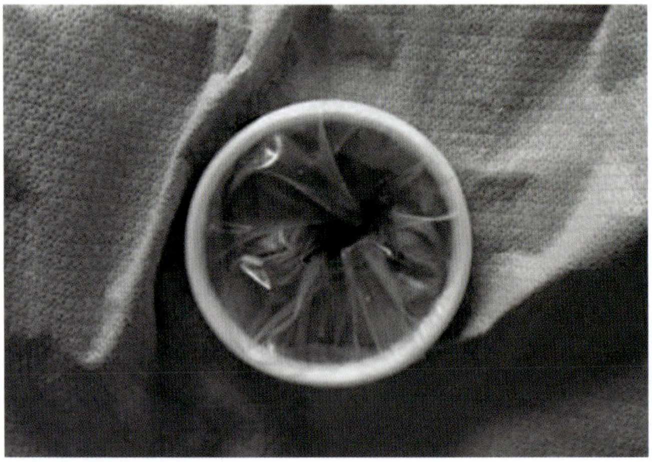

Figure 19.9 Alexis wound retractor resting past the vaginal cuff and on the perineum.

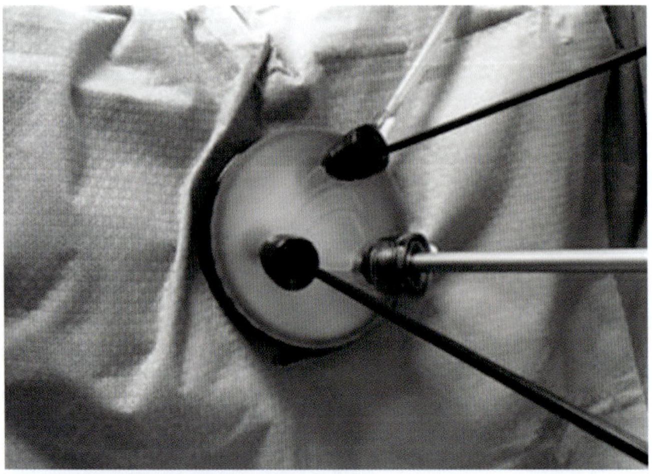

Figure 19.10 GelPOINT advanced-access platform over the Alexis wound retractor in the vagina.

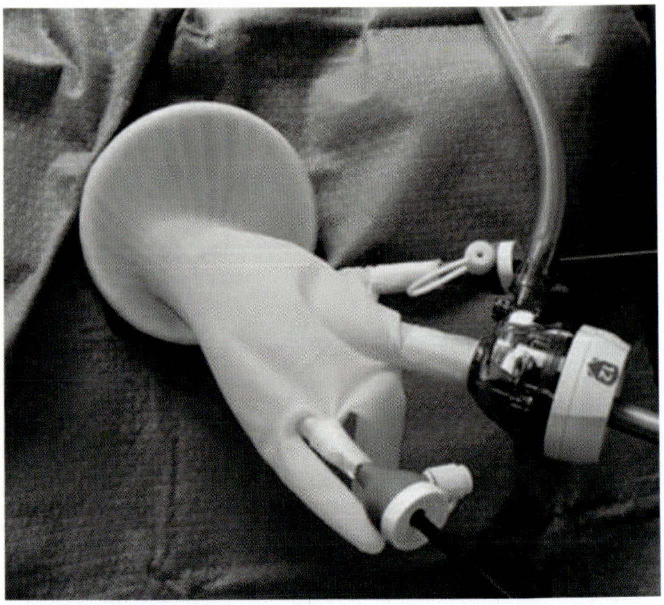

Figure 19.11 Self-constructed glove port.

arm if using a Y-mesh) are then attached to the sacral promontory in the usual fashion. It is critical at this step to consider the location of the L5-S1 intervertebral disc and to avoid entering too deep in order to avoid discitis and other complications [55]. This is especially important as this cephalad view is not the typical surgeon visualization of the sacral promontory. The vaginal cuff is then closed [54].

This area is a growing area of interest, and the description above is just one technique. Hanes has also described an alternative method to a transvaginal sacrocolpopexy utilizing two separate meshes, a long sacral arm and a U-shaped graft that wraps around both the anterior and posterior aspect of the vagina [56,57]. We recommend that surgeons wishing to adopt this technique do so only after achieving clinical excellence in laparoscopic sacrocolpopexy and refining technique with cadaver feasibility. Finally, until vaginal NOTES sacrocolpopexy accumulates more supportive data, it is important to consider the ethical impact of adapting this new technique with input from one's local institutional review board [58].

Summary/Conclusions

It is clear that sacrocolpopexy is not one single procedure – there are dozens of choices that a surgeon must make for each of their patients. Options addressed in this chapter include which type of concurrent hysterectomy to perform and what route of surgery should be utilized, including conventional laparoscopy and robotic assistance. Surgeons have different techniques, and there has yet to be a consensus on many of these choices. However, it is important to think about the potential consequences of each of these options including patient risk, healthcare cost, and prolapse outcomes. As techniques and technology evolve, including transvaginal mesh attachment and vaginal NOTES sacrocolpopexy, it is important that surgeons reflect on their own results to ensure the best care for future patients.

References

1. Moroni RM, Juliato CRT, Cosson M, Giraudet G, Brito LGO. Does sacrocolpopexy present heterogeneity in its surgical technique? A systematic review. Neurourol 2018; 37(8): 2335–45.
2. O'Sullivan OE, Matthews CA, O'Reilly BA. Sacrocolpopexy: is there a consistent surgical technique? Int Urogynecol J 2016; 27(5): 747–50.
3. Cosson M, Rajabally R, Bogaert E, Querleu D, Crepin G. Laparoscopic sacrocolpopexy, hysterectomy, and Burch colposuspension: feasibility and short-term complications of 77 procedures. J Soc Laparoendosc Surg 2002; 6(2): 115–19.
4. Antiphon P, Elard S, Benyoussef A, et al. Laparoscopic promontory sacral colpopexy: is the posterior, recto-vaginal mesh mandatory? Eur Urol 2004; 45(5): 655–61.
5. Gadonneix P, Ercoli A, Salet-Lizee D, et al. Laparoscopic sacrocolpopexy with two separate meshes along the anterior and posterior vaginal walls for multicompartment pelvic organ prolapse. J Am Assoc Gynecol Laparosc 2004; 11(1): 29–35.
6. Higgs PJ, Chua HL, Smith AR. Long-term review of laparoscopic sacrocolpopexy. BJOG 2005; 112(8): 1134–8.
7. Paraiso MFR, Walters MD, Rackley RR, Melek S, Hugney C. Laparoscopic and abdominal sacral colpopexies: a comparative cohort study. J Urol 2006; 175(4): 1438.
8. Rozet F, Mandron E, Arroyo C, et al. Laparoscopic sacral colpopexy approach for genito-urinary prolapse: experience with 363 cases. Eur Urol 2005; 47(2): 230–6.
9. Campbell P, Cloney L, Jha S. Abdominal versus laparoscopic sacrocolpopexy: a systematic review and meta-analysis. Obstet Gynecol Surv 2016; 71(7): 435–42.
10. Paraiso MF, Jelovsek JE, Frick A, Chen CC, Barber MD. Laparoscopic compared with robotic sacrocolpopexy for vaginal prolapse: a randomized controlled trial. Obstet Gynecol 2011; 118(5): 1005–13.
11. Anger JT, Mueller ER, Tarnay C, et al. Robotic compared with laparoscopic sacrocolpopexy a randomized controlled trial. Obstet Gynecol 2014; 123(1): 5–12.
12. De Gouveia De Sa M, Claydon LS, Whitlow B, Dolcet Artahona MA. Robotic versus laparoscopic sacrocolpopexy for treatment of prolapse of the apical segment of the vagina: a systematic review and meta-analysis. Int Urogynecol J 2016; 27(3): 355–66.
13. Callewaert G, Bosteels J, Housmans S, et al. Laparoscopic versus robotic-assisted sacrocolpopexy for pelvic organ prolapse: a systematic review. Gynecol Surg 2016; 13: 115–23.
14. Akl MN, Long JB, Giles DL, et al. Robotic-assisted sacrocolpopexy: technique and learning curve. Surg Endosc 2009; 23(10): 2390–4.
15. Akladios CY, Dautun D, Saussine C, et al. Laparoscopic sacrocolpopexy for female genital organ prolapse: establishment of a learning curve. Eur J Obstet Gynecol Reprod Biol 2010; 149(2): 218–21.
16. Judd JP, Siddiqui NY, Barnett JC, et al. Cost-minimization analysis of robotic-assisted, laparoscopic, and abdominal sacrocolpopexy. J Minim Invasive Gynecol 2010; 17(4): 493–9.
17. Lee RK, Mottrie A, Payne CK, Waltregny D. A review of the current status of laparoscopic and robot-assisted sacrocolpopexy for pelvic organ prolapse. Eur Urol 2014; 65(6): 1128–37.
18. Catanzarite T, Tan-Kim J, Whitcomb EL, Menefee S. Ergonomics in surgery: a review. Female Pelvic Med Reconstr Surg 2018; 24(1): 1–12.
19. Cardenas-Trowers O, Stewart JR, Meriwether KV, Francis SL, Gupta A. Perioperative outcomes of minimally invasive sacrocolpopexy based on route of concurrent hysterectomy: a secondary analysis of the National Surgical Quality Improvement Program Database. J Minim Invasive Gynecol 2019; 27(4): 953–8. https://doi.org/10.1016/j.jmig.2019.08.010
20. Davidson ERW, Thomas TN, Lampert EJ, Paraiso MFR, Ferrando CA. Route of hysterectomy during minimally invasive sacrocolpopexy does not affect postoperative outcomes. Int Urogynecol J 2019; 30(4): 649–55.
21. Gluck O, Blaganje M, Veit-Rubin N, et al. Laparoscopic sacrocolpopexy: a comprehensive literature review on current practice. Eur J Obstet Gynecol Reprod Biol 2020; 245: 94–101.
22. Davenport A, Stark S, Quian A, Sheyn D, Mangel J. A patient-centered approach to refractory overactive bladder and barriers to third-line therapy. Obstet Gynecol 2019; 134(1): 141–8.
23. Deng T, Liao B, Luo D, Shen H, Wang K. Risk factors for mesh erosion after female pelvic floor reconstructive surgery: a systematic review and meta-analysis. BJU Int 2016; 117(2): 323–43.
24. Warner WB, Vora S, Hurtado EA, et al. Effect of operative technique on mesh exposure in laparoscopic sacrocolpopexy. Female Pelvic Med Reconstr Surg 2012; 18(2): 113–17.
25. Osmundsen BC, Clark A, Goldsmith C, et al. Mesh erosion in robotic sacrocolpopexy. Female Pelvic Med Reconstr Surg 2012; 18(2): 86–8.

26. Nosti PA, Carter CM, Sokol AI, et al. Transvaginal versus transabdominal placement of synthetic mesh at time of sacrocolpopexy. Female Pelvic Med Reconstr Surg 2016; 22(3): 151–5.
27. Unger CA, Paraiso MFR, Jelovsek JE, Barber MD, Ridgeway B. Perioperative adverse events after minimally invasive abdominal sacrocolpopexy. Am J Obstet Gynecol 2014; 211(5): 547.e1–8.
28. Wu JM, Wells EC, Hundley AF, et al. Mesh erosion in abdominal sacral colpopexy with and without concomitant hysterectomy. Am J Obstet Gynecol 2006; 194(5): 1418–22.
29. Nosti PA, Lowman JK, Zollinger TW, Hale DS, Woodman PJ. Risk of mesh erosion after abdominal sacral colpoperineopexy with concomitant hysterectomy. Am J Obstet Gynecol 2009; 201(5): 541.e1–4. https://doi.org/10.1016/j.ajog.2009.07.053
30. Marinkovic SP. Will hysterectomy at the time of sacrocolpopexy increase the rate of polypropylene mesh erosion? Int Urogynecol J 2008; 19(2): 199–203.
31. Ehsani N, Ghafar MA, Antosh DD, et al. Risk factors for mesh extrusion after prolapse surgery: a case-control study. Female Pelvic Med Reconstr Surg 2012; 18(6): 357–61.
32. Griffis K, Evers MD, Terry CL, Hale DS. Mesh erosion and abdominal sacrocolpopexy: a comparison of prior, total, and supracervical hysterectomy. J Pelvic Med Surg 2006; 12(1): 25–30.
33. Tan-Kim J, Menefee SA, Luber KM, Nager CW, Lukacz ES. Prevalence and risk factors for mesh erosion after laparoscopic-assisted sacrocolpopexy. Int Urogynecol J. 2011; 22(2): 205–12.
34. Morciano A, Marzo G, Caliandro D, et al. Laparoscopic sacral colpopexy and a new approach to mesh fixation: a randomized clinical trial. Arch Gynecol Obstet 2018; 298(5): 939–44.
35. Tan-Kim J, Nager CW, Grimes CL, et al. A randomized trial of vaginal mesh attachment techniques for minimally invasive sacrocolpopexy. Int Urogynecol J 2015; 26(5): 649–56.
36. Lamblin G, Dubernard G, de Saint Hilaire P, et al. Assessment of synthetic glue for mesh attachment in laparoscopic sacrocolpopexy: a prospective multicenter pilot study. J Minim Invasive Gynecol 2017; 24(1): 41–7.
37. Panel P, Soffray F, Roussillon E, et al. Glue mesh fixation: feasibility, tolerance and complication assessment. Results 24 months after laparoscopic sacrocolpopexy. J Gynecol Obstet Hum Reprod 2017; 46(4): 333–8.
38. Athanasiou S, Grigoriadis T, Chatzipapas I, Protopapas A, Antsaklis A. The vaginally assisted laparoscopic sacrocolpopexy: a pilot study. Int Urogynecol J 2013; 24(5): 839–45.
39. Park AJ, Ridgeway B, Gustilo-Ashby AM, et al. Efficacy of a standardized technique of trans-vaginal entry into the peritoneal cavity for post-hysterectomy vaginal vault suspension. Int Urogynecol J Pelvic Floor Dysfunct 2008; 19(10): 1393–8.
40. Nosti PA, Carter CM, Sokol AI, et al. Transvaginal versus transabdominal placement of synthetic mesh at time of sacrocolpopexy. Female Pelvic Med Reconstr Surg 2016; 22(3): 151–5.
41. Chen Y, Li J, Hua K. Transvaginal single-port laparoscopy pelvic reconstruction with Y-shaped mesh. J Minim Invasive Gynecol 2018; 25(7): 1138–41.
42. Gadonneix P, Ercoli A, Salet-Lizée D, et al. Laparoscopic sacrocolpopexy with two separate meshes along the anterior and posterior vaginal walls for multicompartment pelvic organ prolapse. J Am Assoc Gynecol Laparosc 2004; 11(1): 29–35.
43. Tan-Kim J, Menefee SA, Lippmann Q, et al. A pilot study comparing anatomic failure after sacrocolpopexy with absorbable or permanent sutures for vaginal mesh attachment. Perm 2014; 18(4): 40–4.
44. Bernhardt J, Sasse S, Ludwig K, Meier PN. Update in Natural Orifice Translumenal Endoscopic Surgery (NOTES). Curr Opin Gastroenterol 2017; 33(5): 346–51.
45. Baekelandt J. Total vaginal NOTES hysterectomy: a new approach to hysterectomy. J Minim Invasive Gynecol 2015; 22(6): 1088–94.
46. Baekelandt J, Vercammen J. IMELDA transvaginal approach to ectopic pregnancy: diagnosis by transvaginal hydrolaparoscopy and treatment by transvaginal natural orifice transluminal endoscopic surgery. Fertil Steril 2017; 107(1): e1–e2.
47. Li CB, Hua KQ. Transvaginal natural orifice transluminal endoscopic surgery (vNOTES) in gynecologic surgeries: a systematic review. Asian J 2020; 43(1): 44–51.
48. Oh SH, Park SJ, Lee EJ, Yim GW, Kim HS. Pelvic lymphadenectomy by vaginal natural orifice transluminal endoscopic surgery (vNOTES) for early-stage endometrial cancer. Gynecol Oncol 2019; 153(1): 211–12.
49. Lowenstein L, Baekelandt J, Paz Y, Lauterbach R, Matanes E. Transvaginal natural orifice transluminal endoscopic hysterectomy and apical suspension of the vaginal cuff to the uterosacral ligament. J Minim Invasive Gynecol 2019; 26(6): 1015.
50. Lauterbach R, Matanes E, Amit A, Wiener Z, Lowenstein L. Transvaginal Natural Orifice Transluminal Endoscopic (vNOTES) hysterectomy learning curve: feasibility in the hands of skilled gynecologists. Isr Med Assoc J 2020; 22(1): 13–16.
51. Noblett KL, Murphy M, Guerette N. Natural orifice vaginal sacrocolpopexy (NOVaS): a cadaver feasibility study. Int Urogynecol J 2012; 23(4): 447–52.
52. Chen Y, Li J, Zhang Y, Hua K. Transvaginal single-port laparoscopy sacrocolpopexy. J Minim Invasive Gynecol 2018; 25(4): 585–8.
53. Liu J, Kohn J, Fu H, Guan Z, Guan X. Transvaginal natural orifice transluminal endoscopic surgery for sacrocolpopexy: a pilot study of 26 cases. J Minim Invasive Gynecol 2019; 26(4): 748–53.
54. Jallad K, Walters MD. Natural Orifice Transluminal Endoscopic Surgery (NOTES) in gynecology. Clin Obstet Gynecol 2017; 60(2): 324–9.
55. Good MM, Abele TA, Balgobin S, et al. Preventing L5-S1 discitis associated with sacrocolpopexy. Obstet Gynecol 2013; 121(2 Pt 1): 285–90.
56. Hanes CR, 2nd. Vaginal sacral colpopexy: a natural orifice approach to a gold standard procedure. J Minim Invasive Gynecol 2018; 25(1): 47–52.
57. Hanes CR. Natural orifice sacral colpopexy: a new approach to a time-honored procedure. J Minim Invasive Gynecol 2015; 22(6S): S246–S247.
58. Miller ME, Siegler M, Angelos P. Ethical issues in surgical innovation. World J Surg 2014; 38(7): 1638–43.

Chapter 20

Total Laparoscopic Hysterectomy: Procedure Steps and Evidence

Lisa C Hickman, Katie Propst

Introduction

The first laparoscopic hysterectomy was described by Dr Harry Reich in 1989 [1]. Since that time, the number of laparoscopic hysterectomies performed annually has increased significantly, surpassing the rate of vaginal hysterectomy in 2012 [2]. As of 2010, approximately 40% of hysterectomies were laparoscopic and 46% of these were performed as outpatient surgery [3,4]. Compared to abdominal hysterectomy, laparoscopic hysterectomy has the benefit of faster return to baseline activity, shorter length of hospitalization, and fewer wound infections, with longer operating time and higher rates of lower urinary tract injuries [5]. Compared to vaginal hysterectomy, there was no difference in complications, risk of lower urinary tract injury, blood loss, and length of hospital stay [5]. Rates of cuff dehiscence, conversion to laparotomy, and operating times were increased in the laparoscopic group [6].

There are three primary types of laparoscopic hysterectomy: total laparoscopic hysterectomy, laparoscopic-assisted vaginal hysterectomy, and laparoscopic subtotal hysterectomy (see Chapter 14 for further discussion). A laparoscopic-assisted vaginal hysterectomy differs from a total hysterectomy in that the procedure is performed using both laparoscopic and vaginal access. Laparoscopic portions of the procedure often include ligation and transection of the utero-ovarian ligament, broad ligament, infundibulopelvic ligament when indicated, and possibly the uterine arteries, with the remaining components of the procedure performed vaginally. Staging of laparoscopic hysterectomies has been described, with the term total laparoscopic hysterectomy being reserved when the entire procedure is performed laparoscopically [7].

Indications and Contraindications

Minimally invasive hysterectomy, including laparoscopic, vaginal, and robotic-assisted, should be performed whenever feasible as opposed to open techniques. When a vaginal approach is not feasible, due to factors such as poor uterine decensus or limited vaginal access, a need to evaluate the pelvis for extrauterine disease, suspected extensive adhesive disease, adnexal masses, need for concurrent laparoscopic procedures, or large uterine size, a laparoscopic approach should be considered [8]. Contraindications to laparoscopic hysterectomy according to the American Association of Gynecologic Laparoscopists (AAGL) include individuals with significant cardiopulmonary disease who cannot tolerate the steep Trendelenburg positioning and increased intra-abdominal pressures, or suspicious or known gynaecologic malignancy requiring removal of specimen intact [9]. Additionally, the technical skill required to complete the surgery laparoscopically, which is associated with steep learning curves for the necessary advanced techniques, may preclude the performance of this procedure. Consideration of surgeon training, experience, and volume, as well as hospital factors such as available equipment and support, is important. Lastly, the risks and benefits of the different surgical modalities should be discussed with the patient. The patient's preferences and values should be incorporated as part of shared decision-making for selecting the hysterectomy mode.

For urogynaecologists, the approach to hysterectomy (vaginal versus laparoscopic) is often dictated by the planned approach to pelvic organ prolapse repair. In patients planning native tissue prolapse repair, vaginal approach to hysterectomy is indicated. However, in patients who are undergoing a mesh-augmented abdominal repair, laparoscopic hysterectomy may be indicated. Selection of total laparoscopic hysterectomy versus subtotal laparoscopic hysterectomy depends on patient anatomy, history of cervical disease, abnormal uterine bleeding, and postmenopausal bleeding, risk of vaginal mesh exposure, and surgeon preference. When discussing total versus subtotal hysterectomy, it is important to note that indications for cervical preservation, such as improved bowel, bladder, or sexual function postoperatively, compared to total hysterectomy, have not been validated [10]. Clinical differences between the two techniques, such as modest decreases in blood loss and operating time, do not likely confer significant clinical benefits, however reproductive-aged patients should be counselled about the possibility of postoperative cyclical bleeding when the cervix is preserved [10]. Factors that help to drive selection of a total laparoscopic hysterectomy include patients with increased risk for cervical or uterine pathology (i.e. history of abnormal pap smears or other cervical disease, current abnormal uterine bleeding, current or a history of postmenopausal bleeding), cervical elongation, and increased vaginal length that precludes optimal support without shortening the vagina. Subtotal hysterectomy may be indicated in patients with increased risk of vaginal mesh exposure as a method to decrease this risk or with decreased vaginal length to prevent further shortening of the vagina [11].

Steps of a Laparoscopic Hysterectomy

Preparing and Positioning the Patient

The patient is first placed on an anti-slip pad, which is secured to the operating table, to prevent shifting during the utilization of Trendelenburg positioning during the surgery. Sequential compression stockings should be applied to the lower extremities and activated prior to anaesthesia induction. Once general anaesthesia and intubation have been achieved, the patient should be repositioned in dorsal lithotomy utilizing Allen or Yellow Fin stirrups (Allen Medical Systems, Acton MA). The patient's buttocks should be positioned at the inferior edge of the operating table to permit sufficient vaginal manipulation and access for any planned concurrent vaginal procedures. Care should be taken to ensure the coccyx is padded. The legs should be placed in an anatomic position, ensuring no hyperflexion or hyperextension of the hips or knees. The arms should be tucked in a neutral position at her sides and padding of the extremities should be utilized to prevent both neuropathy and iatrogenic injury with bed position changes. The patient's chest should be strapped to the operating table to prevent intraoperative slippage. An examination under anaesthesia is then performed to confirm preoperative exam findings regarding uterine size, position, and mobility and to assess the adnexa. Hair can be removed with clippers, if necessary. The patient is then prepared, both abdominally and vaginally, and draped.

A foley catheter and uterine manipulator are placed, while the laparoscopic set-up is performed concurrently. If the patient's surgical history is concerning for potential vesicouterine adhesive disease, a three-way foley catheter can be placed to permit bladder backfilling, which can help identify anatomy and facilitate dissection. Regarding uterine manipulators, there are a variety of available manipulators including disposable and reusable options. Features include a cervical cup to assist with the colpotomy, a vaginal balloon to help maintain pneumoperitoneum after colpotomy, and a bedside attachment. Proper placement of the manipulator and cervical cup are vital for facilitating effective uterine manipulation and delineation of the cervicovaginal junction at the time of colpotomy. Alternatively, the uterus can be manipulated by placing instruments through the laparoscopic ports such as a laparoscopic tenaculum or a myoma screw. Ultimately, surgeon preference will dictate the approach to uterine manipulation.

Prior to initiating the laparoscopic entry, one should ensure that a naso- or orogastric tube has been placed by the anaesthesia team with successful decompression of gastric contents. This becomes even more important if a left upper quadrant entry is planned.

Surgical Technique

Obtaining Laparoscopic Entry

With the patient supine, the initial laparoscopic port is placed. Selection of entry method, including optical entry, Veress needle, or open Hassan technique, is at the discretion of the surgeon, with no significant differences in vascular or visceral injury amongst the techniques. Typically, the first port is placed at the umbilicus, where the abdominal wall is thinnest, however this location may need to be modified depending on uterine or pelvic mass size, surgical history, or umbilical hernia. In such cases, performing a supraumbilical port placement or left upper quadrant entry at Palmer's point are good alternatives (see Chapter 5 for further discussion of considerations and technique). After the initial port is properly placed, the abdomen is insufflated with carbon dioxide gas to a pressure of approximately 15 mm Hg. The abdominal contents deep to the initial port placement should be surveyed for injury, followed by a general survey of the anatomy including the upper quadrant organs and appendix. The patient is then placed in Trendelenburg positioning, and the accessory ports are placed under direct visualization. These ports are typically placed in the bilateral lower quadrants 2 cm medial and 2 cm cephalad to the anterior superior iliac spine. This location helps to avoid injury to the ilioinguinal and iliohypogastric nerves. Additionally, the course of the superficial epigastric vessels should be visualized via abdominal wall trans-illumination and the inferior epigastric vessels should be visualized intra-abdominally coursing along the anterior abdominal wall lateral to the medial umbilical ligaments. These structures should be avoided during port placement to prevent injury. A fourth port may be placed lateral to the umbilicus or in the suprapubic region to help with dissection or laparoscopic suturing. The insufflation tubing can be replaced on an upper quadrant port, and a smoke evacuator can be utilized on a lower quadrant port to help maintain visualization or alternatively the plume can be intermittently evacuated.

Surveying the Pelvis

With the patient in Trendelenburg positioning, the pelvic anatomy should be surveyed. If adhesive disease is present, careful lysis should be performed to allow visualization of the surgical field and important anatomic structures. The ureters should be identified bilaterally and their course followed along the pelvic sidewall. The ureters can usually be identified transperitoneally on the pelvic side wall or crossing the pelvic brim over the common iliac artery on the right. If the ureter cannot be visualized, a retroperitoneal dissection can be performed by incising the peritoneum parallel to infundibulopelvic ligament at the pelvic brim. Sharp and blunt dissection can then be used to bring the ureter into view. This dissection can be carried inferiorly as needed. The ureter must be located at the time of ligation and transection of the infundibulopelvic ligament and the uterine arteries.

Managing the Adnexal Structures

Timing of salpingectomy is at the discretion of the surgeon. The fallopian tube is grasped at the fimbriated end and deflected cephalad and medially. Using an electrosurgical or ultrasonic device, the mesosalpinx is transected immediately inferior to the fallopian tube, moving lateral to medial to the level of the cornu. The fallopian tube can either remain attached to the uterus and removed as one specimen or transected just lateral the cornu and removed from the laparoscopic port.

If a salpingo-oophorectomy is planned, the ovary is grasped and deflected medially away from the pelvic side wall. The infundibulopelvic ligament is then ligated and transected using electrosurgery. Ligation should be performed close to the ovary to avoid injury to the pelvic sidewall structures, and the ureter should be visualized at the time of transection. Similar to the fallopian tubes, the ovaries can remain attached to the uterus via the utero-ovarian ligament, or the utero-ovarian ligament can be ligated and transected, freeing the ovary for immediate removal from the abdomen.

Transecting the Round Ligament

The round ligament can be identified by following its course anterolaterally to the inguinal canal. The uterus should be manipulated to the contralateral side to both assist with exposure and place traction on the ligament. Using an electrosurgical or ultrasonic device, the round ligament is ligated and cut in an area free of broad ligament vessels (Figure 20.1).

Developing the Bladder Flap

Transection of the round ligament generally permits access to the anterior leaf of the broad ligament, which is incised in an inferiomedial fashion to create the bladder flap using the cervical cup as a landmark to direct the dissection. Bluntly undermining the peritoneum can permit carbon dioxide gas to enter the areolar, avascular space and help facilitate the dissection. The bladder flap is further developed inferiorly, while upward traction on cervix is placed with the uterus in either the mid-position or retroversion (Figure 20.2). The dissection should mobilize the bladder at least 1 cm inferior to the edge of a cervical cup, if utilized, to ensure adequate cuff closure can be performed in an area free of bladder. When mobilizing the bladder, the presence of perivesicular fat indicates proximity to the bladder and the area should be avoided. If bladder adhesions are encountered, backfilling the bladder and/or performing bladder mobilization from a lateral approach may help guide the surgeon to the correct plane. Use of electrosurgery should be avoided to prevent thermal bladder damage.

Ligating the Cornua

If the ovary is to be left in situ, division of the utero-ovarian ligament is performed (Figure 20.3). The uterus should be deflected towards the contralateral side to help with exposure and traction. The selected location for ligation and transection should be slightly lateral to the cornu in order to avoid bleeding. If the adnexal structures are to be removed attached to the uterus, this step is omitted.

Skeletonizing and Transecting the Uterine Vessels

The posterior leaf of the broad ligament should be dissected in a similar fashion to that described for the anterior leaf. With cephalad traction on the uterus, any remaining tissue overlying the uterine vessels is serially lysed with the uterus deviated towards the contralateral side (Figure 20.4). We prefer to

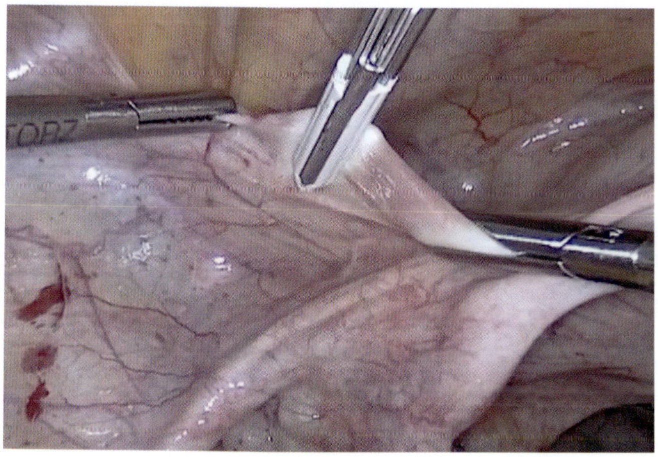

Figure 20.1 Transection of the round ligament using bipolar energy. Photo courtesy of Dr Cara King.

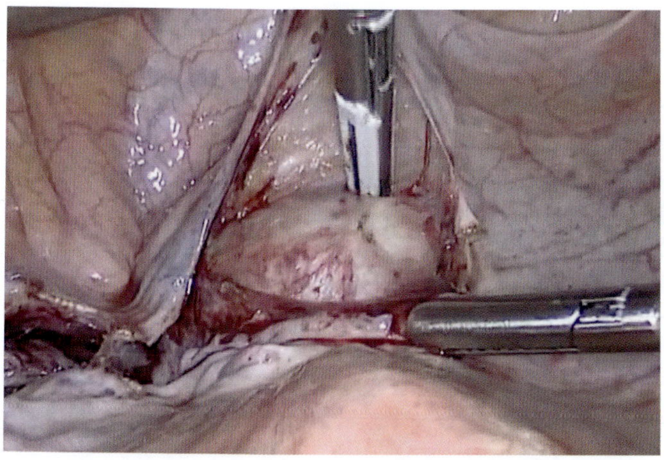

Figure 20.2 Bladder flap development with uterus in midposition. Blunt dissection is being utilized to mobilize the bladder caudad from the cervical cup. Photo courtesy of Dr Cara King.

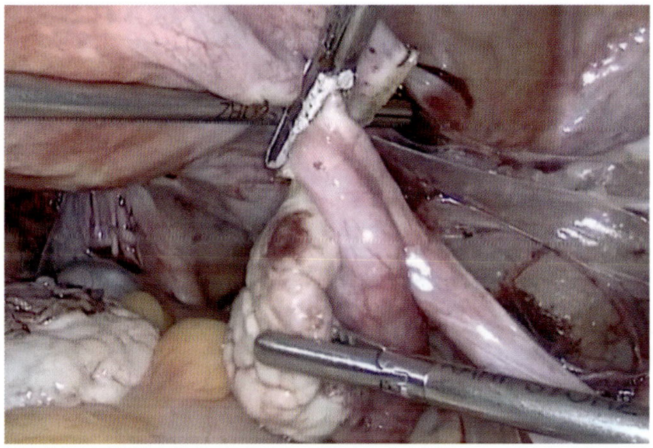

Figure 20.3 Transection of the utero-ovarian ligament and fallopian tube at the cornua using bipolar energy. This can be performed as a part of adnexal sparing surgery or for later removal. Photo courtesy of Dr Cara King.

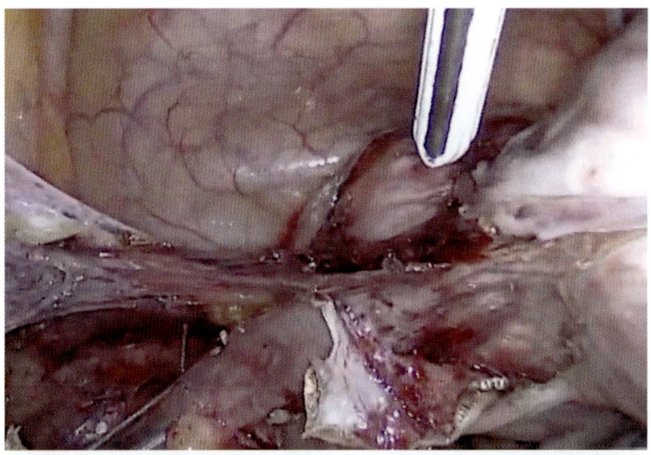

Figure 20.4 Uterine arteries are skeletonized using a combination of bipolar energy and both blunt and sharp dissection. The anterior and posterior peritoneum has been dissected and areolar tissue is freed so that the uterine vessels can be safely transected. Photo courtesy of Dr Cara King.

skeletonize the uterine arteries bilaterally and ensure adequate bladder mobilization away from the uterine arteries prior to ligation and transection. After the ureters are visualized, the uterine vessels can be desiccated at the level of the internal os (Figure 20.5). Desiccation should also be performed above the level of the internal os to limit back bleeding from the uterus. Once electrosurgical ligation is complete, the uterine arteries are transected at the level of the internal cervical os. This pedicle is then lateralized using the same technique so that the colpotomy and subsequent vaginal cuff closure can be performed free of the uterine vasculature.

Performing the Colpotomy

Prior to performing the colpotomy, in addition to ensuring sufficient lateralization of the bilateral uterine artery pedicles, one should also verify that the bladder is mobilized at least 1 cm inferior to the planned colpotomy site. The colpotomy is then performed with monopolar, bipolar, or ultrasonic energy (Figure 20.6a). Cephalad traction on the uterus and cervix should be utilized in order to increase the margin of safety between the dissecting tool and the local anatomy (bladder, bowel, ureter), as well as to preserve the maximum amount of vaginal length. The colpotomy can be started on the anterior or posterior surface, and should be performed in a circumferential fashion, following the cervical cup, if one is being used (Figure 20.6b). Once the uterus and cervix are completely detached, the specimen can be removed through the vagina. If the specimen is enlarged, a contained extraction bag, such as the Applied Medical Alexis Contained Extraction System (Rancho Santa Margarita, CA), can be utilized for vaginal morcellation. Alternatively, extension of a port site or a mini-laparotomy incision can be made for specimen extraction.

Closing the Vaginal Cuff

Approach to vaginal cuff closure is dictated by surgeon preference. Cuff closure can be performed laparoscopically or vaginally using number zero delayed absorbable suture in figure-of-eights or a running fashion, or using a barbed suture in a running fashion (Figure 20.7). If laparoscopic cuff closure is preferred, the suture can be passed through a laparoscopic port incision into the abdomen or through the vagina cuff opening if all ports are 5 mm in size. A pneumo-occluder balloon or surgical glove containing a sponge is placed in the vagina to aid in maintaining pneumopertioneum. Surgical knots can be tied

(a)

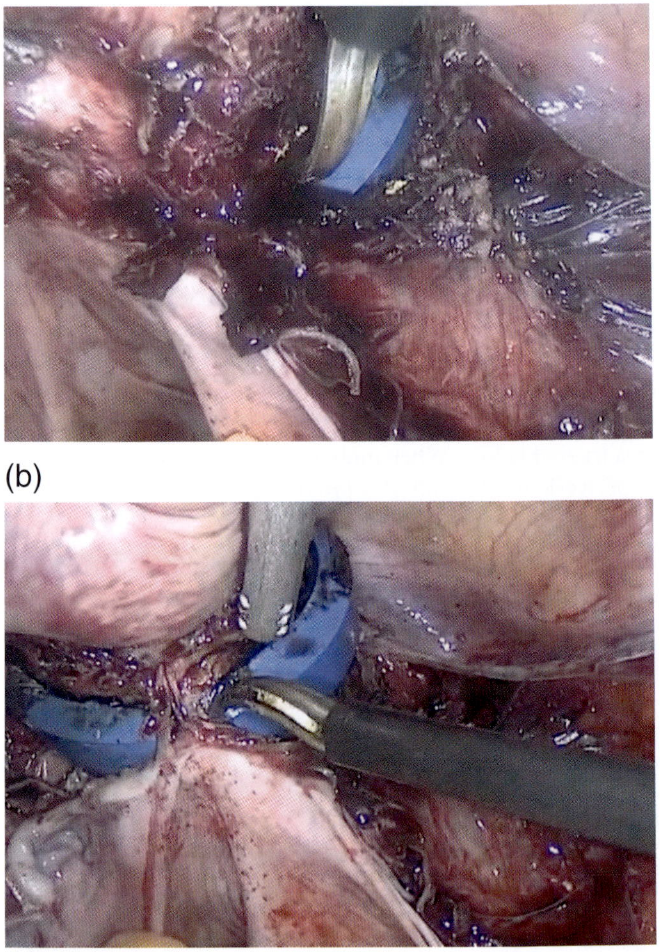

Figure 20.6 (a) Initiation of colpotomy using monopolar energy with uterus on upward traction and deviated to the contralateral side. Blue cervical cup has been identified and can be used as a guide for remainder of colpotomy. (b) Completion of colpotomy after fully circumscribing the cerviovaginal junction along the cervical cup. Photo courtesy of Dr Cara King.

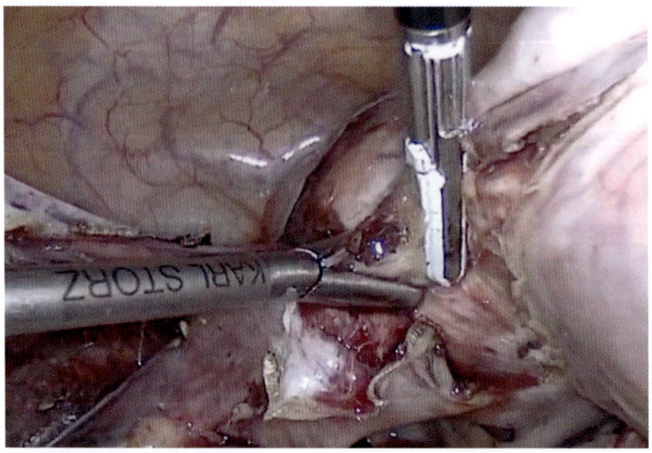

Figure 20.5 The uterine arteries are ligated using bipolar energy prior to transection. Photo courtesy of Dr Cara King.

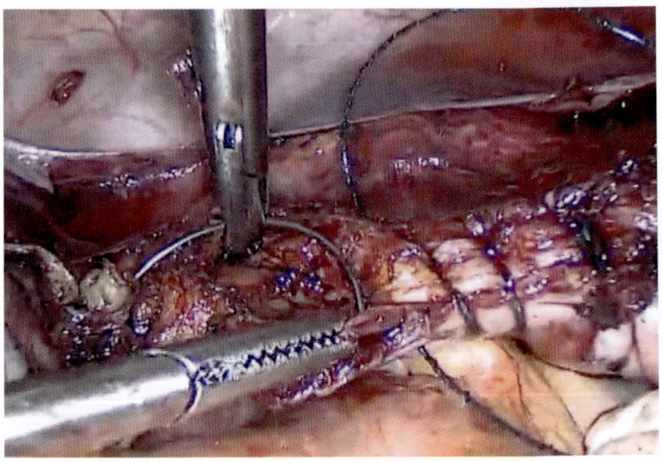

Figure 20.7 Laparoscopic vaginal cuff closure using a barbed suture. Photo courtesy of Dr Cara King.

using intracorporeal technique or extracorporeal technique using a laparoscopic knot pusher. To avoid knot tying, barbed suture or a Lapra-Ty (Ethicon, Inc Cincinnati, Ohio) can be used. After completion of cuff suturing, the needle can either be removed through a 5 mm port incision (after removing the port) or through the 5 mm port after laparoscopically flattening the curve of the needle.

Care must be taken to ensure haemostasis is achieved during cuff closure and that sutures are placed sufficiently from the cuff edge to reduce the risk of cuff dehiscence, especially in light of the thermal spread that occurs when monopolar instruments are utilized to perform the colpotomy.

Supporting the Vaginal Apex

It is well established that performing hysterectomy alone is insufficient for the management of pelvic organ prolapse [12]. Level 1 support (uterosacral and cardinal ligament attachments) is typically compromised during hysterectomy. Procedures to re-establish this support should be considered regardless of whether or not the patient has baseline pelvic organ prolapse in an effort to reduce the risk of future apical support defects [13].

For most urogynaecologists, hysterectomy is performed as a component of the surgical correction of pelvic organ prolapse and often dictates the approach to hysterectomy. In these women, a procedure to restore apical support is indicated and techniques are outlined in other chapters. In women undergoing a total laparoscopic hysterectomy with anterior or posterior prolapse and normal apical support, we recommend consideration of an apical support procedure at the time of hysterectomy. Data on how to manage the apex in this population of women is lacking; however, our preference is to perform uterosacral ligament colpopexy or McCall culdoplasty. For women undergoing a total laparoscopic hysterectomy for indications other that pelvic organ prolapse who have asymptomatic apical prolapse, we typically perform uterosacral ligament or sacrospinous ligament colpopexy. This is important as several studies have demonstrated that women who do not have an apical support procedure at the time of a hysterectomy or prolapse repair are significantly more likely to require a subsequent prolapse repair [14–16]. Similarly, for patients with normal support, but with prolapse risk factors such as family history, increased vaginal parity, other pelvic floor disorders, menopause, and conditions with chronically increased intra-abdominal pressure, we recommend performing an apical support procedure, as this group is known to be at higher risk for future prolapse [16].

In women with normal pelvic support, the best approach to managing the apex is unknown. For patients without a prolapse indication, only 3.1% of women had a concurrent support procedure in a large national database study [17]. While large population-based studies suggest an increased rate of subsequent prolapse in hysterectomized women with non-prolapse surgical indications, factors such as surgical technique utilized, patient characteristics, and duration of follow-up contribute to the heterogeneity in the results and likely the lack of broad clinical utilization of prophylactic apical support procedures [18,19]. In women with normal support, we typically re-attach the uterosacral ligament pedicles to the vaginal cuff. As an alternative, culdoplasty can be performed during this procedure by reefing the peritoneum in the posterior cul-de-sac.

Completing the Procedure

A cystoscopic survey is encouraged to evaluate ureteral patency and ensure that no iatrogenic injuries to the bladder occurred during the procedure; however, the level of available evidence precludes the AAGL from making this a universal recommendation [20]. Haemostasis should be re-evaluated at each of the pedicles prior to concluding the procedure. Insufflation should be decreased and then the pedicles should be re-inspected. All laparoscopic ports greater than 8 mm in size should be closed with a fascial closure device, such as the Carter-Thomason CloseSure System (Inlet Medical, Inc., Eden Prairie, MN) or under direct vision after ports are removed. All instruments are then removed. The abdomen is desufflated and the anaesthesia team is asked to provide three large breaths to evacuate as much of the carbon dioxide gas as possible. Once this is complete, all ports are then removed and a monofilament or braided suture can be used to re-approximate the epithelium at each of the port sites.

Vaginal Assistance for the Laparoscopic Hysterectomy

Laparoscopic-assisted vaginal hysterectomy was first introduced within a year of laparoscopic hysterectomy [21]. While it has similar indications and contraindications to laparoscopic hysterectomy, vaginal assistance may be employed when there is difficulty completing the hysterectomy in its entirety laparoscopically due to anatomic factors or surgeon skill.

Special Laparoscopic Considerations

Abdominal Access

Access to the peritoneal cavity can be gained via open or closed techniques. The open (Hasson) technique involves making an incision in the abdominal wall under direct vision. The fascia is tagged after it is incised, and these tags can be used to aid in fascial closure at the conclusion of the surgery. Once access is gained, the umbilical port is placed, and the abdomen is insufflated. Advantages of the open technique include direct vision of each layer upon entry and that it can be used anywhere on the abdominal wall. The disadvantage is that it takes longer to perform than the closed technique.

Closed technique involves use of the Veress needle to puncture the layers of the abdominal wall to insufflate the abdomen prior to port placement. Once the abdomen is insufflated, laparoscopic ports are placed. The advantage of this technique is rapid access and that it can be used at multiple abdominal sites. The disadvantage is increased risk of major vascular complications.

Patient Body Habitus

When operating on obese patients, the umbilical port should be inserted at a 90-degree angle to the abdominal wall, as compared to a thinner patient for whom the umbilical port should be angled towards the pelvis. The reason for this is two-fold: (1) Vertical port placement reduces tracking of the port in the subcutaneous tissue and (2) there is greater distance between the abdominal wall and the great vessels because the weight of the pannus displaces the umbilicus inferiorly on the abdominal wall. In obese patients, extra-long trocars may also be indicated, whereas in thin patients, the classic ribbed trocars may slip through the fascia, such that a balloon trocar may be helpful.

Complications

Intraoperative and postoperative complications associated with hysterectomy vary based upon a number of factors including surgical approach and technique, patient characteristics, and surgeon experience. The major intraoperative complications include conversion to laparotomy, haemorrhage, and urinary tract, bowel, and nerve injuries. Common postoperative complications include infection, venous thromboembolic events, and vaginal cuff dehiscence [22].

Conversion to Laparotomy

In a large retrospective cohort study of nearly 7,000 patients, conversion to laparotomy during laparoscopic hysterectomy occurred in 3.9% of cases [23]. Risk factors for conversion included presence of adhesive disease, endometriosis of the uterus, fallopian tubes and ovaries, presence of any intraoperative complication (bowel, bladder, ureteral, vascular), unexpected malignancy, and increased operating time (>120 minutes), uterine size (weight >250 g), and estimated blood loss (>100 cc). Higher surgeon volume and robotic assistance were protective in this study.

Haemorrhage

The incidence of haemorrhage during any hysterectomy ranges from 2.0–5.1%, with the greatest blood loss associated with an abdominal approach [22]. Blood loss during laparoscopic hysterectomy is dependent upon a variety of factors including patient-specific (obesity, anticoagulation status) and surgical factors (poor visual exposure, distorted anatomy, enlarged uterus, adhesive disease, surgeon experience). When bleeding does occur, the vascular source should be visualized, such as with the use of a suction device, prior to utilizing either an energy source or a vascular clip. This will ensure that an inadvertent injury to the local anatomy, such as the bowel or ureter, does not occur.

Urinary Tract Injury

Urinary tract injury has been estimated to occur in 1.2–2.6% of laparoscopic hysterectomies [24]. Bladder injury is three-times more common than ureteral injury (0.24% versus 0.08%, respectively). Bladder injuries most often occur during lysis of adhesions and are recognized intraoperatively, whereas most ureteral injuries occur from the use of electrosurgery and are not identified until postoperatively [24]. Intraoperative bladder injuries can be repaired in a two-layer water-tight closure after completion of the hysterectomy. The patient should be managed with continuous bladder drainage for 7–14 days. Use of urinary tract imaging at the time of foley catheter removal, such as with an X-ray cystogram, is at the discretion of the provider, but may not be necessary for the majority of injuries. Management of ureteral injuries is dependent upon the type of injury, location on the ureter, and timing of diagnosis. While no difference in ureteral injury incidence was identified between vaginal and laparoscopic approaches, this may be due to power limitations; in contrast, there was a higher rate of lower urinary tract injuries in laparoscopic compared to abdominal hysterectomy [5].

Bowel Injury

Bowel injuries during hysterectomy were reported to occur with an incidence of 0.34–0.45% in a systematic review by Llarena et al [25]. The majority of injuries (55%) occurred during the initial abdominal access with either a Veress needle or trocar and were managed by laparotomy (80%). Most cases were identified intraoperatively, however 41% were delayed by greater than one day. Not surprisingly, delayed diagnosis was associated with the highest mortality risk (3.2%). The management of bowel injuries depends upon the type of injury, bowel location, and size of the injury. When a bowel injury is suspected or identified, the rest of the bowel typically should be inspected for injury as well. Consultation with a general surgeon or colorectal specialist should be considered when the injury is complex or cannot be repaired primarily.

Nerve Injury

While rare, nerve injuries occur in approximately 0.2–2.0% of hysterectomies [22]. Femoral nerve injury is the most common in pelvic surgery, often associated with self-retaining retractor blades in prolonged abdominal surgeries. Other nerves include iliohypogastric and ilioinguinal nerves, which can be injured with laterally placed laparoscopic ports, and the peroneal nerve, related to poor lower extremity positioning in lithotomy.

Infection

Infection is the most common complication after laparoscopic hysterectomy, with an overall incidence of 9.0% [26]. Infectious aetiologies include vaginal cuff cellulitis, infected haematoma, wound infection, urinary tract infection, and respiratory infection. Numerous factors, including patient- and procedure-related, contribute to the risk of these conditions.

Venous Thromboembolic Event

Venous thromboembolic events (VTE) after hysterectomy occur with an incidence of 2.0–5.1% [22]. Clinical risk factors associated with VTE are well established in the literature [27]. Interestingly, hysterectomy was not found to be an independent risk factor for postoperative VTE after gynaecologic surgery [28]. There is also no difference in VTE incidence amongst the hysterectomy approaches according to the Cochrane meta-analysis [5].

Vaginal Cuff Dehiscence

Vaginal cuff dehiscence after laparoscopic hysterectomy (total and robotic) is associated with an incidence of 1–4.1% [29]. Surgical risk factors include type of incision, cuff closure technique, and surgeon experience. Patient risk factors include factors that impair wound healing and those that increase strain on the vaginal cuff as it heals. Compared to a vaginal cuff closure, laparoscopy is associated with a higher incidence of dehiscence [6]. This typically occurs one to three months after hysterectomy and requires a return to the operating room for surgical management [30].

References

1. Reich H, DeCaprio J, McGlynn F. Laparoscopy hysterectomy. J Gynecol Surg 1989; 5: 213–15.
2. Driessen SRC, Baden NLM, van Zwet EW, Twijnstra ARH, Jansen FW. Trends in the implementation of advanced minimally invasive gynecologic surgical procedures in The Netherlands. J Minim Invasive Gynecol 2015; 22(4): 642–7.
3. Schiavone MB, Herzog TJ, Ananth C V, et al. Feasibility and economic impact of same-day discharge for women who undergo laparoscopic hysterectomy. Am J Obstet Gynecol 2012; 207(5): 382.e1–382.e9.
4. Wright JD, Ananth CV., Lewin SN, et al. Robotically assisted vs laparoscopic hysterectomy among women with benign gynecologic disease. JAMA 2013; 309(7): 689.
5. Aarts JW, Nieboer TE, Johnson N, et al. Surgical approach to hysterectomy for benign gynaecological disease. Cochrane Database Syst Rev 2015; (8): CD003677.
6. Sandberg EM, Twijnstra ARH, Driessen SRC, Jansen FW. Total laparoscopic hysterectomy versus vaginal hysterectomy: a systematic review and meta-analysis. J Minim Invasive Gynecol 2017; 24(2): 206–17.e22.
7. Munro MGPW. A classification system for laparoscopic hysterectomy. Obs Gynecol 1993; 82(4 Pt 1): 624–9.
8. Committee on Gynecologic Practice. Committee Opinion No 701. Obstet Gynecol 2017; 129(6): e155–e159.
9. AAGL Advancing Minimally Invasive Gynecology Worldwide. AAGL position statement: route of hysterectomy to treat benign uterine disease. J Minim Invasive Gynecol 2011; 18(1): 1–3.
10. Lethaby A, Mukhopadhyay A, Naik R. Total versus subtotal hysterectomy for benign gynaecological conditions. Cochrane Database Syst Rev 2012; (4): CD004993.
11. Tan-Kim J, Menefee SA, Luber KM, Nager CW, Lukacz ES. Prevalence and risk factors for mesh erosion after laparoscopic-assisted sacrocolpopexy. Int Urogynecol J 2011; 22(2): 205–12.
12. Committee on Practice Bulletins – Gynecology, American Urogynecologic Society. Practice Bulletin No 185. Obstet Gynecol 2017; 130(5): e234–e250.
13. DeLancey JO. Anatomic aspects of vaginal eversion after hysterectomy. Am J Obstet Gynecol 1992; 166(6 Pt 1): 1717–24; discussion 1724–8.
14. Eilber KS, Alperin M, Khan A, et al. Outcomes of vaginal prolapse surgery among female Medicare beneficiaries: the role of apical support. Obstet Gynecol 2013; 122(5): 981–7.
15. Blandon RE, Bharucha AE, Melton LJ, et al. Incidence of pelvic floor repair after hysterectomy: a population-based cohort study. Am J Obstet Gynecol 2007; 197(6): 664.e1–7.
16. Dällenbach P, Kaelin-Gambirasio I, Dubuisson J-B, Boulvain M. Risk factors for pelvic organ prolapse repair after hysterectomy. Obstet Gynecol 2007; 110(3): 625–32.
17. Ross WT, Meister MR, Shepherd JP, Olsen MA, Lowder JL. Utilization of apical vaginal support procedures at time of inpatient hysterectomy performed for benign conditions: a national estimate. Am J Obstet Gynecol 2017; 217(4): 436.e1–436.e8.
18. Lykke R, Blaakær J, Ottesen B, Gimbel H. Age at hysterectomy as a predictor for subsequent pelvic organ prolapse repair. Int Urogynecol J 2016; 27(5): 751–5.
19. Altman D, Falconer C, Cnattingius S, Granath F. Pelvic organ prolapse surgery following hysterectomy on benign indications. Am J Obstet Gynecol 2008; 198(5): 572.e1–6.
20. AAGL Practice Report. Practice guidelines for intraoperative cystoscopy in laparoscopic hysterectomy. J Minim Invasive Gynecol 2012; 19(4): 407–11.
21. Kovac SR, Cruikshank SH, Retto HF. Laparoscopy-assisted vaginal hysterectomy. J Gynecol Surg 1990; 6(3): 185–93.
22. Clarke-Pearson DL, Geller EJ. Complications of hysterectomy. Obstet Gynecol 2013; 121(3): 654–73.
23. Lim CS, Mowers EL, Mahnert N, et al. Risk factors and outcomes for conversion to laparotomy of laparoscopic hysterectomy in benign gynecology. Obstet Gynecol 2016; 128(6): 1295–305.
24. Wong JMK, Bortoletto P, Tolentino J, Jung MJ, Milad MP. Urinary tract injury in gynecologic laparoscopy for benign indication. Obstet Gynecol 2018; 131(1): 100–8.
25. Llarena NC, Shah AB, Milad MP. Bowel injury in gynecologic laparoscopy. Obstet Gynecol 2015; 125(6): 1407–17.
26. Makinen J, Johansson J, Tomás C, et al. Morbidity of 10 110 hysterectomies by type of approach. Hum Reprod 2001; 16(7): 1473–8.
27. Committee on Practice Bulletins – Gynecology, American College of Obstetricians and Gynecologists. ACOG Practice Bulletin No 84: Prevention of deep vein thrombosis and pulmonary embolism. Obstet Gynecol 2007; 110(2 Part 1): 429–40.
28. Clarke-Pearson DL, DeLong ER, Synan IS, Coleman RE, Creasman WT. Variables associated with postoperative deep venous thrombosis: a prospective study of 411 gynecology patients and creation of a prognostic model. Obstet Gynecol 1987; 69(2): 146–50.
29. Nezhat C, Kennedy Burns M, Wood M, et al. Vaginal cuff dehiscence and evisceration. Obstet Gynecol 2018; 132(4): 972–85.
30. Byrnes JN, Trabuco EC. Evidence basis for hysterectomy. Obstet Gynecol Clin North Am 2016; 43(3): 495–515.

Chapter 21

Vaginal Hysterectomy and Ligamentopexy for Apical Prolapse: Procedure Steps and Evidence

Yara Abdelkhalek, Nikolaus Veit-Rubin, Bruno Deval

Introduction

Pelvic organ prolapse is the downward displacement of the pelvic organs (uterus or vaginal vault, bladder and/or rectum) following a weakness in the pelvic floor support system (levator ani muscles, ligamentous and connective tissue and nerves) [1], and presents as a sensation of vaginal bulge associated with an impairment in urinary, bowel, and/or sexual functions.

It is a condition that affects millions of women worldwide and has an enormous negative impact on their quality of life [2]. According to an analysis of the American database from 2007 to 2011, 13% of women will undergo a surgery for prolapse by the age of 80, and 29% will need another surgery later on for relapse [3]. In this same population, studies expect an increase by 50% in the incidence of pelvic organ prolapse by 2050 along with the increase in life expectancy [4].

Historically, vaginal hysterectomy has been the treatment of pelvic organ prolapse, but the uterus itself is not the cause of this disease, therefore removing it does not correct the defect in the pelvic floor support, which may lead to further recurrences and need for re-interventions thereafter [5,6]. Also, some studies have shown that hysterectomy is associated with a damage to the nerve supply system, causing weakness in the pelvic floor, thus increasing the risk of prolapse recurrence [7].

Therefore, management of pelvic organ prolapse is challenging, with multiple surgical treatments possible and no recommendation on the best approach. Surgical correction of pelvic organ prolapse may be achieved via abdominal or transvaginal procedures.

The transvaginal approach is the most common (80–90%) with high efficacy and low risks [8]. 75% of the British urogynaecology society surgeons consider vaginal hysterectomy the procedure of choice in the case of prolapse [3].

In a dynamic magnetic resonance imaging study, Chen et al identified good apical support as the major element for successful outcomes in prolapse repair [9]. This was confirmed later on by numerous studies [8,10].

Given that the aetiology is defects in native tissue structures (muscles, connective tissue), surgeons started using transvaginal meshes as sustainable treatment for prolapse. In 2011, the US Food and Drug Administration started to raise concerns about the safety of these meshes (erosion, infection, dyspareunia) [11], so alternative options were pursued.

Reconstructive transvaginal surgery with native tissue is an old concept. In 1927, Miller was the first to describe the technique of vaginal vault suspension by plication of the uterosacral ligaments [9].

The support of the vaginal apex derives from the integrity of multiple native tissue structures: the endopelvic fascia and ligaments such as the uterosacral, the cardinal and the rounds ligaments, the retro-vesical and pre-rectal peritoneum [12,13,14].

The uterosacral ligaments are probably the strongest support structure; they consist of large amounts of smooth muscle cells, connective tissue and nerves which provide them with a high stiffness level at low and high deformation compared to the other native tissue structures [12]. Originating from S1-S4 vertebrae, they attach the cervix to the sacrum providing, along with the other structures mentioned above, a good supportive system to the uterus.

In this chapter, we discuss the technique of vaginal hysterectomy with ligamentopexy as a native tissue reconstructive strategy for pelvic organ prolapse.

Epidemiology

Pelvic organ prolapse is a common condition and its incidence is increasing worldwide with the increase in obesity and in women's life expectancy. 40% of women aged 40 years old and above are affected [10] but only 10–20% of them seek medical assistance because early stages of prolapse are usually asymptomatic [11]. Recent studies showed a lifetime risk of surgery for prolapse of 12.6–20% with a risk of re-operation for recurrence of 17–30% [9,15,16,17].

In the US, 300,000 interventions for correction of pelvic organ prolapse are performed annually, with a cost of more than one billion dollars [9], with vaginal hysterectomy being the most common procedure.

Clinical Presentation

Clinically, 40% of women have some degree of pelvic organ prolapse but remain completely asymptomatic [8]. There is no indication for surgical treatment in the case of asymptomatic prolapse. The prolapse usually becomes symptomatic after it reaches the threshold of the hymen [11,13]. The symptoms may vary from mild discomfort to pelvic pressure and sensation of a vaginal bulge [8]. Urinary retention and difficulty to defaecate might also be seen [8].

If the prolapse is protruding beyond the hymen, chronic discharge, ulcerations, and bleeding may be associated [8]. Extreme cases of hydronephrosis and ultimately a renal failure were also described [1].

All these symptoms interfere with women's daily activities and account for major psychological and sexual discomfort, then treatment is mandatory to improve their quality of life.

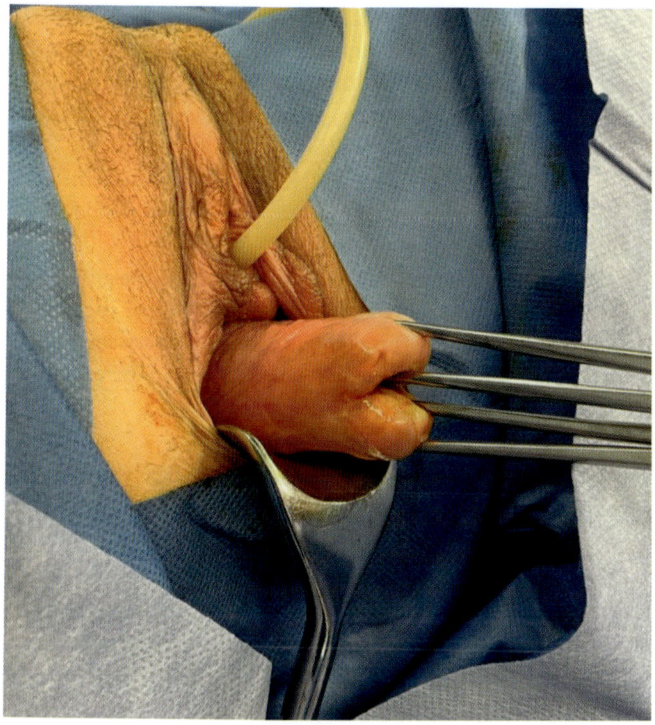

Figure 21.1 Genital prolapse (C+6).

Risk Factors

Many risk factors have been associated with pelvic organ prolapse; they include aging, obesity, parity and childbirth, chronic constipation, connective tissue disorders, family history of prolapse, denervation, and weakness of the pelvic floor [9,11].

Furthermore, the sensibility of the pelvic organs and their connective tissue support to oestrogen means that symptoms of the prolapse usually start after the menopause [9,11].

Candidates for Vaginal Native Tissue Reconstructive Surgery

Pelvic organ prolapse is a common condition that may remain asymptomatic for years. The symptoms usually appear after the prolapse protrudes through the hymen [13].

As we mentioned above, there is no indication for surgical correction of an asymptomatic prolapse.

For bothersome pelvic organ prolapse, conservative or surgical correction must be offered to restore the woman's normal pelvic anatomy, treat urinary, bowel, and sexual dysfunctions, and improve quality of life [5].

The weakness of the level 1 support system, which includes the uterosacral and cardinal ligaments, can cause a uterine prolapse. The general indications for apical prolapse surgical correction are the same as for other compartmental prolapse: any grade 2 or more symptomatic apical prolapse with which conservative treatment no longer works.

There are no guidelines for the surgical management of apical prolapse. Abdominal and transvaginal surgeries are available; native strong connective tissue support (uterosacral and sacrospinous ligament) for suspension of the vaginal vault or use of prosthetic meshes are possible.

The transvaginal approach is reasonable when concomitant vaginal procedure is needed, especially in women who have contraindication for general anaesthesia [11].

All the surgical options must be discussed with the patient along with its risks and outcomes so that the decision can be clearly made.

Vaginal hysterectomy with uterosacral ligament suspension is the most common procedure for correction of apical prolapse [11]. We are going to describe below our surgical technique and its outcomes.

Surgical Technique

- Under general or regional anaesthesia, the patient is placed in dorsal lithotomy position. Proper antibiotics are given according to each hospital guidelines.
- A bladder catheter is inserted.
- Anterior and posterior vaginal retractors are used to expose the cervix.
- Grasp the anterior and posterior lips of the cervix with two Pozzi forceps.
- Draw a circumferential incision of the vaginal mucosa around the cervix.
- Pull the cervix upward, dissect and open the posterior pouch of Douglas. Use scissors instead of electrocautery to avoid any rectal injury.
- Apply a downward traction on the cervix and gently dissect the vesicouterine space to open the anterior cul-de-sac.
- Move the retractors into both spaces created to protect the bladder and the rectum. A vaginal gauze can be used to push back and protect the intestines.
- Clamp the utero-sacral ligament, cut and ligature your first suture. Only delayed absorbable sutures are used along the procedure. We do not recommend the use of non-absorbable sutures because of possible discomfort later on during intercourse [18].
- A second suture is placed on the utero-sacral ligament, this one will allow traction and afterward the suspension of the vaginal vault, so the needle is left in place and the suture is held with a Kocher clamp. Passing the sutures through the vaginal mucosa can aid in the vaginal vault suspension technique later on.
- The cardinal ligament is clamped, cut, and sutured. Avoid any traction on this ligament to prevent any haematoma formation.
- Perform the same steps on the other side.
- Both uterine artery pedicles are then identified, clamped, cut, and sutured. Place your clamps as close as possible to the uterus to avoid any ureteral injury.
- Both utero-ovarian ligaments are clamped, cut, and sutured. The uterus can now be removed.
- Proceed with round ligament identification and suturing on both sides. These ligaments will aid in vaginal vault suspension so keep the needles in place and hold your sutures with straight clamps for traction.
- Before starting the ligamentopexy, you should ensure at this stage a good haemostasis along all the vascular pedicles.

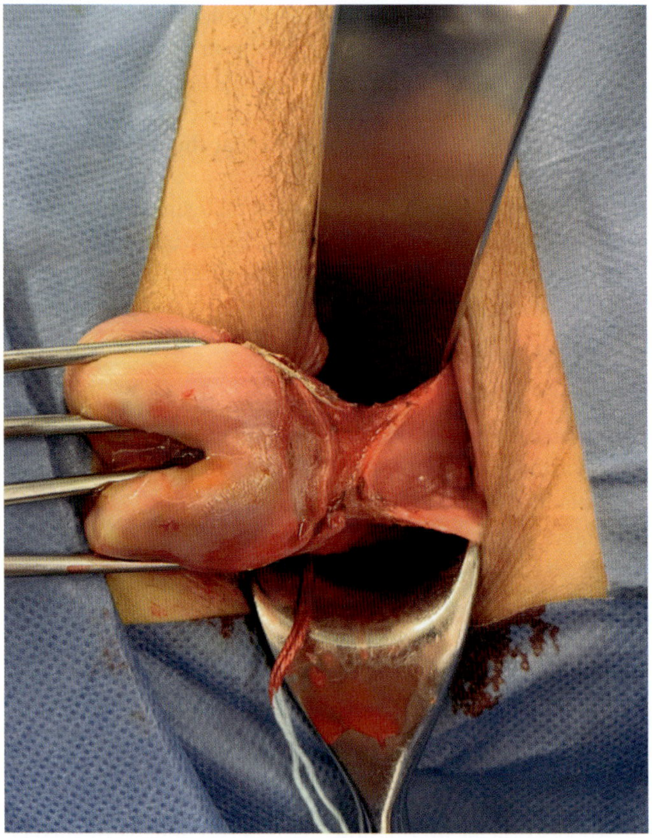

Figure 21.2 Identification of the left utero-sacral ligament.

- Close the posterior vaginal cuff with the posterior peritoneum using a continuous delayed absorbable suture. This allows a reinforcement of the recto-vaginal septum.
- Each suture previously passed through every round ligament is brought out through the contralateral one. Next the sutures are passed in the midline through the anterior then the posterior vaginal wall to fold inside the ligaments.
- Then the uterosacral ligaments are sutured to the anterior and posterior vaginal walls to elevate the vaginal apex toward the sacrum. This allows a continuity between the anterior and posterior vaginal muscularis and the vaginal vault, the key to a successful sustainable repair.
- Mean operative time is 90 minutes [12].
- Vaginal examination is recommended to assess the degree of prolapse repair.
- A vaginal pack is left in place.
- Prophylaxis against thrombosis in needed and non-opioid analgesics usually provide adequate pain relief.
- Vaginal packing and bladder catheter can be removed on day one after the surgery if no bladdery injury occurred, and total hospital stay is around three days. In the case of bladder injury, keep catheterization for five days.
- We recommend abstinence from heavy physical activities for at least six weeks.

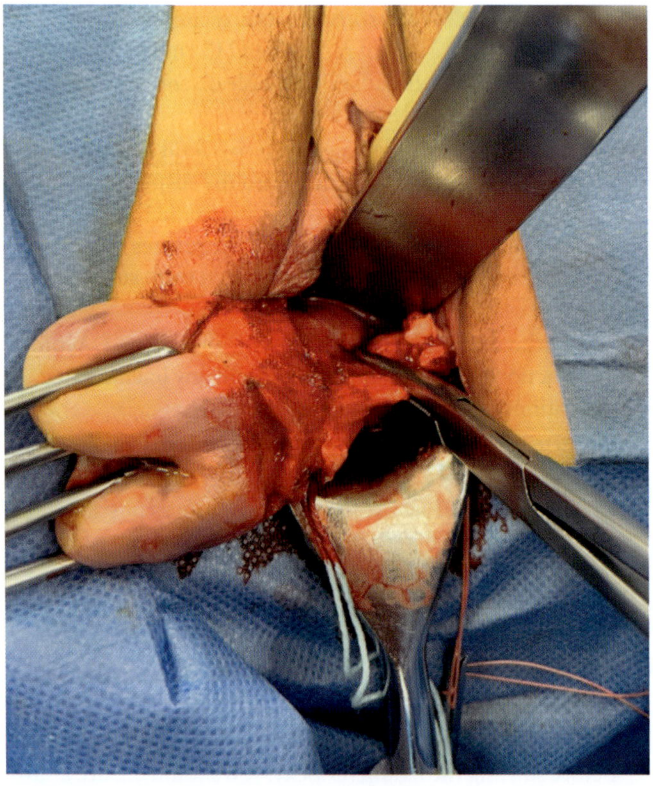

Figure 21.3 Clamping of the left cardinal ligament.

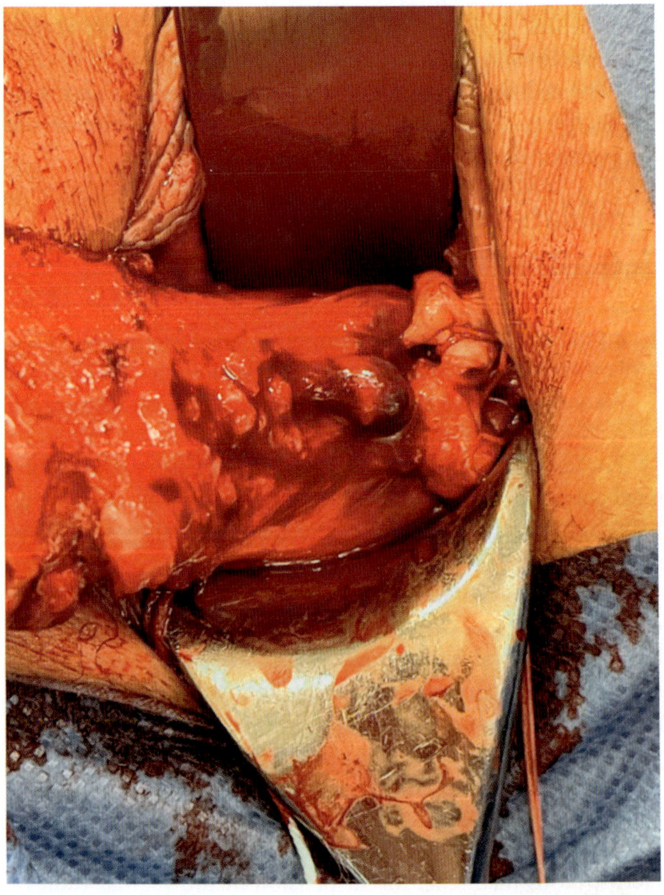

Figure 21.4 Identification of the left uterine pedicle.

(a)

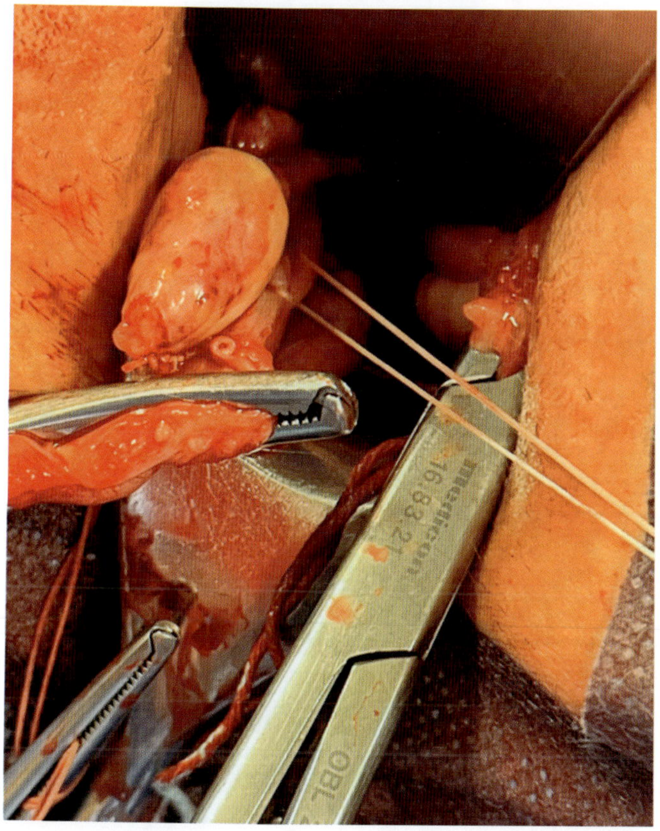

(b)

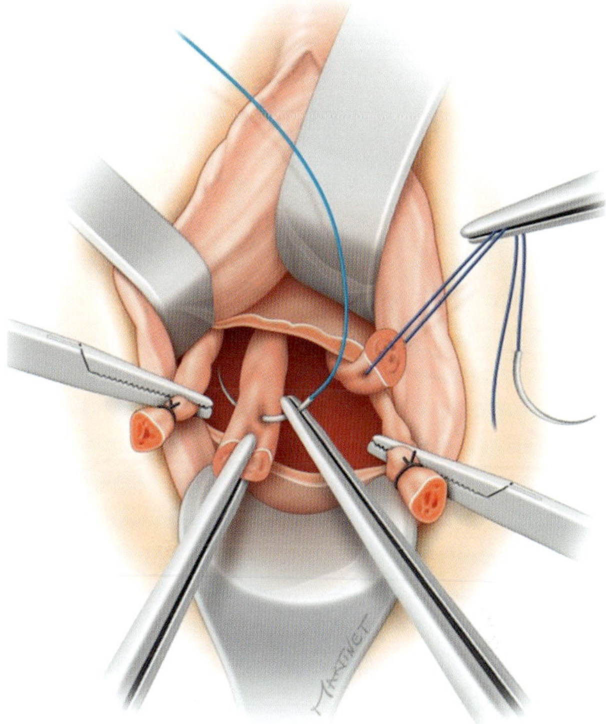

Figure 21.5a Utero-ovarian ligaments clamping on both sides and identification of the right round ligament. On the corresponding Figure 21.5b, clamps are placed on the utero-ovarian ligaments and blue sutures on both round ligaments.

(a)

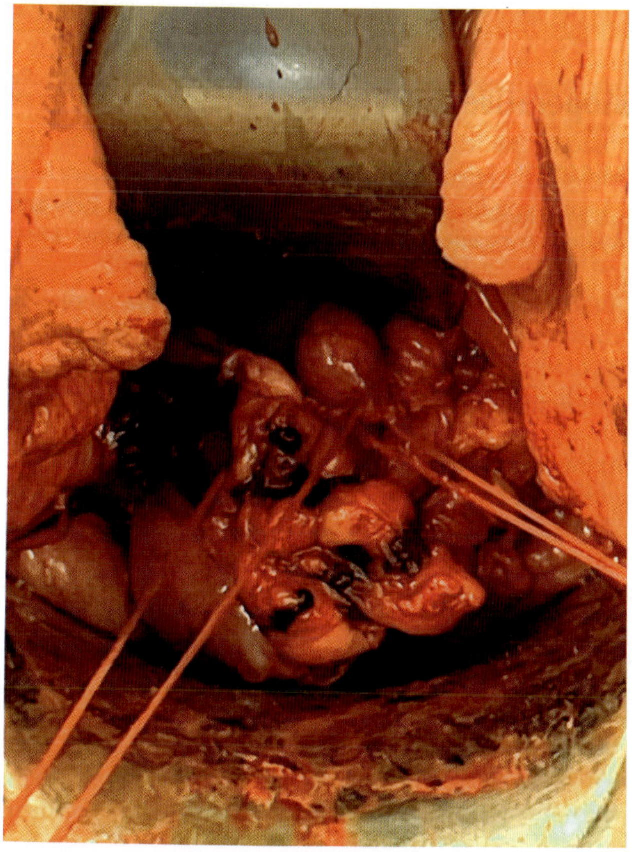

(b)

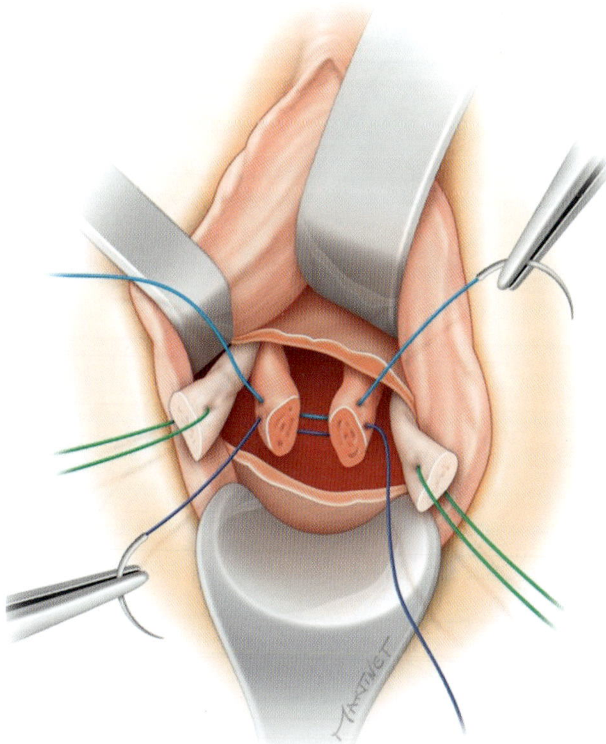

Figure 21.6a Crossing of both round ligaments. On the corresponding Figure 21.6b, blue sutures show the crossing of the round ligaments, green sutures are held on the uterosacral ligaments.

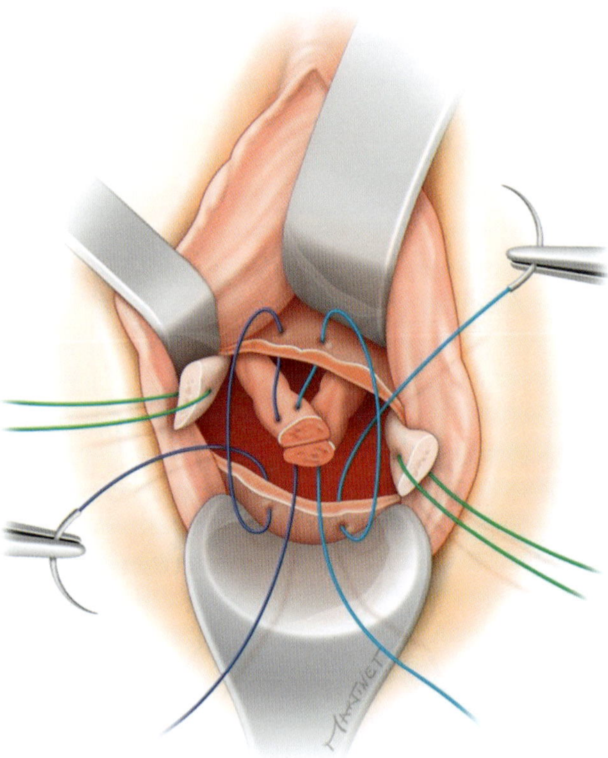

Figure 21.7 Fixation of the round ligaments (blue sutures) on the vaginal vault, in an *in-out* then *out-in* technique.

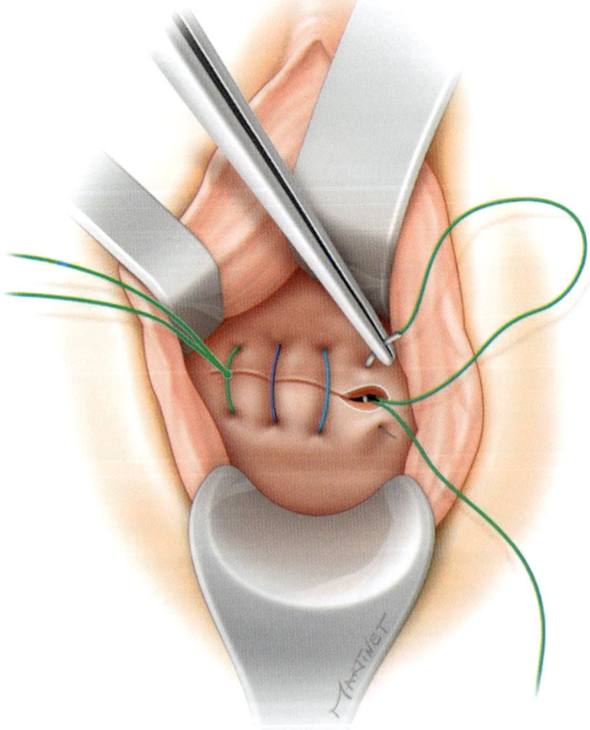

Figure 21.8 Fixation of the uterosacral ligaments (green sutures) on the vaginal vault.

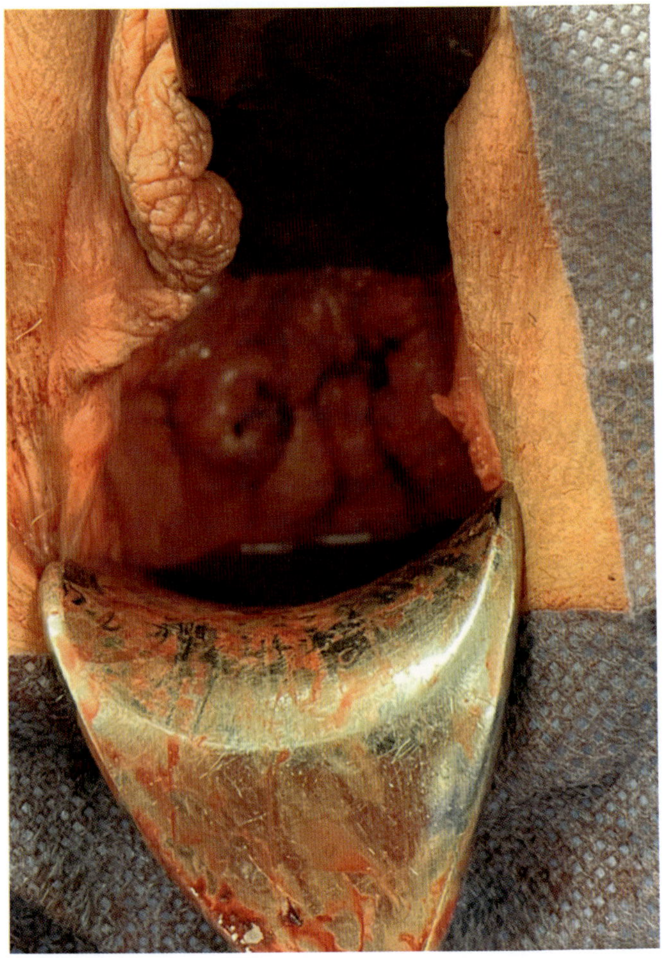

Figure 21.9 Final result with restoration of a normal vaginal length (TVL = –7 cm).

Postoperative Outcomes

Uterosacral ligament suspension for reconstructive transvaginal native tissue repair is a technique that proved its efficacy long ago. A study conducted on over 300 surgeries between 1994 and 1998 showed excellent postoperative anatomic results (87%) [19].

A more recent meta-analysis of 10 observational studies on 930 cases of uterosacral ligament suspension found as well a rate of 98% of anatomic success [10,13,20]. Yet with longer follow-up periods, high rates of recurrence and retreatment were observed (47.5% and 12% at five years respectively) [13,21].

Another recent study conducted on 109 patients found a vaginal length of 9 cm after the surgery [22]. There were no reported episodes of discomfort at the vaginal vault after a follow-up period of 2.8 years [22] compared to dyspareunia frequently observed after vaginal mesh use.

According to this study, although anatomic results tend to diminish over time, they concluded that this technique is associated with high clinical subjective results even after long periods of follow-up (87%) [22].

Several studies compared vaginal hysterectomy with uterosacral ligamentopexy to other techniques of prolapse repair. We are going to discuss below the major comparisons made in recent studies across the literature with both abdominal and vaginal techniques.

The OPTIMAL trial compared the two most common transvaginal native tissue reconstructive techniques for apical prolapse. Nine American medical centres joined, and 374 women were randomized between 2008 and 2013. 188 women underwent correction using uterosacral ligaments [23,24].

After two years of follow-up, anatomic success rates were similar after uterosacral ligament suspension and sacrospinous ligament fixation (64.5% and 63.1% respectively). Likewise, there was no statistical difference in subjective results and adverse outcomes. Re-treatment rates were 5% [24].

The OPTIMAL trial also proved that behavioural therapy with pelvic muscle re-education does not improve long-term outcomes after transvaginal prolapse repair [24]. The Extended OPTIMAL study also compared both techniques mentioned above but had a longer follow-up period. Nine American medical centres joined, and 285 women were randomized between 2008 and 2016 [4].

Although the group of women treated with uterosacral ligament suspension had more vaginal deliveries, after five years of follow-up the study did not show a significant difference in surgical failure of both techniques (61.5% for uterosacral ligament suspension and 70.3% for sacrospinous ligament fixation) [4]. As the OPTIMAL study, E-OPTIMAL showed same anatomic failure rates after behavioural therapy [4]. The median time to anatomic failure after uterosacral ligament suspension was 2.6 years and only 11.9% of participants needed re-operation for recurrence [4].

Despite this evidence, we advise pelvic muscle re-education therapy for all our patients after apical prolapse correction for its better clinical and subjective outcomes according to our experience.

As expected, these two studies showed high anatomic failure rates of native tissue reconstructive transvaginal surgeries, and rates increased with an extended follow-up as well as the need for re-intervention, but they also proved a maintenance of the improvement in the prolapse symptoms, the sexual function, and women's quality of life over time. 56.9% of women treated with uterosacral ligament suspension considered their symptoms 'very much better' and 'much better' after five years of the surgery [4].

One Dutch study conducted on 208 women between 2009 and 2012 also compared these two vaginal techniques. Rates of apical prolapse after vaginal hysterectomy with ligamentopexy were 0–12%, with no significant difference after one year of follow-up [15].

One retrospective study on 248 procedures of uterosacral ligament suspension showed that anatomic failure rates were higher with the delayed absorbable sutures compared to the permanent ones [13,25]. In our practice, we only use delayed absorbable sutures along the procedure. We do not recommend the use of non-absorbable sutures because of possible discomfort during intercourse [18].

A randomized American study was conducted to compare our surgical technique to vaginal mesh hysteropexy. The study was conducted between 2013 and 2015 on 175 women with a follow-up period of three years. It did not prove any statistical difference in failure rates in both groups [3]. Later the US Food and Drug Administration prohibited the use of these transvaginal kits, but the importance of this study remains in the fact that it proves that reconstructive surgery using native tissue can ensure the same outcomes as the prosthetic meshes without any of its related complications.

After the prohibition of vaginal meshes, a recent retrospective study compared our vaginal approach to laparoscopic uterosacral ligament hysteropexy. 159 women were enrolled between 2010 and 2015 and the follow-up lasted about one year [10]. Clinical cure rates and patient satisfaction were similar and very high in both groups (96% versus 98% and 96% versus 95% respectively) [10].

A Cochrane review grouped 30 randomized controlled trials on surgeries for apical vaginal prolapse made on more than 3,000 women [8]. Different surgical techniques were compared, among which we choose to list in the following the comparisons made with our technique.

First, vaginal ligamentopexy was compared to abdominal sacral colpopexy. Six randomized trials were found treating 583 women and with a follow-up period of one to four years. Vaginal ligamentopexy was associated to more symptoms of prolapse (RR 2.11), more recurrence (RR 1.89) and re-interventions (RR 2.28), more stress urinary incontinence (RR 1.86) and dyspareunia (RR 2.53), while quality of life and patient satisfaction were similar in both groups [8]. The advantage of the vaginal approach was the shorter operative time (mean difference of 21.49 minutes) [8].

Then our technique was compared to vaginal mesh for apical prolapse. Six randomized trials were found treating 598 women over a follow-up period of one to three years. There was no statistical difference in terms of prolapse symptoms, recurrent prolapse, or re-intervention between both groups. Native tissue reconstructive surgery was associated with a better satisfaction and quality of life (RR 5.70) [8].

These trials meet the conclusion of the American study mentioned above, but both were conducted on classical vaginal meshes that are nowadays prohibited and yet there is no evidence on the safety of the new lighter meshes available.

Vaginal hysterectomy with ligamentopexy for prolapse repair may not ensure the best anatomical results, but subjective outcomes and women's satisfaction remain very high, years after the intervention. It should be the first-line treatment for every woman presenting with an indication of a vaginal approach surgery. In comparison to other interventions, our technique can be done under regional anaesthesia, it does not require long operative times nor long recoveries, and is probably the least expensive technique.

Another reason to choose our surgical technique is its low complication rates.

Pelvic organ injury can be encountered in 0.4% of cases [13]. A good exposition using vaginal retractors and a vaginal gauze is crucial to avoid injuries to nearby pelvic organs.

Ureteral obstruction is one of the most common complications (1.8–3.2%) [13,24]. The technique of uterosacral ligament suspension implicates passing the sutures throughout the medial part of the ligament. In a cadaver study, the average distance from this suture spot to the ureter was 14 mm [26], which explains the high risks of ureteral damage. Surgeons resort to cystoscopy to avoid this complication. In our technique, we use the suture placed on the uterosacral ligaments during the hysterectomy for the suspension; the suture is placed as close as possible to the uterus to avoid any ureteral damage.

Likewise, sacral nerve entrapment has been seen with deep sutures on the ligaments [13], causing sensory neuropathy in the S2-S3 dermatomes, a complication that is spared by our technique.

Another adverse effect is granulation tissue formation. It is more frequently encountered after vaginal hysterectomy with uterosacral ligament suspension (11% versus 1% after mesh-associated hysteropexy at 12 weeks follow-up) [3]. The E-OPTIMAL trial also demonstrated the higher prevalence of this complication with our technique compared to sacrospinous ligament fixation, and found that it only appeared after a long-term follow-up [4].

Threes studies regrouping 297 women evaluated the effect of vaginal oestrogen after pelvic reconstructive surgeries. Although their evidence quality was poor, it was beneficial in decreasing urinary frequency and urgency and granulation tissue formation in comparison to placebo application [11]. The effect of vaginal oestrogen on prolapse recurrence was uncertain [11] but because it has no adverse effects it can be proposed to women after the surgery.

Furthermore, one retrospective study on pathology findings after hysterectomy with reconstructive surgeries found 2.6% of premalignant and malignant uterine disease, among which 0.3% was of endometrial carcinoma [17].

Symptomatic pelvic organ prolapse requiring surgery affects mainly postmenopausal women. This age group is at higher risk of endometrial cancer, and hysterectomy with apical vault suspension may not only improve women's satisfaction but can save their lives.

Prophylactic Vaginal Suspension

Apical support has been proved to be the major element for prolapse treatment. Some surgeons suggest performing native tissue reconstructive surgery for women undergoing vaginal hysterectomy for other indications.

Until now there is no evidence that ligamentopexy can prevent any future prolapse [27], but it can be proposed to women having asymptomatic prolapse or symptoms of prolapse without any findings on physical examination (grade 2 C) [27].

Do not perform the procedure in women with normal pelvic support on examination (grade 2 C) [27].

References

1. Dwyer L, Keamey R. Conservative management of pelvic organ prolapse. Obstet Gynecol Reprod Med 2017; 28: 1.
2. Biler A, Ertas E, Tosun G, et al. Perioperative complications and short-term outcomes of abdominal sacrocolpopexy, laparoscopic sacrocolpopexy, and laparoscopic pectopexy for apical prolapse. Int Braz J Urol 2018; 44(5): 996–1004.
3. Nager C, Visco A, Richter H, et al. Effect of vaginal mesh hysteropexy vs vaginal hysterectomy with uterosacral ligament suspension on treatment failure in women with uterovaginal prolapse: a randomized clinical trial. JAMA 2019; 322(11): 1054–65.
4. Jelovsek J, Barber M, Brubaker L, et al. Effect of uterosacral ligament suspension vs sacrospinous ligament fixation with or without perioperative behavioral therapy for pelvic organ vaginal prolapse on surgical outcomes and prolapse symptoms at 5 years in the OPTIMAL randomized clinical trial. JAMA 2018; 319(15): 1554–65.
5. Nair R, Nikolopoulos K, Claydon L. Clinical outcomes in women undergoing laparoscopic hysteropexy: a systematic review. Eur J Obstet Gynecol Reprod Biol 2017; 208: 71–80.
6. Faraj R, Broome J. Laparoscopic sacrohysteropexy and myomectomy for uterine prolapse: a case report and review of the literature. J Med Case Rep 2009; 3(99): 1–4.
7. Ijsselmuiden M, Coolen AL, Detollenaere R, et al. Hysteropexy in the treatment of uterine prolapse stage 2 or higher: a multicenter randomized controlled non-inferiority trial comparing laparoscopic sacrohysteropexy with vaginal sacrospinous hysteropexy (LAVA-trial, study protocol). BMC Women's Health 2014; 14: 112.
8. Maher C, Feiner B, Baessler K, et al. Surgery for women with apical vaginal prolapse (Review). Cochrane Database Syst Rev 2016; 10(10): CD012376. https://doi.org/10.1002/14651858.CD012376
9. Enemchukwu E. Transvaginal suture-based repair. Urol Clin N Am 2019; 46: 97–102.
10. Haj-Yahya R, Chill H, Levin G, et al. Laparoscopic uterosacral ligament hysteropexy vs total vaginal hysterectomy with uterosacral ligament suspension for anterior and apical prolapse: surgical outcome and patient satisfaction. JMIG 2020; 27(1): 88–93.
11. Giannini A, Russo E, Gano A, et al. Current management of pelvic organ prolapse in aging women: EMAS clinical guide. Maturitas 2018; 110: 118–23.
12. Novara L, Sgro L, Pecchio S, et al. Transvaginal high uterosacral ligament suspension: an alternative to McCall culdoplasty in the treatment of pelvic organ prolapse. Eur J Obstet Gynecol Reprod Biol 2019; 240: 278–81.
13. Kenton K, Brubaker L, Eckler K. Pelvic organ prolapse in women: surgical repair of apical prolapse (uterine or vaginal vault prolapse). UpToDate 2020. Available at: www.uptodate.com/contents/pelvic-organ-prolapse-in-women-surgical-repair-of-apical-prolapse-uterine-or-vaginal-vault-prolapse#!
14. Graefe F, Marschke J, Dimpfl T, et al. Vaginal vault suspension at hysterectomy for prolapse – myths and facts, anatomical requirements, fixation techniques, documentation and cost accounting. Geburtshilfe Frauenheilkd 2012; 72(12): 1099–106.
15. Detollenaere R, Boon J, Stekelenburg J, et al. Sacrospinous hysteropexy versus vaginal hysterectomy with suspension of the uterosacral ligaments in women with uterine prolapse stage 2 or higher: multicentre randomized non-inferiority trial. BMJ 2015; 351: h3717.
16. Nager C, Grimes C, Nolen T, et al. Concomitant anterior repair, preoperative prolapse severity, and anatomic prolapse outcomes after vaginal apical procedures. Female Pelvic Med Reconstr Surg 2019; 25(1): 22–8.
17. Jelovsek J, Brubaker L, Eckler K. Pelvic organ prolapse in women: choosing a primary surgical procedure. UpToDate

2020. Available at: www.uptodate.com/contents/pelvic-organ-prolapse-in-women-choosing-a-primary-surgical-procedure#!

18. Tan-Kim J, Menefee S, Brubaker L, et al. Prophylactic vaginal apex suspension at the time of hysterectomy. UpToDate 2020. Available at: www.uptodate.com/contents/prophylactic-vaginal-apex-suspension-at-the-time-of-hysterectomy?_escaped_fragment_=
19. Shull B, Bachofen C, Coates K, et al. A transvaginal approach to repair of apical and other associated sites of pelvic organ prolapse with uterosacral ligaments. Am J Obstet Gynecol 2000; 183(6): 1365–73.
20. Margulies RU, Rogers MA, Morgan DM. Outcomes of transvaginal uterosacral ligament suspension: systematic review and metaanalysis. Am J Obstet Gynecol 2010; 202: 124.
21. Jelovsek JE, Barber MD, Brubaker L, et al. Effect of uterosacral ligament suspension vs sacrospinous ligament fixation with or without perioperative behavioral therapy for pelvic organ vaginal prolapse on surgical outcomes and prolapse symptoms at 5 years in the OPTIMAL randomized clinical trial. JAMA 2018; 319: 1554.
22. Marschke J, Pax C, Beilecke K, et al. Vaginal hysterectomy with apical fixation and anterior vaginal wall repair for prolapse: surgical technique and medium-term results. Int Urogynecol J 2018; 29: 1187–92.
23. Barber M, Brubaker L, Menefee S, et al. Operations and pelvic muscle training in the management of apical support loss (OPTIMAL) trial: design and methods. Contemp Clin Trials 2009; 30: 178–89.
24. Barber M, Brubaker L, Burgio K, et al. Comparison of 2 transvaginal surgical approaches and perioperative behavioral therapy for apical vaginal prolapse: the OPTIMAL randomized trial. JAMA 2014; 311(10): 1023–34.
25. Chung CP, Miskimins R, Kuehl TJ, et al. Permanent suture used in uterosacral ligament suspension offers better anatomical support than delayed absorbable suture. Int Urogynecol J 2012; 23: 223.
26. Wieslander C, Roshanravan S, Wai C, et al. Uterosacral ligament suspension sutures: anatomic relationships in unembalmed female cadavers. Am J Obstet Gynecol 2007; 197: 672.e1.
27. AAGL Advancing Minimally Invasive Gynecology Worldwide. AAGL practice report: practice guidelines on the prevention of apical prolapse at the time of benign hysterectomy. J Minim Invasive Gynecol 2014; 21: 715.

Chapter 22

Laparoscopic Ventral Rectopexy for Rectal Prolapse: Steps and Evidence

Yara Abdelkhalek, Ohad Gluck, Bruno Deval

Introduction and Epidemiology

Rectal prolapse is the bulging of the rectum into the digestive lumen and ultimately exteriorization through the anus. It affects approximately 0.5% of the population [1] and women are more frequently affected than men (female to male ratio 6/1), mostly in the elderly [2]. Furthermore, one woman in eight has a mixed rectal and genital prolapse (Figure 22.1) [3]. The true incidence of this disease is unknown because it is often under-reported, especially when associated with faecal incontinence that also affects 1–18% of the general population [4]. Rectal prolapse is associated with major psychological discomfort and embarrassment, so treatment is an option to improve women's quality of life.

Classification and Clinical Presentation

In the first stage of the disease, the prolapse remains in the rectal lumen, then progressively it reaches the anal lumen in stage 2 and finally it exteriorizes in stage 3. Rectal prolapse may involve only the mucosa or all the layers of the rectum [5].

Clinical presentation varies according to the level of protrusion.

In stage 1, the majority of patients remain asymptomatic. Hereafter, with disease progression, symptoms may vary from perineal heaviness, sensation of a lump at the anus, dyschezia, a sense of incomplete evacuation, tenesmus, bleeding or mucosal discharge, and faecal incontinence in 50–80% of cases [2,5,6]. Symptoms may appear after episodes of high abdominal pressure (sneezing, coughing, etc.), on standing position or can persist all the time [2]. Rectal prolapse is usually a chronic illness and clinical features evolve gradually, but cases of urgent diagnosis and treatment have been described in patients with an incarcerated prolapse and rectal ischaemic gangrene [2].

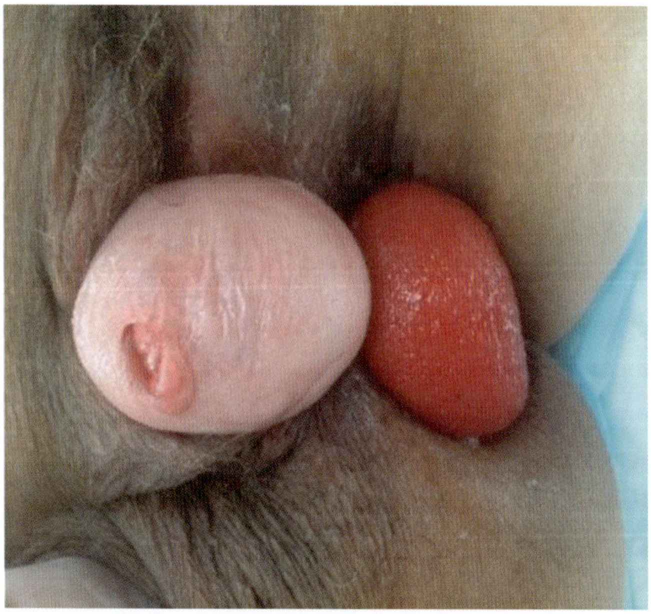

Figure 22.1 Rectal and genital prolapse [9].

Risk Factors

Many risk factors have been associated with rectal prolapse; they include [2,7]:

- Multiple pregnancies
- Vaginal childbirth, especially instrumental deliveries (Forceps)
- High infant birth weight
- Obesity
- Neurologic disorders
- Connective tissue disorders
- Psychiatric illness

Indications

Many surgical techniques can be indicated for the treatment of rectal prolapse. Some are abdominal and others use the perineal approach. Abdominal rectopexy can be performed by open or laparoscopic techniques, using an anterior or a posterior approach. The choice of the appropriate surgical technique for rectal prolapse correction depends on several components.

Ventral mesh laparoscopic rectopexy is indicated for the treatment of full-thickness rectal prolapse of any stage. It consists of anterior mobilization of the rectum with fixation of the mesh on the distal rectovaginal septum then stretching it towards the promontory which allows the elevation of the pelvic floor [8]. With this technique, the dissection plane is maintained anteriorly between the anterior rectal wall and the posterior vaginal wall, in order to spare the hypogastric and the inferior rectal nerves [9]. The aim is to restore normal bowel function by providing anatomical correction using a prosthetic mesh along with maintaining normal innervation to the rectum. [10]. In early-stage disease, dynamic magnetic resonance imaging or defecography may be helpful to confirm the diagnosis. Solitary rectal ulcer syndrome is also an indication for ventral rectopexy. It consists of bleeding, mucosal discharge, and pelvic floor dysfunction [3,10].

Contra-indications

Some conditions constitute a contra-indication for rectopexy; they include [10]:

- Proctitis
- Neurologic disorders or anorectal dyssynergia
- Pelvic tumours
- Pregnancy

Obesity (BMI >35) increases the risks of postoperative infections and long-term recurrence but does not preclude the intervention. Multiple abdominal interventions associated with severe adhesions and respiratory compromise can make the laparoscopic approach unfeasible.

Surgical Technique

Below we outline our technique for ventral mesh rectopexy.

- Under general anaesthesia, the patient is placed in lithotomy position. Proper antibiotics are given according to each hospital's guidelines.
- Bowel preparation is recommended.
- Repeat clinical examination under general anaesthesia to assess the degree of rectal prolapse and to recognize any associated genital prolapse, an indication to perform a hysteropexy during the procedure (Figure 22.1).
- A bladder catheter is inserted along with an optional uterine manipulator to facilitate its mobilization.
- Pneumoperitoneum is created by using a Veress needle entry at Palmer's point.
- Four laparoscopic ports are needed: one umbilical 10 mm port and three 5 mm ports in the supra-pubic, right and left iliac fossa.
- Before starting, perform an adequate evaluation of the abdominal cavity to rule out any pathology that may preclude rectopexy.
- First, the uterus is suspended to the anterior abdominal wall using a long straight needle to expose the uterosacral ligaments.

  If needed, the sigmoid colon is attached to the left lateral abdominal wall using the same technique to allow a better exposure of the posterior pouch of Douglas. Use this method with caution, especially when operating on the elderly or on patients with known history of colonic diverticulosis.
- The first step is the dissection at the level of the promontory. The sacral promontory is identified, as well as all the vital structures nearby (right common iliac vessels, right ureter).
- Start by opening the peritoneum at the level of the promontory. The pre-sacral space is an avascular space, so try to maintain the dissection as close to the midline to prevent any vascular damage. The dissection should not be excessive and must be performed with extreme accuracy to preserve the superior hypogastric plexus below the promontory, thus protecting the autonomic innervation of the pelvic organs. The mean distance between the midsacral promontory and the right hypogastric nerve is 7 mm (0–17 mm) according to a vascular anatomy study conducted of female cadavers [11] (Figures 22.2–22.3).
- A good haemostasis is a must to prevent any possible haemorrhagic complications afterwards. In our practice, we use a harmonic scalpel that allows precise dissection and adequate coagulation.
- The anterior longitudinal ligament is identified; it consists of the solid support to which the uterus will be suspended.
- Initiate two stiches on the anterior longitudinal ligament using a non-absorbable Mersuture 2.0 to fix later on the meshes. Do not knot your threads at this point.
- Dissection of the peritoneum is continued towards the right uterosacral ligament.
- The second step is the recto-vaginal space dissection. A malleable retractor is inserted in the posterior vaginal fornix as well as a Hegar dilator in the anus to facilitate the dissection of the recto-vaginal space.
- Meticulous dissection over a distance of 10 cm following the posterior vaginal wall is done, to prevent any rectal/

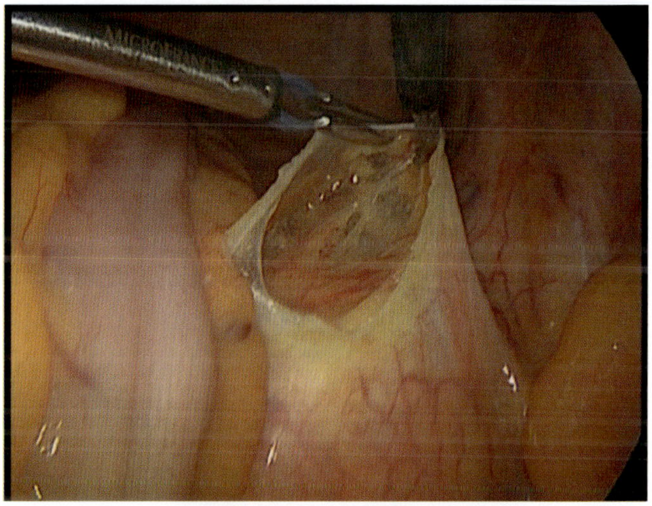

Figure 22.2 Peritoneum opening at the level of the promontory [9].

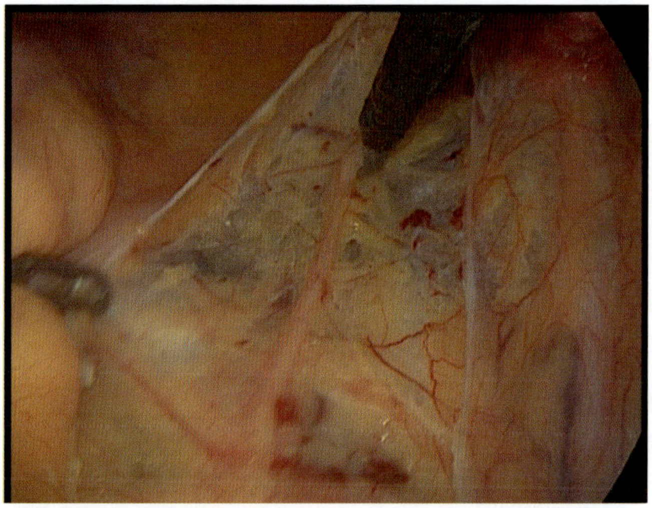

Figure 22.3 Peritoneal dissection [9].

bowel injury, which consistutes a contra-indication to the use of the mesh afterwards (Figures 22.4–22.5).

- The third step consists of mesh fixation on the rectum. From a polypropylene 30 x 30 cm mesh, the rectal mesh is drawn and cut in a rectangular 4 x 15 cm shape.
- The mesh is introduced into the abdominal cavity and fixed to the anterior rectal wall using at least six non-absorbable sutures of Mersuture 2.0 (Figures 22.6–22.7).
- Attention is needed to avoid folding and wrinkling of the mesh.
- At this stage, if genital prolapse is present, a concomitant hysteropexy can be performed which is described in Chapter 20.
- The next step is the fixation of the mesh on the sacrum. The mesh is stretched towards the sacral promontory where it is anchored using ProTack, then sutured using the two knots initiated there before (Figures 22.8–22.9).
- Avoid any excessive tension on the mesh which may lead to dyschezia and constipation later on.
- Cut any extra portion of the mesh, then last step is the closure of the peritoneum to completely cover it.

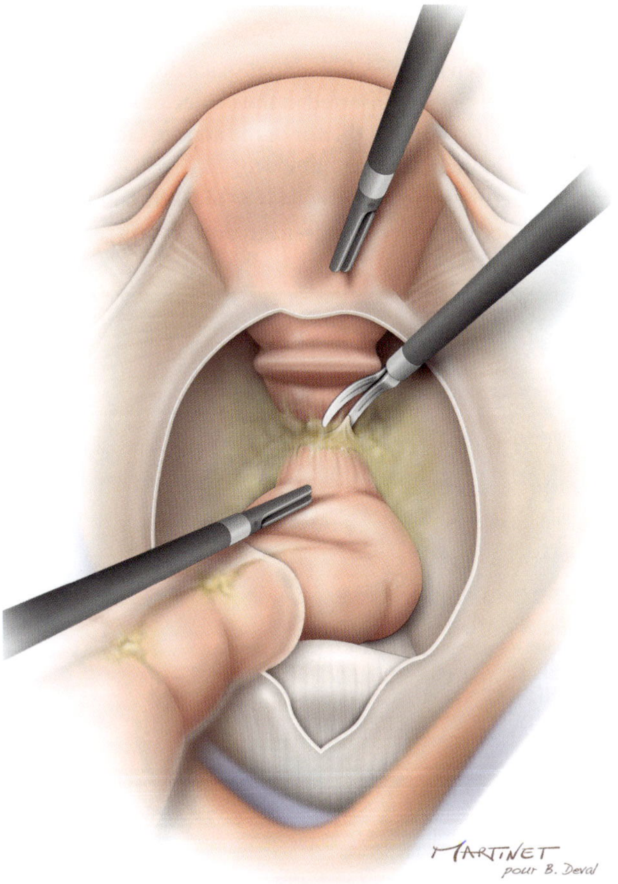

Figure 22.4 Recto-vaginal space dissection [9].

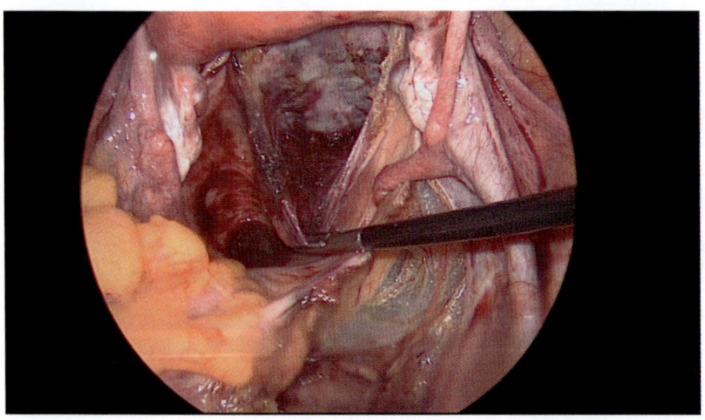

Figure 22.5 Recto-vaginal space dissection [9].

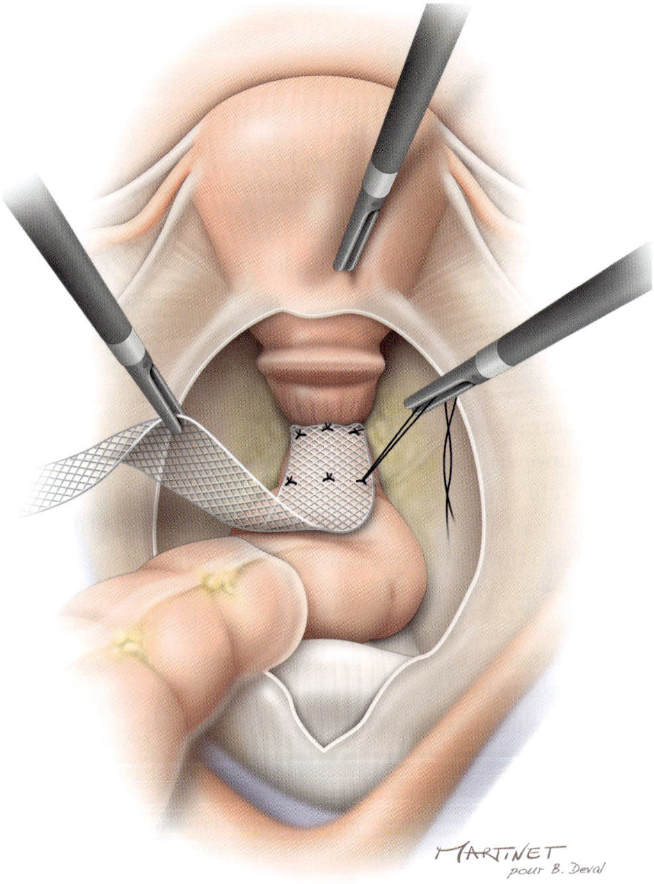

Figure 22.6 Mesh fixation on the rectum [9].

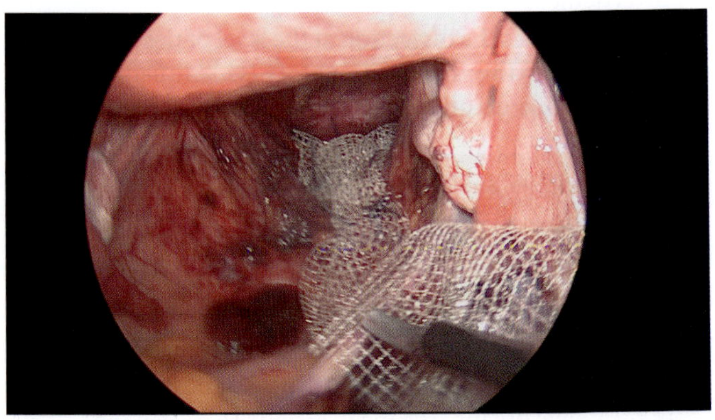

Figure 22.7 Mesh fixation on the rectum [9].

- No surgical drain is usually needed.
- Remove all laparoscopic ports and close the wounds.
- Clinical examination is recommended to assess the degree of prolapse repair.
- Mean operative time is 90 minutes, depending on the surgeon's experience.
- Non-opioid analgesics usually provide adequate pain relief.
- Bladder catheter can be removed on day one after the surgery if no bladdery injury occurred, and total hospital stay is around two to three days. In the case of bladder injury, keep catheterization for five days.

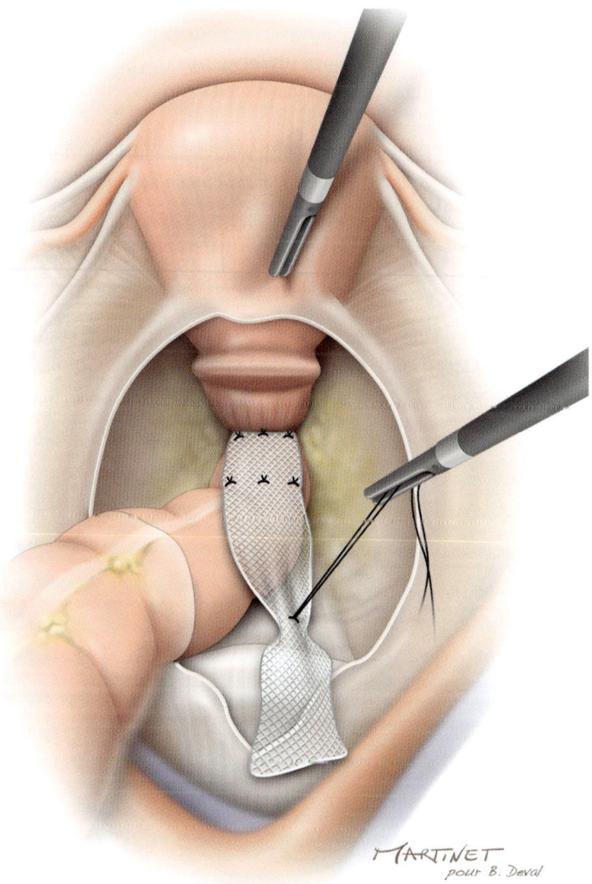

Figure 22.8 Mesh fixation on the promontory [9].

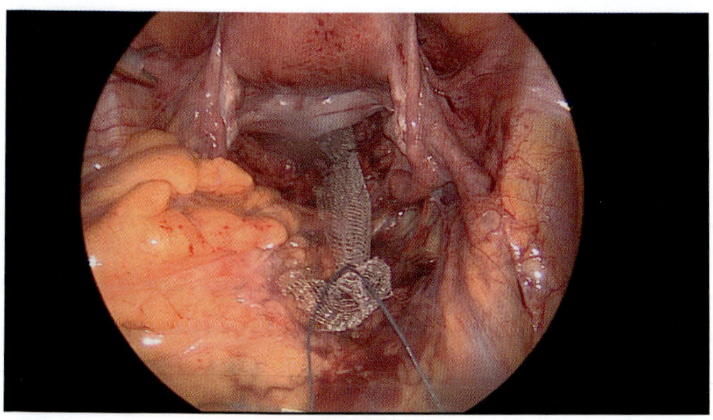

Figure 22.9 Mesh fixation on the promontory [9].

- We recommend avoidance of constipation and abstinence from heavy physical activities for at least six weeks.

Results

The laparoscopic approach of ventral rectopexy is associated with better postoperative outcomes (less pain, faster discharge) and most importantly the same rates of recurrence compared to the open abdominal technique [6,12]. Studies showed high rates of functional improvement (74–91%) and low rates of recurrence (2–8%) [10,13]. Higher rates of relapse were observed in the male population [13]. Despite the fact that postoperative defaecatory disorders can be common (40% of constipation [2]) 60% of patients reported an improvement in faecal incontinence after the intervention [14]. Five years follow-up studies showed less than 5% of relapse associated with improvement in the bothersome symptoms (faecal incontinence, dyschezia) [10]. Moreover, 10 years follow-up studies have shown 3–4% of recurrence [7,15] and 4.6% of mesh-related complications [1]. Furthermore, one woman in eight has a mixed rectal and genital prolapse [3]. In these cases, the laparoscopic ventral rectopexy should be associated to hysteropexy according to the surgical technique described in the appropriate chapter before. The combined surgery has the same rate of long-term recurrence compared to the isolated correction of rectal prolapse [3].

Other studies also proved identical low rates of recurrence regardless of the stage of the prolapse or its association with a genital prolapse as we mentioned above [13].

Complications

Complications are uncommon, with rates quoted from 2–16% of cases [12]. Major complications are infection, erosion, and mesh extrusion. The surgical technique along with the size and type of the prosthetic mesh may influence the development of these complications. Prosthetic mesh has 0–12% risk of erosion compared to 0% with the biological implants [12]. Also in the prosthetic group, type 1 meshes with pore size >75 micron are associated with the lowest risk of erosion. For laparoscopic ventral rectopexy, the ideal mesh type has not been determined yet [9].

Patient-related factors such as smoking, diabetes, or corticosteroids use may also increase the risk of complications, as well as some surgical issues (pelvic haematoma, rectal bowel injury, full thickness transfixing sutures, excessive mesh stretching) [9]. Mesh erosion may cause bleeding, mucosal or purulent discharge, and dyschezia. Extreme cases of extrusion of the mesh through the anus have been described [12]. Other possible complications are spondylodiscitis, post incisional hernia, bladder or bowel injury, pelvic haematoma, and bowel obstruction. Closure of the peritoneum above the mesh is essential to reduce risks of bowel obstruction [7].

Conclusion

Rectal prolapse is a common condition that is associated with many bothersome symptoms and major psychological discomfort and embarrassment. Laparoscopic ventral rectopexy is a reconstructive pelvic surgery technique that can be performed by visceral surgeons as well as gynaecologists in colorectal and pelvic floor clinics to improve women's quality of life.

References

1. Bordeianou L, Paquette I, Johnson E, et al. Clinical practice guidelines for the treatment of rectal prolapse. Dis Colon Rectum 2017; 60: 1121e31.
2. MacKay G, Dorrance H, Molloy R, O'Dwyer P, (eds.). Anorectal disorders. In *Colorectal Surgery.* Oxford Specialist Handbooks in Surgery. Oxford University Press: 2011; 249e83.
3. Slawik S, Soulsby R, Carter H, Payne H, Dixon AR. Laparoscopic ventral rectopexy, posterior colporrhaphy and vaginal sacrocolpopexy for the treatment of recto-genital prolapse and mechanical outlet obstruction. Colorectal Dis 2008; 10(2): 138–43.
4. Lehur P, Wong M. Incontinence. In: Phillips R, Clark S, eds. *A Companion to Specialist Surgical Practice in Colorectal Surgery*. 5th edn. Elsevier Saunders: 2014; 167e83.
5. Proctor V, Harikrishnan A. Rectal prolapse and surgery for faecal incontinence. Intest Surg II 2020; 38: 6.
6. Boons P, Collinson R, Cunningham C, et al. Laparoscopic ventral rectopexy for external rectal prolapse improves constipation and avoids de novo constipation. Colorectal Dis 2010; 12(6): 526–32.
7. Fearnhead N. Functional problems and their surgical management. In: Phillips R, Clark S, eds. *A Companion to Specialist Surgical Practice in Colorectal Surgery*. 5th edn. Elsevier Saunders: 2014; 184e201.
8. Tou S, Brown SR, Nelson RL. Surgery for complete (full-thickness) rectal prolapse in adults. Cochrane Database Syst Rev 2015. Available from:www.cochranelibrary.com/cdsr/doi/10.1002/14651858.CD001758.pub3/full?highlightAbstract ¼withdrawn%7Crectal%7Cprolapse%7Cprolaps [last accessed 1 November 2021].
9. Gluck O, Blaganje M, Deval B. How I do … Laparoscopic ventral rectopexy using a synthetic mesh. Gynecologie Obstertrique Fertilite & Senologie 2019; 47: 753–6.
10. Mercer-Jones MA, D'Hoore A, Dixon AR, et al. Consensus on ventral rectopexy: report of a panel of experts. Color Dis 2014; 16(2): 82–8.
11. Wieslander CK, et al. Vascular anatomy of the presacral space in unembalmed female cadavers. Am J Obstet Gynecol 2006; 195: 1736.
12. Patil NS, Saluja SS, Mishra PK, et al. Intrarectal migration of mesh following rectopexy: case series and review of literature. Int J Surg 2015; 20(2015): 145–8.
13. Mackenzie H, Dixon AR. Proficiency gain curve and predictors of outcome for laparoscopic ventral mesh rectopexy. Surgery (United States) 2014; 156(1): 158–67.
14. Parchment-Smith C. Abdomen. In: Parchment-Smith C, ed. *Essential Revision Notes for Intercollegiate MRCS Book 2.* Pastest: 2006; 1e445.
15. Garland B. Ventral mesh rectopexy: is this the new standard for surgical treatment of pelvic organ prolapse? Dis Colon Rectum 2014; 57: 1446e7.

Chapter 23

Hysterectomy versus Uterine Preservation in the Management of Uterine Prolapse

Vladimír Kališ, Zdeněk Rušavý, Khaled M Ismail

Introduction

The Uterus and Womanhood

Am I a woman? Isn't having a uterus the very definition of womanhood?

Lossie, 50, president and CEO of Beautiful You MRKH (Mayer-Rokitansky-Kuster-Hauser Syndrome) Foundation

Although it does not seem to be Lossie's view, based on the published article [1], nevertheless, for some women this might be what they actually believe in.

Clinicians practising cross-cultural medicine soon realize the variation in perception of the uterus amongst women from different cultures and backgrounds. One can reflect on a consultation with a nulliparous woman in her twenties who was adamant she wanted a hysterectomy for pelvic pain, followed by a consultation with a multiparous woman in her early forties with large multiple fibroids, menorrhagia, and anaemia, who did not wish to even discuss hysterectomy as an option. However, these varying views might not be necessarily cultural but rather individual. Indeed, Solbraekke and Bondevik undertook in-depth interviews with a cohort of Norwegian women exploring their accounts of hysterectomy [2]. In their study, two contradictory storylines stood out: Some women considered that by performing a hysterectomy *'They have removed what made me a woman'* versus *'Without a uterus, I feel more like a woman'*. In their conclusion, the researchers acknowledged the diversity in the way women experience hysterectomy and its importance to better understand the ways in which such a procedure impacts on women as human beings. They concluded that this is essential to developing a more cultural-competent healthcare service.

The uterus has the one major role of keeping the baby safe inside until childbirth. However, because of several biological, cultural, religious, ethical, and/or philosophical reasons, the uterus can be very important for their own perception of womanhood. In some societies, hysterectomized women feel inferior, mainly because of the negative approach of men and other non-hysterectomized women towards them [3,4]. It has been suggested that up to 42% of women feel that the uterus is an important contributor to their sense of self [5–9]. Korbly et al [6] and Urdzík et al [8] reported that the vast majority of women in this group favoured the choice of uterine preservation rather than hysterectomy.

The Uterus and Sexual Quality of Life

The perception of sexual satisfaction depends on the interaction of several complex contributing factors [10]. Positive contributing factors include a healthy relationship with one's partner, good general health of both partners, no life stresses, and no financial worries [11]. The relative importance of these factors is difficult to quantify, nevertheless, it seems higher than that of hysterectomy [12]. The results of studies comparing the effect of hysterectomy on the frequency of sexual intercourse, sexual desire, sexual arousal, and orgasm are contradictory, and the summary of evidence is inconclusive.

Views about the uterus and its role in women's lives have changed over time. In ancient times, the uterus was believed to have a major role in female physical and mental well-being and was responsible for emotional instability. Indeed, in 370 BC, Hippocrates stated that 'Women are subject to intermittent agitations which make their way from the head to the uterus whence they are expelled' – probably the first description of premenstrual syndrome [14]. For centuries, removal of the uterus was believed to cure emotional instability in women. Views about the uterus have changed in the twentieth century, when it was suggested that it was involved in the process of orgasm. It was believed that removal of the uterus could lead to female sexual dysfunction in women who experience uterine orgasm. Historically, the uterus has been regarded as a sexual organ, a source of energy and vitality, and a maintainer of youth and attractiveness. Since such beliefs may still prevail, women may feel that their sexuality may be affected by hysterectomy [15]. The importance of the uterus in sexual life quality has been questioned in studies demonstrating no difference in sexual functions in women after hysterectomy compared to those who have uterine sparing procedures e.g. hysteroscopic endometrial ablation in case of dysfunctional bleeding [16] or uterine artery embolization for uterine fibroids [17].

It has been suggested that the uterus plays a role in vaginal lubrication during intercourse [13]. This is plausible because, apart from absence of cervical mucus production, hysterectomy may lead to a reduction of vaginal lubrication due to damage to innervation and vascular supply of the upper third of the vagina [15]. It has also been reported that shortening of the vagina, along with pain in the surgical incision scars, may contribute to dyspareunia [18,19]. When performing total hysterectomy, part of the vaginal vault is removed or lost during closure of the vaginal apex. According to a Turkish study, all 15 (5.1%) women with *de novo* post-hysterectomy dyspareunia had the total vaginal length (TVL) shortened ≥2 cm when compared to preoperative TVL [20]. This shortening is not supposed to happen in uterine saving techniques.

Information about sexual functioning is often gathered during consultation or as part of quality-of-life (QoL) questionnaires addressing sexuality. In a recent study by Bradford et al on 204 participants, 41.2% of women experienced at least one negative sexual outcome after hysterectomy; the most common were deterioration of sexual desire (36.8%) and lack of vaginal lubrication (33.2%) [21].

In contrast, a review of the literature has shown that in the short term, sexual function either improves or does not change in most women after hysterectomy for benign indication, irrespective of the route [15]. Several explanations were provided. Removal of the uterus may eliminate or reduce dyspareunia or dysmenorrhoea, thus improving quality of life with a positive influence on sexual function. Relief from fear of unwanted conception, freedom from vaginal bleeding, improved physical well-being, and oestrogen replacement therapy were also stated as possible reasons [15].

In this context, it is imperative to take into account the underlying condition for which the hysterectomy was performed. In the case of malignant condition, the issue of sexuality is more complex. Cancer treatment modalities including radical surgery, chemotherapy, and radiation, together with patient and partner psychosocial issues, can all influence sexual function [22]. However, pelvic organ prolapse (POP) surgery generally has a positive impact on global sexual function [19,23]. Satisfaction in most patients may be due to complete relief of no longer feeling a vaginal bulge, improving self-image, and absence of pain [24]. Despite the fact that hysterectomy during POP repair reduces vaginal length, it does not seem to adversely affect sexual function. This can be explained by the improvement in symptoms of vaginal bulging with POP repair, which are known to negatively impact on sexual function [119].

Hysterectomy and Ovarian Function

Hysterectomy might have a detrimental effect on ovarian function. If performed premenopausally, women report more climacteric complaints, mainly hot flushes and the decrease of vaginal lubrication compared with their contemporaries [25–27]. In a German study, 26.1% of premenopausal women registered signs of ovarian failure after hysterectomy [28]. There was a significantly higher decrease in anti-müllerian hormone levels (p<.001) and the hormone was not detectable in more women one year after hysterectomy compared to controls (p=.02) [29].

Furthermore, due to a variety of reasons, including hormonal changes, it is increasingly recognized that a certain proportion of women develop depression after hysterectomy for benign condition. In a study by Yen et al [30], the incidence of *de novo* major depressive disorder shortly after hysterectomy was 7.7%. These women also reported worse sexual function and body image [30].

Hysterectomy and Risk of Uterine Cancer

Endometrial cancer is the third most frequent female malignancy, following breast and colo-rectal cancers. In spite of the fact that the signs and symptoms of this condition, i.e. abnormal bleeding, tend to present early, many of these are fairly common in non-malignant conditions like polyps. Endometrial polyps are reported to have a background prevalence of 8–13%, with a higher frequency in older age [31,32]. Abnormal bleeding occurs in 10–11% of postmenopausal women [33,34]. All these women need to undergo a clinical and ultrasonographic examination with a high possibility of endometrial sampling or hysteroscopy for optimal assessment. It is estimated that 25% of these women will be subsequently diagnosed with a premalignant or malignant lesion [31,35], which is usually treated with hysterectomy. Furthermore, the diagnostic process has to be repeated if recurrent bleeding occurs.

Hysterectomy and Pelvic Organ Prolapse Repair

The impact of hysterectomy on the anatomic and functional results of POP surgery has been studied for many years. There is high-level evidence that abdominal and laparoscopic sacrocolpopexy (LSC) result in better anatomical outcome compared to sacrospinous ligament fixation and transvaginal mesh insertion [36]. Non-hysterectomized women with POP who are considered suitable for a laparoscopic procedure have several options to choose from: laparoscopic sacro-hysteropexy (LSH), laparoscopic supra-cervical (subtotal) hysterectomy and sacrocervicopexy (LSCH+LSC), or total laparoscopic hysterectomy and laparoscopic sacro-colpopexy (TLH+LSC).

Removing periods and their associated symptoms, together with the need to use contraception, and minimizing the cost and time required for some of the gynaecological screening programmes might be perceived, by some women, as pros for hysterectomy, even in the absence of an abnormality or indication. While in contrast, their felt sense of womanhood, self-esteem, concern about impact on sexual function, or concern about the potential for using hormone replacements, might be the reasons why other women are against the procedure. Therefore, women's personal views play a part in their decision-making process about hysterectomy. In contrast, clinicians are expected to undertake surgical procedures only if indicated and justifiable, yet the same patient might be offered a hysterectomy by one gynaecologist and recommended uterine preservation by the other. In the following sections we will present why some clinicians and women might argue for and against hysterectomy at the time of laparoscopic reconstructive POP surgery.

Opinion A: Hysterectomy in Pelvic Organ Prolapse Repair

Why Some Professionals Are Pro Hysterectomy

Pelvic Organ Prolapse Repair Surgical Outcomes

By definition, POP involves the vagina as well as other pelvic organs, most frequently the uterus. The prolapsed cervix is traumatized by occasional or even permanent irritation and contamination with the external environment. Hence, chronic POP may result in local ischaemia with subsequent development of cervical decubitus ulcer. The concomitant conditions (tissue atrophy, oedema, and vessel congestion) contribute to tissue fragility; superficial ulceration with subsequent bleeding and infection [37,38]. Indeed, a degree of cervicitis has been identified in 100% of advanced POP patients [38]. A positive relation was found between the number and size of decubitus ulcers and POP-Q stage [39]. Despite appropriate care, healing of such lesions can take months [37]. Some clinicians believe that a hysterectomy with sufficient circumcision of the decubitus ulcer margin might accelerate the management of these chronically ill women.

Vaginal hysterectomy with uterosacral ligament suspension has been the traditional approach in surgical POP management. The efficacy of this procedure for the correction of apical compartment prolapse was reported to be 92.8% at a five-year follow-up [40]. There is also the perception that uterine preservation would increase the risk of POP recurrence. A large population-based study (on > 90,000 women) found that concomitant hysterectomy at the time of index POP repair, regardless of type of former as well as recurrent defect, reduced the risk of POP recurrence (OR 0.7) up to seven years. In this study, it was reported that the risk of repeat POP surgery at five years was 8.1–9.0% in the concomitant hysterectomy groups versus 11.3–15.0% in the non-hysterectomy group ($p<.001$) [41]. Moreover, it has been reported that women who had a hysterectomy for benign, non-POP indication seemed to be at a much lower risk of developing POP requiring repair after their hysterectomy [42]. It is also recognized that the size of the cervix might significantly affect POP staging [43,44]. Cervical elongation has been reported in 22–85% of women undergoing POP surgery depending on whether the elongation was based on actual length or the ratio of uterine body to cervix [43,44,45]. The size of the uterus might also adversely affect the outcome of POP surgery. If performing laparoscopic hysteropexy, the presence of a bulky uterus makes the dissection of the rectovaginal space, fixation to the sacral bone or promontory, and peritoneal closure technically demanding and can significantly prolong operative time.

Finally, removing the uterus provides better access to suspensory structures e.g. higher level of the uterosacral ligaments, sacrospinous ligament, or arcus tendineous fasciae pelvis. Furthermore, it has been reported that there is a markedly increased number of concomitant procedures in association with uterine sparing procedures. In a study by Pan et al [46], in 31% there were additional procedures associated with uterine preservation (trachelectomy, cervical cone biopsy, cervical or endometrial polyp removal, tubal ligation, myomectomy). These additional procedures may increase the risk of peri- or postoperative complications.

There is always a risk of mesh exposure after any surgery where mesh is used. This risk is reported to range from 2.3–2.7% [47,48]. However, in several studies comparing LSH versus TLH+LSC, the only mesh exposure occurred in the LSH group [46,49,50]. Moreover, a more recent study reported equal mesh exposure rates in each group [51].

Pelvic Organ Prolapse Repair Clinical Outcomes

There is not enough evidence regarding the long-term impact of LSH [52]. In contrast, the long-term results of sacrocolpopexy with concomitant hysterectomy or sacrocolpopexy after previous hysterectomy are available and may be provided to women at the time of their counselling.

Bedford et al [53] found a significantly higher recurrence rate in the apical compartment in laparoscopic uterosacral ligament suspension hysteropexy group (24% versus 13%, $p=.03$) as well as the higher rate of overall recurrence (53% versus 38%, $p=.02$) up to three years after surgery.

Unlike other researchers [49,50,54], Pan et al found a higher failure rate in the LSH group, where symptomatic prolapse was found in 16% after LSH versus none after TLH + LSC ($p=.01$) [46]. However, Gagyor et al [51] found a higher rate of recurrent cystoceles after LSH compared to TLH + LSC (21.1% versus 5.2%). A similar trend was observed in a study by Illiano et al [50], where the correction rates for anterior compartment defect were 92.6% after LSH and 96.4% after TLH+LSC. The explanation could be the asymmetry in the size of compartment defect where large anterior and apical defects co-exist with much smaller posterior defect. This asymmetry can be balanced by creating a *de novo* vaginal apex from the superior part of the anterior vaginal wall in case of sacrocolpopexy, however, this step is challenging when performing hysteropexy [55].

A 10–20% difference ($p=.003$) in overall ultrasonographic criteria for a proper mesh placement favouring TLH + LSC over LSH was noticed. This was mainly because of the regularity in shape of the inserted mesh and its folding rate [51]. Thus, to our knowledge, there is no study favouring anatomic outcomes of endoscopic hysteropexy compared to laparoscopic hysterectomy with sacrocolpopexy.

In a study by Illiano et al the bladder storage symptoms resolved in 83.8% after LSH compared to 88.3% of women after TLH+LSC [50]. Sexual outcome measured by the increment of FSFI was lower after LSH than after TLH + LSC (18.8 versus 23.2) [50].

Subjective satisfaction rate was reported to be 92% after LSH versus 100% after TLH + LSC ($p<.001$) [46]. While, at one year, 86.8% of women who had an LSH reported that their symptoms were much or very much better compared to 94.8% treated with TLH + LSC [51].

Symptomatic prolapse was also reported to be higher after LSH (16%) versus none following TLH + LSC ($p=.01$) [46]. Furthermore, *de novo* stress urinary incontinence developed more commonly after sacrohysteropexy (37.9% versus 21.7%) [51].

Perceived Impact on the Woman's Quality of Life

Current practice expects clinicians to give equal weight to patient reported outcomes as they traditionally did to clinical outcomes. Urogynaecology is one of the subspecialties at the forefront of this approach where clinicians have to rely on QoL measures to assess the impact of the condition and interventions on women and utilize this information to facilitate the patient's decision-making process [56].

The overall risk of complications during or after hysterectomy at POP repair is minimal, since the removal of a normal sized uterus is a safe and, relatively, fast procedure [52]. The safety of laparoscopic hysterectomies has been demonstrated in a large population-based study [57].

Although there is a paucity of information regarding the impact of hysterectomy versus uterine preservation on QoL in the short- and long-term, there is a perception amongst some clinicians that a hysterectomy can have several positive effects [8]. Cessation of menstrual loss, particularly if heavy or associated with dysmenorrhoea, reducing or removing completely the need for some screening check-ups and the use of contraception and its potential side-effects. There is also evidence that sexuality can be positively changed after hysterectomy for benign conditions [15]. A comprehensive review by Thakar reported no change or even improvement in sexual function after hysterectomy [15]. While an RCT on a population of women with abnormal bleeding revealed statistically significant differences in the hysterectomy group in terms of sexual desire in the short- and long-term [58]. Similarly, other RCTs revealed a significant increase in frequency of intercourse and decrease in deep dyspareunia a year after total or subtotal hysterectomy [59,60]. Moreover, a study by Flory et al [61] found a consistent reduction in abdominal pain and improvement in sexual functioning after laparoscopic hysterectomy compared to controls. There is also evidence that hysterectomy can have a positive impact on a woman's mental health. A meta-analysis by Darwish [62] found that symptoms of depression were significantly reduced after hysterectomy. An RCT by Thakar [60] found a significant improvement in seven out of eight QoL subscales and in three out of four psychological measures after hysterectomy.

Mitigating the Risk of Future Uterine Pathology

When considering that POP repair is a procedure affecting functional and often subjective outcomes where repeated surgery decreases the chance of improvement, the general philosophy of POP surgery is to reconstruct the pelvic floor structures in a way that no future additional repair would be needed. With uterine preserving surgery, there is always a risk of future hysterectomy because of future uterine pathology requiring such a procedure for their management. Although for the vast majority of women, a hysterectomy at the time of POP surgery will entail removing a healthy organ, there is a small, but real possibility that the seemingly normal uterus is in fact pathological. In studies in women undergoing POP and concomitant hysterectomy, 15 – 48% of specimens had evidence of other benign gynaecological pathologies like myomas, and 18–40% had adenomyosis [31,63–65]. More significantly, several studies found that the risk of unrecognized high-grade premalignant cervical lesion is present in 0.3% of unsuspected hysterectomy samples [64–67,71] (Table 23.1). Furthermore, unsuspected atypical hyperplasia and/or endometrial cancer were accidently found in 1.3% and 0.3% postmenopausal and premenopausal women respectively [64–71] (Table 23.2). Additionally, and as stated in the introduction to this chapter, there is always the risk of developing *de novo* pre-cancerous or malignant pathology in the future requiring a hysterectomy. Apart from the risk of surgery posed by the previous POP repair and the impact of surgery on the repair integrity, there is also the issue of a serious pathology that could have otherwise been avoided.

Table 23.1 Incidence of concomitant cervical pathology

	Menopausal status	Group size, [N]	CIN I, [N] (%)	CIN II/III, [N] (%)	Cancer, [N] (%)	≥ CIN II, [N] (%)
Frick et al [65]	Pre- and postmenopausal	629	2 (0.3%)	0	0	0
Renganathan et al [71]	Premenopausal	165	NS	NS	0	Non-calculable
	Postmenopausal	352	NS	NS	0	Non-calculable
Wan et al [64]	Pre- and postmenopausal	640	4 (0.6%)	1 (0.2%)	0	1 (0.2%)
Grigoriadis et al [66]	Premenopausal	58	0	0	0	0
	Postmenopausal	275	3 (0.9%)	1 (0.3%	1 (0.3%)	2 (0.6%)
Mizrachi et al [67]	Premenopausal	59	0	0	0	0
	Postmenopausal	608	0	3 (0.4%)	0	3 (0.4%)
Total		**2269**	**9 (0.4%)**	**5 (0.2%)**	**1 (0.4%)**	**6 (0.3%)**

Table 23.2 Incidence of concomitant uterine pathology

	Menopausal status	Group size, [N]	US provided	Complex hyperplasia	Atypical hyperplasia	Uterine malignangy	Total
Renganathan et al [71]	Premenopausal	165	Selective US	NS	NS	0	Non-calculable
	Postmenopausal	352	Selective US	NS	NS	4 (1.1%)	
Wan et al [64]	Premenopausal	87	Selective US and sampling	NS	3 (1.7%)	0	6 (3.4%)
	Postmenopausal	553	Selective US and sampling	NS		3 (1.7%)	

Table 23.2 (cont.)

	Menopausal status	Group size, [N]	US provided	Complex hyperplasia	Atypical hyperplasia	Uterine malignangy	Total
Ackenbom et al [68]	Premenopausal	220	NS	7 (0.6%)		3 (0.3%)	10 (0.8%)
	Postmenopausal	976	NS				
Frick et al [65]	Premenopausal	178	NS	0	0	0	0
	Postmenopausal	466	NS	3 (0.5%)	7 (1.1%)	2 (0.3%)	12 (2.6%)
Ramm et al [70]	Premenopausal	255	Selective US	NS	0	0	0
	Postmenopausal	453	Selective US	NS	1 (0.2%)	5 (1.1%)	6 (1.3%)
Andy et al [69]	Premenopausal	117	Selective US	0	0	0	0
	Postmenopausal	207	Selective US	1 (0.5%)*	1 (0.5%)	0	2 (1.0%)
Grigoriadis et al [66]	Premenopausal	58	Yes	1 (1.7%)	1 (1.7%)	0	2 (3.4%)
	Postmenopausal	275	Yes	3 (1.1%)	0	0	3 (1.1%)
Mizrachi et al [67]	Premenopausal	59	Yes	0	0	0	0
	Postmenopausal	608	Yes	0	2 (0.3%)	1 (0.2%)	3 (0.5%)
Total	**Premenopausal**	**667**	**N/A**	**1 (0.15%)**	**1 (0.15%)**	**0**	**2 (0.3%)**
	Postmenopausal	**2009**	**N/A**	**7 (0.3%)**	**11 (0.5%)**	**8 (0.4%)**	**26 (1.3%)**

*atypia non-assessable; NS not stated

What Are Women's Views about Hysterectomy?

When it comes to a decision about hysterectomy as part of POP management in women who have not completed their families, fertility is considered important or very important in 57% and 30% of women respectively [5]. Hence, in women who might wish to get pregnant in the future, uterine-saving techniques are definitely the preferred option. However, the median age of women undergoing laparoscopic POP repair is ≥ 55 [46,49,53,54,72]. In a study by Gagyor et al [51], four out of five women undergoing a variant of laparoscopic sacro-colpopexy for a uterovaginal prolapse were > 50 years of age. Irrespective of preserving fertility, several studies report that the majority of women in their cohorts seemed to prefer hysterectomy. It is reported that nearly 70% of women prefer hysterectomy at the time of POP surgery [7,8]. Several factors have been suggested as reasons for such preference, such as eliminating the need for contraception or ending menstruation [5,8].

It is important to recognize that for the vast majority of women (98–100%), the doctor's opinion is important to help them make a decision [5,8]. Moreover, their decision is very much influenced by the information provided. One of the main determinants of women's choice about whether to spare or remove the uterus at the time of POP surgery is the postoperative outcome. Urdzík et al conducted a survey among female gynaecologists about their personal views regarding uterine preservation versus hysterectomy at the time of POP management in response to different hypothetical scenarios [8]. In this study, more than 80% of respondents who originally preferred hysteropexy changed their opinion when informed that the outcome might be better after a hysterectomy, resulting in more than 90% of survey participants choosing a concomitant hysterectomy [8]. Another important factor that influences women's views is the risk of surgical complications [5,7,8]. The risk of fatal or serious long-term complication can never be absolutely eliminated. However, with a reported mortality rate after laparoscopic hysterectomy of 1:6,814 and after laparoscopic sacrocolpopexy of 1:1,246, the majority of women would be fairly reassured to aim for a concomitant hysterectomy [73]. A third and important factor to be taken into account is the woman's expectations after surgery, with the majority of women expecting a significant improvement in their QoL [5].

Opinion B: Why Uterine Preservation in Pelvic Organ Prolapse Repair?

Why Some Professionals Are Pro Uterine Preservation

Generally, POP occurs secondary to macroscopic or microscopic injuries to the pelvic floor connective tissue (ligaments, endopelvic fascia), musculature (levator ani complex), and/or neural structures. The concept that the uterus plays a negligible role in POP causation has been postulated for decades [74,75]. Based on an anatomic study by DeLancey, the integrity of the endopelvic fascia and of the uterosacral/cardinal ligaments' complex, as the main supporting structure for uterus and vaginal vault, is essential [75]. Indeed, the long-term composite anatomical failure after vaginal hysterectomy, in spite of concomitant uterosacral ligament suspension, occurs in up to 50% of cases [40,76,77]. Moreover, there are studies suggesting that a hysterectomy, performed for other gynaecological reasons, might be a predisposing factor for POP development [77,78].

Pelvic Organ Prolapse Repair Surgical Outcomes

It is postulated that removing the uterus at the time of LSC facilitates the procedure and accessibility. However, when considering the average operative time (between 2–3.5 hours) and mean blood loss (≤250 ml), the differences were not clinically significant between the different LSC variants [46,51,53]. Moreover, in the study by Gagyor et al [51], there was only one (2.3%) postoperative Clavien-Dindo grade ≥2 complication in each of their study groups (LSC with uterine sparing and LSC with concomitant hysterectomy), indicating that the risk of serious complications is low and similar between POP repair, irrespective of how the uterus is managed.

With a TLH+LSC, the opening of the vaginal vault increases the risk of mesh exposure (up to 8%) [79,80]. Moreover, ascending postoperative infections are reported to range from 0.9–4.3% while the risk of any cuff complication varied between 4.7–9.8% depending on type of closure [81].

In case of LSCH+LSC, morcellation of the uterine corpus and/or adnexa is often necessary. As there is always a small risk of unrecognized concomitant precancerous or cancer lesion (Tables 23.1 and 23.2) or sarcoma, a morcellation might contribute to the spread of this disease and impair the prognosis [82,83]. Moreover, there is the added risks of visceral and vascular injuries [84], iatrogenic dissemination of endometriosis (1.4%), adenomyosis (0.5%), and myoma (0.9%) [85]. Therefore, in perimenopausal and postmenopausal age, an endometrial biopsy is highly recommended before surgery with planned morcellation [83].

Furthermore, two large population-based studies found major complication rates after laparoscopic hysterectomy ranging from 4.1–4.3%, while the overall complications proportion was 12.1–15.4% [86,87]. These data may be acceptable in case of a uterine abnormality, however, any complication is difficult to accept or justify when the organ removed was healthy in the first place.

There is still a dearth of literature on pregnancy after hysteropexy and the long-term outcomes. However, the preliminary data are reassuring [88–90].

Pelvic Organ Prolapse Repair Clinical Outcomes

A wide variety of hysteropexy approaches has been described in the literature. Currently, no systematic reviews or guidelines regarding choice of hysteropexy type exist [91]. Interpretation and synthesis of results of various studies on its efficacy is challenging due to the heterogeneity of research methods used to investigate these surgeries.

A meta-analysis of Meriwether et al included nine non-randomized studies concerning abdominal POP surgery with the median follow-up between 12 and 39 months. They found no significant difference between women where the uterus was preserved and the concomitant hysterectomy group in terms of both subjective resolution in POP symptoms and objective success of POP treatment [92]. However, in their meta-analysis, the authors combined both open and laparoscopic approaches and did not differentiate between total and subtotal hysterectomies.

There is a paucity of research regarding the importance of hysterectomy in laparoscopic POP surgery. A limited number of studies comparing laparoscopic sacrocolpopexy with hysterectomy and hysteropexy were published with contradictory conclusions [46,50,51]. Pan et al demonstrated significantly higher subjective satisfaction rate in the concomitant laparoscopic hysterectomy cohort (92.3% versus 100%; p<0.001) after a mean follow-up of 33 months. The POP-Q scores improved significantly in both groups postoperatively. There was no difference in the anatomical cure rate, however, the postoperative PFIQ-7 and PFDI-20 scores were significantly better in the group after hysterectomy. The authors concluded that TLH+LSC offers a higher subjective satisfaction rate and improvement in symptom severity and QoL, while also eliminating the risk of future intervention required for uterine or cervical pathology. Based on their results, the authors recommended that postmenopausal patients and perimenopausal patients who no longer desired fertility should be encouraged to consider concomitant hysterectomy with laparoscopic sacrocolpopexy [46]. However, a more recent prospective study comparing laparoscopic sacrocolpopexy with hysterectomy and LSH did not replicate these results in a longer follow-up (median follow-up 65.3 months). The authors demonstrated comparable long-term results regarding prolapse resolution, functional outcomes, and global patient satisfaction in both procedures [50]. Concurrently, a study by Gagyor et al demonstrated no statistically significant differences in any of the patient reported outcomes (PFDI) at one year after the surgery [51].

Subtotal and total hysterectomies are frequently reported together. A small study comparing LSCH+LSC or TLH+LSC showed no difference in postoperative POP-Q measurements and PFDI-20 results at 12 months after the surgery [93]. On the contrary, three studies with a 12-month follow-up have demonstrated superior subjective and objective success rate after LSCH+LSC versus LSH [51,72,94].

Laparoscopic lateral suspension is a safe and feasible alternative to sacrocolpopexy avoiding difficult dissection of the promontory. A recent retrospective study has shown that the uterine-preserving approach appears to result in better anatomic outcome for the anterior compartment (98.7% versus 94.6%, p=0.02), better subjective outcome (83.5% versus 72.8%, p=0.04), and higher patient satisfaction one year after the surgery [95]. However, this difference could have been due to the differences in the implanted material.

Overall, the efficacy of laparoscopic POP surgery either associated with hysterectomy or uterine preservation is high in most studies. Although some short-term follow-up studies report better outcomes of concomitant hysterectomy [46,94], these were not demonstrated at longer follow-up [50].

Perceived Impact on the Woman's Quality of Life

Management of any urogynaecological symptom involves the assessment of the impact of the disease and the interventions on the woman's QoL. It is highly unlikely that POP would threaten a woman's life [96]. Furthermore, QoL is a highly individual, complex issue. Moreover, the woman has the right to choose which overall QoL variables are important for her and which are less [56].

With the exception of transplantation of the uterus [97,98] or surrogacy [99], hysterectomy terminates any chance for future conception. While this might be acceptable for peri- and postmenopausal women, it can pose a dilemma for women in reproductive age. Nowadays, in several countries around the globe, childbearing is postponed for a variety of reasons [100]. Moreover, it is reported that the relatively higher fragility of partnership is another contributing factor as to why a woman might decide to restart a family in a new relationship [101]. Hence, it is sometimes difficult to exclude the possibility that the woman might change her mind and renew her desire for another baby.

Furthermore, the view of deferring POP surgery until family completion is sometimes unrealistic and unjustifiable, particularly when considering the impact of POP on the woman's QoL, her sexual life, and the burden of the problem in general when taking into account the substantial proportion of her life living with such a problem. Indeed, the youngest patient to undergo hysteropexy was 28 [102].

It is also important to consider that one of the basic pillars of medical ethics is the principle of '*primum non nocere*'. Indeed, 22% of Dutch women reported that the risk of peri- or postoperative complications related to an unnecessary hysterectomy was the main reason why they opted for uterine preservation [103].

Hysterectomy might have a detrimental effect on ovarian and sexual function. A large population study by McPherson et al including more than 11,000 women revealed that at five-years follow-up for dysfunctional uterine bleeding, the rate of psychosexual problems was significantly higher after hysterectomy compared to transcervical endometrial resection [104]. The ORs for hysterectomy (where at least one ovary remained) compared to transcervical endometrial resection were: 1.35 for extreme loss of libido, 1.26 for extreme difficulty in sexual arousal, and 1.51 for vaginal dryness [104]. These results are consistent with another study reporting that up to 37% of women suffered deterioration in their sexual life [16]. Finally, it is increasingly recognized that a certain proportion of women develop depression after hysterectomy for benign condition. In a study by Yen et al [30], the incidence of *de novo* major depressive disorder shortly after hysterectomy was 7.7%. These women also reported worse sexual functions and body image [30].

Risk of Uterine Pathology Later in Life

Based on data from the American Cancer Society, the risk for endometrial cancer within a woman's lifespan is 1/33, while the risk of cervical cancer is 1/159 [105]. The statistical risks of dying from these tumors are 1/159 and 1/455 respectively [105]. Furthermore, these risks can be substantially decreased if women with higher risk are excluded [52].

Moreover, it must be stressed that there are other oncological entities that are equally or even more common and which have worse prognosis compared to uterine cancers, nevertheless, these organs are not *electively* removed during the context of another surgery in low-risk populations. See Table 23.3. Indeed, only 18% from the whole cohort of Dutch women reported favouring a hysterectomy because of the risk of endometrial cancer [103].

Table 23.3 Risk of some malignancies within a woman's lifespan (adapted from the American Cancer Society [105])

Tumour	Risk of diagnosis		Risk of death	
Bladder	1.2 %	1/85	0.4 %	1/286
Breast	12.8 %	1/8	2.6 %	1/39
Colon and rectum	4.1 %	1/25	1.7 %	1/60
Leukaemia	1.3 %	1/78	0.7 %	1/147
Lung and bronchus	6.1 %	1/17	4.5 %	1/22
Pancreas	1.6 %	1/63	1.4 %	1/74

What Are Women's Views about Hysterectomy?

There are only a few studies focusing on women's preferences [5-9,103]. In a survey from the north-east region of the US, 60% of women with POP preferred uterine preservation during POP surgery [5]. Moreover, in the scenario that uterine preservation might show potentially inferior outcome, 46% of these women still opted for uterine-saving operation [5]. In another survey from all four major US regions, 36% of women preferred uterine preservation [6]. This number increased to 46% in cases where uterine preservation showed superior outcome. However, in the reverse scenario, 21% of women still remained in the uterine preservation group [6]. In another study by Wong et al, 31% of Hispanic women, mainly from a low social and educational level, opted for uterine preservation [7].

In Europe, based on the concept that hysteropexy was equally efficient, a Dutch survey found that 43% of all (54% of premenopausal and 37% of postmenopausal) women preferred uterine-saving approaches [103]. Another recent study dealing with impact of cultural background on the opinion of women regarding sparing of the uterus in POP surgery revealed that 40% of German-speaking and 54% of Russian-speaking women preferred uterine sparing. The uterus was more important for sexuality, partnership, and body image in Russian-speaking patients [106].

A multicentric European survey of female gynaecologists [8] found that if postmenopausal, still 37.7% of respondents would choose uterine preservation surgery. Knowledge of the risk of diagnosis of different cancers (Table 23.3) did not change the proportion of women preferring uterine-sparing surgery [8].

It is reported that up to 42% of women feel the uterus is an important contributor to their sense of self [5-9]. In this group, the choice for uterine preservation was reported to be 8.8-fold higher than hysterectomy (44% versus 5%) in a study by Korbly et al [6] and 4.7-fold higher (57.9% versus 22.8%) in a study by Urdzík et al [8].

It has also been shown that a woman who is more actively involved in the decision-making process chooses more frequently uterine preservation surgery ($p=.03$) [5]. These women show better satisfaction with their doctor but also a higher satisfaction with the outcome [107,108]. The active patients feel less severe discomfort ($p=.04$), higher recession of symptoms ($p=.008$), and more significant overall improvement ($p=.04$) [109].

Women with an active approach are usually younger, seek more information, and are generally more likely to accept innovative interventions compared to what is considered old or traditional [110]. FitzGerald et al reported that 79% of women from a urogynaecological population evaluated the new technique as better [111]. Since hysteropexy of any kind can be considered a novelty, it may be better accepted by these women.

Women commonly express apprehension that hysterectomy might impair their emotional status, body image, sense of womanhood, or QOL in general [5,9,112–114]. Mainly women of fertile age feel to be defeminized following hysterectomy [9,28]. A survey by van IJsselmuiden et al [103] revealed that 22% of women chose a uterus-saving approach because they wanted to preserve body completeness as much as possible. Moreover, just 4% of women expect that concomitant hysterectomy at the time of POP surgery might improve their body image versus 18% that presume getting better after uterine-sparing POP surgery [103]. Sexual function seems to be one of the important factors for women when it comes to deciding whether to spare or remove their uterus [5,8,112–114]. Interestingly, only 1/25 women deem that hysterectomy during POP repair might improve their sexuality versus 1/8 after uterine-sparing POP surgery [103].

Conclusion

Pelvic organ prolapse is, still, the most common indication for hysterectomy in postmenopausal women. Techniques involving subtotal or total hysterectomy were historically used most frequently for symptomatic uterine prolapse treatment [115]. In the past decade, increased worldwide interest, advances in the knowledge of pelvic organ support, and development of reconstructive surgical techniques have led to a significant rise in uterine-sparing surgery. Although there is still an ongoing debate whether the uterus should be preserved or removed, the current trend in favour of uterine preservation techniques is obvious [103,116,117]. However, the literature is limited and full of contradictions, making it difficult for clinicians to offer evidence-based advice and for women to make an informed choice [50]. Counselling regarding managing the uterus at the time of POP repair must be individualized for each patient and should include the woman's preferences, clinical efficacy, functional outcome, perioperative morbidity, surgical access, treatment of any concomitant uterine disease, cost, and surgeon's skills [92].

The type of surgery offered, information given, and decision made by the patient largely depend on the view of the professional expert [5,8]. Therefore, it is the doctor´s utmost responsibility to stick with the main ethical principles: respect for autonomy, nonmaleficence, beneficence, and justice. Until now, some surgeons may have not routinely offered uterine preserving POP surgery because of practice patterns, skill, reimbursement, or concern about prolapse recurrence [92]. A study assessing change in practice patterns amongst urogynaecologists reported a significantly positive trend towards uterine preservation surgery over time regardless of gender and volume of surgeries. Nevertheless, overall, uterine preservation surgery was more frequently performed in younger patients, by younger and more experienced surgeons in high-volume hospitals [117].

Many clinicians' views are influenced by traditional beliefs coming from classical prolapse surgery. The introduction of uterine preservation into patient counselling before POP surgery may add another layer of complexity when ensuring that women are provided with suitable options for their POP surgery [92,118]. Women are frequently equipped with easily accessible information from publicly available media resources and expect to be the final decision-makers in this process. Therefore, we concur with the view that the proper urogynaecological approach to the patient is, first and foremost, to respect their autonomy and choices while providing an up-to-date professional account of the problem [56].

Undergoing a hysterectomy is not always an easy decision for many women, especially in the absence of a uterine pathology. Culture, level of education, and social status can play a major role in determining the importance of uterine preservation [6,110]. It has been reported that women with a higher education level were more likely to ask for hysteropexy compared to those with high school education or less. Women with a higher income were more likely to choose uterine preservation. Those who believed the uterus was important for a sense of self were also more likely to opt for uterine preservation [6].

The menopausal status seems to be a significant factor in the decision-making process. Women who were premenopausal were twice as likely to ask for uterine preservation [6]. Sexuality is a highly individual issue, however, generally, post-menopause, its importance in woman's QoL assessment gradually decreases compared to the risk of future malignancy, repeated medical check-ups, repeated surgery due to the failure of the original operation, etc. [120–123].

A survey among women with prolapse seeking medical care conducted by Good et al has shown that 47% of women disagreed with the statement that the uterus was important for sex and most women did not believe that the uterus was important for a sense of self (60%) [9]. The majority also disagreed with the statement that hysterectomy would make them feel less feminine (64%) and that hysterectomy would make them feel less whole (67%) [9]. Hence, a woman's preference about uterine management in POP surgery is based on the interaction of multiple factors that are individually and differently weighted by each woman, making the decision totally unique for her at the time of counselling.

However, in addition to the aforementioned personal factors that contribute to the ultimate decision about uterine sparing or not, one important determinant of such a choice is the quoted clinical and functional outcomes in relation to both surgical alternatives. A survey of preferences regarding hysterectomy for the treatment of uterovaginal prolapse has shown that a majority of all participants would decline a hysterectomy if presented with an equally efficacious POP repair alternative [5]. Another multicentre, cross-sectional study found that a higher proportion of women with prolapse symptoms examined for urogynaecologic evaluation preferred uterine preservation (36% versus 20%) assuming comparable efficacy. A more recent survey study from the Netherlands has also shown that, assuming functional and anatomical outcomes after hysterectomy and uterus-preserving surgery were equal, more women expressed preference for uterus preservation compared to hysterectomy (43% versus 27%) [103]. On the contrary, if concomitant hysterectomy was deemed superior, the decrease in persistent preference of uterine preservation was 40% in the general population

[6]. Furthermore, this decrease (the conversion from originally pro uterus approach to pro hysterectomy approach) was more than 80% if the patient herself was a female gynaecologist [8]. Thus, in this scenario, finally, only 8.8% of female gynaecologists still opted for uterine-sparing surgery [8]. Therefore, it is imperative to focus on the refinement of surgical technique in order to increase the efficiency of uterine-saving POP reconstruction procedures.

It is our duty as healthcare providers in general and urogynaecologists in particular to ensure that this information is provided in a clear, equitable, and non-biased way ensuring that lack of evidence of effectiveness does not equate to evidence of ineffectiveness.

Traditionally, severe uterine prolapse was treated by removal of the uterus with concomitant pelvic reconstruction. However, the evolution in anatomical knowledge and surgical techniques makes the need for hysterectomy at least questionable [117]. The final decision may depend on multiple factors, e.g. patient preference, female autonomy, desire to preserve uterus, sexuality, expert opinions, hospital factors, risks of surgical complication, and risks of malignancy [110]. Women nowadays are increasingly more likely to opt for uterus-preserving POP surgery [6,8,103]. Nonetheless, uterine preservation techniques are not suitable for all women and contraindications are to be respected.

Box 23.1 Suggested Points to Consider and Discuss with Women at the Time of Pelvic Organ Prolapse Surgery Counselling

1. Is the uterus important for the woman's sense of self or for sexuality?
2. Is she considering pregnancy/would she be happy with permanent sterilization?
3. Is menstruation desired/troublesome to her?
4. Is she afraid of hysterectomy adverse outcome?
5. What is the woman's general level of psychological well-being?
6. Is the statistical prevalence of concomitant/future premalignant or malignant uterine disease acceptable when compared to other cancer risks?
7. If premenopausal, is the risk of future menstrual disorders acceptable?
8. In case of (future) hormonal substitution would she prefer oestrogen replacement treatment (ERT) (as opposed to hormonal replacement treatment (HRT) or none)?
9. Is the continuation of routine screening acceptable?
10. Are there any contraindications of uterine preservation?

References

1. Barnes Z. You Don't Need a Uterus to Be a Woman. Self – Sexual & Reproductive Health. Available from: Published 2018. www.self.com/story/being-a-woman-uterus [last accessed 2 November 2021].
2. Solbrække KN, Bondevik H. Absent organs—present selves: exploring embodiment and gender identity in young Norwegian women's accounts of hysterectomy. Int J Qual Stud Health Wellbeing 2015; 10(1): 26720.
3. Marván ML, Catillo-López RL, Ehrenzweig Y, Palacios P. Psychological meaning of a woman with a hysterectomy among Mexican physicians and women. Women Health 2012; 52(7): 658–78.
4. Marván ML, Quiros V, López-Vázquez E, Ehrenzweig Y. Mexican beliefs and attitudes toward hysterectomy and gender-role ideology in marriage. Health Care Women Int 2012; 33(6): 511–24.
5. Frick AC, Barber MD, Paraiso MFR, et al. Attitudes toward hysterectomy in women undergoing evaluation for uterovaginal prolapse. Female Pelvic Med Reconstr Surg 2013; 19(2): 103–9.
6. Korbly NB, Kassis NC, Good MM, et al. Patient preferences for uterine preservation and hysterectomy in women with pelvic organ prolapse. Am J Obstet Gynecol 2013; 209(5): 470.e471–470. e476.
7. Wong K, Jakus-Waldman S, Yazdany T. Patient beliefs regarding hysterectomy in women seeking surgery for pelvic organ prolapse: findings in a predominantly Hispanic population. Female Pelvic Med Reconstr Surg 2014; 20(5): 267–71.
8. Urdzík P, Kalis V, Blaganje M, et al. Pelvic organ prolapse and uterine preservation: a survey of female gynecologists (POP-UP survey). BMC Women's Health. 2020; 20(1): 241.
9. Good MM, Korbly N, Kassis NC, et al. Prolapse-related knowledge and attitudes toward the uterus in women with pelvic organ prolapse symptoms. Am J Obstet Gynecol 2013; 209(5): 481. e481–481. e486.
10. Barber MD, Visco AG, Wyman JF, et al. Sexual function in women with urinary incontinence and pelvic organ prolapse. Obstet Gynecol 2002; 99(2): 281–9.
11. Darling CA, McKoy Smith YM. Understanding hysterectomies: sexual satisfaction and quality of life. J Sex Res 1993; 30(4): 324–35.
12. Farrell SA, Kieser K. Sexuality after hysterectomy. Obstet Gynecol 2000; 95(6): 1045–51.
13. Hasson HM. Cervical removal at hysterectomy for benign disease. Risks and benefits. J Reprod Med 1993; 38: 781–90.
14. O'Brien PS, Ismail KM. History of premenstrual disorders. The Premenstrual Syndromes: PMS and PMDD. Informa Healthcare: 2007; 1–8.
15. Thakar R. Is the uterus a sexual organ? Sexual function following hysterectomy. Sexual Med Rev 2015; 3(4): 264–78.
16. Alexander DA, Naji AA, Pinion SB, et al. Randomised trial comparing hysterectomy with endometrial ablation for dysfunctional uterine bleeding: psychiatric and psychosocial aspects. BMJ 1996; 312(7026): 280–4.
17. Hehenkamp WJ, Volkers NA, Bartholomeus W, et al. Sexuality and body image after uterine artery embolization and hysterectomy in the treatment of uterine fibroids: a randomized comparison. Cardiovasc Intervent Radiol 2007; 30 (5): 866–75.
18. Thakar R. Dispelling the myth—does hysterectomy cause pelvic organ dysfunction? BJOG 2004; 111: 20–3.
19. Espuña M, Puig M, Carmona F. De novo dyspareunia after pelvic organ prolapse surgery. Gynecol Surg 2010; 7(3): 217–25.
20. Polat M, Kahramanoglu I, Senol T, et al. Comparison of the effect of laparoscopic and abdominal hysterectomy on lower urinary tract function, vaginal length, and dyspareunia: a randomized clinical trial. J Laparoendosc Adv Surg Tech 2016; 26 (2): 116–21.

21. Bradford A, Meston C. Sexual outcomes and satisfaction with hysterectomy: influence of patient education. J Sex Med 2007; 4(1): 106–14.
22. Sadovsky R, Basson R, Krychman M, et al. Cancer and sexual problems. J Sex Med 2010; 7(1): 349–73.
23. Shatkin-Margolis A, Pauls RN. Sexual function after prolapse repair. Curr Opin Obstet Gynecol 2017; 29(5): 343–8.
24. Pons ME. Sexual health in women with pelvic floor disorders: measuring the sexual activity and function with questionnaires—a summary. Int Urogynecol J 2009; 20(1): 65–71.
25. Oldenhave A, Jaszmann LJ, Everaerd WTA, Haspels AA. Hysterectomized women with ovarian conservation report more severe climacteric complaints than do normal climacteric women of similar age. Am J Obstet Gynecol 1993; 168(3): 765–71.
26. Moorman PG, Myers ER, Schildkraut JM, et al. Effect of hysterectomy with ovarian preservation on ovarian function. Obstet Gynecol 2011; 118(6): 1271.
27. Farquhar CM, Sadler L, Harvey SA, Stewart AW. The association of hysterectomy and menopause: a prospective cohort study. BJOG 2005; 112(7): 956–62.
28. Rannestad T. Hysterectomy: effects on quality of life and psychological aspects. Best Pract Res Clin Obstet Gynaecol 2005; 19(3): 419–30.
29. Trabuco EC, Moorman PG, Algeciras-Schimnich A, Weaver AL, Cliby WA. Association of ovary-sparing hysterectomy with ovarian reserve. Obstet Gynecol 2016; 127(5): 819.
30. Yen J-Y, Chen Y-H, Long C-Y, et al. Risk factors for major depressive disorder and the psychological impact of hysterectomy: a prospective investigation. Psychosomatics 2008; 49(2): 137–42.
31. Anastasiadis P, Koutlaki N, Skaphida P, et al. Endometrial polyps: prevalence, detection, and malignant potential in women with abnormal uterine bleeding. Eur J Gynaecol Oncol 2000; 21(2): 180–3.
32. Dreisler E, Stampe Sorensen S, Ibsen P, Lose G. Prevalence of endometrial polyps and abnormal uterine bleeding in a Danish population aged 20–74 years. Ultrasound Obstet Gynecol 2009; 33(1): 102–8.
33. Astrup K, Olivarius NdF. Frequency of spontaneously occurring postmenopausal bleeding in the general population. Acta Obstet Gynecol Scandi 2004; 83(2): 203–7.
34. Sheikh MA, Althouse AD, Freese KE, et al. USA endometrial cancer projections to 2030: should we be concerned? Future Oncol 2014; 10(16): 2561–8.
35. Begum J, Samal R. A clinicopathological evaluation of postmenopausal bleeding and its correlation with risk factors for developing endometrial hyperplasia and cancer: a hospital-based prospective study. J Mid-life Health 2019; 10(4): 179.
36. Maher CM, Feiner B, Baessler K, Glazener CM. Surgical management of pelvic organ prolapse in women: the updated summary version Cochrane review. Int Urogynecol J 2011; 22(11): 1445.
37. Abdullah B, Khong SY, Tan PC. Oestrogen-soaked vaginal packing for decubitus ulcer in advanced pelvic organ prolapse: a case series. Int Urogynecol J 2016; 27(7): 1057–62.
38. Awale R, Isaacs R, Singh S, Mandrelle K. Uterine prolapse: should hysterectomy specimens be subjected for histopathological examination? J Mid-life Health 2017; 8(4): 179.
39. Deshpande HG, Madkar CS, Kiwalkar SR. Relationship of decubitus ulcer on cervix in pelvic organ prolapse with pop-q staging. J Obstet Gynecol India 2019; 69(3): 266–71.
40. Schulten SF, Detollenaere RJ, Stekelenburg J, et al. Sacrospinous hysteropexy versus vaginal hysterectomy with uterosacral ligament suspension in women with uterine prolapse stage 2 or higher: observational follow-up of a multicentre randomised trial. BMJ 2019; 366: l5149.
41. Dallas K, Elliott CS, Syan R et al. Association between concomitant hysterectomy and repeat surgery for pelvic organ prolapse repair in a cohort of nearly 100,000 women. Obstet Gynecol 2018; 132(6): 1328–36.
42. Dällenbach P, Kaelin-Gambirasio I, Dubuisson J-B, Boulvain M. Risk factors for pelvic organ prolapse repair after hysterectomy. Obstet Gynecol 2007; 110(3): 625–32.
43. Nosti PA, Gutman RE, Iglesia CB, et al. Defining cervical elongation: a prospective observational study. J Obstet Gynaecol Canada 2017; 39(4): 223–8.
44. Mothes AR, Mothes H, Fröber R, Radosa MP, Runnebaum IB. Systematic classification of uterine cervical elongation in patients with pelvic organ prolapse. Eur J Obstet Gynecol Reprod Biol 2016; 200: 40–4.
45. Hsiao S-M, Chang T-C, Chen C-H, et al. Risk factors for coexistence of cervical elongation in uterine prolapse. Eur J Obstet Gynecol Reprod Biol 2018; 229: 94–7.
46. Pan K, Cao L, Ryan NA, Wang Y, Xu H. Laparoscopic sacral hysteropexy versus laparoscopic sacrocolpopexy with hysterectomy for pelvic organ prolapse. Int Urogynecol J 2016; 27(1): 93–101.
47. Stepanian AA, Miklos JR, Moore RD, Mattox TF. Risk of mesh extrusion and other mesh-related complications after laparoscopic sacral colpopexy with or without concurrent laparoscopic-assisted vaginal hysterectomy: experience of 402 patients. J Minim Invasive Gynecol 2008; 15(2): 188–96.
48. Ganatra AM, Rozet F, Sanchez-Salas R, et al. The current status of laparoscopic sacrocolpopexy: a review. Eur Urol 2009; 55(5): 1089–105.
49. Costantini E, Porena M, Lazzeri M, et al. Changes in female sexual function after pelvic organ prolapse repair: role of hysterectomy. Int Urogynecol J 2013; 24(9): 1481–7.
50. Illiano E, Giannitsas K, Costantini E. Comparison between laparoscopic sacrocolpopexy with hysterectomy and hysteropexy in advanced urogenital prolapse. Int Urogynecol J 2020; 5: 1–6.
51. Gagyor D, Kalis V, Smazinka M, et al. Pelvic organ prolapse and uterine preservation: a case control study (POP-UP study). BMC Womens Health 2021; 21(1): 72.
52. Gutman RE. Does the uterus need to be removed to correct uterovaginal prolapse? Curr Opin Obstet Gynecol 2016; 28(5): 435–40.
53. Bedford ND, Seman EI, O'Shea RT, Keirse MJ. Effect of uterine preservation on outcome of laparoscopic uterosacral suspension. J Minim Invasive Gynecol 2013; 20(2): 172–7.
54. Rosen DM, Shukla A, Cario GM, Carlton MA, Chou D. Is hysterectomy necessary for laparoscopic pelvic floor repair? A prospective study. J Minim Invasive Gynecol 2008; 15(6): 729–34.
55. Kalis V, Rusavy Z, Ismail KM. Laparoscopic sacrohysteropexy: the Pilsner modification. Int Urogynecol J 2020; 31(6): 1277–80.

56. American College of Obstetricians and Gynecologists. ACOG Committee Opinion. Surgery and patient choice: the ethics of decision making. Obstet Gynecol 2003; 102(5 Pt 1): 1101.
57. Settnes A, Topsoee MF, Moeller C, et al. Reduced complications following implementation of laparoscopic hysterectomy: a danish population-based cohort study of minimally invasive benign gynecologic surgery between 2004 and 2018. J Minim Invasive Gynecol 2019; 27(6): 1344–53.
58. Kuppermann M, Varner RE, Summitt Jr RL, et al. Effect of hysterectomy vs medical treatment on health-related quality of life and sexual functioning: the medicine or surgery (Ms) randomized trial. JAMA 291(12): 1447–55.
59. Thakar R, Ayers S, Clarkson P, Stanton S, Manyonda I. Outcomes after total versus subtotal abdominal hysterectomy. New Engl J Med 2002; 347(17): 1318–25.
60. Thakar R, Ayers S, Georgakapolou A, et al. Hysterectomy improves quality of life and decreases psychiatric symptoms: a prospective and randomised comparison of total versus subtotal hysterectomy. BJOG 2004; 111(10): 1115–20.
61. Flory N, Bissonnette F, Amsel RT, Binik YM. The psychosocial outcomes of total and subtotal hysterectomy: a randomized controlled trial. J Sex Med 2006; 3(3): 483–91.
62. Darwish M, Atlantis E, Mohamed-Taysir T. Psychological outcomes after hysterectomy for benign conditions: a systematic review and meta-analysis. Eur J Obstet Gynecol Reprod Biol 2014; 174: 5–19.
63. Genc M, Celik E, Eskicioglu F, et al. The relationship between uterine prolapse and premalignant endometrial pathology. Clin Exp Obstet Gynecol 2016; 43 (4): 500–3.
64. Wan OY, Cheung RY, Chan SS, Chung TK. Risk of malignancy in women who underwent hysterectomy for uterine prolapse. Austr N Z J Obstet Gynaecol 2013; 53(2): 190–6.
65. Frick AC, Walters MD, Larkin KS, Barber MD. Risk of unanticipated abnormal gynecologic pathology at the time of hysterectomy for uterovaginal prolapse. Am J Obstet Gynecol 2010; 202(5): 507.e501–507. e504.
66. Grigoriadis T, Valla A, Zacharakis D, Protopapas A, Athanasiou S. Vaginal hysterectomy for uterovaginal prolapse: what is the incidence of concurrent gynecological malignancy? Int Urogynecol J 2015; 26(3): 421–5.
67. Mizrachi Y, Tannus S, Bar J, et al. Unexpected significant uterine pathological findings at vaginal hysterectomy despite unremarkable preoperative workup. IMAJ 2017; 19(10): 631.
68. Ackenbom MF, Giugale LE, Wang Y, Shepherd JP. Incidence of occult uterine pathology in women undergoing hysterectomy with pelvic organ prolapse repair. Female Pelvic Med Reconstr Surg 2016; 22(5): 332–5.
69. Andy UU, Nosti PA, Kane S, et al. Incidence of unanticipated uterine pathology at the time of minimally invasive abdominal sacrocolpopexy. J Minim Invasive Gynecol 2014; 21(1): 97–100.
70. Ramm O, Gleason JL, Segal S, Antosh DD, Kenton KS. Utility of preoperative endometrial assessment in asymptomatic women undergoing hysterectomy for pelvic floor dysfunction. Int Urogynecol J 2012; 23(7): 913–17. https://doi.org/10.1007/s00192-012-1694-2
71. Renganathan A, Edwards R, Duckett JR. Uterus conserving prolapse surgery what is the chance of missing a malignancy? Int Urogynecol J 2010; 21(7): 819–21. https://doi.org/10.1007/s00192-010-1101-9
72. Saliba E, Nisolle M, Tchente C, De Landsheere L. Do we need to perform systematic supracervical hysterectomy during laparoscopic sacrocolpopexy? Gynecologie, obstetrique, fertilite & senologie 2019; 47(7–8): 549–54. https://doi.org/10.1016/j.gofs.2019.04.007
73. Behbehani S, Suarez-Salvador E, Buras M, Magtibay P, Magrina J. Mortality rates in benign laparoscopic and robotic gynecologic surgery: a systematic review and meta-analysis. J Minim Invasive Gynecol 2020; 27(3): 603–12.e601. https://doi.org/10.1016/j.jmig.2019.10.005
74. Bonney V. The principles that should underlie all operations for prolapse. BJOG 1934; 41(5): 669–83.
75. DeLancey JO. Anatomic aspects of vaginal eversion after hysterectomy. Am J Obstet Gynecol 1992; 166(6): 1717–28.
76. Blandon RE, Bharucha AE, Melton III LJ et al. Incidence of pelvic floor repair after hysterectomy: a population-based cohort study. Am J Obstet Gynecol 2007;197(6): 664.e661–664. e667.
77. Forsgren C, Lundholm C, Johansson AL, et al. Vaginal hysterectomy and risk of pelvic organ prolapse and stress urinary incontinence surgery. Int Urogynecol J 2012; 23(1): 43–8. https://doi.org/10.1007/s00192-011-1523-z
78. Blandon RE, Bharucha AE, Melton LJ, et al. Risk factors for pelvic floor repair after hysterectomy. Obstet Gynecol 2009; 113(3): 601–8. https://doi.org/10.1097/AOG.0b013e3181998998
79. Wu JM, Wells EC, Hundley AF, et al. Mesh erosion in abdominal sacral colpopexy with and without concomitant hysterectomy. Am J Obstet Gynecol 2006; 194(5): 1418–22.
80. Costantini E, Mearini L, Bini V, et al. Uterus preservation in surgical correction of urogenital prolapse. Eur Urol 2005; 48(4): 642–9.
81. Uccella S, Malzoni M, Cromi A, et al. Laparoscopic vs transvaginal cuff closure after total laparoscopic hysterectomy: a randomized trial by the Italian Society of Gynecologic Endoscopy. Am J Obstet Gynecol 2018; 218(5): 500.e501–500.e513
82. Halaska MJ, Haidopoulos D, Guyon F, et al. European society of gynecological oncology statement on fibroid and uterine morcellation. Int J Gynecol Cancer 2017; 27(1): 189–92.
83. Halaska MJ, Gracia M, Laky R, Zapardiel I. Morcellation of the uterus: is there any place? Curr Oncol Rep 2020; 22(7): 68.
84. Milad MP, Milad EA. Laparoscopic morcellator-related complications. J Minim Invasive Gynecol 2014; 21(3): 486–91.
85. Tulandi T, Leung A, Jan N. Nonmalignant sequelae of unconfined morcellation at laparoscopic hysterectomy or myomectomy. J Minim Invasive Gynecol 2016; 23(3): 331–7.
86. Settnes A, Moeller C, Topsoee MF, et al. Complications after benign hysterectomy, according to procedure: a population-based prospective cohort study from the Danish hysterectomy database, 2004–2015. BJOG 2020; 127(10): 1269–79.
87. Brummer TH, Jalkanen J, Fraser J, et al. FINHYST, a prospective study of 5279 hysterectomies: complications and their risk factors. Hum Reprod 2011; 26(7): 1741–51. https://doi.org/10.1093/humrep/der116
88. Jefferis H, Price N, Jackson S. Pregnancy following laparoscopic hysteropexy-a case series. Gynecol Surg 2017; 14(1): 16. https://doi.org/10.1186/s10397-017-1017-1
89. Pandeva I, Mistry M, Fayyad A. Efficacy and pregnancy outcomes of laparoscopic single sheet mesh sacrohysteropexy. Neurourol 2017; 36(3): 787–93. https://doi.org/10.1002/nau.23026
90. Adegoke TM, Vragovic O, Yarrington CD, Larrieux JR. Effect of pregnancy on uterine-sparing pelvic organ prolapse repair.

Int Urogynecol J 2020; 31(3): 657–62. https://doi.org/10.1007/s00192-019-04179-2

91. Meriwether KV, Balk EM, Antosh DD, et al. Uterine-preserving surgeries for the repair of pelvic organ prolapse: a systematic review with meta-analysis and clinical practice guidelines. Int Urogynecol J 2019; 30(4): 505–22.
92. Meriwether KV, Antosh DD, Olivera CK, et al. Uterine preservation vs hysterectomy in pelvic organ prolapse surgery: a systematic review with meta-analysis and clinical practice guidelines. Am J Obstet Gynecol 2018; 219(2): 129–46. e122.
93. Ko YC, Yoo E-H, Han GH, Kim Y-M. Comparison of sexual function between sacrocolpopexy and sacrocervicopexy. Obstet Gynecol Sci 2017; 60(2): 207–12.
94. Gracia M, Perelló M, Bataller E, et al. Comparison between laparoscopic sacral hysteropexy and subtotal hysterectomy plus cervicopexy in pelvic organ prolapse: a pilot study. Neurourol 2015; 34(7): 654–8.
95. Veit-Rubin N, Dubuisson J, Constantin F, et al. Uterus preservation is superior to hysterectomy when performing laparoscopic lateral suspension with mesh. Int Urogynecol J 2019; 30(4): 557–64.
96. Lucassen EA, la Chapelle CF, Krouwel E, Groeneveld M. Renal failure caused by severe pelvic organ prolapse. BMJ Case Rep 2019; 12(7): e229318.
97. Flyckt R, Falcone T, Quintini C, et al. First birth from a deceased donor uterus in the United States: from severe graft rejection to successful cesarean delivery. Am J Obstet Gynecol 2020; 223(2): 143–51.
98. Brännström M, Dahm-Kähler P, Kvarnström N,et al. Live birth after robotic-assisted live donor uterus transplantation. Acta Obstet Gynecol Scand 2020; 99(9): 1222–9.
99. Phillips AM, Magann EF, Whittington JR, Whitcombe DD, Sandlin AT. Surrogacy and pregnancy. Obstet Gynecol Surv 2019; 74(9): 539–45. https://doi.org/10.1097/ogx.0000000000000703
100. Mills M, Rindfuss RR, McDonald P, Te Velde E. Why do people postpone parenthood? Reasons and social policy incentives. Hum Reprod Update 2011; 17(6): 848–60.
101. Eurostat. (2020). Marriage and divorce statistics. Available from: https://ec.europa.eu/eurostat/statistics-explained/index.php/Marriage_and_divorce_statistics#Fewer_marriages.2C_more_divorce [last accessed 2 November 2021].
102. Kalis V, Smazinka M, Rusavy Z, et al. Laparoscopic sacrocolpopexy as the mainstay management for significant apical pelvic organ prolapse (LAP) study. Eur J Obstet Gynecol Reprod Biol 2020; 244: 60–5. https://doi.org/10.1016/j.ejogrb.2019.10.049
103. Van IJsselmuiden MN, Detollenaere RJ, Gerritse MB et al. Dutch women's attitudes towards hysterectomy and uterus preservation in surgical treatment of pelvic organ prolapse. Eur J Obstet Gynecol Reprod Biol 2018; 220: 79–83.
104. McPherson K, Herbert A, Judge A, et al. Psychosexual health 5 years after hysterectomy: population-based comparison with endometrial ablation for dysfunctional uterine bleeding. Health Expect 2005; 8(3): 234–43.
105. Society TAC. (2020). Lifetime Risk of Developing or Dying from Cancer. Available from: www.cancer.org/cancer/cancer-basics/lifetime-probability-of-developing-or-dying-from-cancer.html [last accessed 2 November 2021].
106. Lyatoshinsky P, Fünfgeld C, Popov A, et al. Pelvic organ prolapse patients' attitudes and preferences regarding their uterus: comparing German- and Russian-speaking women. Int Urogynecol J 2019; 30(12): 2077–83. https://doi.org/10.1007/s00192-019-03918-9
107. Joosten EA, DeFuentes-Merillas L, de Weert GH, et al. Systematic review of the effects of shared decision-making on patient satisfaction, treatment adherence and health status. PsychotherPsychosom 2008; 77(4): 219–26. https://doi.org/10.1159/000126073
108. Truglio-Londrigan M, Slyer JT, Singleton JK, Worral P. A qualitative systematic review of internal and external influences on shared decision-making in all health care settings. JBI Libr Syst Rev 2012; 10(58): 4633–46. https://doi.org/10.11124/jbisrir-2012-432
109. Brody DS, Miller SM, Lerman CE, Smith DG, Caputo GC. Patient perception of involvement in medical care: relationship to illness attitudes and outcomes. J Gen Intern Med 1989; 4(6): 506–11. https://doi.org/10.1007/bf02599549
110. Anglim B, O'Sullivan O, O'Reilly B. How do patients and surgeons decide on uterine preservation or hysterectomy in apical prolapse? Int Urogynecol J 2018; 29(8): 1075–9.
111. FitzGerald MP, Elliott C, Brubaker L. New vs old: descriptors can affect patients' surgical preferences. Am J Obstet Gynecol 2008; 199(5): 476.e471–473. https://doi.org/10.1016/j.ajog.2008.03.055
112. Flory N, Bissonnette F, Binik YM. Psychosocial effects of hysterectomy: literature review. J Psychosom Res 2005; 59(3): 117–29.
113. Bachmann GA. Psychosexual aspects of hysterectomy. Women's Health Issues 1990; 1(1): 41–9.
114. Sloan D. The emotional and psychosexual aspects of hysterectomy. Am J Obstet Gynecol 1978; 131(6): 598–605.
115. Wilcox LS, Koonin LM, Pokras R, et al. Hysterectomy in the United States, 1988–1990. Obstet Gynecol 1994; 83(4): 549–55.
116. Khan AA, Eilber KS, Clemens JQ, et al. Trends in management of pelvic organ prolapse among female Medicare beneficiaries. Am J Obstet Gynecol 2015; 212(4): 463.e461–463.e468.
117. Lin Y-L, Lo T-S, Long C-Y, et al. Time-frame comparison of hystero-preservation in the surgical treatment of uterine prolapse: a population-based nation-wide follow-up descriptive study, 2006–2013 versus 1997–2005. Int Urogynecol J 2020; 31(9): 1839–50.
118. Greene KA, Wyman AM, Scott LA, et al. Evaluation of patient preparedness for surgery: a randomized controlled trial. Am J Obstet Gynecol 2017; 217(2): 179.e171–179. e177.
119. Lowenstein L, Gamble T, Sanses TV, et al. Changes in sexual function after treatment for prolapse are related to the improvement in body image perception. J Sex Med 2010; 7(2): 1023–8.
120. Thornton K, Chervenak J, Neal-Perry G. Menopause and sexuality. Endocrinol Metab Clin North Am 2015; 44(3): 649–61.
121. Hoffe S, Balducci L. Cancer and age: general considerations. Clin Geriatr Med 2012; 28(1): 1–18.
122. Brijoux T, Woopen C, Zank S. Multimorbidity in old age and its impact on life results. Z Gerontol Geriatr 2021; 54(Suppl 2): 108–13.
123. de S Santos Machado V, Valadares AL, Costa-Paiva LH, et al. Aging, obesity, and multimorbidity in women 50 years or older: a population-based study. Menopause 2013; 20(8): 818–24.

Chapter 24

Laparoscopic Hysterectomy: Total or Subtotal Debate

Kim WM van Delft, Steven ES Koops

Introduction

The total hysterectomy via laparotomy has been performed for centuries. The first subtotal hysterectomy, leaving the cervix in situ, was described in 1843 by Charles Clay. Gynaecological surgeons sometimes prefer this method as some believe that it may have a positive impact on pelvic floor functions.

In 1989, the total laparoscopic hysterectomy was firstly introduced [1], with the main advantage of shorter hospital stay, quicker recovery, and better cosmetic results; however laparoscopic hysterectomy took longer to perform [2]. Initially, the complication rate was higher when comparing laparoscopic hysterectomy with abdominal hysterectomy [2]. However, recent literature revealed a lower complication rate of laparoscopic hysterectomy in experienced hands 0.5–1.7% [3,4,5,6], and less readmissions due to adhesions [7].

Learning Curve for Laparoscopic Hysterectomy

A learning curve of about 25 cases of laparoscopic hysterectomy was found for gynaecological surgeons with large laparoscopic experience [2,8]. A suggestion of a mentorship programme, including tailor-made learning moments, has been developed to teach the surgical procedure [8]. Two large Finnish cohort studies also found that with an increase of surgical experience and a national learning curve, the number of complications decreased [4,6]. After reviewing all literature, Aarts et al in their Cochrane review concluded that there is no clear number of laparoscopic hysterectomy procedures one must have performed, before having passed the learning curve phase [9].

A retrospective single centre study among two gynaecological surgeons analysed the learning curve effect and found a plateau was reached after the first 75 cases [10]. This resulted in a significant reduction of operating time (76 minutes versus 69 minutes), and non-significant reduction in complication rate (8% to 4.7%) [10]. The authors suggest that this additional number needed for the learning curve and the somewhat larger percentage of complications could be due to more difficult cases, i.e. larger uteri and higher BMI [10]. In 2002, a learning curve study including analysis of complications in 1,647 cases, revealed a lower complication rate with increasing laparoscopic experience [11].

Current Indication Laparoscopic Hysterectomy

Laparoscopic hysterectomy is nowadays indicated for benign cases after failed conservative therapy, such as cases of menstrual bleeding disorders, uterine myomas, adenomyosis, and endometrial hyperplasia. Furthermore, another requirement to choose for laparoscopic hysterectomy is when vaginal hysterectomy is not expected to be successful due to intra-abdominal adhesions, a large uterus, or insufficient uterine descent on preoperative clinical examination [12].

The first laparoscopic subtotal hysterectomy was described in 1991 by Semm [13]. In 2014, the AAGL presented a concise report on the impact of laparoscopic subtotal versus total hysterectomy on complications and pelvic floor dysfunction, concluding that there was not much good quality data at that point in time [14]. These days, practice patterns still vary among gynaecological surgeons. However, to be able to make reliable comparisons between surgeons and surgical procedures, it is important to perform case-mix correction and to use uniform outcome definitions [15].

A Cochrane review analysed nine randomized controlled trials (RCTs) with a total of 1,553 women to compare subtotal versus total hysterectomy [16]. Their conclusions are based on abdominal procedures, as the quality of the laparoscopic research studies was not strong enough to give reliable recommendations [16]. The authors found no evidence on urinary, bowel, or sexual function between abdominal total and subtotal hysterectomy in the short- and long-term (up to nine years post-surgery) [16]. Only perioperative data differed significantly; there were no clinically relevant differences in peri-operative data [16].

This chapter will describe the techniques of total and subtotal laparoscopic hysterectomy as well as the possible complications of both procedures. Furthermore, the impact of retaining the cervix on pelvic floor dysfunction will be covered, such as pelvic organ prolapse, urinary problems, defaecatory problems, and sexual function.

Surgery

Positioning

Prior to booking of a laparoscopic hysterectomy, women should provide informed consent, after receiving counselling about the risks of the procedure. In the operating theatre, the time-out procedure is performed with the entire team, prior to induction. Women receive a single dose of antibiotics prior to incision. The patient is placed in dorsal lithotomy position under general anaesthesia, intubated, and often with a nasogastric tube, according to local protocol. The arms are arranged alongside the body, and are well protected, which enables the gynaecological surgeon to stand close to the operating table. For the usage of extreme Trendelenburg, to be able to move the bowels out of Douglas, the patient is placed on an anti-slip mattress, to prevent sliding downwards during the procedure. An alternative could be shoulder support; however, pressure could become too much, with possible neurological and/or musculoskeletal injuries as a consequence. With the use of a good anti-slip mattress the shoulder supports can be avoided, even for extreme Trendelenburg position.

The patient is then placed at the edge of the table, lying on the tip of the os coccyx. The legs will be put in stirrups, semi-flexed. Desinfection occurs according to local protocol, both vagina and abdomen. A transurethral catheter, as well as a uterine manipulator, are placed.

Trocars

The position of the trocars is dependent on the gynaecological surgeon's preferences and the size of the uterus. Usually, the camera is placed in a subumbilical port. However, if the uterus is large, or if the distance between symphysis and umbilic is short, a trocar can be placed in the midline between xiphoid and umbilicus for the laparoscopic camera.

Once entry to the abdominal cavity is obtained, and the ports are placed, the gynaecological surgeon assesses the entire abdomen, including upper abdominal cavity. The uterus and ovaries are inspected to judge access, mobility, and the possibility to successfully remove the uterus (and possibly tubes and ovaries) per laparoscope.

Subsequently, two lateral ports are placed under direct vision, on either side lateral of the arteria epigastrica inferior, at least 6 cm lateral to the midline. They should be placed medial and superior to the anterior superior iliac spine to avoid the ilioinguinal and iliohypogastric nerves that run along the lateral border of the psoas muscle. A third accessory port is then placed in the midline, slightly higher than both lateral ports, to create as much workspace as possible. Care must be taken that the distance between the camera and the accessory ports is at least 8 cm.

The size of the ports depends on the instruments available.

Uterus Manipulator

Using a uterus manipulator will help greatly to visualize and mobilize the different structures near the uterus. Correct use of a manipulator will help to expose the tissues, and to have the operating trocars free during the procedure to work on the removal of the uterus:

- Mobilization of the uterus towards anteversion, retroversion, lateral, inside
- Visualization of the vaginal fornices and keeping them away from the ureter
- Sealing of the pelvic abdomen while opening the vagina
- Visualization of the vaginal cuff and sealing of the pelvic abdomen while closing the vagina

The more difficult the hysterectomy is, the more beneficial a uterus manipulator will be. There are a variety of uterus manipulators available; most of them have different sizes depending on the measurement of the uterine cavity and the cervix. Very sophisticated uterine manipulators can be steered by voice, implying that they are expensive. But most are handled by the bed-side assistant.

Technique of Laparoscopic Total Hysterectomy

Round Ligaments

The procedure usually starts with coagulation and division of the round ligaments on either side of the uterus. To do so, the surgeon grasps the round ligament at one-third of the uterine side and creates traction towards the pelvic side wall and upwards. The uterus is moved, with the aid of a uterus manipulator, to the opposite direction to create workspace. The round ligament is coagulated using bipolar forceps and cut through. The anterior and posterior peritoneal layers of the broad ligament will become visible. The surgeon will work on the uterine side to make his way towards the bladder by undermining, coagulating if necessary, and cutting the anterior peritoneal layer of the broad ligament very superficially. The undermining process can be performed by placing two instruments in the pouch under the anterior peritoneal layer and by spreading the instruments towards ventral and caudal. The intra-abdominal CO_2, together with the traction, will open up the space. The same procedure is carried out at the other side, after moving the uterus to the other direction. The dissection stops around 1 cm from the midline.

Vesico-uterine Pouch

The uterus will be pushed upwards and retroverted. The first assistant will grasp the pre-vesical peritoneum and the uterine serosa and move the grasped structures towards ventral. By using the scissors to cut strictly perpendicular to the uterus, the bladder will be dissected from the uterus, avoiding a bladder lesion. After the first incision, the plane of the vesicovaginal dissection is reached, following which blunt dissection of the bladder is carried out towards the base of the bladder. If necessary, bladder pillars are coagulated separately. Extra caution should be warranted if the patient has had a caesarean section in the past.

Broad Ligaments

After careful dissection of the bladder, the posterior part of the broad ligament can be fenestrated on either side, by moving the uterus towards anteversion, by blunt dissection, or can be divided. Following this, the surgeon enters two instruments into the opening and widens the opening by divergent traction. Creating this window will help to skeletonize the utero-ovarian ligament or infundibulopelvic ligament and ensure lateral movement of the ureter towards the pelvic side wall.

The Adnexa

The opening of the peritoneum is extended to the suspensory ligament of the ovary on either side. Because of the created fenestration, the ureter has been displaced towards the external pelvic wall laterally. However, we would still advise to carefully examine the course of the ureter prior to dissecting the suspensory ligament of the ovary. When in any doubt after the surgery about the ureters, cystoscopy is advised to ensure both sides produce urine.

When the adnexa are to be left in situ, both ligaments of the ovarium proprium are coagulated bipolar and cut through. When the adnexa are to be removed, both suspensory ligaments of the ovary are coagulated bipolar and cut through, under direct visualization of the ureter on either side. This division should be performed close to the ovaries because the ligament retracts after division. One should ensure haemostasis carefully before carrying on with the procedure.

Opportunistic Salpingectomy

There is a growing amount of scientific evidence that an opportunistic salpingectomy will lower the rate of ovarian cancer. The distal fallopian tubes were found to be strongly associated in early stages of high-grade serous ovarian cancer in a low-risk population [17,18]. The American College of Obstetricians and Gynecolgists therefore recommend the consideration of an opportunistic bilateral salpingectomy at the time of tubal sterilization or hysterectomy [19]. Recently a Cochrane systematic review was published to assess safety of opportunistic salpingectomy during hysterectomy [20]. The authors conclude that the evidence was low [20]. No difference in adverse events were noted, with a very low number of events in women undergoing a hysterectomy [20]. The authors do warn that the onset of menopause could be somewhat earlier, around 20 months, which is not clinically relevant [20]. However, long-term follow-up and data for young pre-menopausal women are missing [20].

We feel, considering the evidence, the option of a bilateral salpingectomy should be discussed with all patients undergoing a hysterectomy.

The Uterine Artery

Careful approach to the uterine arteries is essential to separate the uterine artery from the ureter. The first step is dissection from lateral towards the cervix on the posterior side of the uterus, for which the uterus is manipulated ventrally. The parametrium is coagulated using the bipolar forceps, whilst applying traction to the posterior peritoneum. Step by step the forceps moves towards the base of the uterine artery, where it can be seen as a meandering vessel. Subsequently, the peritoneum is coagulated and divided to create space posteriorly. One continues towards the uterosacral ligament, and when the cardinal ligament is coagulated and cut, usually the base of the uterine artery will be visible. The next step is to move to the front, by retroverting the uterus and to push it upwards. The tissue in front of the uterine artery, starting at the bladder pillars, is coagulated and divided. Finally, the uterine pedicle stands out lateral of the uterine isthmus, surrounded by vaginal fornices. Again, before coagulating and cutting the uterine artery, the ureter must be visible as well, to ensure that the ureter won't be damaged. The same technique is performed on the contralateral side. The surgeon puts traction on the uterus via the stump of the round ligament. When both uterine pedicles are clearly visible, they can be coagulated bipolar on the ascending part perpendicular to the cervix and cut.

When the uterine vessels are secured safely, the surgeon will dissect anterior and posterior to lower the pedicle of the uterine artery beyond the boundary of the vaginal fornix. In this manner, the uterine artery is safely secured before opening the vagina.

Opening the Vagina

The vagina will be opened through 360 degrees. One can start either anterior or posterior. The instrument used can coagulate bipolar in combination with scissors, or one can choose a monopolar hook or scissors. It is important to follow the shape of the uterus manipulator, which is folded over the cervix, and to stay interiorly from the uterus manipulator. In this way, the resection is just around the cervix, and not too much of the vaginal walls will be resected and vaginal length will be preserved. A normal-sized uterus can be removed through the colpotomy by drawing it back in the vagina. If the uterus is too large, it can be hemidissected or morcellated depending on the preference of the surgeon, and of course only in case of a benign uterus (see section on morcellation at subtotal hysterectomy).

Closing the Vagina

The vagina can be closed using the vaginal route or the laparoscopic route. When chosen for the laparoscopic route, it is important to restore the pneumoperitoneum after removal of the uterus. Suturing is often performed using a V-loc suture 0 or 1, which does not need tying the knot due to barbs. The needle and thread will be passed from one side of the vagina to the other side in a continuous fashion. It is important to grasp sufficient bites of the anterior as well as the posterior vaginal wall to cover all small vessels to create total haemostasis. One should take into account that the camera magnifies the image and that too small bites often occur when in the learning phase. If no continuous suture with barbs is available, one can use a normal thread, for example vicryl 0 or vicryl 1. When the suture is brought into the abdominal cavity, be aware that the needle, after closing the vaginal cuff, should fit through the trocard, to take it out of the abdomen.

To possibly prevent apical prolapse in the future, the sacro-uterine ligaments can be fixed on the vaginal top, after careful assessment that no ureter is involved. However, in women with an indication for uterine removal not related to pelvic organ prolapse, suspension of the sacro-uterine ligaments is not standard practice.

Following all laparoscopic procedures, the abdominal cavity will have to be checked on haemostasis. Haemostasis should be checked when the intra-abdominal pressure is lowered. Finally, the laparoscopic instruments should be removed under direct vision to ensure adequate haemostasis. The pelvic fascia of ports larger than 10 mm need to be closed to prevent herniation.

Technique of Laparoscopic Subtotal Hysterectomy

Intraoperative technical considerations regarding subtotal hysterectomy include the level of cervical amputation and the removal of the uterus.

Cervical Amputation

Laparoscopic subtotal hysterectomy is performed similarly to total laparoscopic hysterectomy up to the sealing of the uterine vessels. After the uterine vessels are secured, the cervix is transected at the level of the internal cervical ostium, the presumed junction of the endometrium and cervical columnar epithelium [14]. An anatomic landmark can be the level of uterosacral ligaments and their attachment to the uterus. The uterine manipulator, if used, needs to be removed prior to cervical amputation. Amputation of the cervix may be performed using 'cold' instruments, or ultrasonic or electrosurgical instruments [14]. Special devices have been used, specifically developed for this procedure, leading to a reduction in procedure time, without difference in complications [21]. For example, a loop wire can be used [21]. This wire is placed around the cervix at the level of the isthmus, just under the level of the coagulated uterine vessels [21]. A monopolar coagulation mode is applied while the loop is pulled backward, resulting in separation of the corpus uteri from the cervix [21]. Any residual bleeding from the cervical stump is treated with bipolar coagulation. The epithelial lining of the upper part of the cervical canal is desiccated to destroy the entire endometrial surface [21]. The peritoneum is advised to be closed over the cervix. This can be achieved in the same way as the closure of the vaginal cuff, using a continuous V-loc thread with barbs 0 or 1, or vicryl 0 or 1 interrupted sutures.

Uterine Removal

Following laparoscopic subtotal hysterectomy, the uterus used to be removed either via posterior colpotomy or via intra-abdominal morcellation, depending on the judgment of the gynaecological surgeon as to what would be the best route. However, for the morcellation, restrictions have been made by the US Food and Drug Administration (FDA) in 2014 to decrease the risk of dissemination of malignant tissue due to intra-abdominal morcellation of unexpected malignancies. The incidence of unexpected malignancies in cases of uterine fibroids was: 2.8 (95% CI: 1.8–4.5) per 1,000 persons for uterine sarcoma and 2.0 (95% CI: 1.1–3.8) per 1,000 persons for leiomyosarcoma. These translate to an unsuspected uterine sarcoma in 1 in 352 women and an unsuspected LMS in 1 in 498 women undergoing hysterectomy or myomectomy for presumed benign leiomyoma [22].

However, more recent studies have shown different, lower, numbers. Brölman and his steering committee concluded a prevalence of uterine sarcoma in presumed myomas of 0.014–0.45% [23]. Furthermore, they conclude that there is not enough evidence to predict the risk for an individual woman [23]. In their proposed flow chart, they suggest counselling against morcellation, in case of necrosis and high vascularity seen on transvaginal ultrasound, a single fibroid larger than 8 cm, elevated blood lactate dehydrogenase (LDH) level, and postmenopausal women [23]. Another study created a hypothetical cohort of 100,000 premenopausal women to study the differences in complications after laparoscopic morcellation of a uterus myomatosus versus abdominal removal of the same uterus [24]. The decision analysis predicted fewer overall deaths using the laparoscopic route versus the abdominal route. Furthermore, women in the laparoscopic group had less complications and more quality-adjusted life years [24]. Parasitic myomas could develop after morcellation of a myoma, and they could result in abdominal and pelvic pain [25]. In their systematic review, van der Meulen et al included 44 studies, in which a total number of 69 women were found with parasitic myomas, giving an overall incidence of parasitic myomas after laparoscopic morcellation of 0.12–0.95% [25].

Unfortunately, following the FDA warning, the incidence of open abdominal hysterectomy increased, with indeed an increase in major and minor peri- and postoperative complications, as studies in a cohort of over 75,000 women in the US have shown [26]. These authors suggest that the increased risk of complications should be balanced against the relatively small risk of an unexpected malignancy and parasitic myomas, spread through the abdomen following morcellation [26].

Current guidelines suggest the use of in-bag intra-abdominal morcellation to have the advantage of an entire laparoscopic procedure, with probably a reduced possibility of intra-abdominal spread of a possible unexpected malignancy, although this has not been proven yet [12,27,28,29]. A survey in the US revealed that the reason for not using a morcellator anymore was lack of availability, due to the ban in 50% of cases [30]. However, in a survey amongst gynaecologists from the UK, most of the doctors do not use an intra-abdominal bag for tissue retrieval when using morcellation techniques for leiomyomas [31]. The disadvantage of the in-bag morcellation technique is that it can be quite time-consuming. Data on safety and complications of in-bag morcellation are scarce.

Differences between Laparoscopic Total and Subtotal Hysterectomy

Complication Rate

The AAGL, as well as a recent systematic review, stated that there is no evidence that laparoscopic subtotal hysterectomy is safer than laparoscopic total hysterectomy [14,32].

Though, the incidence of minor and severe complications differs among the different studies. Donnez et al separated laparoscopic subtotal (n=1,613) versus total (n=1,577) hysterectomy and found a similar number of complications in both groups: minor complications 1–1.1% and major complications 0.4–0.5% [5]. However, a recent national guideline has shown that the risk to undergo a severe complication was 4.5% following laparoscopic total hysterectomy (n=3,222), versus 1.8% following laparoscopic subtotal hysterectomy (n=3,901), which was not significant [27]. The risk of a mild complication was 4.1% following laparoscopic total hysterectomy (n=3,222), versus 1.6% following laparoscopic subtotal hysterectomy (n=3,901), which again was not significant [27]. These mild complications include fewer bladder lesions, fewer haematomas, fewer local infections, and less vaginal cuff dehiscence [27,33,34,35].

There were no significant differences in vascular injury, bowel injury (0.2–0.5%), or ureteric injury (0.1–0.3%) between laparoscopic total versus subtotal hysterectomy [5,27,32,36]. Following laparoscopic subtotal hysterectomy, the incidence of bladder injury was lower (OR 4.01 [1.79; 8.99]), between 0.25–0.75% [5,27,34,36]. There was no difference in urinary retention following the two types of laparoscopic hysterectomy [27].

Intraoperative outcomes between laparoscopic subtotal versus laparoscopic total hysterectomy were similar with regards to blood loss, postoperative hospital stay, readmission rates, and febrile morbidity [14,32].

In most studies, the time of the surgical procedure for laparoscopic hysterectomy is not of clinically relevant difference to the laparoscopic total hysterectomy. The recent systematic review found a shorter operative time for subtotal hysterectomy, both in the abdominal and in the laparoscopic subtotal hysterectomy group (13 minutes less surgical time), although not all included studies were powered to analyse this [32]. Interestingly, operative times for subtotal hysterectomy had a very wide range: 47–181 minutes [14], probably depending on the experience of the gynaecologic laparoscopy surgeon and the difficulty of the cases. This difference can be even larger due to the extra time in-bag morcellation takes.

Another possible complication of a laparoscopic procedure is the conversion to a laparotomy, which can be strategic or due to complications. The incidence of a conversion to laparotomy ranges from 0.03%–6.6% [5,10,27,33]. A recent Cochrane review analysing high-quality studies decided on the percentage of 2.4% for laparoscopic hysterectomy [9]. The number of conversions to laparotomy was lower for laparoscopic subtotal hysterectomy, 3.6% following laparoscopic total hysterectomy versus 2.5% following laparoscopic subtotal hysterectomy [27].

A study with 122 women revealed that, following laparoscopic subtotal hysterectomy, women improved on their short-term physical component score (3–4 weeks) and a better quality of life score, without any difference in pain, nausea, or return to normal daily activities [37]. A recent systematic review found no differences in return to daily activities [32]. At 12 months postoperatively, a similar postoperative improvement in quality of life was found[38].

The incidence of intermittent postoperative vaginal bleeding was 2% in a retrospective study with 400 women [14,36]. Burning of the residual endometrium intracervical does not always prevent spotting for pre-menopausal patients [14,36]. The re-operation rate for cervical removal was 2.2–2.7% in two studies, encompassing almost 400 women within 12 months following subtotal hysterectomy [33,39]. Regarding cyclical bleeding, this was less frequent following laparoscopic hysterectomy compared to abdominal hysterectomy, with a trend towards less cyclical bleeding following laparoscopic total hysterectomy when compared to subtotal hysterectomy (5% versus 18%) [32]. The results of this systematic review are mainly based on a large cohort study (one-year follow-up), regardless of intraoperative cervical treatment [40]. In this cohort, women with vaginal bleeding were less satisfied with the result of their surgery, which should be taken into consideration when counselling women [40].

Endometrial malignancy may still develop following subtotal hysterectomy, and therefore hormone replacement therapy should be considered carefully in women with perimenopausal symptoms, with the avoidance of an oestrogen-only therapy [14,28].

Furthermore, women will have to be reminded of the need for cervical PAP smear testing when the cervix is left in situ.

Some studies report on an increased incidence of pelvic pain, due to endometriosis, following laparoscopic hysterectomy, without a difference between subtotal or total hysterectomy (1.4%) [41].

Impact on Pelvic Floor Dysfunction

Initial thoughts on the advantages of performing subtotal hysterectomy instead of total hysterectomy were a reduction of the impact on bladder function, due to less damage to nerves and blood vessels around the bladder and ureters. These theoretical advantages have not been demonstrated in clinical studies comparing open abdominal subtotal versus open abdominal total hysterectomy [14,16]. Furthermore, sexual and bowel function do not improve when performing open abdominal subtotal versus total hysterectomy [16].

At the time of the report of the American Association of Gynecologic Laparoscopists, regarding practice guidelines for laparoscopic subtotal/supracervical hysterectomy (LSH) there were no robust and strong data available regarding the impact of laparoscopic subtotal versus total hysterectomy on pelvic floor dysfunction [14]: no difference in bladder function, no difference in pelvic organ prolapse, no difference in bowel function, some small differences in sexual outcome in the short-term unfortunately in poorer quality studies [14]. The authors therefore state that based on those data, they could not provide strong recommendations to perform subtotal hysterectomy to possibly reduce the incidence of pelvic floor dysfunction [14].

It appears that much of the information regarding laparoscopic subtotal hysterectomy is missing, as it is often not clear from the cases [42] or the literature what type of laparoscopic hysterectomy is performed. This is a real omission, as it does not help to answer our question of whether to perform subtotal or total laparoscopic hysterectomy. We would encourage doctors and researchers to specify the type of laparoscopic hysterectomy performed in their research.

When studying the latest evidence, there appears to be a little more evidence to support clinical advice on whether or not to leave the cervix in situ in case of a laparoscopic hysterectomy for benign indications.

In their systematic review, Aleixo et al aimed to define a difference in pelvic floor dysfunction following laparoscopic total versus subtotal hysterectomy in the long-term (> 5 years) [43]. However, these authors found no laparoscopic studies that could answer their research question and therefore presented again on the differences between abdominal total versus subtotal hysterectomy [43]. Unfortunately, the included studies were of poorer quality: not blinded and large loss to follow-up [43]. Their conclusions, however, were a lower risk of (stress) urinary incontinence following total abdominal hysterectomy [43]. Other outcomes, such as urinary frequency, urge incontinence, incomplete bladder emptying, pelvic organ prolapse, incontinence of stool, and constipation were not significantly different between abdominal total versus subtotal hysterectomy in the long-term [43]. Although not supported by evidence, the authors speculate that the lack of a difference in pelvic organ prolapse could be that following a hysterectomy, suspension sutures are performed, which would not be the case following subtotal hysterectomy [43]. Another recent review, trying to answer the outcome on urinary function after total versus subtotal hysterectomy, again could not find any studies following laparoscopic total versus subtotal hysterectomy [44].

Sexual Function

A recent systematic review could not find data on dyspareunia or sexual satisfaction when comparing laparoscopic total versus subtotal hysterectomy [32]. The authors concluded that studies analysing abdominal total versus subtotal hysterectomy did not show a difference [32]. A non-RCT did show some data regarding differences in sexual function between laparoscopic total versus subtotal hysterectomy. Following subtotal hysterectomy, sexual activities were resumed sooner (36 (SD 11) days versus 48 (SD 9) days, but overall no differences in quality of sex life were found [34,37,38]. One study found significantly more dyspareunia following total laparoscopic hysterectomy (20%) versus subtotal laparoscopic hysterectomy (10%), with no preoperative data available [35].

Sexuality was considered more important in women choosing to undergo subtotal hysterectomy [45]. From a questionnaire study it appeared that patients' expectations regarding sexual functioning following hysterectomy might have influenced their choice for subtotal hysterectomy [45]. In the same group of women, sexual functioning improved in most women following hysterectomy, especially in patients with lower quality of sexuality prior to surgery [46]. The preservation of the cervix resulted in more improvement of sexual functioning three months following surgery, but not at six or 12 months [46].

Pelvic Organ Prolapse

Certainly, prolapse is more likely to re-occur in women when the indication for index surgery was pelvic organ prolapse irrespective of route of hysterectomy [14]. In a prospective study, no difference in preoperative pelvic organ prolapse was found in a cohort of women undergoing laparoscopic total versus subtotal hysterectomy [38]. 12 months following surgery, an asymptomatic pelvic organ prolapse grade 1 was found more often following laparoscopic total hysterectomy (32% versus 5%), which is not of clinical significance [38]. In the past, again there have been no data that support the theory that subtotal hysterectomy will prevent women from pelvic organ prolapse [16].

Conclusions

The indication for a laparoscopic hysterectomy can be made when the uterus needs to be removed, but vaginal hysterectomy is not possible.

The surgical procedure of a laparoscopic subtotal hysterectomy has become a little more complicated due to in-bag morcellation, since evidence has emerged regarding the possible spread of an unknown malignancy through the abdominal cavity.

The overall complication rates do not differ much between total laparoscopic hysterectomy versus subtotal hysterectomy. The risks of morcellation, persistent vaginal bleeding, as well as the need for cervical cytology must be discussed with the individual woman. The option of performing concurrent opportunistic bilateral salpingectomy to reduce the chances of ovarian cancer should be discussed with all patients undergoing a hysterectomy for benign indication.

The option of a subtotal hysterectomy can be discussed in the light of a possible advantage on sexual functioning, mainly in the short-term. However, little evidence is available that laparoscopic subtotal hysterectomy results in more stress urinary incontinence. Other than that, until now, no significant differences are found regarding influence on pelvic floor dysfunction, such as micturition, bowel function, and pelvic organ prolapse. These results related to laparoscopic hysterectomy are similar to results from the past related to abdominal hysterectomy.

References

1. Reich H, DeCaprio J, McGlynn F. Laparoscopic hysterectomy. J Gynecol Surg 1989; 5(2): 213–16.
2. Garry R, Fountain J, Mason S, et al. The eVALuate study: two parallel randomised trials, one comparing laparoscopic with abdominal hysterectomy, the other comparing laparoscopic with vaginal hysterectomy. BMJ 2004; 328(7432): 129.
3. Mettler L, Ahmed-Ebbiary N, Schollmeyer T. Laparoscopic hysterectomy: challenges and limitations. Minim Invasive Ther Allied Technol 2005; 14(3): 145–59.
4. Brummer TH, Seppälä TT, Härkki PS. National learning curve for laparoscopic hysterectomy and trends in hysterectomy in Finland 2000–2005. Hum Reprod 2008; 23(4): 840–5.
5. Donnez O, Jadoul P, Squifflet J, Donnez J. A series of 3190 laparoscopic hysterectomies for benign disease from 1990 to 2006: evaluation of complications compared with vaginal and abdominal procedures. BJOG 2009; 116(4): 492–500.
6. Mäkinen J, Brummer T, Jalkanen J, et al. Ten years of progress–improved hysterectomy outcomes in Finland 1996–2006: a longitudinal observation study. BMJ Open 2013; 3(10): e003169.
7. Krielen P, Stommel MWJ, Pargmae P, et al. Adhesion-related readmissions after open and laparoscopic surgery: a retrospective cohort study (SCAR update). Lancet 2020; 395(10217): 33–41.
8. Twijnstra AR, Blikkendaal MD, Kolkman W, et al. Implementation of laparoscopic hysterectomy: maintenance of skills after a mentorship program. Gynecol Obstet Invest 2010; 70(3): 173–8.
9. Aarts JW, Nieboer TE, Johnson N, et al. Surgical approach to hysterectomy for benign gynaecological disease. Cochrane Database Syst Rev 2015; (8): CD003677.
10. Terzi H, Biler A, Demirtas O, et al. Total laparoscopic hysterectomy: analysis of the surgical learning curve in benign conditions. Int J Surg 2016; 35: 51–7.
11. Wattiez A, Soriano D, Cohen SB, et al. The learning curve of total laparoscopic hysterectomy: comparative analysis of 1647 cases. J Am Assoc Gynecol Laparosc 2002; 9(3): 339–45.
12. ACOG.Committee opinion. Choosing the route of hysterectomy for benign disease. Published 2017.
13. Semm K. Hysterectomy via laparotomy or pelviscopy. A new CASH method without colpotomy. Geburtshilfe Frauenheilkd 1991; 51(12): 996–1003.
14. American Association of Gynecologic Laparoscopists. AAGL practice report: practice guidelines for laparoscopic subtotal/supracervical hysterectomy (LSH). J Minim Invasive Gynecol 2014; 21: 9–16.
15. Driessen SR, Sandberg EM, la Chapelle CF, et al. Case-mix variables and predictors for outcomes of laparoscopic hysterectomy: a systematic review. J Minim Invasive Gynecol 2016; 23(3): 317–30.

16. Lethaby A, Mukhopadhyay A, Naik R. Total versus subtotal hysterectomy for benign gynaecological conditions. Cochrane Database Syst Rev 2012; (4): CD004993.
17. Piek JM, van Diest PJ, Zweemer RP, et al. Dysplastic changes in pro-phylactically removed Fallopian tubes of women predisposed to developing ovarian cancer. J Pathol 2001; 195: 451–6.
18. Kindelberger DW, Lee Y, Miron A, et al. Intraepithelial carcinoma of the fimbria and pelvic serous carcinoma: evidence for a causal relationship. Am J Surg Pathol 2007; 31: 161–9.
19. Committee on Gynecologic Practice. Committee opinion no. 620: salpingectomy for ovarian cancer prevention. Obstet Gynecol 2015; 125: 279–81.
20. van Lieshout LAM, Steenbeek MP, De Hullu JA, et al. Hysterectomy with opportunistic salpingectomy versus hysterectomy alone. Cochrane Database Syst Rev 2019; 8: CD012858.
21. Erian J, El-Toukhy T, Chandakas S, Theodoridis T, Hill N. One hundred cases of laparoscopic subtotal hysterectomy using the PK and Lap Loop systems. J Minim Invasive Gynecol 2005; 12(4): 365–9.
22. US Food and Drug Administration. FDA warning morcellation. Published 2014. Available from: www.fda.gov/media/88703/download [last accessed 2 November 2021].
23. Brölmann H, Tanos V, Grimbizis G, et al. European Society of Gynaecological Endoscopy (ESGE) steering committee on fibroid morcellation. Options on fibroid morcellation: a literature review. Gynecol Surg 2015; 12(1): 3–15.
24. Siedhoff MT, Wheeler SB, Rutstein SE, et al. Laparoscopic hysterectomy with morcellation vs abdominal hysterectomy for presumed fibroid tumors in premenopausal women: a decision analysis. AJOG 2015; 212(5): 591.e1–8.
25. Van der Meulen JF, Pijnenborg JM, Boomsma CM, et al. Parasitic myoma after laparoscopic morcellation: a systematic review of the literature. BJOG 2016; 123(1): 69–75.
26. Multinu F, Casarin J, Hanson KT, et al. Practice patterns and complications of benign hysterectomy following the fda statement warning against the use of power morcellation. JAMA Surg. 2018; 153(6): e180141.
27. Sandberg EM, Hehenkamp WJK, Geomini PM, et al. Laparoscopic hysterectomy for benign indications: clinical practice guideline. Arch Gynecol Obstet 2017; 296(3): 597–606.
28. Sloth SB, Schroll JB, Settnes A, et al. Systematic review of the limited evidence for different surgical techniques at benign hysterectomy: a clinical guideline initiated by the Danish Health Authority. Eur J Obstet Gynecol Reprod Biol 2017; 216: 169–77.
29. Royal College of Obstetricians and Gynaecologists. Consent Advice No. 13. Morcellation for Myomectomy or Hysterectomy. Published 2019.
30. Nezhat F, Apostol R, Greene AD, Pilkinton ML. To morcellate or not to morcellate: a cross-sectional survey of gynecologic surgeons. JSLS 2017; 21(1): e2016.00092. https://doi.org/10.4293/JSLS.2016.0009
31. Sankaran S, Brown A, Kent A, Odejinmi F. Laparoscopic specimen retrieval and attitudes towards morcellation: a questionnaire survey of gynaecology consultants in the United Kingdom. J Obstet Gynaecol 2019; 39(3): 345–8.
32. Aleixo GF, Fonseca MCM, Bortolini MAT, et al. Total versus subtotal hysterectomy: systematic review and meta-analysis of intraoperative outcomes and postoperative short-term events. Clin Ther 2019; 41(4): 768–89.
33. Bardens D, Solomayer E, Baum S, et al. Comparison of total and supracervical laparoscopic hysterectomy for benign disease in a collective of 200 patients. J Gynecol Surg 2012; 28(5): 333–7.
34. Brucker S, Rothmund R, Krämer B, et al. Cervical detachment using monopolar supraloop electrode versus monopolar needle in laparoscopic supracervical hysterectomy (lsh): an interventional, comparative cohort study. Geburtshilfe Frauenheilkd 2013; 73(11): 1121–7.
35. Saccardi C, Gizzo S, Noventa M, et al. Subtotal versus total laparoscopic hysterectomy: could women sexual function recovery overcome the surgical outcomes in pre-operatory decision making? Arch Gynecol Obstet 2015; 291(6): 1321–6.
36. Erian J, Hassan M, Pachydakis A, et al. Efficacy of laparoscopic subtotal hysterectomy in the management of menorrhagia: 400 consecutive cases. BJOG 2008; 115(6): 742–8.
37. Einarsson JI, Suzuki Y, Vellinga TT, et al. Prospective evaluation of quality of life in total versus supracervical laparoscopic hysterectomy. J Minim Invasive Gynecol 2011; 18(5): 617–21.
38. Berner E, Qvigstad E, Myrvold AK, Lieng M. Pain reduction after total laparoscopic hysterectomy and laparoscopic supracervical hysterectomy among women with dysmenorrhoea: a randomised controlled trial. BJOG 2015; 122(8): 1102–11.
39. Boosz A, Lermann J, Mehlhorn G, et al. Comparison of re-operation rates and complication rates after total laparoscopic hysterectomy (TLH) and laparoscopy-assisted supracervical hysterectomy (LASH). Eur J Obstet Gynecol Reprod Biol 2011; 158(2): 269–73.
40. Borendal Wodlin N. Intraoperative cervical treatment does not affect the prevalence of vaginal bleeding 1 year postoperatively after subtotal hysterectomy. A register study from the Swedish National Register for Gynecological Surgery. Acta Obstet Gynecol Scand 2017; 96(12): 1430–7.
41. Okaro EO, Jones KD, Sutton C. Long term outcome following laparoscopic supracervical hysterectomy. BJOG 2001; 108(10): 1017–20.
42. Huang CC, Lo TS, Huang YT, et al. surgical trends and time frame comparison of surgical types of hysterectomy: a nationwide, population-based 15-year study. J Minim Invasive Gynecol 2020; 27(1): 65–73.e1.
43. Aleixo GF, Fonseca MCM, Bortolini MAT, Brito LGO, Castro RA. Pelvic floor symptoms 5 to 14 years after total versus subtotal hysterectomy for benign conditions: a systematic review and meta-analysis. Int Urogynecol J 2019; 30(2): 181–91.
44. Longo PS, Borbily LV, Glina FPA. Urinary incontinence following subtotal and total hysterectomy: a systematic review. Einstein (Sao Paulo) 2019; 17(2): eRW4320.
45. Berlit S, Lis S, Jürgens S, et al. Postoperative sexual functioning in total versus subtotal laparoscopic hysterectomy: what do women expect? Arch Gynecol Obstet 2017; 296(3): 513–18.
46. Berlit S, Tuschy B, Wuhrer A, et al. Sexual functioning after total versus subtotal laparoscopic hysterectomy. Arch Gynecol Obstet 2018; 298(2): 337–44.

Chapter 25

Evidence-based Approach to Concomitant Incontinence Surgery at the Time of Sacrocolpopexy

Mugdha Kulkarni, James Alexander, Anna Rosamilia

Introduction

Stress urinary incontinence (SUI) is the involuntary loss of urine on exertion (e.g. sporting activities, or on sneezing or coughing) [1]. About 40% of women with pelvic organ prolapse (POP) will complain of stress urinary incontinence [2]. SUI and POP have similar pathophysiology and arise due to pelvic floor dysfunction [3]. Women with preoperative SUI are at highest risk of ongoing SUI after prolapse repair surgery [2,4]. Up to 30% of continent women develop *de novo* (new onset) SUI postoperatively, and this is highest in women with the preoperative finding of occult SUI [5–7]. Occult SUI is a sign observed after the reduction of co-existent prolapse [1]. This is predominantly thought to be due to kinking of the urethra from the prolapse.

The relationship between SUI and POP informs different treatment algorithms including correction of both conditions at the same time or in a staged manner. In addition, the occurrence of new onset SUI after prolapse correction is a major source of dissatisfaction. There is widespread variation in practice geographically.

In addition, the type of POP surgery may have a variable impact on correction of SUI or the subsequent development of *de novo* SUI. For instance, transvaginal mesh anchored anterior and apical repairs were associated with a higher rate of new onset SUI compared with native tissue repair [8]. Performing an incontinence procedure for the treatment or prevention of SUI at the time of POP surgery involves finding a balance between the benefit of combination surgery versus the potential complications of additional surgery and adverse events such as overactive bladder or voiding dysfunction. Potential mesh complications from mid-urethral synthetic sling (MUS), in the order of 1–3%, also needs to be addressed in counselling. In addition, there are considerations about the comparative cost of staged or concomitant approach.

The main options for incontinence surgery are retropubic urethropexy (commonly referred to as colposuspension or Burch colposuspension), mid-urethral sling (MUS – often referred to in the literature by the market name, TVT or TOT – meaning tension-free vaginal tape or transobturator tape), autologous fascial sling, or an intraurethral bulking agent [9]. The most accepted minimally invasive sacral colpopexy (SCP) utilizes mesh which is usually polypropylene, or Dynamesh™ (a combination of Polyvinylidene fluoride and polypropylene). There are recent reports of autologous fascia lata as the graft material also being used in addition to the use of cadaveric fascia lata in the past [10]. The graft material utilized may influence the patient's choice of incontinence procedure in terms of their comfort with a concomitant polypropylene mid-urethral sling. There is limited data on the SUI outcomes of laparoscopic or robotic SCP and a concomitant incontinence procedure. There is a large study with extended follow-up addressing open sacral colpopexy and colposuspension which will be described in detail. The majority of studies addressing POP repair and concomitant incontinence procedures are for vaginal repairs and some of this data will also be presented. The most common concomitant incontinence surgeries are the mid-urethral sling or retropubic urethropexy.

Overview of Incontinence Procedures

The literature on concomitant incontinence surgery reflects the general trends that were seen when mid-urethral slings overtook the colposuspension as the most common female incontinence surgery by 2004. Cochrane reviews, meta-analyses, and large databases have reported on comparisons in cure and complications between different procedures. Recent trends showing decreased rates of MUS and of incontinence surgery overall in some countries has in large part been attributed to transvaginal mesh litigation. No doubt this will also have an effect on concomitant incontinence surgery but perhaps less so in the context of laparoscopic sacral colpopexy which also utilizes mesh.

The Cochrane review on open retropubic colposuspension, published in 2017, concluded that this was an effective treatment modality for SUI, with an overall continence rate of 85% to 90% at one year and 70% at five years. Colposuspension was associated with a higher risk of POP compared to sling surgery but a lower risk of voiding dysfunction compared to traditional sling surgery [11].

The Cochrane review on laparoscopic colposuspension published in 2019 found that this surgery had a similar subjective cure rate at 18 months compared with open colposuspension but had a lower risk of perioperative complications and similar or higher rates of bladder perforation. There was also little difference between laparoscopic colposuspension and tension-free vaginal tape (TVT) for subjective cure at 18 months, although there may be an increased re-operation risk with the colposuspension and a similar risk of perioperative complications. The review commented on the wide confidence intervals for this comparison. *De novo* detrusor overactivity and voiding dysfunction rates were similar across all three surgeries, also with wide confidence intervals [12].

The Cochrane review on mid-urethral sling published in 2017 had included 81 trials and a total of 12,113 women until 2014, which represents the most studied procedure for SUI. This study concluded that more than 80% of women were cured or significantly improved with either retropubic or transobturator mid-urethral sling for up to five years after surgery [13].

The metanalysis performed by Fusco et al [14] included 28 randomized controlled trials (RCTs) and 15,855 subjects. Women receiving MUS had significantly higher overall (OR 0.59, p = 0.0003) and objective (OR 0.51, p = 0.001) cure rates than those receiving Burch colposuspension (open and laparoscopic). Women undergoing MUS and pubovaginal slings had similar cure rates. Patients treated with a retropubic MUS had higher subjective (OR 0.83, p = 0.03) and objective (OR 0.82, p = 0.01) cure rates than those receiving transobturator slings. The latter had a lower risk of intraoperative bladder or vaginal perforation, pelvic haematoma, urinary tract infections, and voiding dysfunction symptoms.

Morling et al [15] reported adverse events including readmission after MUS and colposuspension surgery between 1997 and 2016 in 16,660 women having primary surgery in Scotland; 79% of the women had MUS. Compared with open colposuspension, MUS had a lower risk of immediate complications (adjusted relative risk [aRR] 0·44) and subsequent prolapse surgery (aRR 0·30), and a similar risk of further incontinence surgery (aRR 0·90) and later complications (aRR 1·12).

Techniques for different incontinence procedures including retropubic urethropexy, mid-urethral sling, pubovaginal sling and bulking agents have been described in a recent International Urogynecology Association (IUGA) terminology document [9].

Preoperative Evaluation with Urodynamic Assessment

There are recommendations that women with high-grade pelvic organ prolapse should ideally undergo preoperative multichannel urodynamic assessment with prolapse reduction [16,17]. It is claimed that this will help assess the presence of occult SUI and detrusor function although the role of urodynamic assessment in the management of stress urinary incontinence has been questioned in recent European and US literature [18,19].

Visco et al assessed reduction testing in stress-continent women undergoing (open) sacrocolpopexy in the Colpopexy and Urinary Reduction Efforts (CARE) randomized surgical trial [6,20]. They assessed whether stress leakage during urodynamic testing with prolapse reduction predicted postoperative stress incontinence. Preoperatively, only 12 of 313 (3.7%) subjects demonstrated urodynamic stress incontinence (USI) without prolapse reduction. However, 19% of subjects reported symptomatic stress incontinence at baseline. Preoperative detection of USI with prolapse reduction at 300 ml was seen with pessary in 6% (5 of 88); by manual reduction in 16% (19 of 122); by forceps reduction in 21% (21 of 98); by swab reduction in 20% (32 of 158); and with the use of a speculum in 30% (35 of 118). They found that overall, 27% of stress continent women leaked with reduction testing using these different techniques. The swab had the highest positive predictive value of 70% compared to other methods which ranged from 50–55%; this difference was not statistically significant. Postoperative SUI was higher after positive preoperative reduction testing. However, the predictive value of a preoperative urodynamic assessment was limited as a negative test was associated with 38% of subjects experiencing postoperative SUI in the SCP alone group and 21% in the SCP with Burch colposuspension group.

The urodynamic assessment may also demonstrate voiding dysfunction and bladder overactivity. Both of these findings are associated with pelvic organ prolapse and may resolve after prolapse correction.

A subsequent study by Elser et al was a retrospective series of 441 women who had undergone laparoscopic sacral colpopexy (concomitant hysterectomy in 35%, anterior repair in 18%, and posterior repair in 31%). All women had preoperative urodynamic assessment; 20% had urodynamic or occult stress urinary incontinence and 16% had voiding dysfunction. Women with urodynamic or occult stress incontinence had a concomitant incontinence procedure with either Burch colposuspension (23%) or MUS (77%). At a mean of 46 weeks follow-up, the 'any incontinence' rate was 13% for all women [21]. These authors recommended an approach guided by urodynamic assessment and treating only women with overt or occult SUI with concomitant SUI surgery.

Approach to Treatment

Based on history, examination, and urodynamic assessment, women undergoing sacral colpopexy (SCP) can be classified into the following:

a. Stress continent or asymptomatic women without occult SUI
b. Asymptomatic women with occult SUI
c. Women with overt SUI

Stress Continent or Asymptomatic Women without Occult Stress Urinary Incontinence

The largest study to address this was the CARE study with three-month outcome results reported in 2006 by Brubaker et al; 157 women were assigned to concomitant open Burch colposuspension and 165 to open sacral colpopexy alone. There was less postoperative stress incontinence in the Burch group (34% versus 57%) compared to the SCP alone group (P<0.001). Urge incontinence was similar at 33% and 38%, respectively. Bothersome stress incontinence was reported by 25% of SCP alone group versus 6% with concomitant Burch (P<0.001). There was no difference in serious adverse events judged to be plausibly related to the Burch surgery (4.5% versus 3%, p=0.24) though specific outcomes such as cystotomy, UTI, and voiding dysfunction were not published.

Two years after surgery, 42% and 58% of women in the Burch and SCP, and the SCP alone groups, respectively, met the stress incontinence endpoint (presence of symptoms or positive cough stress test or interval treatment for stress incontinence, P=.020). The apex was well supported (point C within 2 cm of total vaginal length) in 95% of women, and this was not affected by concomitant Burch (P=.18). There was a trend toward fewer urgency symptoms in the Burch group (32% versus 45% no

Burch, P=.085). Twenty participants experienced mesh or suture erosion with no difference between the groups.

Nygaard et al described the long-term outcomes of the CARE trial with median follow-up of seven years. The estimated probability of SUI in the SCP and Burch group was 0.62 versus 0.77 for ASC alone. The time to surgical failure for SUI was 3.1 versus 0.9 years, respectively. Complications specific to Burch surgery were not reported.

A smaller randomized controlled trial by Costantini et al reported on long-term outcomes of Burch colposuspension in continent women at the time of open abdominal sacrocolpopexy for stage 3 or greater POP [22]. Sixty-six continent women (negative for SUI: subjective, objective, and occult) were randomly assigned to SCP and Burch colposuspension or SCP alone. At median follow-up of eight years, 29% (9 of 31) in the Burch group were incontinent compared with 15% (5 of 31) in the SCP only group (p=0.55).

The Cochrane review in 2018 summarizes that the two abovementioned RCTs produced results in different directions with a very wide confidence interval. The difference between groups in rates of subjective postoperative SUI had a RR 1.31 [8].

A small series of 53 women with no SUI or occult SUI on urodynamic assessment before surgery had laparoscopic sacral colpopexy (LSCP) with no incontinence procedure. Twenty months after their surgery, 13% developed *de novo* SUI at a median of two months after surgery. The five-year SUI-free survival rate after LSCP was 86% [23].

The authors' practice is to counsel regarding the possibility of occult stress incontinence occurring in 10–20% after sacral colpopexy in the continent patient and to offer urodynamic assessment preoperatively if the patient desires it. The authors' may perform paravaginal repair following sacral colpopexy to correct residual cystocele. If this were a surgeon's practice, it may provide similar outcome in terms of stress urinary incontinence to retropubic urethropexy although this has not been assessed in a clinical trial.

Women with Occult Stress Urinary Incontinence

The majority of occult SUI studies are based on vaginal POP repair with concomitant MUS procedure.

In the OPUS trial by Wei et al [24], 337 women without symptoms of SUI were randomized to vaginal repair alone or vaginal repair with mid-urethral sling (MUS). Thirty-three percent of the participants had occult SUI. At three months, 24% in the sling group compared to 49% in the no sling group had urinary incontinence (UI) ($p<0.001$). At 12 months, SUI was present in 27% and 43% of patients in the sling and no sling groups, respectively ($P = 0.002$). The number needed to treat with a sling to prevent one case of urinary incontinence at 12 months was 6.3. The rate of bladder perforation was higher in the sling group (6.7% versus 0%), as were rates of urinary tract infection (31% versus 18.3%), major bleeding complications (3.1% versus 0%), and incomplete bladder emptying six weeks after surgery (3.7% versus 0%) ($P \leq 0.05$ for all).

Schierlitz et al [25], conducted a RCT comparing retropubic MUS at the time of POP repair in women asymptomatic for USI who had stress urinary incontinence without reduction or occult SUI on prolapse reduction at the time of urodynamic assessment. The prevalence of combined urodynamic SUI and occult SUI was 17%. Forty-three women were randomized to POP repair without sling and 37 with sling. Urodynamic assessment was repeated six months following surgery in 60 of the participants (27 TVT and 33 no TVT). Twelve subjects (5 TVT and 7 no TVT) declined as they were asymptomatic and 8 (5 TVT and 3 no TVT) failed to attend. Four of 27 (15%) of the TVT group had USI compared with 22 out of 33 (66%) in the no TVT group with an ARR of 52% ($p < 0.001$). However, in these 26 women, four out of four (100%) in the TVT group and 18 out of 22 (81%) in the no TVT group reported no incontinence symptoms, ARR 18% ($p = 0.40$).

At six months, an interval sling was performed in 3 of 43 (7%) of the no TVT and none of the TVT group; by two years, the rate was 4 of 43 (9%) and none, respectively. By four years, 6 of 43 (14%) had an interval sling in the first group versus none in the TVT group. The number needed to treat to prevent an interval mid-urethral sling was between 6 and 11[26].

A subgroup analysis of the CARE trial by Visco et al reported a prevalence of occult SUI of 27%. Postoperative SUI in the ASC with Burch group was 32% compared to 58% in the ASC only group in those with OSI.

All women undergoing pelvic organ prolapse should be informed of the risk of occult stress incontinence in the order of 10–20%. If occult stress incontinence is confirmed, a discussion regarding the advantages and disadvantages of concomitant incontinence surgery takes place which needs to take into account the risks including those of mid-urethral sling if that is appropriate. The number needed to treat is based mainly on vaginal prolapse surgery and is of the order of six slings inserted to prevent one interval sling.

Women with Overt Stress Urinary Incontinence

In a multicentre, prospective RCT, women with POP and SUI were randomized to have a MUS at the time of POP vaginal repair (87 participants) or three months later (94 participants). Borstad et al found that women in the concomitant sling group had higher cure of SUI compared to the delayed group. However, 27% were also cured after POP surgery alone [27].

Costantini et al compared ASC with Burch colposuspension versus without Burch colposuspension in women with POP and UI. There was no significant difference between the two groups at a follow-up of 82 months. However, the sample size was small: 47 in total and included women with SUI, mixed urinary incontinence (MUI), or occult SUI [28]. The 2018 Cochrane review states that an additional Burch colposuspension probably has little or no effect on postoperative SUI at one year (RR 1.38), OAB symptoms (RR 0.85), or voiding dysfunction (RR 0.96), based on this only available study [8].

The same authors concluded that in women with POP and SUI (symptomatic or occult), a concurrent MUS probably reduces postoperative SUI and should be discussed in counselling. It might be feasible to postpone the MUS and perform a delayed (two-stage) incontinence procedure, if required.

In a series of women undergoing robotic SCP + TVT for preoperative stress incontinence, Osmundsen et al [29] demonstrated a continence failure rate of 20% (n=77) which was defined as a positive CST at 12 months. This was compared to 8% failure rate in aggregate recent trials where prolapse was absent. In this study, 50% also underwent hysterectomy. Satisfaction remained high, with 83% of patients happy or very happy (PGI-I). Positive CST was associated with lower satisfaction. Repeat TVT was performed in 4.5% and one subject required sling release.

The authors' approach is to advise concomitant incontinence surgery with sacral colpopexy in women with bothersome stress incontinence and assess these women with urodynamic work-up including with prolapse reduction. The type of incontinence surgery depends on clinical and urodynamic features and patient preference.

One-step versus Two-step (Staged) Surgery

A survey of members of the American Urogynecological Society (AUGS), which included 15 surgeons from outside of the US, was conducted post publication of the CARE trial to determine the utilization of the prophylactic Burch procedure with abdominal sacrocolpopexy in 2008. Forty-two per cent of clinicians surveyed would not perform an incontinence procedure at the time of SCP in a woman without symptoms of SUI [30].

Clancy et al conducted an observational study comparing surgical complications of women having minimally invasive SCP with concomitant incontinence procedure. Of 7,097 participants, 2,433 underwent concomitant incontinence surgery. The majority of these procedures were mid-urethral slings (2,408). Apart from longer operating time and increased likelihood of urinary tract infection (UTI) there were no differences in composite outcome of surgical complications [31].

Christmann-Schmid et al [32] performed a prospective study of 75 women where laparoscopic SCP was performed with or without concomitant MUS insertion in women who had POP stage ≥ 2 and overt (n=62) or occult SUI (n=13). Concurrent hysterectomy was performed in 48 women. Of the 62 women who chose LSCP alone, 69% had no SUI postoperatively. None of 13 women who had MUS had SUI postoperatively. It is reasonable to conclude that a two-step approach will reduce some unnecessary surgical treatment.

In addition, a prospective study by Kummeling et al set out to illustrate urodynamic changes as a result of LSCP alone. Forty-two patients undergoing LSCP consented to pre- and postoperative urodynamic evaluation. LSCP corrected prolapse in all 42 patients at six months after surgery. In the absence of concomitant incontinence surgery, the first desire to void was significantly increased and maximal detrusor pressure at voiding phase was significantly decreased. Irritative and storage voiding symptoms, and detrusor overactivity, were also decreased. There were no adverse urodynamic findings identified. The median bother score of stress incontinence (range; 0–100) was 17 (0–83) preoperatively and 0 postoperatively (0–67) but this was not significant (p=0.1) [33].

The author's practice is to discuss the merits of one-step versus two-step staged surgery. Planned two-step staged surgery most often occurs in the setting of urodynamic assessment showing significant voiding dysfunction in addition to stress urinary incontinence. The voiding dysfunction is most often due to the prolapse and will likely resolve with prolapse correction. It is however potentially problematic to perform incontin ence surgery such as midurethral or other sling in this situation so this may be deferred for three months.

Table 25.1

Author	Year	Study design	Population	N	Median follow-up (months)	Group(s)	Result
Brubaker et al* [34]	2008	RCT	Stress-continent	302	24	ASC + BC vs ASC alone	SUI in 32% vs 45%
Nygaard et al* [35]	2013	RCT	Stress-continent	215	84	ASC + BC vs ASC alone	SUI in 62% vs 77% UI in 75% vs 81%
Costantini et al ^ [36]	2007	RCT	Stress-continent	66	39.5	ASC + BC vs ASC alone	SUI 26% vs 3% UI 35% vs 9%
Costantini et al^ [22]	2011	RCT	Stress-continent	62	97	ASC + BC vs ASC alone	SUI 22% vs 6% UI 28% vs 16%
Costantini et al§ [28]	2008	RCT	Urinary incontinent	47	48	ASC + BC vs ASC alone	SUI 33% vs 39% UI 54% vs 39%
Costantini et al§ [37]	2012	RCT	Urinary incontinent	45	66	ASC + BC vs ASC alone	SUI 30% vs 27% UI 57% vs 41%
Cosson et al [38]	2002	Retrospective case series	Reported SUI	74	11	LSC + BC	Re-operation for two patients due to SUI
Zhao et al [39]	2020	Retrospective case series	Positive CST or USI	47	14	RSC + BC	3 of 29 Burch colposuspension required MUS for recurrent SUI

*^§ *Denotes results that were from the same trials at different time points.*

Concomitant Colposuspension versus Mid-urethral Synthetic Sling

Trabuco et al [40] conducted an RCT comparing Burch colposuspension versus MUS with concomitant SCP. Of the 133 women included, 56 underwent MUS and 57 Burch colposuspension. All women had either symptomatic SUI, stress-predominant mixed urinary incontinence, or OSI. At six-month follow-up, there was no difference in overall and stress specific UI between the two groups. The MUS group did however report greater satisfaction (78% compared with 57%; P=0.04) and were more likely to report successful SUI surgery (71% compared with 50%; P=0.04)) [40,41]. The same study group [40] showed that at two-year follow-up, retropubic mid-urethral sling resulted in higher stress-specific continence rates than Burch retropubic urethropexy (70% (40 of 57) versus 45% (25 of 56) P=.006). Overall continence was higher in the sling group at one year (49% (28 of 57) versus 29% (16 of 56), P=.03) but not at two years (47% (27 of 57) versus 32% (18 of 56), P=.10). There were no differences in prolapse recurrence, voiding dysfunction, antimuscarinic medication use, or patient satisfaction.

Lazarou et al performed a retrospective cohort study of 117 women who underwent ASC with Burch (n=60) or TOT (n=57). All women had preoperative SUI by either subjective measures, positive CST, or urodynamic assessment. The TOT group had lower rates of postoperative SUI (TOT 12.5%, Burch 30%, OR = 0.15, 95% CI 0.04, 0.62). There were no differences in intra- and postoperative complications including estimated blood loss, duration of procedure, and length of hospital stay. Although not significant, the Burch group trended toward a higher rate of reoperation for persistent/recurrent SUI (Burch 25%, TOT 12%, p = 0.078) [42].

Moon et al also concluded in a retrospective review that compared with Burch, TOT was associated with shorter hospital stay and operating time, and less urinary retention, *de novo* urgency, and recurrent SUI. The cure rate was higher in the TOT group (98.3% versus 69.7%, p<0.001) [43].

Patel et al conducted a retrospective chart review of 150 subjects with abdominal sacral colpopexy comparing the outcome of concomitant Burch colposuspension versus mid-urethral sling. One hundred and fifteen had SUI preoperatively; 48 with overt SUI and 34 with occult SUI had concomitant Burch, and 22 with overt and four with occult SUI had concomitant MUS. At median follow-up of eight months, 10% (15 of 150) of all subjects had SUI; 10 of the Burch group, none of the TVT group, and five *de novo*. Of these, 47% went on to have further surgery. Subjects with preoperative SUI who had a Burch were more likely to have postoperative SUI than those who had a TVT (10 versus 0, p = 0.007) [44].

Concomitant Fascial Sling

There are no published trials of women undergoing minimally invasive SCP with concomitant fascial sling.

Tubre et al performed a retrospective, single institution, single surgeon review of women who underwent open SCP (n=152) and concomitant sling procedure for overt or occult SUI. They compared synthetic MUS (retropubic, n=58, and transobturator,n=45) to autologous rectus fascial sling (n=49) [47]. No difference in SUI cure rates or sling revision surgery were observed, including after stratification for overt and occult SUI. Quality of life indices improved for all groups. There was no evidence of a difference in postoperative complications between sling types. Overall, 22 patients were discharged with an indwelling catheter (two for bladder injury). Four (two in the fascial sling group, one in the retropubic group, one in the transobturator group) required intermittent self-catheterization beyond 30 days.

Table 25.2

Author	Year	Study design	Population	N=	Median follow-up (months)	Group(s)	Result
Trabuco et al [40]	2018	RCT	Stress incontinent	133	24	ASC + BC vs ASC + MUS	Objective/subjective stress cure in 70% vs 45%; UI cure in 32% vs 47%
Jeon et al [45]	2014	Prospective observational study	Stress continent and incontinent	223 (SCP + TOT = 124)	14	LSC (n=34) or ASC (n=189) + TOT if USI	No TOT – 29% with SUI or received incontinence surgery. TOT – 5%
Osmundsen et al [29]	2015	Prospective observational study	Stress incontinent	77	12	RSC + TVT	Continence failure rate 20%
Botros et al [46]	2014	Prospective observational study	Stress incontinent	101	12	RSC + SIS	Objective cure 90%; subjective cure 87%
Lazarou et al (42)	2019	Retrospective cohort	Stress incontinent	117		ASC + BC vs ASC + TOT	SUI 30% vs 12.5%; re-operation 25% vs 12%
Moon et al [43]	2011	Retrospective cohort	Stress incontinent	109	24months (BC), 12 months (TOT)	ASC + BC vs ASC + TOT	Cure 70% vs 98%

Concomitant Urethral Bulking Agent or Artificial Urinary Sphincter

To the best of our knowledge, there are no trials or reported cohort studies of SCP with urethral bulking agent or with artificial urinary sphincter.

Cost Effectiveness of Concomitant Incontinence Surgery

In 2013, Richardson et al [48], using decision analysis modelling, compared the cost-effectiveness during a one-year postoperative period of three treatment approaches including:

1. abdominal sacrocolpopexy alone with deferred option for mid-urethral sling
2. abdominal sacrocolpopexy with universal concomitant mid-urethral sling
3. preoperative urodynamic study for selective mid-urethral sling

Using published data, they modelled the probabilities of stress urinary incontinence after abdominal sacrocolpopexy with or without mid-urethral sling, the predictive value of urodynamic study to detect occult stress urinary incontinence, and the likelihood of complications after mid-urethral sling. Costs were derived from Medicare 2010 reimbursement rates. They found that universally performing mid-urethral sling at abdominal sacrocolpopexy was the most cost-effective approach, with an incremental cost per quality-adjusted life-year gained of $2,867 compared to abdominal sacrocolpopexy alone. Preoperative urodynamic study was more costly and less effective than universally performing intraoperative mid-urethral sling.

This paper was published in 2013 and utilizes data from 2010 which was the peak prevalence of mid-urethral sling surgery and predates the second FDA update on transvaginal mesh surgery in 2011. Also, it is based on US costing, which may not be generalizable to other countries. A re-evaluation of this costing modelling, taking into account the costs of sling complication management in the order of 1–3% and litigation costs may substantially change the conclusion.

Conclusion

Current evidence is limited when making a conclusive decision regarding concomitant procedure for urinary incontinence at the time of SCP. Simplistically, the addition of an incontinence procedure decreases the rate of subsequent stress urinary incontinence, however, the number needed to treat is a complicated discussion. Needless to say, the decision should be individualized, after appropriate preoperative assessment (understanding the limitations of this) and discussion with the patient. The choice of incontinence procedure will depend on patient preference for mesh or non-mesh incontinence surgery, and concomitant or staged surgery and other factors such as surgeon expertise.

The authors' local practice is to perform urodynamic assessment in women with bothersome stress urinary incontinence and offer concomitant incontinence surgery; to inform stress continent women of the risk of occult stress urinary incontinence of the order of 10–20% and offer urodynamic assessment to those women. If positive, the discussion becomes one of the number needed to treat occult stress incontinence. The authors' practice is to not mandate universal preoperative urodynamic assessment in stress continent women prior to sacral colpopexy.

Large, well designed, and powered RCTs in the future may change this approach.

References

1. Haylen BT, de Ridder D, Freeman RM, et al. An International Urogynecological Association (IUGA)/International Continence Society (ICS) joint report on the terminology for female pelvic floor dysfunction. Int Urogynecol J 2010; 21(1): 5–26.
2. Lensen EJ, Withagen MI, Kluivers KB, Milani AL, Vierhout ME. Urinary incontinence after surgery for pelvic organ prolapse. Neurourol Urodyn 2013; 32(5): 455–9.
3. Hilton P, Dolan LM. Pathophysiology of urinary incontinence and pelvic organ prolapse. BJOG 2004; 111(Suppl 1): 5–9.
4. van der Ploeg JM, van der Steen A, Oude Rengerink K, van der Vaart CH, Roovers JP. Prolapse surgery with or without stress incontinence surgery for pelvic organ prolapse: a systematic review and meta-analysis of randomised trials. BJOG 2014; 121(5): 537–47.
5. Borstad E, Rud T. The risk of developing urinary stress-incontinence after vaginal repair in continent women. A clinical and urodynamic follow-up study. Acta Obstet Gynecol Scand 1989; 68(6): 545–9.
6. Brubaker L, Cundiff GW, Fine P, et al. Abdominal sacrocolpopexy with Burch colposuspension to reduce urinary stress incontinence. N Engl J Med 2006; 354(15): 1557–66.
7. Ennemoser S, Schonfeld M, von Bodungen V, et al. Clinical relevance of occult stress urinary incontinence (OSUI) following vaginal prolapse surgery: long-term follow-up. Int Urogynecol J 2012; 23(7): 851–5.
8. Baessler K, Christmann-Schmid C, Maher C, et al. Surgery for women with pelvic organ prolapse with or without stress urinary incontinence. Cochrane Database Syst Rev 2018; 8: CD013108.
9. Joint Writing Group of the American Urogynecologic Society and the International Urogynecological Association. Joint report on the terminology for surgical procedures to treat stress urinary incontinence in women. Int Urogynecol J 2020; 31(3): 465–78.
10. Culligan PJ, Lewis C, Priestley J, Mushonga N. Long-term outcomes of robotic-assisted laparoscopic sacrocolpopexy using lightweight Y-mesh. Female Pelvic Med Reconstr Surg 2020; 26(3): 202–6.
11. Lapitan MCM, Cody JD, Mashayekhi A. Open retropubic colposuspension for urinary incontinence in women. Cochrane Database Syst Rev 2017; 7(7): CD002912.
12. Freites J, Stewart F, Omar MI, Mashayekhi A, Agur WI. Laparoscopic colposuspension for urinary incontinence in women. Cochrane Database Syst Rev 2019; 12(12): CD002239.
13. Ford AA, Rogerson L, Cody JD, Aluko P, Ogah JA. Mid-urethral sling operations for stress urinary incontinence in women. Cochrane Database Syst Rev 2017; 7(7): CD006375.
14. Fusco F, Abdel-Fattah M, Chapple CR, et al. Updated systematic review and meta-analysis of the comparative data on colposuspensions, pubovaginal slings, and midurethral tapes in

the surgical treatment of female stress urinary incontinence. Eur Urol 2017; 72(4): 567–91.

15. Morling JR, McAllister DA, Agur W, et al. Adverse events after first, single, mesh and non-mesh surgical procedures for stress urinary incontinence and pelvic organ prolapse in Scotland, 1997–2016: a population-based cohort study. Lancet 2017; 389(10069): 629–40.
16. Winters JC, Dmochowski RR, Goldman HB, et al. Urodynamic studies in adults: AUA/SUFU guideline. J Urol 2012; 188(6 Suppl): 2464–72.
17. Nambiar AK, Lemack GE, Chapple CR, Burkhard FC, European Association of Urology. The role of urodynamics in the evaluation of urinary incontinence: The European Association of Urology Recommendations in 2016. Eur Urol 2017; 71(4): 501–3.
18. Nager CW, Brubaker L, Litman HJ, et al. A randomized trial of urodynamic testing before stress-incontinence surgery. N Engl J Med 2012; 366(21): 1987–97.
19. van Leijsen SA, Kluivers KB, Mol BW, et al. Value of urodynamics before stress urinary incontinence surgery: a randomized controlled trial. Obstet Gynecol 2013; 121(5): 999–1008.
20. Visco AG, Brubaker L, Nygaard I, et al. The role of preoperative urodynamic testing in stress-continent women undergoing sacrocolpopexy: the Colpopexy and Urinary Reduction Efforts (CARE) randomized surgical trial. Int Urogynecol J Pelvic Floor Dysfunct 2008; 19(5): 607–14.
21. Elser DM, Moen MD, Stanford EJ, et al. Abdominal sacrocolpopexy and urinary incontinence: surgical planning based on urodynamics. Am J Obstet Gynecol 2010; 202(4): 375 e1–5.
22. Costantini E, Lazzeri M, Bini V, et al. Pelvic organ prolapse repair with and without prophylactic concomitant Burch colposuspension in continent women: a randomized, controlled trial with 8-year followup. J Urol 2011; 185(6): 2236–40.
23. Misraï V, Rouprêt M, Cour F, Chartier-Kastler E, Richard F. De novo urinary stress incontinence after laparoscopic sacral colpopexy. BJU Int 2008; 101(5): 594–7.
24. Wei JT, Nygaard I, Richter HE, et al. A midurethral sling to reduce incontinence after vaginal prolapse repair. N Engl J Med 2012; 366(25): 2358–67.
25. Schierlitz L, Dwyer PL, Rosamilia A, et al. Pelvic organ prolapse surgery with and without tension-free vaginal tape in women with occult or asymptomatic urodynamic stress incontinence: a randomised controlled trial. Int Urogynecol J 2014; 25(1): 33–40.
26. Walsh C, Dwyer P, Rosamilia A, et al. 41st Annual Meeting – Cape Town, South Africa August 4 – 5, 2016. Int Urogynecol J 2016; 27(1): 19–149.
27. Borstad E, Abdelnoor M, Staff AC, Kulseng-Hanssen S. Surgical strategies for women with pelvic organ prolapse and urinary stress incontinence. Int Urogynecol J 2010; 21(2): 179–86.
28. Costantini E, Lazzeri M, Bini V, et al. Burch colposuspension does not provide any additional benefit to pelvic organ prolapse repair in patients with urinary incontinence: a randomized surgical trial. J Urol 2008; 180(3): 1007–12.
29. Osmundsen B, Gregory WT, Denman MA, et al. Tension-free vaginal tape failure after robotic sacrocolpopexy and tension-free vaginal tape for concomitant prolapse and stress incontinence. Female Pelvic Med Reconstr Surg 2015; 21(5): 244–8.
30. Aungst MJ, Mamienski TD, Albright TS, Zahn CM, Fischer JR. Prophylactic Burch colposuspension at the time of abdominal sacrocolpopexy: a survey of current practice patterns. Int Urogynecol J Pelvic Floor Dysfunct 2009; 20(8): 897–904.
31. Clancy AA, Mallick R, Breau RH, Khalil H, Hickling DR. Complications after minimally invasive sacrocolpopexy with and without concomitant incontinence surgery: A National Surgical Quality Improvement Program (NSQIP) database study. Neurourol Urodyn 2018; 37(7): 2234–41.
32. Christmann-Schmid C, Bruehlmann E, Koerting I, Krebs J. Laparoscopic sacrocolpopexy with or without midurethral sling insertion: is a two-step approach justified? A prospective study. Eur J Obstet Gynecol Reprod Biol 2018; 229: 98–102.
33. Kummeling MT, Rietbergen JB, Withagen MI, Mannaerts GH, van der Weiden RM. Sequential urodynamic assessment before and after laparoscopic sacrocolpopexy. Acta Obstet Gynecol Scand 2013; 92(2): 172–7.
34. Brubaker L, Nygaard I, Richter HE, et al. Two-year outcomes after sacrocolpopexy with and without Burch to prevent stress urinary incontinence. Obstet Gynecol 2008; 112(1): 49–55.
35. Nygaard I, Brubaker L, Zyczynski HM, et al. Long-term outcomes following abdominal sacrocolpopexy for pelvic organ prolapse. JAMA 2013; 309(19): 2016–24.
36. Costantini E, Zucchi A, Giannantoni A, et al. Must colposuspension be associated with sacropexy to prevent postoperative urinary incontinence? Eur Urol 2007; 51(3): 788–94.
37. Costantini E, Lazzeri M, Bini V, et al. Pelvic organ prolapse repair with and without concomitant Burch colposuspension in incontinent women: a randomised controlled trial with at least 5-year followup. Obstet Gynecol Int 2012; 2012: 967923.
38. Cosson M, Rajabally R, Bogaert E, Querleu D, Crépin G. Laparoscopic sacrocolpopexy, hysterectomy, and Burch colposuspension: feasibility and short-term complications of 77 procedures. JSLS 2002; 6(2): 115–19.
39. Zhao Y, Martin BS. Robotic-assisted laparoscopic sacrocolpopexy: initial Canadian experience. Can Urol Assoc J 2020; 14(6): E257–E263. https://doi.org/10.5489/cuaj.6121
40. Trabuco EC, Linder BJ, Klingele CJ, et al. Two-year results of Burch compared with midurethral sling with sacrocolpopexy: a randomized controlled trial. Obstet Gynecol 2018; 131(1): 31–8.
41. Trabuco EC, Klingele CJ, Blandon RE, et al. Burch retropubic urethropexy compared with midurethral sling with concurrent sacrocolpopexy: a randomized controlled trial. Obstet Gynecol 2016; 128(4): 828–35.
42. Lazarou G, Minis E, Grigorescu B. Outcomes of stress urinary incontinence in women undergoing TOT versus Burch colposuspension with abdominal sacrocolpopexy. Int Urogynecol J 2019; 30(2): 245–50.
43. Moon YJ, Jeon MJ, Kim SK, Bai SW. Comparison of Burch colposuspension and transobturator tape when combined with abdominal sacrocolpopexy. Int J Gynaecol Obstet 2011; 112(2): 122–5.
44. Patel M, O'Sullivan D, Tulikangas PK. Is Burch or mid-urethral sling better with abdominal sacral colpopexy? Int Urogynecol J Pelvic Floor Dysfunct 2009; 20(7): 787–90.

45. Jeon MJ, Kim JY, Moon YJ, Bai SW, Yoo EH. Two-year urinary outcomes of sacrocolpopexy with or without transobturator tape: results of a prolapse-reduction stress test-based approach. Int Urogynecol J 2014; 25(11): 1517–22.
46. Botros C, Lewis C, Culligan P, Salamon C. A prospective study of a single-incision sling at the time of robotic sacrocolpopexy. Int Urogynecol J 2014; 25(11): 1541–6.
47. Tubre RW, Padmanabhan P, Frilot CF, 2nd, Porta W, Gomelsky A. Outcomes of three sling procedures at the time of abdominal sacral colpopexy. Neurourol Urodyn 2017; 36(2): 482–5.
48. Richardson ML, Elliott CS, Shaw JG, et al. To sling or not to sling at time of abdominal sacrocolpopexy: a cost-effectiveness analysis. J Urol 2013; 190(4): 1306–12.

Chapter 26

Management of the Posterior Compartment in Laparoscopic Urogynaecology: Role of Rectopexy, Vaginal Rectocele Repair, and Perineorrhaphy

Angela S Yuan, Sarah A Vogler

Introduction

Approximately one-third of surgeries performed for pelvic organ prolapse in the US include procedures on the posterior vaginal wall [1]. Structural defects of the posterior compartment include rectocele, enterocele, and sigmoidocele. Rectoceles can manifest as an asymptomatic bulge, or with bothersome symptoms such as pelvic pressure, constipation, faecal seepage or urgency, and defaecatory dysfunction. In the evaluation of these symptoms, additional problems such as rectal prolapse or rectal intussusception may be discovered. It is important to develop a good understanding of the anatomy, pathophysiology, and work-up of these conditions prior to proceeding with surgical management. While pelvic organ prolapse and rectal prolapse have historically been treated as separate problems, patients in whom these issues co-exist will ideally benefit from a multidisciplinary team approach. The following chapter will address management of the posterior compartment and is tailored to readers from both urogynaecology and colorectal surgery backgrounds.

Anatomy and Pathophysiology

Anatomy of the Posterior Compartment and Pathogenesis of the Rectocele

Pelvic organ support is divided into an anterior compartment, containing the bladder and urethra, and a posterior compartment, containing the rectum and anus. The two compartments are separated by the vagina and uterus, which comprises the middle compartment. The endopelvic fascia is a layer comprised of collagen, smooth muscle, elastin, and fibrovascular elements. The fascia is arranged as a continuous sheet that covers the levator ani muscles and pelvic viscera. Together, the endopelvic fascia and levator ani muscles provide support to the pelvic organs.

Normal anatomic support of the posterior vaginal wall is divided into DeLancey's three levels. The upper portion of the posterior vaginal wall (level 1) is suspended to the pelvic wall by the uterosacral-cardinal ligament complex. The middle portion of the posterior vaginal wall (level 2) is attached on either side of the rectum to the inner surface of the pelvic diaphragm by a sheet of endopelvic fascia. These endopelvic fascial sheets prevent ventral movement of the posterior vaginal wall. The urogenital diaphragm and the perineal body provide support to the lower part of the vagina (level 3).

Normally, the puborectalis muscle is in a tonic state of contraction. As a result, the anterior and posterior vaginal walls are in contact with one another, balancing anterior and posterior pressures with little to no stress on level 2 endopelvic fascial supports. The force is carried by the levator ani muscles and perineal body, which are in a horizontal plane. When the puborectalis muscle is relaxed or damaged, the vaginal canal opens, and support is required from the connective tissues in level 2. Defects in mid-vaginal support can give rise to a rectocele. Separation of the distal posterior vaginal wall from the perineal body can give rise to a distal rectocele or perineocele. This condition must be addressed by reuniting the separated fibres of the perineal body and reattaching the perineal body to the level 2 supports.

Rectal Prolapse: Definitions and Pathogenesis

Rectal prolapse and rectal intussusception (occult rectal prolapse) are pelvic floor conditions that share a common aetiology and risk factors with rectoceles. Complete rectal prolapse is a full-thickness, circumferential protrusion of the rectum through the anus. Prolapse of the rectal mucosa only is referred to as rectal mucosal prolapse. Rectal intussusception is the 'telescoping' of the rectal wall on itself without protrusion through the anus, and is also called occult rectal prolapse. Rectal intussusception is believed to be the precursor to full thickness rectal prolapse. Although not all cases of rectal intussusception will develop into overt rectal prolapse, this progression has been described and studied [2–3].

The annual incidence of rectal prolapse, most common in elderly women, is estimated at 2.5 per 100,000 people [4]. Risk factors for rectal prolapse are summarized in Table 26.1 [5–10]. Long-standing straining and prior obstetric injury are believed to cause pudendal nerve damage, thereby gradually weakening the levator ani muscles and eventually the anal sphincter [11]. This theory underlies the findings of levator ani avulsion and genital hiatal widening that have been observed in women with rectal intussuception [10] and prolapse [12].

Anatomic features generally associated with rectal prolapse include weakness of the levator ani and anal sphincter muscles, an abnormally deep and wide cul-de-sac, and laxity or loss of the sacral attachments to the rectum [12]. In 1968, Broden and Snellman confirmed that rectal prolapse represented a circumferential intussusception through the use of cineradiography [13].

Table 26.1 Risk factors for rectal prolapse

• Age ≥ 50 years	• Prior pelvic surgery
• Female gender	• Irritable bowel syndrome
• Multiparity	• Spinal cord abnormalities
• Obstetric injury	• Cystic fibrosis
• Chronic straining	• Malnutrition
• Chronic constipation	• Psychiatric illness

Clinical Presentation

Symptoms associated with posterior compartment prolapse include splinting (manual pressure applied to the vagina, rectum, or perineum to assist defaecation), pelvic pressure or heaviness, constipation, defaecatory dysfunction with incomplete defaecation, sexual dysfunction, and faecal incontinence [14]. Digital splinting along the posterior vaginal wall can assist some women in daefecation by maintaining support within the rectovaginal septum.

It is critical to characterize constipation symptoms described by women because a rectocele can be present within two broad categories of constipation symptoms – obstructive defaecation secondary to muscle dyssynergia versus muscle weakness. Those patients with dyssynergia tend to have a well-defined puborectalis muscle along the posterior rectal wall and relatively high anal sphincter tone. They will present with symptoms of excessive straining, hard consistency of the stools, feeling of incomplete emptying, or infrequent stools. This clinical picture of pelvic floor muscle dyssynergia is frequently seen in combination with slow-transit constipation. In this category of patients, rectoceles (and the associated symptoms) are best treated with a bowel regimen to improve stool consistency and regularity, and pelvic floor physical therapy and biofeedback to improve pelvic muscle coordination and thus aid in defaecation. Conversely, patients who have a rectocele and profoundly weak muscles (puborectalis and anal sphincter complex) can also present with outlet obstructive symptoms. The rectal wall collapsing along the rectocele due to loss of muscle support may trap stool within a distal rectal pocket, which can lead to the feeling of incomplete bowel evacuation or post-defaecatory soiling. In both categories of obstructive defaecation, patients will describe a feeling of incomplete defaecation with most bowel movements.

Issues with sexual function are common among women with pelvic floor disorders. One study noted that dyspareunia was present in 87% of women with symptomatic rectoceles (n=68), and showed statistically significant improvement after native tissue rectocele repair in sexual desire, satisfaction, and pain [15], as assessed by the Female Sexual Function Index [16].

Faecal incontinence is common in patients with pelvic organ prolapse and urinary incontinence, occurring in approximately 15–17% of women [17–18]. The relationship between these conditions is understandable, given their shared pathogenesis, namely, pelvic floor damage and pudendal nerve injury [17]. Studies have not consistently demonstrated a linear relationship between the severity of posterior vaginal wall prolapse and faecal incontinence symptoms [17]. However, studies have shown a linear relationship between depth of rectal intussusception and increasing severity of faecal incontinence and decreasing anal sphincter tone [20]. Faecal incontinence associated with pelvic organ prolapse tends to be due to a combination of incomplete defaecation from rectal collapse and anal sphincter weakness.

The most common presentation of rectal prolapse is the presence of a rectal tissue protruding through the anus. Rectal prolapse is also associated with the passage of blood and/or mucus per rectum. About 50–75% of patients with rectal prolapse report faecal incontinence, and 24–50% of patients report constipation [21]. Patients with rectal intussusception may present with anorectal pain, obstructed defaecation, and incomplete bowel evacuation, as well as the symptoms seen in overt rectal prolapse [21].

Multi-disciplinary Approach to the Management of Concomitant Rectal and Pelvic Organ Prolapse

Patients with combined vaginal and rectal prolapse should be offered multi-disciplinary pelvic floor evaluation and combined surgery. Doing so avoids unnecessary delays in care and fragmentation of surgical treatment which can result in suboptimal outcomes. Combined surgery allows for complete pelvic floor repair with a single recuperation period and is associated with higher patient satisfaction and cost savings [22]. A multidisciplinary pelvic floor clinic is offered at our institution, and patients presenting with a combination of bowel, prolapse, and/or urinary complaints are assessed by a urogynaecologist and colorectal surgeon during a joint encounter. In addition to patient convenience, this combined clinic permits direct communication between the urogynaecologist and colorectal surgeon to decide on evaluation and treatment planning. Where this clinical model is not available, urogynaecologists should strive to identify appropriate patients for referral to colorectal surgery, and vice versa.

Evaluation of the Patient

History

The first step in evaluating these patients is to take a comprehensive history, with special attention given to bowel and dietary habits, urinary function, and pelvic symptoms. It is important to inquire about symptoms related to urinary incontinence, as well as anterior compartment and vaginal vault/uterine prolapse, as pelvic floor support defects typically do not occur in isolation. Patients with combined rectal and pelvic organ prolapse should have a multi-disciplinary approach to their evaluation and management. A directed medical history should also be performed to assess for risk factors for posterior wall and rectal prolapse such as obstetric history, previous pelvic surgeries, prior prolapse history and management, and past colonoscopy findings. History of sexual dysfunction should be elicited, as patients will often not voluntarily disclose this information unless directly asked. The use of standardized, validated bowel and urinary function and quality-of-life questionnaires should be considered at the time of initial assessment.

Physical Exam

Posterior compartment prolapse is typically assessed with the patient in dorsal lithotomy or semi-recumbent position. The woman may also be examined in standing position, especially if the degree of prolapse visualized in lithotomy is not consistent with the patient's description. The severity of prolapse is evaluated by visualizing the vaginal wall using a single blade of a bivalve speculum or a Sims speculum. The patient is asked to perform a Valsalva manoeuvre or cough during the exam. Staging of the prolapse is performed with the Pelvic Organ Prolapse-Quantification (POP-Q) system, which uses objective measurements against defined reference points in the vaginal canal [23]. Evaluation of all three compartments (anterior, apical, and posterior) should be performed so that the prolapse can be appropriately addressed during surgery.

The perineal body should also be examined during a Valsalva manoeuvre to assess for perineal descent. Convexity or bulging of the perineum may be visualized. This clinical finding results from the loss of continuity between the perineal body (level 3) from the suspensory support of the vaginal apex (level 1). Perineal descent is usually a consequence of chronic straining causing progressing weakening to the pelvic floor supports and stretching of the pudendal nerve [24]. It can be seen in women with faecal incontinence and rectal prolapse [24].

A rectovaginal exam should be performed to evaluate the posterior vaginal wall and perineal body. A rectocele is confirmed if the area of posterior vaginal wall bulging on speculum exam correlates with that on rectovaginal exam. An enterocele should be suspected if loops of small bowel are palpated. Standing position may augment detection of an enterocele by shifting bowel into the enterocele sac. Findings may be correlated with defecography and should be re-evaluated intraoperatively to ensure that an enterocele, if indeed present, is addressed.

The anorectal exam can be performed with the patient in dorsal lithotomy but is more typically done in left lateral decubitus or prone jack knife (knee-chest) positions. The choice of position should be based on the examiner's preference and ability in which to obtain an effective examination. A visual inspection of the perianal skin is performed first to assess for skin changes, scars or prior trauma, external skin tags or haemorrhoids, fissures, and fistulas.

The diagnosis of rectal prolapse is made by clinical inspection of the patient while straining. If the rectal prolapse cannot be elicited while on the examination table, the patient should be examined while squatting or sitting over a commode. The examiner can use a mirror when examining in this position to identify the concentric rings of rectal mucosa protruding through the anus. If this is unsuccessful, the patient can be asked to bring a photograph of their findings.

A digital rectal exam is important to assess the anal sphincter. The sphincter is assessed for tone at rest and during squeeze, as well as for symmetry, attenuation, or disruption. The patient should be asked to Valsalva during the exam in order to mimic defaecation and allow for assessment of normal relaxation of the pelvic floor muscles. The rectovaginal exam, as described above, can be performed at the time of the digital rectal exam to minimize patient discomfort.

Anorectal Testing

The tools used to investigate anorectal disorders include both anatomic and functional testing. Not every test is necessary for each patient or each disorder. A complete history and physical examination will help to decide which investigations are necessary. Commonly used tests, their indications, and procedural steps are detailed below.

Defecography

Defecography is a dynamic radiologic study examining the anatomic and functional changes of the pelvic organs during defaecation. Imaging contrast is inserted into the vagina and the rectum, and the patient is asked to evacuate the contrast during the examination. Oral contrast may be administered 45–60 minutes prior to the study for opacification of the small bowel to facilitate visualization of an enterocele. Defecography can be achieved by the use of fluoroscopy or dynamic magnetic resonance imaging (MRI). The advantages and disadvantages of each imaging modality are depicted in Table 26.2.

While not required for the diagnosis of overt rectal prolapse, defecography is still necessary to determine presence or degree of rectal intussusception, extent of multicompartment pelvic organ prolapse and patient's ability to appropriately coordinate pelvic floor muscles during defaecation.

During defecography, the anorectal angle (ARA) and anorectal junction (ARJ) are measured (Figure 26.1). The ARA is measured between the longitudinal axis of anal canal and the posterior rectal line, parallel to the longitudinal axis of the rectum. Its average value at rest is approximately 90 degrees. The ARA is an indirect marker of puborectalis activity, becoming more acute during contraction, and more obtuse during relaxation. The ARJ is the uppermost point of the anal canal and is measured in reference to a fixed bony landmark, such as the bi-ischiatic line (line drawn between the ischial tuberosities) or the pubococcygeal line (line between the inferior border of the symphysis pubis and tip of the coccyx). The craniocaudal migration of the ARJ represents the elevation and descent of the pelvic floor.

The patient is evaluated in three phases: rest, evacuation, and recovery. Normal findings are as follows: During rest, the ARA is about 90 degrees. During voluntary squeezing, the ARA becomes more acute (about 75 degrees) and the ARJ migrates cranially. When the patient is asked to strain to evacuate, the

Table 26.2 Comparison of defecography by fluoroscopy versus dynamic magnetic resonance imaging

	Fluoroscopy	MRI
Advantages	- Natural/upright position during evacuation - Easily available with fluoroscopic equipment - Low cost	- Clear images of pelvic compartments and musculature - Exact radiographic measurements - No radiation exposure
Disadvantages	- Imprecise image quality to assess muscle integrity - Radiation exposure	- Unnatural position/ lying supine or lateral during evacuation - High cost

ARA widens and the ARJ migrates caudally; less than 3.5 cm of caudal migration relative to resting position is considered normal. During evacuation, the anal canal widens and the anorectum is seen funnelling. The ARA increases with relaxation of the anal sphincter and puborectalis. The rectum should completely evacuate the contrast, with collapse of the rectal walls. Once active straining ceases, the rectum returns to its original resting position.

Rectocele

On defecography, a rectocele is represented by an outpouching of the anterior rectal wall with displacement of the vaginal lumen during straining and defaecation. An example is depicted in Figure 26.2. Small rectoceles are detected in approximately 80% of asymptomatic controls [25]. Rectoceles demonstrating contrast retention have been found in women who report complete defaecation [26]. Therefore, radiologic findings should be interpreted cautiously. Fluoroscopically detected rectoceles larger than 2 cm correlate strongly with presence of advanced stage (stage 2–3) rectoceles on examination [27]. While defecography provides a useful adjunct in the detection of posterior vaginal wall prolapse, it should not be used in place of physical examination.

Rectal Intussusception and Rectal Prolapse

Rectal intussusception and external rectal prolapse can be demonstrated on defecography during straining or defaecation. Figure 26.3 depicts examples of rectal intussusception and external rectal prolapse. The presence of an infolding of the rectal wall measuring ≥3 mm thickness seen during straining is consistent with intussusception. Grading of the rectal intussusception on defecography is done with the Oxford Rectal Prolapse Grading System (Table 26.3).

Anorectal Manometry

Anorectal manometry can be performed to evaluate sphincteric function in patients with faecal incontinence, constipation, obstructed defaecation, and anorectal pain. A pressure-sensitive probe, which has a balloon at its tip, is inserted into the patient's rectum and used to measure pressures along the length of the anal canal. Previous position statements provide guidance on techniques and data reporting [28–30]. Standard measurements obtained from anorectal manometry include resting pressure, squeeze pressure, length of the high-pressure zone, rectal sensation, recto-anal inhibitory reflex, and the balloon expulsion test. Normal values for these measurements depend greatly on the utilized equipment and protocol [31–32], with consideration given to the variability that is seen in gender, parity, and age [30].

Table 26.3 Oxford Rectal Prolapse Grading System

Rectal Intussusception	Radiologic Characteristics of Rectal Prolapse
I (low grade)	Descends to proximal limit of rectocele
II (low grade)	Descends into level of rectocele, but not into anal canal
III (high grade)	Descends into proximal anal canal
IV (high grade)	Descends into distal anal canal
Rectal Prolapse	
V (overt rectal prolapse)	Protrudes out of anal canal

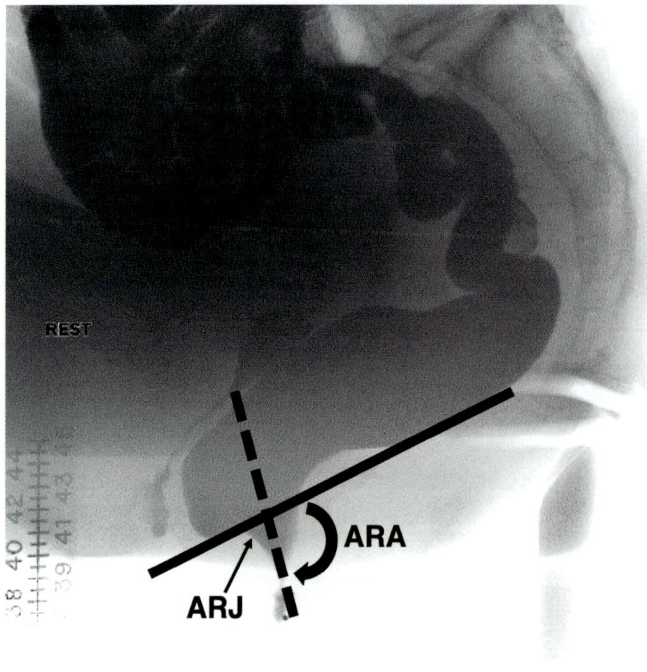

Figure 26.1 Anorectal angle (ARA) and anorectal junction (ARJ) on fluoroscopic defecography at rest.

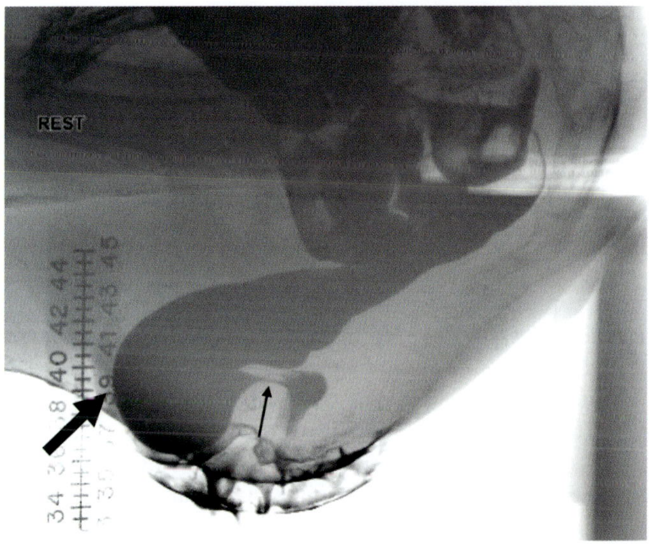

Figure 26.2 Rectocele on fluoroscopic defecography.

To perform the test, the patient is positioned in left lateral decubitus. A lubricated manometry probe is inserted into the anal canal, and a few minutes are allowed to pass while the anal sphincter returns to its basal state. The probe is kept stationary during the duration of the test to avoid excitatory stimuli.

Next, resting and squeeze pressures are measured. Resting pressure is assessed over at least 20 seconds. The internal anal sphincter accounts for approximately 85% of anal canal resting tone. Decreased resting pressure suggests isolated internal anal sphincter dysfunction. The patient is then asked to squeeze their anal sphincter and to maintain each squeeze for 30 seconds. The

(a)

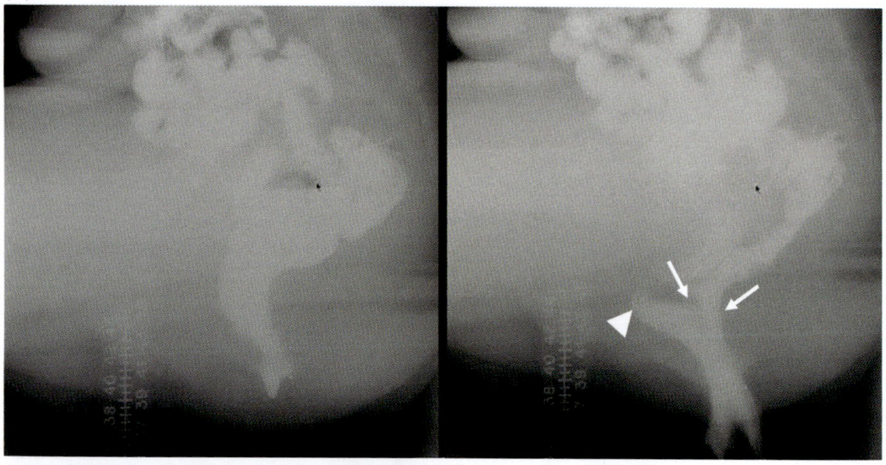

(b)

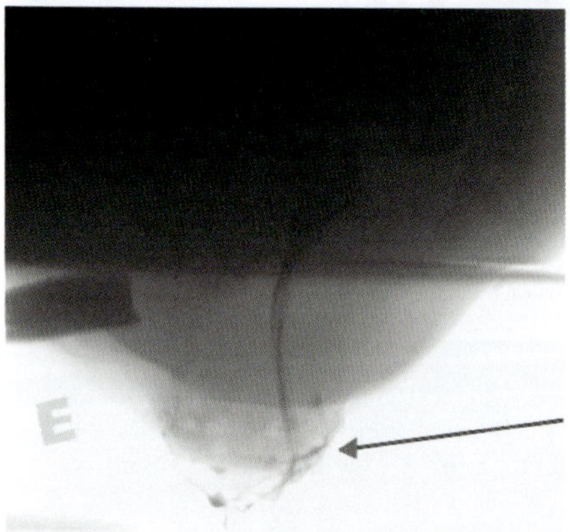

Figure 26.3 (a) Rectal intussusception on fluoroscopic defecography and (b) external rectal prolapse.

external anal sphincter (and puborectalis muscle) are responsible for the voluntary control of faecal continence. Decreased squeeze pressure suggests external anal sphincter dysfunction. Patients who have rectal prolapse may exhibit decreased squeeze pressures from stretching of the external anal sphincter [33], and in late-stage cases may also show low resting pressures due to weakening of the internal anal sphincter [34].

The patient is then asked to cough. This manoeuvre measures the recto-anal pressure changes during an abrupt change in intra-abdominal pressure, which induces reflex contraction of the external anal sphincter. This reflex screens for damage to the sacral reflex arc. Next, the patient is asked to push to simulate evacuation. Normal defaecation requires a coordinated effort involving increased rectal pressure along with relaxation of the anal sphincters and pelvic floor muscles. Anorectal manometry in patients with defaecatory disorders may demonstrate impaired relaxation or inappropriate contraction of the pelvic floor muscles, in addition to inadequate rectal pressures during simulated evacuation.

The balloon is then distended with a small volume to induce the recto-anal inhibitory reflex (RAIR). This is a normal response in which the internal anal sphincter transiently relaxes in response to sudden rectal distension. The role of the RAIR is believed to allow sampling of rectal contents by sensory receptors on the anal canal, helping to differentiate gas from stool and distinguish solid from liquid stool. This reflex plays a role in the continence mechanism and is absent in patients with Hirschsprung's disease or Chagas disease.

Anorectal sensation is assessed by distending the balloon with incremental volumes, and the volumes are recorded when the patient experiences first constant sensation, desire to defaecate, and maximum tolerated volume. Patients with rectal hypersensitivity exhibit lower than expected values during rectal distension. This can be seen in patients with urge faecal incontinence, irritable bowel syndrome, and inflammatory conditions or post-radiation changes to the rectum. Patients with higher-than-expected volumes exhibit decreased sensation with rectal filling and may suffer from faecal incontinence resulting from overfilling. This faecal overflow incontinence can be seen in patients with long-standing constipation.

Lastly, the patient is asked to attempt to push out the balloon while sitting, and the ability and time taken to expel the balloon from the rectum is recorded. This test is useful in the evaluation of patients with constipation, as it can demonstrate obstructive defaecation due to pelvic floor muscle dyssynergia.

Electromyography

Electromyography (EMG) is used to evaluate the activity of the external anal sphincter and puborectalis muscles. It is incredibly helpful in the evaluation of obstructed defaecation and constipation. Biofeedback treatment may directly incorporate EMG for muscle retraining and to monitor response to therapy.

Electromyography is performed with three different types of electrodes: needle, surface, or anal plug. Needle electrodes are considered the most accurate method, as the electrodes are inserted directly into the muscle, but these are rarely used due to obvious discomfort. Surface electrodes, which are taped to the skin, are better tolerated by patients. During testing, the patient is asked to squeeze, relax, and push. The EMG should show an increase in electrical activity with squeeze and return to baseline with relaxing. EMG activity with squeeze is decreased in patients with nerve injury or stretch. During defaecation, EMG activity should be close to zero. Patients with pelvic floor dyssynergia may demonstrate high EMG activity during defaecation due to paradoxic puborectalis contraction.

Management of Posterior Vaginal Wall and Rectal Prolapse

Medical Management

Rectoceles

Symptomatic rectoceles can be conservatively managed with the use of pessaries or pelvic floor muscle exercises. Pessaries are effective in relieving symptoms of pelvic organ prolapse and pelvic floor dysfunction [35], including bowel complaints [36]. Patients with advanced rectoceles may not have success with ring support pessaries, in particular. In a prospective study of over 600 women with symptomatic prolapse, the presence of a leading posterior compartment prolapse was a predictor for unsuccessful fitting of ring with support pessary, but not for Gellhorn pessary [37].

Pelvic floor physical therapy aims to increase the strength of pelvic floor muscles and thereby improve pelvic organ support. A meta-analysis of over 2,300 patients found that women who received pelvic floor muscle training showed a greater subjective improvement in prolapse symptoms compared to controls [38]. Nevertheless, advanced prolapse is unlikely to resolve with physical therapy alone.

Rectal Prolapse

There have been no studies that directly compare surgical and medical management of rectal prolapse. Medical management does not definitively treat the condition, but should be offered to patients to mitigate symptoms prior to surgery, or to patients who decline or cannot undergo surgery due to comorbid conditions. Conservative management should be targeted toward improvement of specific symptoms, namely, constipation and faecal incontinence. Ensuring adequate fluid and fibre intake is essential.

Indications for Surgical Management

The goal of a rectocele repair is to relieve symptoms caused by a structural problem of the posterior vaginal wall, with the primary technical goal of restoring normal anatomy. The decision to pursue surgical management of symptomatic rectoceles should be a shared decision made between the patient and her surgeon after comprehensive counselling about all management options, with consideration given to the patient's age, severity of symptoms, degree of bother, medical comorbidities, and prior treatments. Choice of surgical procedure should address all significant support defects, as failure to correct these at the time of surgery can lead to progression or recurrence of rectocele.

Surgery is usually required to correct rectal prolapse, and unnecessary delays in surgery should be avoided to prevent prolapse and/or incontinence from worsening. For patients with rectal intussusception due to pelvic floor weakness, surgery is most likely to benefit patients whose intussusception is high-grade [39] and associated with faecal incontinence or enterocele [40–41]. Significant improvement in faecal incontinence has been reported in 38–80% of patients who underwent surgical repair of an associated rectal intussusception [41–42].

Conversely, studies evaluating surgical repair of rectal intussusception in obstructed defaecation syndrome (ODS) due to dyssynergia were disappointing due to low success rates and worsening of symptoms [43–45]. Surgical treatment of rectal intussusception in patients with high tone in the puborectalis or anal sphincter, and with dyssynergia should be avoided as surgery can actually increase tension and stiffen movement. Advances in dynamic pelvic floor imaging with defecography and more sophisticated manometry testing has facilitated identification of patients who have ODS secondary to dyssynergia. Thus, avoidance of surgery in this patient population is better determined.

Surgical Techniques

Surgical correction of rectal prolapse can be performed through an abdominal or perineal approach. Transabdominal procedures include rectopexy with or without concomitant sigmoid resection, and ventral mesh rectopexy. Transperineal procedures include perineal rectosigmoidectomy (Altmeier procedure) or rectal mucosal resection with muscular plication (Delorme procedure). Choice of route depends on patient factors including age, medical comorbidities, ability to tolerate pneumoperitoneum and steep Trendelenburg, prior surgical procedures, as well as the decision to use mesh.

Abdominal procedures generally involve mobilization of the rectum and suspension of the rectum to the sacral promontory with either sutures or mesh. A shift toward minimally invasive approaches by either traditional or robotic-assisted laparoscopy has occurred over the past couple of decades and has been well-studied [46], leading to fewer postoperative complications and shorter hospital stay than open procedures [47]. The choice of conventional over robotic-assisted laparoscopy depends primarily on surgeons' preferences, expertise, and institutional availability. A meta-analysis of ventral rectopexy comparing robotic and traditional laparoscopy showed no strong benefit of one approach over the other [48].

Reconstructive procedures for pelvic organ prolapse can be performed either through a vaginal or abdominal/minimally invasive approach. Most commonly, a combined, minimally invasive abdominal mesh sacrocolpopexy and ventral rectopexy is performed for women with concomitant pelvic organ and rectal prolapse. These procedures can typically correct posterior compartment prolapse, but a concurrent posterior colporrhaphy and perineorrhaphy may also be performed for more severe prolapse. The following section will describe these procedures in greater detail.

Combined Laparoscopic Mesh Sacrocolpopexy and Ventral Rectopexy

Preoperative Preparation

The decision to use mechanical bowel preparation prior to surgery should be made between the urogynaecologist and colorectal surgeon. For most urogynaecologists, bowel preparation is not necessary, but colorectal surgeons may prefer to implement this in order to avoid retracting on and manoeuvring the rectum that is potentially full of stool.

Operative Set-up

The patient is placed on a non-slip pad in dorsal lithotomy position using Yellofin® (Allen Medical Systems, Acton, MA) stirrups. Arms are tucked bilaterally, with care to ensure neurologically neutral positioning and adequate padding of bony prominences. The patient's buttocks should be positioned at the inferior edge of the operating table to permit sufficient vaginal manipulation and access for any planned concurrent vaginal procedures. The chest is secured to prevent intraoperative slippage. The abdomen, vagina, and perineum are prepped and draped. Intravenous antibiotics are administered for prophylaxis.

A Foley catheter is placed to drain the bladder; a three-way Foley catheter should be considered in the event that backfilling the bladder is needed to facilitate the vesicovaginal or vesicouterine dissection. A uterine manipulator is placed if a hysterectomy is planned. A nasogastric or orogastric tube should be inserted prior to laparoscopic entry.

Procedure Steps

Laparoscopic entry is obtained with a Veress needle, direct vision, or open (Hasson) technique depending on the surgeon's preference.

During conventional laparoscopy, four trocars are placed: a 5-mm umbilical trocar, a 5-mm left lower quadrant trocar, and two trocars in the right lower quadrant (5 mm and 8–12 mm).

During robotic-assisted surgery, five trocars are placed. For the da Vinci Xi® platform (Intuitive Surgical Inc., Sunnyvale, CA), we utilize four robotic ports (8 mm) and one accessory port (8–12 mm) all placed above the level of the umbilicus, spaced 8 cm apart in a straight line. Body habitus and prior abdominal surgery may require modification of the placement. Robotic ports 1 and 2 are placed to the left of the umbilicus, port 3 is placed directly above the umbilicus, and port 4 is placed to the right of the umbilicus. The accessory port is placed on the patient's right side, at the level or slightly inferior to the umbilicus. The robot is docked in standard fashion. A 30-degree robotic laparoscopic is loaded into robotic arm 3 and targeting is performed with visualization of the pelvis. Small bowel grasping forceps are loaded into arm 1, fenestrated bipolar forceps into arm 2, and monopolar scissors are inserted into arm 4.

The patient is placed in steep Trendelenburg, and the small bowel and sigmoid colon are brought out of the pelvis. Adhesiolysis is performed as necessary to restore normal anatomy.

At this point, a supracervical hysterectomy is performed by the urogynaecologist in the standard fashion, if indicated. The uterine corpus is left in the upper abdomen and retrieved within a bag through an extended umbilical incision after completion of the remainder of the procedure.

The sacral promontory is visualized. Prior to beginning the presacral dissection, the surgeon identifies the common iliac vessels and the right ureter. The dissection is begun by elevating and incising the overlying peritoneum approximately halfway between the rectal mesentery and the right ureter. The retroperitoneal fat is dissected off until the anterior longitudinal ligament of the sacrum can be visualized. Care should be taken to avoid the middle sacral artery, hypogastric nerves, and the left common iliac vein, which courses underneath and medial to the left common iliac artery.

The peritoneum is then opened in continuation along the right side of the rectum for creation of flaps that will be used later to cover the mesh. The dissection is not continued posteriorly, and the lateral ligaments of the rectum are left intact.

The colorectal surgeon proceeds with dissection of the rectovaginal septum, which is facilitated with retraction from an EEA sizer in the vagina. The dissection proceeds to the level of the pelvic floor, with exposure of the levator ani muscles bilaterally. The urogynaecologist then proceeds with the vesicovaginal dissection to the level of the trigone (see Figure 26.7).

We typically use two pieces of lightweight polypropylene mesh and affix one piece to the anterior vagina and the other to the levator muscles and anterior rectal wall and then to the posterior vagina. Both pieces are brought together to the sacrum in a Y-configuration. We measure the rectal width at the level of the levator ani muscles using a ruler placed through the accessory port (Figure 26.4). The posterior piece of mesh is then fashioned in a T-shape (see Figure 26.5), with the distal width of the mesh cut to match the rectal width, and the proximal width cut to 4 cm. The mesh is sutured by the colorectal surgeon to the levator ani muscles adjacent to the rectum bilaterally using two 2–0 delayed absorbable or permanent sutures. This step serves as a laparoscopic technique for rectocele repair. Then, using seromuscular bites, the mesh is attached to the anterior rectum using ten to twelve 2–0 delayed absorbable sutures (see Figure 26.5). The urogynaecologist then attaches the same piece of mesh to the posterior vagina using approximately six 2–0 delayed absorbable sutures. The other piece of mesh is sutured to the anterior vagina with four to six 2–0 delayed absorbable sutures (Figure 26.8).

Next, both pieces of mesh are brought to the sacrum at the level of S1. The vagina should be displaced cephalad using the EEA sizer but without tension from the mesh (Figure 26.9). Conversely, enough tension should be created on the anterior rectum from the posterior mesh such that small 'ripples' can be

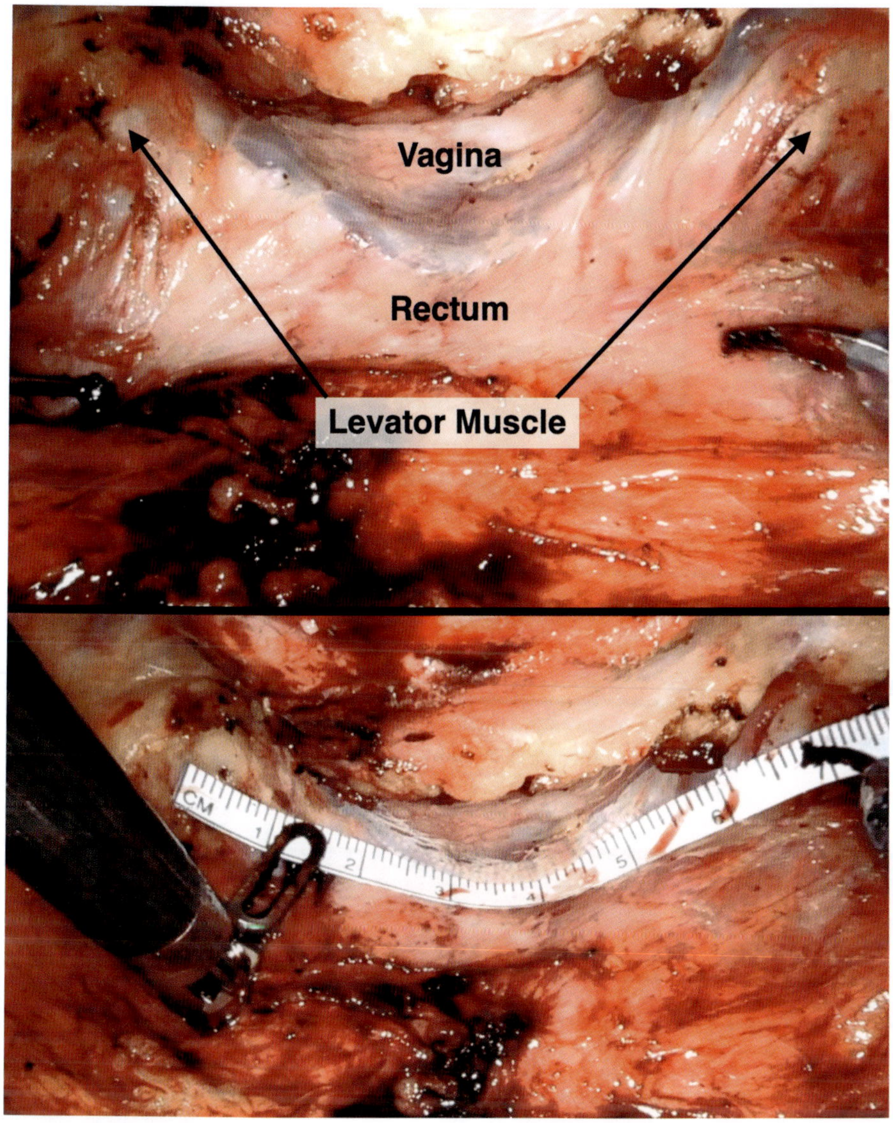

Figure 26.4 Measurement of levator width.

visualized between the sutures and rectum (see Figure 26.6). These 'ripples' will settle once the mesh has been secured to the sacrum and vaginal retraction has been removed. Both pieces of mesh are secured to the anterior longitudinal ligament of the sacrum using at least two 0- or 2–0 permanent sutures. Examination is performed to evaluate prolapse correction and exclude suture perforation of the vaginal epithelium.

Lastly, the peritoneum is closed over the mesh (Figure 26.10). Secure bites of only the peritoneal edges are taken to ensure that the right ureter is not kinked or injured. A cystoscopy is performed at the end of the procedure to evaluate ureteral patency and bladder injury.

Vaginal Procedures

Transvaginal Rectocele Repair

The two primary methods of transvaginal rectocele repair are the traditional posterior colporrhaphy and the site-specific repair. In a prospective randomized trial of 106 patients comparing traditional colporrhaphy, site-specific repair and site-specific repair with graft augmentation, anatomic and functional outcomes were not significantly different between posterior colporrhaphy and site-specific repair groups [49].

Posterior Colporrhaphy

Allis clamps are placed to demarcate the proximal and distal borders of the rectocele and to assist with countertraction. If a perineorrhaphy is also planned, additional clamps are placed along the hymen and on the perineal body. Injection of lidocaine with dilute epinephrine or vasopressin below the vaginal epithelium assists in hydrodissection and haemostasis. A vertical incision is made along the midline of the vaginal epithelium, extending the incision to an area superior to the rectocele defect. If performing a perineorrhaphy, an inverted triangle- or diamond-shaped portion of perineal skin can be excised with the scalpel; if the introitus is already narrow, the surgeon can continue the vertical incision through the perineal skin instead. The posterior vaginal epithelium is dissected sharply off the underlying fibromuscularis until the levator muscles are encountered bilaterally. Dissection should stay close to the vaginal

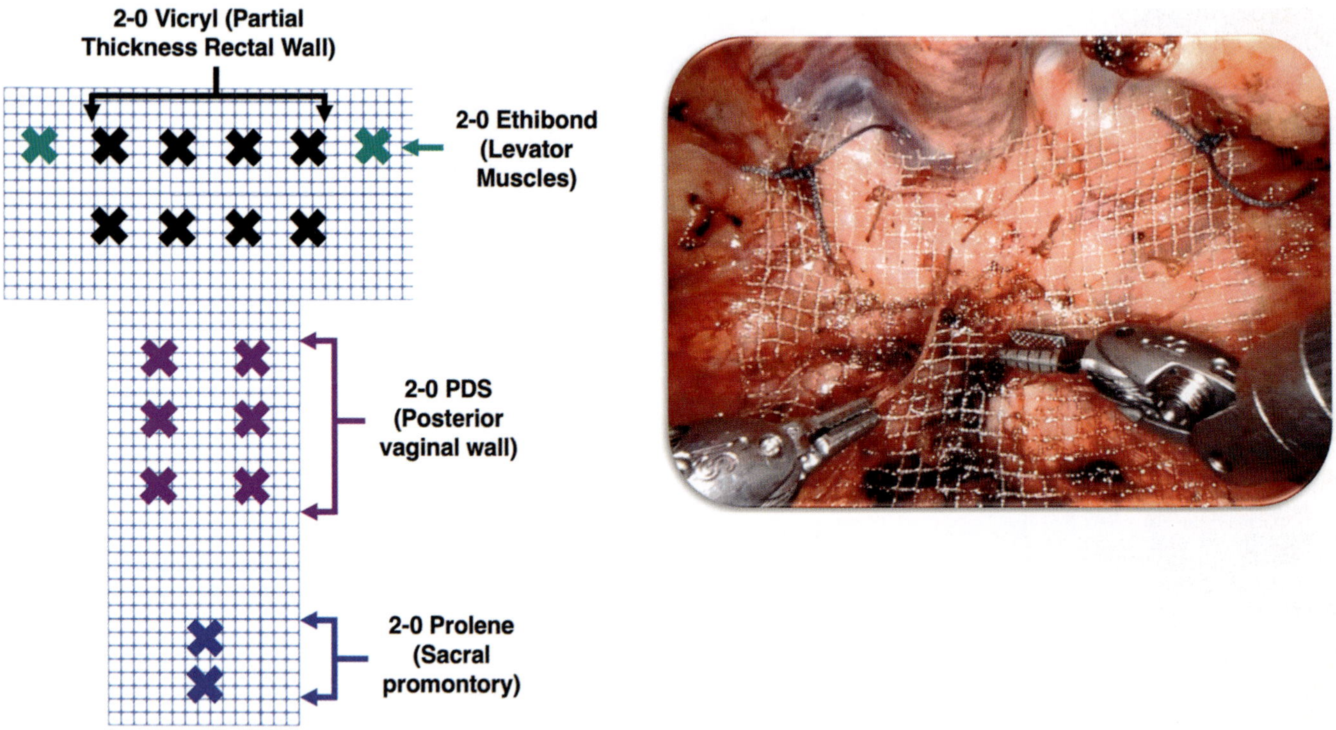

Figure 26.5 Fashioning of ventral rectopexy mesh (length, shape) and sites of mesh fixation during ventral rectopexy (diagram and in-situ photo).

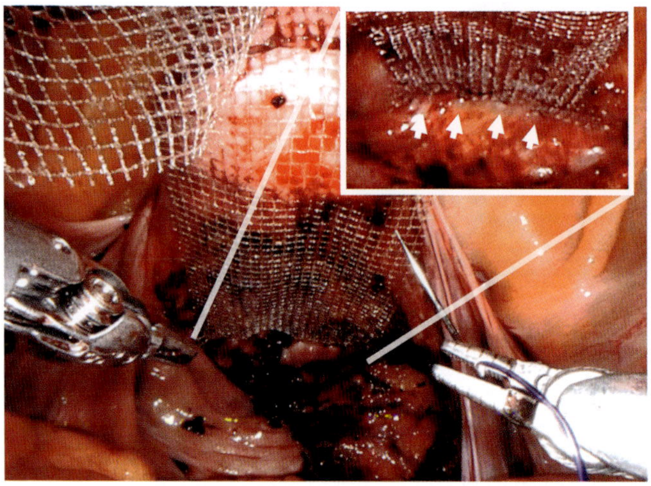

Figure 26.6 Tensioning of rectum after rectopexy mesh attachment as seen during posterior vaginal wall mesh fixation.

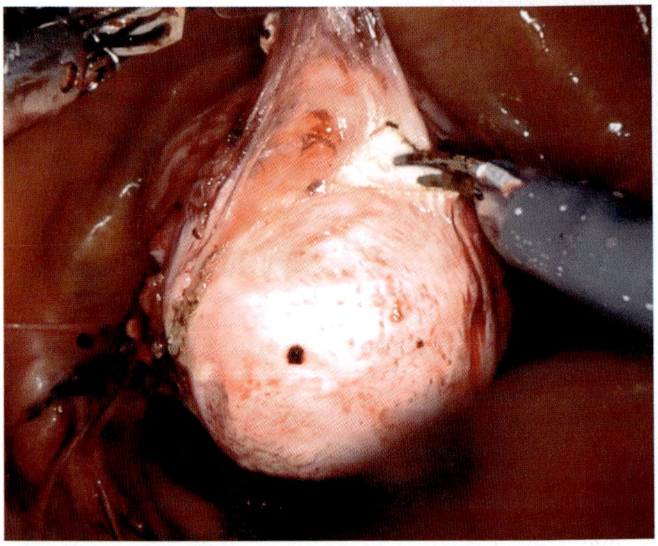

Figure 26.7 Anterior vaginal dissection.

epithelium to avoid injury to the rectum. The fibromuscularis is then plicated in the midline with interrupted transverse or vertical 2–0 delayed absorbable sutures, beginning proximally until the hymen is reached. Care should be taken to ensure continuity between each plication suture, as ridging of the posterior vaginal wall can occur otherwise, which may cause dyspareunia. A rectal exam is performed to rule out injury to the rectum and to confirm there are no areas of weakness requiring further sutures. It is important to reattach the rectovaginal fascia to the perineal body when separation is observed. A perineorrhaphy is performed next, as detailed below.

The vaginal epithelium is trimmed only if necessary and closed with a running 2–0 delayed absorbable suture. Care should be taken to avoid excessive trimming as this can result in dyspareunia and pain from excessive traction and scarring. The vaginal calibre at the conclusion of the colporrhaphy should be at least three fingerbreadths in sexually active women.

Site-Specific Defect Repair

This technique is based on the assumption that there are specific tears in the rectovaginal fascia that allow the rectum to herniate into the vagina. These defects can occur as isolated defects or a

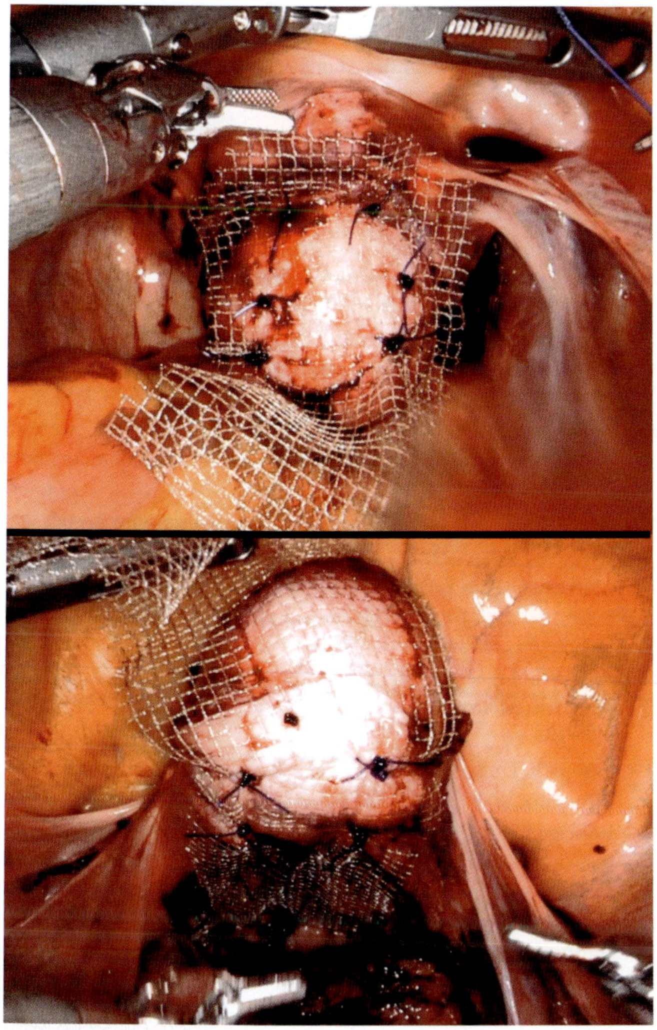

Figure 26.8 Anterior and posterior vaginal wall mesh fixation.

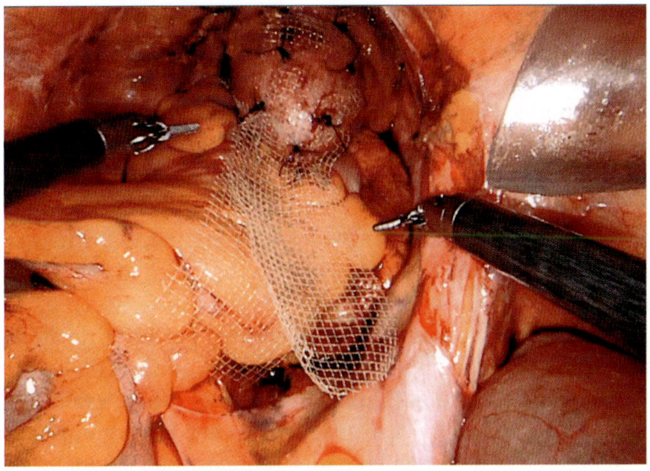

Figure 26.9 Cephalad displacement of vagina during sacral mesh fixation.

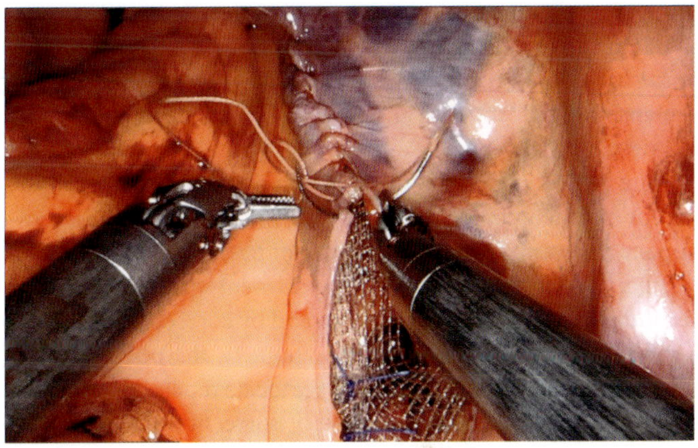

Figure 26.10 Complete reperitonealization of mesh.

combination of defects in the lateral, distal, midline, or proximal portions of the posterior vagina.

The vaginal epithelium is incised in a similar manner as described above, and dissected off the fibromuscularis laterally to the endopelvic fascial attachment of the posterior vaginal wall to the arcus tendineus fasciae pelvis and arcus tendineus fasciae rectovaginalis. The surgeon places a gloved digit from their nondominant hand into the rectum to localize the defects, and irrigation may be used to facilitate this process. Defects in the posterior vaginal wall and perineal body are individually isolated and repaired with interrupted 2–0 or 0- delayed absorbable sutures. Repeat rectal examination should confirm repair of the rectocele. The vaginal epithelium is closed as described above.

Perineorrhaphy

Perineorrhaphy is performed at the time of transvaginal rectocele repair when there is separation of the perineal body. The perineal skin is denuded or incised in the midline as described above. The perineal skin is sharply dissected off the perineal body. The bulbocavernosus and transverse perinei muscles are plicated in the midline with an interrupted 0-absorbable suture. A perineorrhaphy can benefit patients in whom there is a gaping genital introitus, but care should be taken to avoid excessive constriction of the introitus which can result in dyspareunia.

Surgical Outcomes

Laparoscopic ventral mesh rectopexy was first described by D'Hoore and Pennickx in 2004 [50]. A study by their group of 919 patients with rectal prolapse and intussusception who underwent laparoscopic ventral mesh rectopexy, with median follow-up of 34 months, demonstrated postoperative resolution of faecal incontinence and obstructed defaecation symptoms in 80.2% and 74.3% of patients [42]. A total of 68 patients (7.4%) developed recurrence. Acceptable complication rates were also noted; mesh-related complications were recorded in 4.6% of patients, including vaginal mesh erosion in 1.3%. In a randomized controlled trial comparing laparoscopic ventral mesh rectopexy to laparoscopic posterior suture rectopexy with six-year follow-up, ventral mesh rectopexy was demonstrated to be superior in improving constipation, obstructed defaecation, and quality of life scores [51].

Several nonrandomized observational studies have reported promising anatomic and functional medium- and long-term outcomes for combined sacrocolpopexy and ventral rectopexy [52–55]. Cohort sizes ranged from 51 to 110 patients. Median follow-up in these studies ranged from 12.5 to 54 months. Perioperative complications were seen in 13.7–32.7% of patients, and mesh-related complications were rare. Significant improvements in faecal incontinence, constipation, and quality-of-life scores were seen. Recurrence of rectal prolapse was seen in 5–13.5% of patients [52,55], whereas recurrence of pelvic organ prolapse was reported in 4–8.5% of women [54–55].

The decision to perform a concomitant posterior repair at the time of sacrocolpopexy is controversial. In the Colpopexy and Urinary Reduction Efforts (CARE) trial, which evaluated the role of Burch colposuspension in women undergoing sacrocolpopexy, 29% of women underwent posterior vaginal wall repair (i.e. colporrhaphy, perineorrhaphy, or sacrocolpoperineopexy) [56]. Although women who received posterior vaginal procedures had more baseline obstructive defaecatory symptoms compared to women who did not, a similar rate in improvement of bowel symptoms was seen between groups [56]. In observational studies of sacrocolpopexy without posterior colporrhaphy, the rate of recurrence of posterior prolapse ranged from 8% at one-year [57] to 57% at two-years follow-up [58].

The indications and outcomes of a posterior colporrhaphy and/or perineorrhaphy at the time of a combined sacrocolpopexy and ventral rectopexy have not been thoroughly investigated. Arguably, posterior compartment defects are often secondary to loss of apical support, and by correcting the apical support during abdominal sacrocolpopexy, the posterior wall can be restored without a separate rectocele repair. Defaecatory symptoms may improve as a result of correction of co-existing rectal prolapse or intussusception. Furthermore, the distal extent to which mesh is attached along the posterior vagina and anterior rectum during ventral rectopexy may correct outlet dysfunction without the need of a perineorrhaphy. Additional studies are needed to answer these questions.

Conclusions

In summary, rectal prolapse can occur to varying degrees that range from full thickness to short segment intussusception. Similarly, there is variation in the size and clinical impact of posterior vaginal wall defects. These anatomic defects tend to occur in combination. Patient outcomes and satisfaction can be optimized by identifying and treating these problems in a multidisciplinary setting. Pelvic floor physiology testing with defecography and manometry can facilitate accurate diagnosis and treatment planning. Multi-disciplinary surgical repairs are increasing in frequency as more clinicians work closely with colleagues of other subspecialties. Studies focused on these combined repairs continue to show promising results with significant improvement in symptoms of constipation, incontinence, and incomplete defaecation. Minimally invasive surgical techniques improve the ease with which multi-disciplinary surgery can be performed.

References

1. Guzman Rojas R, Kamisan Atan I, et al. The prevalence of abnormal posterior compartment anatomy and its association with obstructed defecation symptoms in urogynecological patients. Int Urogynecol J 2016; 27(6): 939–44.
2. Sun C, Hull T, Ozuner G. Risk factors and clinical characteristics of rectal prolapse in young patients. J Visc Surg 2014; 151(6): 425–9.
3. Wijffels NA, Collinson R, Cunningham C, et al. What is the natural history of internal rectal prolapse? Colorectal Dis 2010; 12(8): 822–30.
4. Kairaluoma MV, Kellokumpu IH. Epidemiologic aspects of complete rectal prolapse. Scand J Surg 2005; 94(3): 207–10.
5. Bordeianou L, Paquette I, Johnson E, et al. Clinical practice guidelines for the treatment of rectal prolapse. Dis Colon Rectum 2017; 60(11): 1121–31.
6. Goldstein SD, Maxwell PJ. Rectal prolapse. Clin Colon Rectal Surg 2011; 24(1): 39–45.
7. Marceau C, Parc Y, Debroux E, et al. Complete rectal prolapse in young patients: psychiatric disease a risk factor of poor outcome. Colorectal Dis 2005; 7(4): 360–5.
8. Kulczycki LL, Shwachman H. Studies in cystic fibrosis of the pancreas; occurrence of rectal prolapse. N Engl J Med 1958; 259: 409–12.
9. Farouk R, Duthie GS. Rectal prolapse and rectal invagination. Eur J Surg 1998; 164(5): 323–32.
10. Rodrigo N, Shek KL, Dietz HP. Rectal intussusception is associated with abnormal levator ani muscle structure and morphometry. Tech Coloproctol 2011; 15(1): 39–43.
11. Neill ME, Parks AG, Swash M. Physiological studies of the anal sphincter musculature in faecal incontinence and rectal prolapse. Br J Surg 1981; 68: 531–6.
12. Muir EG. Treatment of complete rectal prolapse in the adult. *Prolapse of the Rectum: Proceedings of the Royal Society of Medicine* 1962; 55: 1086–7.
13. Broden G, Snellman B. Procidentia of the rectum studied with cineradiography. Dis Colon Rectum 1968; 11: 330–47.
14. Weber AM, Walters MD, Ballard LA, et al. Posterior vaginal prolapse and bowel function. Am J Obstet Gynecol 1998; 179(6 Pt 1): 1446–50.
15. Brandner S, Monga A, Mueller MD, et al. Sexual function after rectocele repair. J Sex Med 2011; 8(2): 583–8.
16. Rosen R, Brown C, Heiman J, et al. The Female Sexual Function Index (FSFI): a multidimensional self-report instrument for the assessment of female sexual function. J Sex Marital Ther 2000; 26(2): 191–208.
17. Jackson SL, Weber AM, Hull TL, et al. Fecal incontinence in women with urinary incontinence and pelvic organ prolapse. Obstet Gynecol 1997; 89(3): 423–7.
18. Roberts RO, Jacobsen SJ, Reilly WT, et al. Prevalence of combined fecal and urinary incontinence: a community-based study. J Am Geriatr Soc1999; 47(7): 837–41.
19. Bordeianou L, Paquette I, Johnson E, et al. Clinical practice guidelines for the treatment of rectal prolapse. Dis Colon Rectum 2017; 60(11): 1121–31.
20. Hawkins AT, Olariu AG, Savitt LR, et al. Impact of rising grades of internal rectal intussusception on fecal continence and symptoms of constipation. Dis Colon Rectum 2016; 59(1): 54–61.

21. Dvorkin LS, Knowles CH, Scott SM, et al. Rectal intussusception: characterization of symptomatology. Dis Colon Rectum 2005; 48(4): 824–31.
22. Kapoor DS, Sultan AH, Thakar R, et al. Management of complex pelvic floor disorders in a multidisciplinary pelvic floor clinic. Colorectal Dis 2008; 10(2): 118–23.
23. Bump RC, Mattiasson A, Bø K, et al. The standardization of terminology of female pelvic organ prolapse and pelvic floor dysfunction. Am J Obstet Gynecol 1996; 175(1): 10–17.
24. Ho YH, Goh HS. The neurophysiological significance of perineal descent. Int J Colorectal Dis 1995; 10(2): 107–11.
25. Shorvon PJ, McHugh S, Diamant NE, et al. Defecography in normal volunteers: results and implications. Gut 1989; 30: 1737–49.
26. Kenton K, Shott S, Brubaker L. The anatomic and functional variability of rectoceles in women. Int Urogynecol J Pelvic Floor Dysfunct 1999; 10(2): 96–9.
27. Wallace SL, Torosis M, Rogo-Gupta L. Does rectocele on defecography equate to rectocele on physical examination in patients with defecatory symptoms? Female Pelvic Med Reconstr Surg 2019 (online). https://doi.org/10.1097/SPV.0000000000000719
28. Rao SS, Azpiroz F, Diamant N, et al. Minimum standards of anorectal manometry. Neurogastroenterol Motil 2002; (5): 553–9.
29. Barnett JL, Hasler WL, Camilleri M. American Gastroenterological Association medical position statement on anorectal testing techniques. Gastroenterology 1999; 116(3): 732–60.
30. Carrington EV, Heinrich H, Knowles CH, et al. The international anorectal physiology working group (IAPWG) recommendations: standardized testing protocol and the London classification for disorders of anorectal function. Neurogastroenterol Motil 2020; 32(1): e13679.
31. Rao SS, Hatfield R, Soffer E, et al. Manometric tests of anorectal function in healthy adults. Am J Gastroenterol 1999; 94(3): 773–83.
32. Oblizajek NR, Gandhi S, Sharma M, et al. Anorectal pressures measured with high-resolution manometry in healthy people - Normal values and asymptomatic pelvic floor dysfunction. Neurogastroenterol Motil 2019; 31(7): e13597.
33. Prichard DO, Lee T, Parthasarathy G, et al. High-resolution anorectal manometry for identifying defecatory disorders and rectal structural abnormalities in women. Clin Gastroenterol Hepatol 2017; 15(3): 412–20.
34. Harmston C, Jones OM, Cunningham C, et al. The relationship between internal rectal prolapse and internal anal sphincter function. Colorectal Dis 2011; 13(7): 791–5.
35. Fernando RJ, Thakar R, Sultan AH, et al. Effect of vaginal pessaries on symptoms associated with pelvic organ prolapse. Obstet Gynecol 2006; 108(1): 93–9.
36. Brazell HD, Patel M, O'Sullivan DM, et al. The impact of pessary use on bowel symptoms: one-year outcomes. Female Pelvic Med Reconstr Surg 2014; 20(2): 95–8.
37. Ma C, Xu T, Kang J, et al. Factors associated with pessary fitting in women with symptomatic pelvic organ prolapse: a large prospective cohort study. Neurourol Urodyn 2020; 39(8): 2238–45.
38. Li C, Gong Y, Wang B. The efficacy of pelvic floor muscle training for pelvic organ prolapse: a systematic review and meta-analysis. Int Urogynecol J 2016; 27(7): 981–92.
39. D'Hoore A. Fine-tuning indications for laparoscopic ventral mesh rectopexy. Tech Coloproctol 2017; 21(8): 593–4.
40. McCue JL, Thomson JP. Rectopexy for internal rectal intussusception. Br J Surg 1990; 77(6): 632–4.
41. Briel JW, Schouten WR, Boerma MO. Long-term results of suture rectopexy in patients with fecal incontinence associated with incomplete rectal prolapse. Dis Colon Rectum 1997; 40(10): 1228–32.
42. Consten EC, van Iersel JJ, Verheijen PM, et al. Long-term outcome after laparoscopic ventral mesh rectopexy: an observational study of 919 consecutive patients. Ann Surg 2015; 262(5): 742–7.
43. Christiansen J, Zhu BW, Rasmussen OO, et al. Internal rectal intussusception: results of surgical repair. Dis Colon Rectum 1992; 35(11): 1026–8.
44. Sielezneff I, Malouf A, Cesari J, et al. Selection criteria for internal rectal prolapse repair by Delorme's transrectal excision. Dis Colon Rectum 1999; 42(3): 367–73.
45. Graf W, Karlbom U, Påhlman L, et al. Functional results after abdominal suture rectopexy for rectal prolapse or intussusception. Eur J Surg 1996; 162(11): 905–11.
46. Senagore AJ. Management of rectal prolapse: the role of laparoscopic approaches. Semin Laparosc Surg 2003; 10: 197–202.
47. Tou S, Brown SR, Nelson RL. Surgery for complete (full-thickness) rectal prolapse in adults. Cochrane Database Syst Rev 2015; (11): CD001758.
48. Ramage L, Georgiou P, Tekkis P, et al. Is robotic ventral mesh rectopexy better than laparoscopy in the treatment of rectal prolapse and obstructed defecation? A meta-analysis. Tech Coloproctol 2015; 19: 381–9.
49. Paraiso MF, Barber MD, Muir TW, Walters MD. Rectocele repair: a randomized trial of three surgical techniques including graft augmentation. Am J Obstet Gynecol 2006; 195(6): 1762–71.
50. D'Hoore A, Penninckx F. Laparoscopic ventral recto(colpo) pexy for rectal prolapse: surgical technique and outcome for 109 patients. Surg Endosc 2006; 20(12): 1919–23.
51. Hidaka J, Elfeki H, Duelund-Jakobsen J, et al. Functional outcome after laparoscopic posterior sutured rectopexy versus ventral mesh rectopexy for rectal prolapse: six-year follow-up of a double-blind, randomized single-center study. EClinicalMedicine 2019; 16: 18–22.
52. Slawik S, Soulsby R, Carter H, et al. Laparoscopic ventral rectopexy, posterior colporrhaphy and vaginal sacrocolpopexy for the treatment of recto-genital prolapse and mechanical outlet obstruction. Colorectal Dis 2008; 10(2): 138–43.
53. Watadani Y, Vogler SA, Warshaw JS, et al. Sacrocolpopexy with rectopexy for pelvic floor prolapse improves bowel function and quality of life. Dis Colon Rectum 2013; 56(12): 1415–22.
54. van Iersel JJ, de Witte CJ, Verheijen PM, et al. Robot-assisted sacrocolporectopexy for multicompartment prolapse of the pelvic floor: a prospective cohort study evaluating functional and sexual outcome. Dis Colon Rectum 2016; 59(10): 968–74.

55. Jallad K, Ridgeway B, Paraiso MFR, et al. Long-term outcomes after ventral rectopexy with sacrocolpo- or hysteropexy for the treatment of concurrent rectal and pelvic organ prolapse. Female Pelvic Med Reconstr Surg 2018; 24(5): 336–40.
56. Bradley CS, Nygaard IE, Brown MB, et al. Pelvic Floor Disorders Network. Bowel symptoms in women 1 year after sacrocolpopexy. Am J Obstet Gynecol 2007; 197(6): 642.e1–8.
57. Guiahi M, Kenton K, Brubaker L. Sacrocolpopexy without concomitant posterior repair improves posterior compartment defects. Int Urogynecol J Pelvic Floor Dysfunct 2008; 19(9): 1267–70.
58. Baessler K, Schuessler B. Abdominal sacrocolpopexy and anatomy and function of the posterior compartment. Obstet Gynecol 2001; 97(5 Pt 1): 678–84.

Chapter 27

The Role of Meshes in the Treatment of Female Pelvic Organ Prolapse

Yara Abdelkhalek, Christian Phillips, Bruno Deval

Introduction

Pelvic organ prolapse (POP) is a condition that affects millions of women worldwide and causes an enormous negative impact on their quality of life [1]. Two-thirds of parous women have evidence of prolapse on examination [2], but while the majority are asymptomatic, others suffer from heavy physical, social, and psychological limitations [3].

Since the late 1990s there has been a significant increase in the number of procedures for stress urinary incontinence and uterovaginal prolapse involving the use of polypropylene mesh. This was initially made popular by the retropubic transvaginal tape procedure, pioneered by Ulf Ulmsten, for stress urinary incontinence and then extended to the transobturator tapes. Transvaginal mesh for vaginal prolapse became popular in the last decade, especially with the advent of commercially produced 'kit form' vaginal mesh procedures. Abdominal polypropylene mesh is also utilized in sacrocolpopexy and sacrohysteropexy. The advances in laparoscopic surgery have led to an increase in the popularity of sacrocolpopexy in abdominal placement of mesh laparoscopically. In this chapter we will discuss the indications of reconstructive native tissue and prosthetic meshes related pelvic surgeries along with their complications in order to settle the issue of meshes in female POP treatment.

The Concept

Pelvic organ prolapse is a common condition and its incidence is increasing with the increase in female life expectancy. The traditional approach for repair in women with either prolapse or stress urinary incontinence (SUI) utilizes the patient's native tissues.

Along with obstetric injury, many studies have attributed pelvic floor dysfunction to deficient collagen [4] which may account for native tissue reconstructive procedures having been associated with higher objective failure rates and increased risks of recurrence [5,6]. Some studies have also suggested higher failure rates can occur in native tissue repair due to variations in surgical technique [7]. One should note that although objective failure rates may seem high after native tissue repair, subjective improvement perceived by patients is often reported as very high [8].

Classification of Meshes

Weakened native tissue can be augmented by an implanted material. Typically these have been in two types: biological materials which are typically referred to as 'grafts' and synthetic materials, referred to as 'mesh'

Biological Grafts

Autologous Grafts

Autologous grafts are harvested from the patient's own tissues; most commonly the rectus sheath and fascia lata [9,10]. The most significant risk is potential donor site morbidity (wound infection, scar, nerve damage, and hernia) [11].

Allografts

Allografts are tissues/grafts harvested from cadavers that have been sterilized and undergone a process to remove immunogenic material. In theory, the use of allografts avoids the morbidity associated with harvesting the tissue, reducing risks of haematoma and hernia.

Xenografts

Xenografts consist of acellular extracts of collagen, harvested from nonhuman donors; usually porcine or bovine.

Biological grafts were popular in the 1990s but their use declined due to concerns of theoretical infectious disease transmission and poor long-term results. A study of women with stage 2 or greater anterior compartment prolapse randomized to synthetic mesh, biological mesh, or native tissue repair, followed up for two years, showed women in the biological mesh group had a significantly higher objective failure rate compared with those in the synthetic mesh group (46% versus 18%, $P = 0.015$) [12]. A 2016 Cochrane review found insufficient evidence to compare biological grafts with native tissue repair [13]. The PROSPECT study evaluated 368 women undergoing primary anterior or posterior repair augmented with porcine acellular collagen matrix, porcine small intestinal submucosa, or bovine dermal grafts. Two-year follow-up demonstrated women in the graft group were significantly more likely to report symptoms of prolapse than women who underwent standard native tissue repair [14].

Synthetic Mesh

Transvaginal mesh can either be sutured across a fascial defect as an 'inlay', surround the vagina as a 'total mesh', or be inserted into pelvic spaces with a 'mesh kit'.

Synthetic Absorbable/Partially Absorbable Mesh

Synthetic absorbable mesh is typically composed of polyglactin or polyglycolic acid and undergoes replacement by collagen-rich connective tissue. Animal models of hernia repair using

Table 27.1 The four types of synthetic mesh

Type of mesh		
Type 1	>75 µm	Prolene® (Ethicon, Somerville, NJ)
Type 2	<10 µm	GORE-TEX® (GORE, Flagstaff, AZ),
Type 3	>75 µm	GORE-TEX® (GORE, Flagstaff, AZ),
Type 4	<1 µm	Not used in vaginal prolapse surgery

absorbable mesh have demonstrated poor long-term tensile strength and early recurrence [15,16]. To date, there is insufficient evidence to support the use of partially absorbable synthetic mesh in POP repair [17,18].

Synthetic Non-absorbable Mesh

Synthetic non-absorbable mesh avoids the risk of infectious disease transmission posed by biological grafts and provides a more durable graft than absorbable mesh. However, synthetic meshes pose the risk of reaction by the host to the foreign body, as well as related infection, mesh contracture, and exposure. Synthetic meshes are classified into four types due to pore size and properties, outlined below (Table 27.1) [19]:

The pore size affects both the density and flexibility of the mesh as well as the host response to the mesh. The majority of current meshes utilized for pelvic floor repair are type 1 macroporous polypropylene with a pore size greater than 75 µm which allows infiltration of fibroblasts, blood vessels, collagen fibres, and macrophages, which promotes tissue incorporation and reduces infection risks.

Approval of Mesh in Pelvic Reconstructive Surgery

In the mid-1990s, several meshes gained US Food and Drug Administration (FDA) approval for inguinal hernia repair [19]. In 1996, Boston Scientific obtained FDA approval for their ProtoGen mesh for the treatment of SUI, under the FDA 510(k) clause. This stated that if manufacturers could demonstrate that their product was 'substantially equivalent' to an existing approved device and 'at least as safe', it would not require further testing and could be approved. Using the FDA 510(k) clause, many vaginal tapes and vaginal mesh 'kits' were introduced in the early 2000s and numerous surgeons performed the procedures with very little formal training or expertise in pelvic floor reconstruction. Mesh-related pelvic floor reconstructive surgery is a complex procedure necessitating years of training and probably not all the surgeons were adequately qualified, thus a perfect storm of over-adoption of new technology and lack of expertise was inevitably going to result in complications [3].

Certainly, the idea of introducing a prosthetic support to enhance the patient's weak native pelvic tissues would seem a reasonable hypothesis, however in retrospect, this was introduced too early, with little/no long-term follow-up on safety and efficacy data, no formal training strategy, and no governance in place for auditing of outcomes or complications.

Despite anatomical improvements following vaginal mesh insertion, dyspareunia and pelvic pain were major postoperative complaints along with mesh exposure [13]. A cross-sectional media analysis of 42 articles studying transvaginal meshes showed 71% of patients expressed regret about their surgery [20].

The Food and Drug Administration released the first notification about transvaginal mesh safety in 2008 and then banned its selling and distribution in the US in 2019 [3]. Concerns started to emerge around the medium- to long-term complications that could occur from tapes and vaginal meshes. The Scottish Mesh Group lobbied and the Scottish parliament banned the use of the mesh in Scotland and this was followed by similar demands in different countries for the withdrawal of mesh. On 10 July 2018, the UK government suspended the use of vaginally placed mesh (mid-urethral slings and transvaginal mesh). The use of abdominal mesh was still permitted in the UK under 'high vigilance', provided certain parameters were followed [21]. Additionally, the Scottish and Australian governments banned reconstructive mesh-related transvaginal procedures in 2016 and 2017 respectively [22].

Most publications, especially regarding adverse events following mesh insertion, have not distinguished between the different types and routes of mesh insertion/operations and grouped all 'mesh procedures' (mid-urethral slings, transvaginal mesh, and abdominally placed mesh) as the same entity. Moreover, managing complications such as mesh erosion and long-term groin pain also pose dilemmas for the clinician with variable outcomes in symptom relief, subsequent urinary function, and patient satisfaction [23,24]. Sub-urethral slings for stress urinary incontinence and vaginal mesh for pelvic organ prolapse have often been grouped together as 'vaginal meshes', thus confusion around the related complications of each type exists [25]. The VIGI-MESH register, which includes pelvic reconstructive surgeries from 19 centres across France, shows that the procedure associated with the highest rate of re-operation is the sub-urethral sling [25]. Although there are high levels of satisfaction amongst women following a mid-urethral sling, a proportion of women also developed significant complications which has led to increased lobbying from affected patient groups [20,25].

The Cost

Pelvic organ prolapse is a common condition, with a quarter of a million reconstructive interventions being performed annually in the US [5, 6], with projections of approximately seven million being performed annually by the year 2030 [5]. Re-operation rates after recurrence are estimated between 13–25% [6]. Furthermore, complications and the resulting litigation also pose a significant burden on the health economy. In 2012, a case against Avaulta Plus transvaginal mesh cost the company 5 million dollars, and in the US so far, 160,000 lawsuits have cost more than four billion dollars [3]. Therefore, appropriate counselling, joint decision-making, and consent regarding the decision and selection of either a mesh or native tissue reconstructive procedure, according to each patient's personal priorities and characteristics, is essential to mitigate burden on healthcare systems.

Postoperative complications result from a multifactorial combination. Mesh properties play an important role in the postoperative outcome, as well as the patient's characteristics and surgical technique [5]. Some of the lessons learned from vaginal mesh could be useful when considering abdominally placed mesh. These include mesh factors, patient factors, and surgical factors.

Mesh Factors

As previously outlined, non-absorbable microporous (>75 Ug) polypropylene mesh is usually preferred for pelvic reconstructive surgeries [27]. The density and pore size of the mesh is an important criteria in mesh selection due to its ability to be incorporated into the patient's tissue with the minimal of host reaction [5,25,27].

Common postoperative complications include pain, dyspareunia, infection, bleeding, mucosal or purulent discharge, and erosion. These complications result from chronic inflammation and smooth muscle thinning and atrophy caused by the stress-shielding of the mesh on the vagina.

Patient Factors

Patient-related risk factors for postoperative complications, notably mesh exposure, are:

- Postoperative active sex life (OR 11.89) [28]
- Concomitant hysterectomy (OR 3.72 to 5.17) [5]
- Smoking (OR 3.1 to 3.7) [5]
- Diabetes [29]
- Corticosteroids [29]

Surgical Factors

Pelvic reconstructive surgery is a complex procedure that requires an adapted training. Studies have shown that mesh exposure rates were lower when performed by surgeons with higher volume and greater experience in pelvic floor reconstructive surgery [3]. According to the Collège National des Gynécologues et Obstétriciens Français (CNGOF) recommendations, surgeons qualified to perform this type of intervention should be experts in this field and demonstrate a complication rate inferior to 5% and a load of at least 20 procedures per year [25]. Abdominally placed mesh also poses similar risks. With the advent of laparoscopic mesh procedures, the learning curve is extremely long. Higher risks due to diversity in surgical technique can lead to crimpling, overtightening, and poor choice of suture, increasing the risk of dyspareunia, erosion, and mesh constriction, if not performed with adequate care and ability [26].

Safety and Efficacy of Abdominally and Laparoscopically Placed Mesh

In addition to vaginally placed mesh, mesh is used in open and laparoscopic surgery to restore atomy after apical prolapse. Apical prolapse encompasses uterine and vaginal vault prolapse, defined as descent of the uterus or vaginal vault (post-hysterectomy) [30].

Sacrocolpopexy has long been regarded as the gold standard for post-hysterectomy vault prolapse, but uterine-sparing surgery for prolapse has become more popular and good medium-term outcomes have been shown following laparoscopic sacrohysteropexy (LSH). LSH has benefits both in terms of medium-term outcomes and intraoperative complications when compared to hysterectomy [31]. The true prevalence of post hysterectomy vault prolapse is unknown, but it is quoted as 0.2% to 43% [32]. Sacrocolpopexy is associated with lower awareness of prolapse, recurrence, need for repeat surgery, and postoperative stress urinary incontinence when compared to a variety of vaginal interventions [33]. Laparoscopic sacrocolpopexy (LSC) is equally effective as abdominal sacrocolpopexy (ASC), giving 90% anatomical cure [34] but the minimal access technique reduces blood loss and length of hospital stay [35].

Concerns regarding the use of vaginal mesh for prolapse has led to questions about the safety and efficacy of abdominally placed mesh. Surgical morbidity, as well as medium- and long-term deleterious sequelae from vaginal mesh, appears higher than initially thought. The main long-term complications for ***vaginal mesh*** have proven to be mesh exposure or pain [36,37].

When placed abdominally for apical prolapse, mesh exposure can be either into the vagina, or into an abdominal viscus. The rate of mesh erosion in ASC is quoted as 2–11%, with the risk of serious complication being 2% [38]. Vaginal mesh exposure following LSC was found to be 0.7% in one study [39] and 2% in another [40]. Long-term follow-up of laparoscopic sacrohysteropexy (LSH) found a 1.8% complication rate and no cases of mesh exposure [41].

Apical prolapse encompasses uterine and vaginal vault prolapse; defined as descent of the uterus or vaginal vault (post-hysterectomy) [30]. It is a common presenting complaint in the gynaecology clinic and appropriate long-term management is paramount. When conservative measures fail and patients ask for surgery, all surgical options should be considered.

At the time of writing this chapter, in the UK, transabdominal placement of mesh (LSC/LSH or Ventral Mesh Rectopexy (VMR)) is permitted, but procedures are categorized under 'high vigilance', with strict guidance on governance surrounding the surgery. Thus long-term evidence on the safety and efficacy of abdominally placed mesh is imperative.

Safety Data

Complications can be separated into perioperative and longer term.

Jefferis et al performed a retrospective case note review of 507 women who had LSH with three-month routine follow-up [41]. Intraoperative complications were rare, with one intraoperative bladder injury and three incidences of haemorrhage. Long-term complications were mainly three cases of bowel adhesions requiring re-laparoscopy. The cases of bowel obstruction were managed with adhesiolysis and re-peritonization, and the surgical approach was adapted subsequently to involve routine mesh re-peritonization There were no vaginal mesh erosions. Seventeen patients had their LSH abandoned due to anatomical variants.

Roovers et al looked at the safety of open sacrohysteropexy compared with vaginal hysterectomy [42]. They reported a 2% risk of intraoperative complications (one patient required blood transfusion due to haemorrhage) and a 24% risk of perioperative complications, however it should be noted that the majority of these were as a consequence of open rather than laparoscopic route for surgery (lower urinary tract symptoms (LUTS) (eight women), fever (three women), and vault abscess (two women)). Two women (4.8%) developed infections of the mesh implant requiring hospital admission. Importantly, there was no difference in the rate of complication between these women and those who underwent vaginal hysterectomy.

Daniels et al reported a case series of LSH with three-month follow-up. They also reported a low complication profile with a 2.2% risk of wound infections, 2.9% risk of vaginal infection, 2.9% risk of pain, and 0.7% risk of bleeding [43]. Pandeva et al reviewed the notes of 159 patients with up to two-years follow-up [44]. They reported two cases of bowel obstruction that required repeat surgery giving a risk of 1.3%.

Nightingale et al reported up to 10-year experience of LSC and LSH (median six years) (22 patients also had concomitant VMR) [45]. One-hundred-and-twelve patients were invited for follow-up examination, of which 93 attended, and, for the remainder of patients, information was obtained from case note review or questionnaires. They too demonstrated a low intraoperative complication rate. The only intraoperative complication involving injury to a viscera was the single bladder injury, which gives an intraoperative complication rate of <1%. Two cases were converted to laparotomy for technical reasons. There were no cases of bowel injury or major blood loss, which confirms that laparoscopy and abdominally placed mesh for prolapse is a safe operation. They reported a mesh exposure rate of 2.6%. No asymptomatic mesh erosions were identified on clinical examination. This may suggest that long-term follow-up to assess mesh exposure rates may not require face-to-face review and examination. The only significant long-term mesh complication was bowel obstruction from a segment of small bowel adherent to the mesh after LSH. This case was early in the learning curve of the surgeon and the technique of covering the entirety of the mesh had been improved in the later cases.

In summary, both open and laparoscopic sacrocolpopexy and sacrohysteropexy appear safe in the short- and long-term. Perioperative complications are greater when open procedures are performed due to the risks around laparotomy. Visceral injury is higher when performed laparoscopically, put still relatively low. Longer-term complications are mainly mesh exposure which is extremely low (1–3%) and bowel obstruction due to adhesions between the bowel and mesh, which is reduced significantly when the mesh is completely covered when re-peritonealization is performed at the initial surgery. Unlike vaginal mesh kits, pain was not a common short- or long-term problem after abdominally placed mesh.

Efficacy Data

LSC is considered gold standard for the management of post-hysterectomy vault prolapse and has been shown to be superior to vaginal sacrospinous fixation and vaginal meshes [32, 33]. The subjective cure rate for LSH and LSC ranges in the literature from 79% to 96% depending on the scale used in some studies [39,40,41,46,47,48,49,50]. Sarlos et al reviewed 68 (out of 101) women with examination and questionnaires and a further 17 with questionnaires only, five years following LSC [46]. They reported a 83.8% success rate (no prolapse) five years after sacrocolpopexy. There were six cases of anterior, four posterior, and one apical prolapse. Nightingale et al reported 97% had stage 1 or less apical prolapse, 96% stage 1 or less for posterior compartment prolapse and 66% anterior compartment prolapse following LSC or LSH [45]. It should be noted that of those, 16 had subsequent anterior colporrhaphy and two posterior colporrhaphy before final follow-up.

Jefferis et al reported a re-operation rate for POP of 87.7% with a mean elevation of POP-Q point C of 7.9 cm [41]. Fourteen women (2.8%) underwent a subsequent apical procedure and for 10 of these women, this was simply a laparoscopic plication of the in-situ hysteropexy mesh. A further 36 women (7.1%) underwent colporrhaphy following LSH. With respect to PGI-I data, available for 404 patients, 93.8% (n=367) described their prolapse as 'much better' or 'very much better'.

Daniels et al reported a subjective cure rate of 84%, although no validated measure was used, and an objective cure rate of 80% at 12 months [43]. Lone et al found that at two-years follow-up, laparoscopic sacrohysteropexy was equally effective subjectively compared with vaginal hysterectomy [50]. The VUE study was a pragmatic study assessing different techniques for management of apical prolapse (post-hysterectomy vault prolapse or uterine prolapse) [51]. The study was a pragmatic study so had great heterogeneity in surgeries performed. However, at one-year follow-up there was no difference in safety, efficacy, complications, or patient-recorded outcomes between either the vaginal or abdominal approaches.

In conclusion, there is no advantage to using mesh for primary prolapse repair. There is little evidence to support biological meshes but synthetic type 1 macroporous polypropylene mesh may have a role in patients with recurrent prolapse. If utilized, patients need careful counselling regarding outcomes, complications, and evidence regarding that particular mesh/procedure. There have been significant shortcomings in launch and rollout of vaginal mesh. Clinicians need to identify which patients may benefit and which may be at greater risk of complications. Surgery should only be performed by clinicians with extensive experience in pelvic floor reconstructive surgery and adequate volume of work to maintain skills. Laparoscopic abdominal mesh placement has benefits over vaginal mesh, with better outcomes and fewer complications, but does require significant expertise and has a longer learning curve to become proficient. The lessons learnt from mesh use and mis-use have demonstrated the need for clinicians to audit their outcomes, and some countries are now mandating registries/databases to document and record complications and outcome measures.

References

1. Biler A, Ertas E, Tosun G, et al. Perioperative complications and short-term outcomes of abdominal sacrocolpopexy, laparoscopic sacrocolpopexy, and laparoscopic pectopexy for apical prolapse. Int Braz J Urol 2018; 44(5): 996–1004.
2. Vergeldt T, Weemhoff M, Inthout J, et al. Risk factors for pelvic organ prolapse and its recurrence: a systematic review. Int Urogynecol J 2015; 26: 1559–73.

3. Resel Folkersma L, Vozmediano Chicharro R, González López R, et al. Consenso de la Asociación Española de Urología sobre el uso de mallas en la cirugía del prolapso de órganos pélvicos. Actas Urol Esp 2020; 44(8): 529–34. https://doi.org/10.1016/j.acuro.2020.04.007
4. Phillips CH, Anthony F, Benyon C, Monga AK. Urogynaecology: collagen metabolism in the uterosacral ligaments and vaginal skin of women with uterine prolapse. *BJOG* 2006; 113(1): 39–46.
5. Jens-Eric W. A comparison of the use of mesh to native tissue in the management of vaginal vault prolapse. Best Prac Res Clin Obstet Gynecol 2019; 54: 73–88.
6. Gonzalez Palanca SJ, Gonzalez Veiga EJ, Palmeiro Fernandez G, et al. Long-term results of genital prolapse surgery with polypropylene mesh. Actas Urol Esp 2019; 43(5): 254–61.
7. Laso-Garcia I, Rodriguez-Cabello M, Jimenez-Cidre M, et al. Prospective long-term results, complications and risk factors in pelvic organ prolapse treatment with vaginal mesh. Eur J Obstet Gynecol Reprod Biol 2017; 211: 62–7.
8. Kapoor DS, Nemcova M, Pantazis K, et al. Reoperation rate for traditional anterior vaginal repair: analysis of 207 cases with a median 4-year follow-up. Int Urogynecol J 2010; 21(1): 27–31.
9. Albo ME, Richter HE, Brubaker L, et al. Burch colposuspension versus fascial sling to reduce urinary stress incontinence. N Engl J Med 2007; 356: 2143–55.
10. Walter AJ, Hentz JG, Magrina JF, Cornella JL. Harvesting autologous fascia lata for pelvic reconstructive surgery: techniques and morbidity. Am J Obstet Gynecol 2001; 185: 1354–8.
11. Birch C, Fynes MM. The role of synthetic and biological prostheses in reconstructive pelvic floor surgery. Curr Opin Obstet Gynecol 2002; 14: 527–35.
12. Menefee SA, Dyer KY, Lukacz ES, et al. Colporrhaphy compared with mesh or graft-reinforced vaginal paravaginal repair for anterior vaginal wall prolapse: a randomized controlled trial. Obstet Gynecol 2011; 118: 1337–44.
13. Maher C, Feiner B, Baessler K, et al. Transvaginal mesh or grafts compared with native tissue repair for vaginal prolapse. Cochrane Database Syst Rev 2016; (2): CD012079.
14. Glazener CM, Breeman S, Elders A, et al. Mesh, graft, or standard repair for women having primary transvaginal anterior or posterior compartment prolapse surgery: two parallel-group, multicentre, randomised, controlled trials (PROSPECT). Lancet 2017; 389: 381–92.
15. Barbolt TA. Biology of polypropylene/polyglactin 910 grafts. Int Urogynecol J Pelvic Floor Dysfunct 2006; 17(Suppl 1):S26–30.
16. Tyrell J, Silberman H, Chandrasoma P, Niland J, Shull J. Absorbable versus permanent mesh in abdominal operations. Surg Gynecol Obstet 1989; 168: 227–32.
17. Rudnicki M, Laurikainen E, Pogosean R, et al. Anterior colporrhaphy compared with collagen-coated transvaginal mesh for anterior vaginal wall prolapse: a randomised controlled trial. BJOG 2014; 121: 102–10.
18. Rudnicki M, Laurikainen E, Pogosean R, et al. A 3-year follow-up after anterior colporrhaphy compared with collagen-coated transvaginal mesh for anterior vaginal wall prolapse: a randomised controlled trial. BJOG 2016; 123: 136–42.
19. Campbell P, Jha S, Cutner A. Vaginal mesh in prolapse surgery. Obstet Gynaecol 2018; 20(1): 49–56.
20. Ray S, Clifton M, Koo K. Inaccuracies in news media reporting about the 2019 US food and drug administration ban on transvaginal mesh for pelvic organ prolapse repair. Urology 2021; 150: 194–200.
21. UK Government. Pause on the use of vaginally inserted surgical mesh for stress urinary incontinence. Available from: www.gov.uk/government/news/pause-on-the-use-of-vaginally-inserted-surgical-mesh-for-stress-urinary-incontinence [last accessed 4 November 2021].
22. Mikhail S, Maher C. Surgical pathway for the treatment of pelvic organ prolapse. Obstet Gynecol Reprod Med 2018; 28: 4.
23. Matthews CA. No evidence-based recommendations exist for optimal management of pelvic mesh complications. BJOG 2020; 127(1): 36.
24. Duckett J, Bodner-Adler B, Rachaneni S, Latthe P. Management of complications arising from the use of mesh for stress urinary incontinence—International Urogynecology Association Research and Development Committee opinion. Int Urogynecol J 2019; 27: 1–5.
25. Cosson M, Fernandez H. Peut-on encore utilizer des prostheses par voie vaginale dans le traitement des prolapses? Gynecologie Obstetrique Fertilite & Senologie 2019; 47: 487–8.
26. Claerhout F, Verguts J, Werbrouck E, et al. Analysis of the learning process for laparoscopic sacrocolpopexy: identification of challenging steps. Int Urogynecol J 2014; 25(9): 1185–91.
27. Richter L, Sokol A. Pelvic organ prolapse – vaginal and laparoscopic mesh: the evidence. Obstet Gynecol Clin North Am 2016; 43(1): 83–92. https://doi.org/10.1016/j.ogc.2015.10.004
28. Dong S, Zhong Y, Chu L, et al. Age-stratified analysis of long-term outcomes of transvaginal mesh repair for treatment of pelvic organ prolapse. Int J Gynecol Obstet 2016; 135(1): 112–16.
29. Gluck O, Blaganje M, Deval B. How I do … Laparoscopic ventral rectopexy using a synthetic mesh. Gynecologie Obstertrique Fertilite & Senologie 2019; 47: 753–6.
30. Haylen BT, De Ridder D, Freeman RM, et al. An International Urogynecological Association (IUGA)/International Continence Society (ICS) joint report on the terminology for female pelvic floor dysfunction. Int Urogynecol J 2010; 21: 5–26. https://doi.org/10.1007/s00192-009-0976-9
31. Meriwether K V, Antosh DD, Olivera CK, et al. Uterine preservation vs hysterectomy in pelvic organ prolapse surgery: a systematic review with meta-analysis and clinical practice guidelines. Am J Obstet Gynecol 2018; 219(2): 129–46.e2.
32. Toozs-Hobson P, Boos K, Cardozo L. Management of vaginal vault prolapse. BJOG 1998; 105: 13–17. https://doi.org/10.1111/j.1471-0528.1998.tb09343
33. Maher C, Feiner B, Baessler K, et al. Surgery for women with apical vaginal prolapse. Cochrane Database Syst Rev 2016. Cochrane Database Syst Rev 2016; 10(10): CD012376. https://doi.org/10.1002/14651858.CD012376
34. Royal College of Obstetricians and Gynaecologists. Post-Hysterectomy Vaginal Vault Prolapse. Green-top Guideline No. 46. Published July 2015. Available from: www.rcog.org.uk/globalassets/documents/guidelines/gtg-46.pdf [last accessed 4 November 2021].
35. Freeman RM, Pantazis K, Thomson A, et al. A randomised controlled trial of abdominal versus laparoscopic sacrocolpopexy for the treatment of post-hysterectomy vaginal vault prolapse: LAS study. Int Urogynecol J Pelvic Floor Dysfunct 2013; 24: 377–384. https://doi.org/10.1007/s00192-012-1885-x
36. National Health Service Scotland. The Scottish Independent Review of the Use, Safety and Efficacy of Transvaginal Mesh Implants in the Treatment of Stress Urinary Incontinence and Pelvic Organ Prolapse in Women Final Report. Published 2017.

37. US Food and Drug Administration. Urogynecologic Surgical Mesh Implants. Available from: www.fda.gov/medical-devices/implants-and-prosthetics/urogynecologic-surgical-mesh-implants [last accessed 4 November 2021].
38. Abrams P, Cardozo L, Khoury S, Wein A. Incontinence: 5th International Consultation on Incontinence. Published 2012.
39. Baines G, Price N, Jefferis H, et al. Mesh-related complications of laparoscopic sacrocolpopexy. Int Urogynecol J 2019; 30: 1475–81. https://doi.org/10.1007/s00192-019-03952-7
40. Orhan A, Ozerkan K, Vuruskan H, et al. Long-term follow-up of laparoscopic sacrocolpopexy: comparison of two different techniques used in urology and gynecology. Int Urogynecol J 2019; 30: 623–32. https://doi.org/10.1007/s00192-018-03858-w
41. Jefferis H, Price N, Jackson S. Laparoscopic hysteropexy: 10 years' experience. Int Urogynecol J 2017; 28: 1241–8. https://doi.org/10.1007/s00192-016-3257-4
42. Roovers JPW, van der Vaart CH, van der Bom JG, et al. A randomised controlled trial comparing abdominal and vaginal prolapse surgery: effects on urogenital function. BJOG 2004; 111(1): 50–6.
43. Daniels S, Robson D, Palacz M, et al. Success rates and outcomes of laparoscopic mesh sacrohysteropexy. Austr N Z J Obstet Gynaecol 2020; 60(2): 244–9.
44. Pandeva I, Mistry M, Fayyad A. Efficacy and pregnancy outcomes of laparoscopic single sheet mesh sacrohysteropexy. Neurourol 2017; 36(3): 787–93.
45. Nightingale G, Phillips C. Long-term safety and efficacy of laparoscopically placed mesh for apical prolapse. Int Urogynecol J 2020; 10: 1–7.
46. Sarlos D, Kots LV, Ryu G, Schaer G. Long-term follow-up of laparoscopic sacrocolpopexy. Int Urogynecol J Pelvic Floor Dysfunct 2014; 25: 1207–12. https://doi.org/10.1007/s00192-014-2369-y
47. Higgs PJ, Chua HL, Smith ARB. Long term review of laparoscopic sacrocolpopexy. BJOG 2005; 112: 1134–8. https://doi.org/10.1111/j.1471-0528.2005.00646.x
48. Ganatra AM, Rozet F, Sanchez-Salas R, et al. The current status of laparoscopic sacrocolpopexy: a review. Eur Urol 2009; 55: 1089–105.
49. Granese R, Candiani M, Perino A, et al. Laparoscopic sacrocolpopexy in the treatment of vaginal vault prolapse: 8 years' experience. Eur J Obstet Gynecol Reprod Biol 2009; 146(2): 227–31.
50. Lone F, Curnow T, Thomas SA. Laparoscopic sacrohysteropexy versus vaginal hysterectomy for uterovaginal prolapse using validated questionnaires: 2-year prospective study. Int Urogynecol J 2018; 29(1): 71–9.
51. Glazener C, Constable L, Hemming C, et al. Two parallel, pragmatic, UK multicentre, randomised controlled trials comparing surgical options for upper compartment (vault or uterine) pelvic organ prolapse (the VUE Study): study protocol for a randomised controlled trial. Trials 2016; 17: 441. https://doi.org/10.1186

Chapter 28

The Rise of Robotic Surgery in Benign Gynaecology

Viviana Casas-Puig, Lisa Hickman

Introduction

Advances in minimally invasive surgery have had a tremendous impact on the field of gynaecology. The introduction and application of laparoscopic technology resulted in significant patient benefits such as decreased blood loss, less postoperative pain, shorter length of hospital stay, earlier return to baseline function, and improved cosmesis compared to an abdominal approach [1]. Over time, these patient benefits have fuelled the adoption of conventional laparoscopy by gynaecologic surgeons; however, technical drawbacks inherent to this approach such as decreased dexterity, tremor amplification, instrument rigidity, increased surgeon strain, and a prolonged learning curve have precluded more widespread use among the broader gynaecologic surgical community [2].

Although originally developed to provide remote surgical care in the battlefield, robotic technology was introduced to hospital systems as a tool to facilitate laparoscopic surgery in 1999. Following the approval of the da Vinci Surgical System (Intuitive Surgical, Inc., Sunnyvale, CA) by the US Food and Drug Administration (FDA) in 2005 for use in gynaecologic surgery, more rapid adoption of this technique ensued. This was likely driven by the unique advantages of the robotic system, including enhanced three-dimensional visualization of the surgical field, improved dexterity with wristed instruments featuring seven degrees of freedom, and tremor-filtering technology [3]. Additionally, the learning curve for robotic surgery seemed to be less steep compared to conventional laparoscopy, thereby allowing surgeons to learn a minimally invasive skillset at a much more rapid pace [3]. As such, the robotic platform enabled gynaecologists to perform minimally invasive surgery on patients who would have otherwise undergone an open procedure. The features of the robotic platform also seemed to overcome previously claimed limitations of conventional laparoscopy. Not surprisingly, between 2010 and 2017, the field of gynaecology witnessed the second fastest growth in surgical robotic case volume (123,000 to 252,000), behind general surgery [4].

Common applications of the robotic platform in benign gynaecologic surgery include procedures such as hysterectomy, sacrocolpopexy, myomectomy, endometriosis, and adnexal surgery. However, the most common robotic technology application has been for the performing hysterectomy in the setting of benign gynaecologic disease. By 2010, robotic-assisted laparoscopy was utilized in 10% of all hysterectomies performed in the US, and 25% of hysterectomies performed in hospitals offering this platform [5].

Low-certainty data supports the safety and efficacy of robotic-assisted procedures such as hysterectomy and sacrocolpopexy. However, in the hands of experienced surgeons, perioperative outcomes are comparable to those reported for conventional laparoscopy, and superior to those with laparotomy [6].

The objectives of this chapter are to review the facets of robotic-assisted surgery, including the indications, operating room set-up, basic technique, and both advantages and disadvantages. Furthermore, we will highlight the available evidence on robotic technology for minimally invasive benign hysterectomy and sacrocolpopexy for the treatment of pelvic organ prolapse.

Indications

The decision to perform robotic procedures for the treatment of benign gynaecologic disease is multifactorial. Generally, the choice of surgical route or approach is determined by equipment availability, surgeon and patient preferences, and the surgeon's skillset. Furthermore, patient-specific considerations such as obesity, past surgical history with the concern of pelvic adhesive disease, enlarged pathology, and/or anticipation of high surgical case complexity may influence the decision to choose robotic surgery over other modalities [7]. While the advantages and proposed benefits of robotic technology on the obese and morbidly obese patient populations are well-established in the oncology literature, only low-quality data supports this observation for patients with benign gynaecologic disease [1].

The American College of Obstetricians and Gynecologists Committee Opinion Number 810 on *Robot-assisted surgery for noncancerous gynecologic conditions* calls for surgeon consideration of robotic technology utilization based on the likelihood of improved outcomes compared with other surgical approaches, due to the complexity of the case or patient factors, with appropriate consideration of costs [1]. Patients scheduled for gynaecologic procedures of short duration with low complexity such as tubal ligation, simple ovarian cystectomy, surgical management of tubal ectopic pregnancy, bilateral salpingo-oophorectomy, bilateral salpingectomy, diagnostic laparoscopy, or other surgeries when diagnosis is unknown, are unlikely to benefit from robotic-assisted surgery. Due to a lack of advantages and potential disadvantages, both the American College of Obstetricians and Gynecologists and the Society of Gynecologic Surgeons recommends against the use of robotic technology for these procedures [1].

Robotic System Equipment

The da Vinci® robotic system is currently the only FDA-approved robotic technology for performing gynaecologic procedures. Four generations of the da Vinci® Surgical System exist, and each system is composed of a patient cart, surgeon console, and vision cart. The operative component of the da Vinci® Si patient cart supports three instrument arms and a camera arm. Generally, the first and second robotic arms of the Si Surgical System are used to perform the surgical procedure (operative arms), while the third arm is used for retraction. The newest generation of the da Vinci® Surgical System, the Xi platform, offers multi-quadrant access and higher versatility for various surgical procedures. Unlike the da Vinci® Si System, the Xi platform allows placement of the camera on any robotic arm (Figure 28.1).

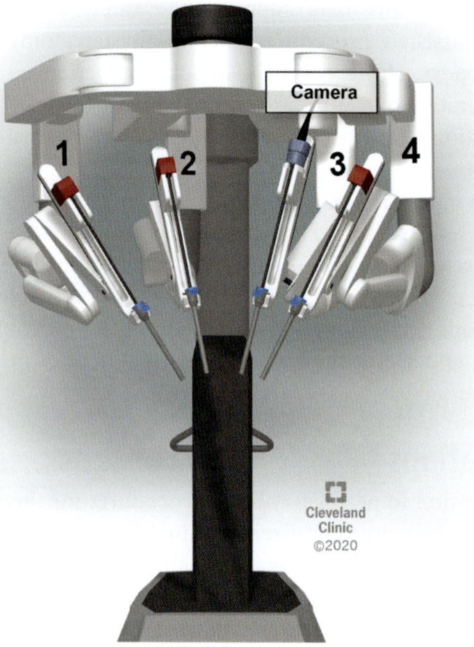

Figure 28.1 Robotic Xi System 'pre-docking'.

The surgeon console for both generations is composed of a stereoscopic viewer through which the surgeon views the operative field, two master controllers, and foot pedals which facilitate selection of the preferred energy source and movement of the camera (Figure 28.2). A toggle side switch allows the surgeon to alternate between operating instruments. The surgeon's thumb and index fingers are placed in the master controllers, and both finger and wrist motion are translated into precise, fine, tremor-filtered movements at the EndoWrist® instrument tips. Lastly, the vision cart provides a three-dimensional, high definition view of the surgical field, and allows for telestration, where the surgeon may utilize the touch screen to point out critical anatomy and/or next steps on the monitor to guide a trainee sitting on the console (Figure 28.3). Additionally, the dual console system provides an excellent opportunity for teaching, whereby the surgeon operates in parallel with the trainee. Instrument control can be exchanged between the consoles, and the master controllers, when not in use, can be utilized for telestration, thereby enhancing a trainee's educational experience.

Operating Room Set-up: Patient Positioning, Port Placement, and Robot Docking

Figure 28.4 demonstrates the operating room set-up for robotic-assisted gynaecologic surgery. The surgical team is composed of the anaesthesiologist at the head of the operating table, the robotic surgeon(s) at the surgeon console, a bedside assistant on

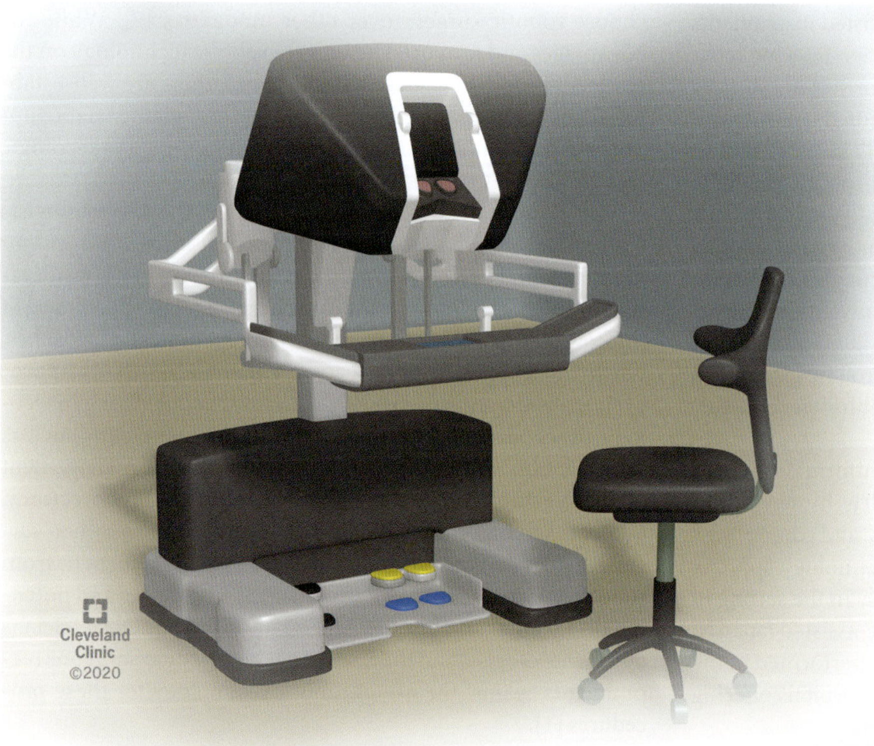

Figure 28.2 Surgeon console.

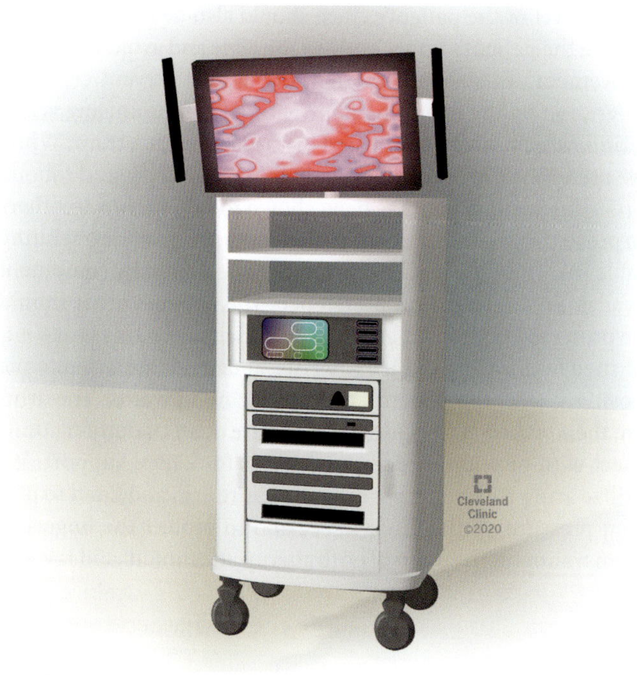

Figure 28.3 Vision cart.

the patient's right side, a vaginal assistant at the foot of the table, a scrubbed surgical technician, and a circulating nurse. Vaginal instruments such as dilators, retractors, end-to-end anastomosis sizers, and uterine manipulators are kept on a designated vaginal table, accessible to the vaginal assistant. A separate surgical table is utilized for the placement of clean laparoscopic and robotic instruments, suture, and/or implants, and a large Mayo tray is utilized for the cystoscopic equipment. The vision cart is strategically placed on the patient's left side, slightly proximal to the robotic cart, ensuring that the bedside assistant has optimal visualization of the operative field through the monitor. Another monitor should be available at the patient's right side to ensure the vaginal assistant has optimal visualization as well.

Patient Positioning

Proper patient positioning is one of the most critical factors to ensure a safe and successful robotic procedure. Safe patient positioning focuses on preventing patient cephalad sliding and avoiding pressure on nerves and bony prominences [8]. Patients should be positioned in dorsal low lithotomy to optimize visualization of the pelvic structures and allow access to the vagina and rectum either for retraction, manipulation,

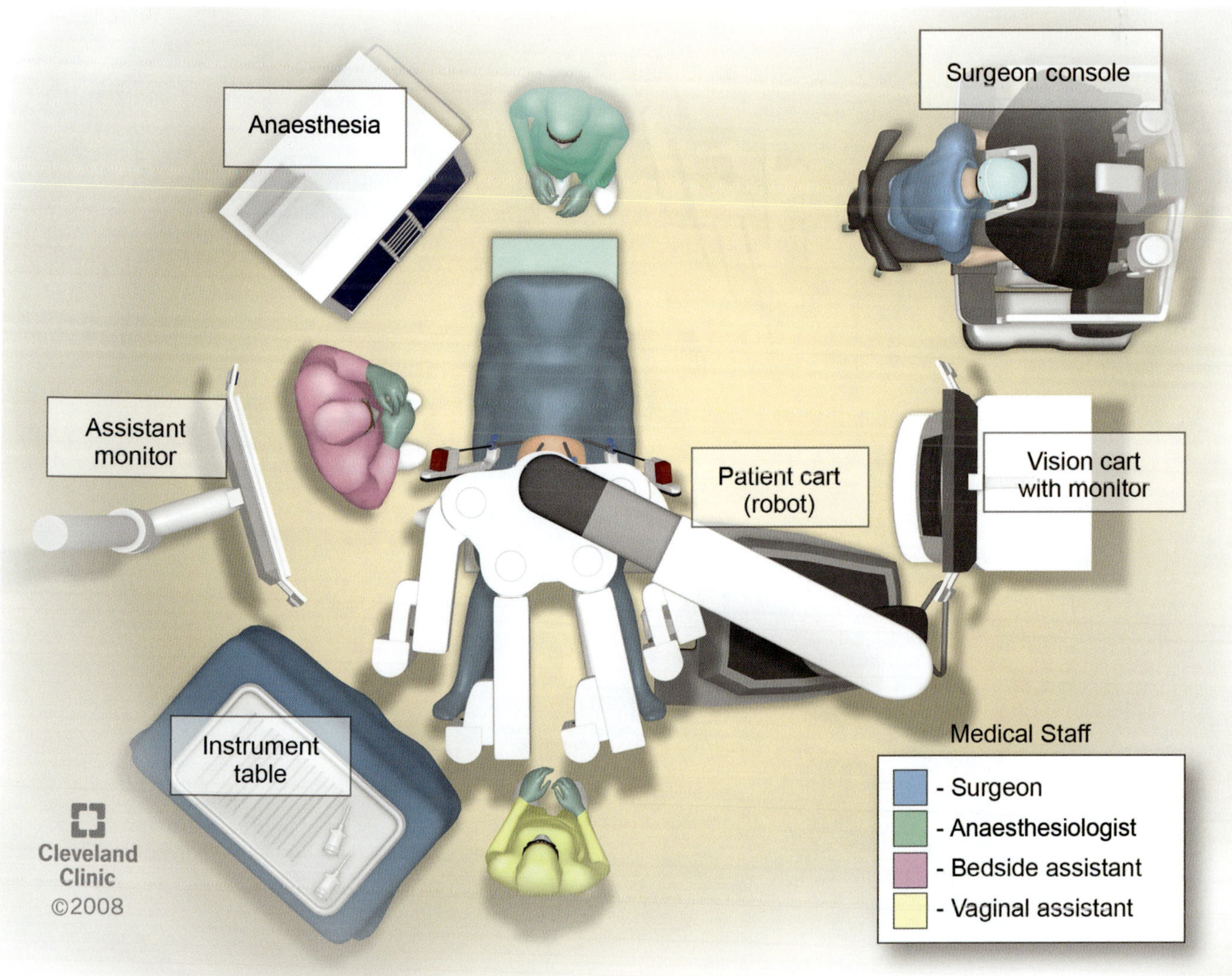

Figure 28.4 Operative set-up 'overview'.

periodic examination throughout the procedure, and/or concurrent vaginal surgery. We recommend the use of Allen® or Yellowfin® (Allen Medical Systems, Acton, MA) stirrups for patient positioning, ensuring the legs are not hyperflexed or extended at the hip or knee (Figure 28.5). Generous padding of all bony prominences should be undertaken to prevent nerve compression injuries. The patient's head should be supported and both eyes covered to minimize the risk of corneal abrasions. The patient should be positioned such that the buttocks are slightly inferior to the end of the table, without compromising support of the sacrum. The patient should be secured to the table so she may be placed in steep Trendelenburg position without cephalad slipping. A variety of devices exist to prevent cephalad patient slide including memory foam (Pink Pad, Xodus Medical, New Kensington, PA), egg crate foam, gel pad (AliGel™ OR Overlay Pad, AliMed, Inc. Dehdam, MA), and surgical bean bag (Olympic Vac-Pac™ Marlin Medical, Bayswater North, VIC, Australia). A padded strap or silk tape with padding at the level of the patient's chest should also be used to further secure the patient's upper body to the table and avoid unwanted movement. This should be tight enough to prevent cephalad migration on the operating table without compromising ventilation, which can be confirmed by the anaesthesia team. While we prefer the use of memory foam for laparoscopic and robotic procedures, no device has been shown to be superior to others in preventing nerve injury or patient migration on the operating table [8]. Thus, device selection should be driven by equipment availability and surgeon preference. The patient's arms should be protected with foam and tucked at her sides. This is accomplished by ensuring the arms, wrists, and hands are in anatomic position, with the patient's thumbs facing upwards. The arms are then tucked at her sides with the use of an underlying draw sheet with or without sled arm boards for lateral support. We utilize arm protectors spanning the entire arm and hand to prevent pressure on the ulnar nerve and to protect the fingertips from trauma at the point of both stirrup attachment and the foot

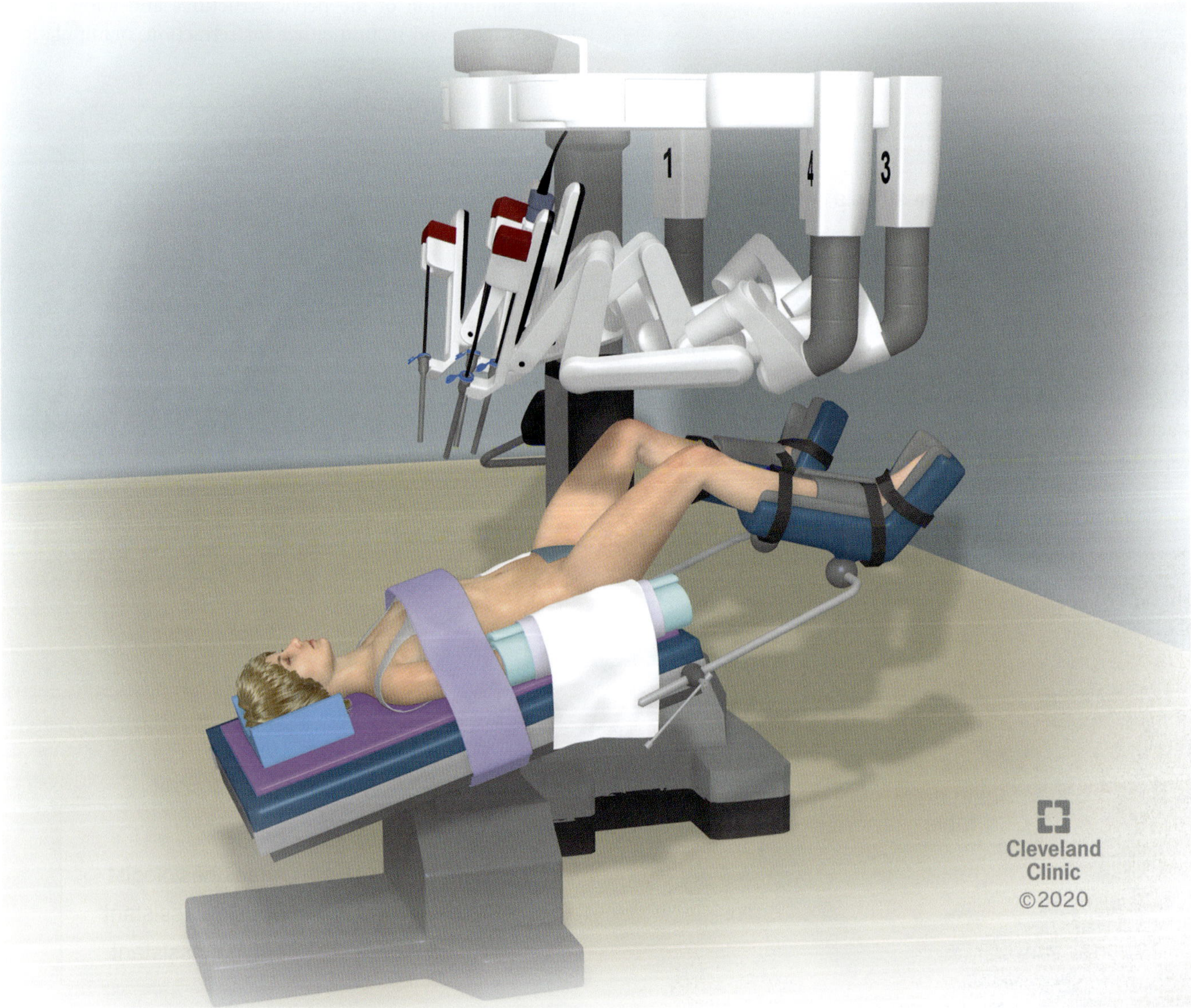

Figure 28.5 Patient positioning.

of the bed. After arm tucking, integrity of the IV lines should be confirmed with the anaesthesia team. An orogastric tube is placed by the anaesthesia team to decompress the stomach, and a Foley catheter is inserted under sterile conditions prior to initiating the gynaecologic procedure.

Robotic and Accessory Port Placement

Proper port placement is essential for facilitating robotic-assisted laparoscopic procedures in gynaecology. This configuration may vary based on the patient's anatomy, uterine size, provider preference, and planned procedure. Universal considerations include careful angulation of each trocar during port placement to ensure adequate articulation of the robotic arms during surgery. Additionally, sufficient distance between the trocars is necessary to prevent robotic arm collision, ideally keeping a 9 cm distance between ports. Robotic ports should also be placed such that its remote centre, indicated by a thick, distal black line on the cannula, lies within the muscle layer of the abdomen. This technology aims to minimize the force applied to the abdominal wall with robotic arm movements. For hysterectomy and pelvic organ prolapse procedures, such as sacrocolpopexy, placement of five ports is typically necessary. While multiple port configurations are described in the literature, we recommend placement of trocars in a 'Z' configuration on the abdomen if using the da Vinci® Si System (Figure 28.6), or in a slightly curved line, or modified 'arc' configuration, when using the Xi system (Figure 28.7). When using the da Vinci® Si robotic platform, placement of a 12 mm trocar is necessary in the umbilicus for the robotic laparoscope. Depending on the patient's surgical history and likelihood of encountering adhesions, a left upper quadrant, or an open entry technique, such as the Hasson, may be more appropriate. Otherwise, we routinely place a 5 mm optic trocar housing a 0-degree laparoscope through a 5 mm umbilical incision to gain entry. Following confirmation of intraperitoneal entry, the pneumoperitoneum is achieved with CO_2 gas, and the upper abdomen is carefully inspected. The patient is then placed in steep Trendelenburg position to move the bowels cephalad and optimize visualization of the pelvis for additional trocar placement. Two 8 mm robotic ports are placed 9 cm lateral, and either slightly superior or inferior to the umbilicus. A third 8 mm robotic port is placed in the mid-axillary line on the left side and an 8 mm or 10 mm assistant port is placed 9 cm lateral and inferior to the right-sided robotic port. Lastly, the 5 mm umbilical port is removed and replaced with a 12 mm trocar under direct visualization. Unlike the Si Surgical System, the Xi platform permits umbilical entry with the use of an optical 8 mm robotic port that is placed under direct visualization with a 0-degree, 5 mm laparoscope. This feature of the Xi System, along with the availability of a smaller (8 mm) lens camera, avoids the need for replacement of the umbilical trocar with a larger port. It also confers the advantage that the fascia need not be repaired at the conclusion of the surgery. Another accessory unique to the Xi system is the reusable robotic Hasson trocar which can be utilized if the surgeon anticipates adhesive disease on initial entry.

While the use of an 8 mm assistant port allows the introduction of suture with SH needles and does not require fascial closure at the completion of the procedure, a 10 mm port allows the passage of larger needles but requires a fascial closure. We prefer the use of an 8 mm assistant port as it safeguards patients against postoperative myofascial abdominal pain due to inadvertent nerve injury and reduces the risk of port-site hernia if proper closure is not achieved. All trocars should be placed under direct visualization to avoid vascular and visceral injury. Refer to Chapter 4 for a detailed description of relevant abdominopelvic anatomy and key anatomic landmarks during port placement.

Robot Docking and Instrumentation

Once all ports are properly placed, one must identify and remove any obstacles in the path of bringing the patient cart to the operating table. Robot docking is the process whereby all robotic arms are attached to the robotic ports on the patient's abdomen. Various robot docking techniques have been

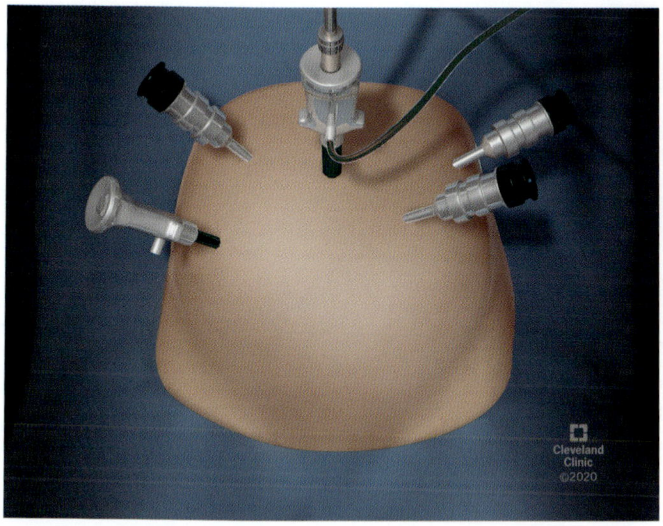

Figure 28.6 Port placement – Z configuration.

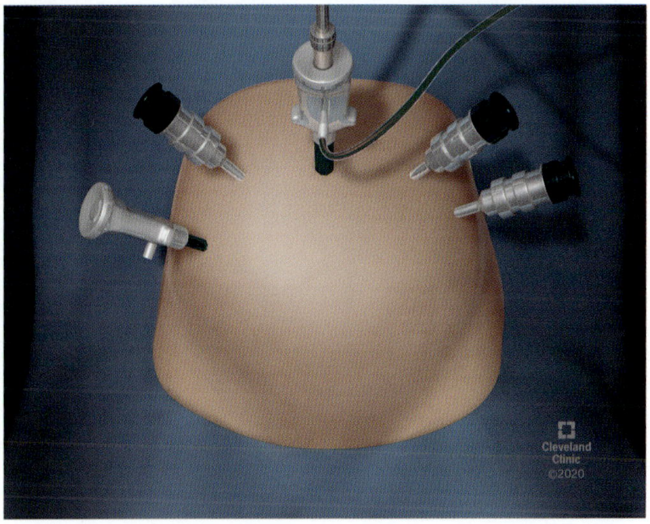

Figure 28.7 Port placement – arc configuration

described in the literature. For the purposes of benign gynaecologic surgery including hysterectomy and both pelvic organ prolapse and anti-incontinence surgery, we recommend side docking either in a parallel fashion or at a 45-degree angle to the operative table on the patient's left side. We prefer parallel docking, which is accomplished by placing the leading edge of the patient cart along the edge of the operative table on the patient's left side. The patient cart is then carefully advanced until the camera arm reaches the umbilical port. The camera arm is affixed first followed by the other robotic arms. The fourth robotic arm (arm 3 in the da Vinci® Si System), which is the most lateral arm on the patient's left side, should be affixed last as it should be angled in a horizontal plane, parallel to the floor. All instrument arms are affixed to their respective ports, or cannulas, with the use of a port clutch button. Great care must be taken to position the arms for optimal triangulation, thereby minimizing robotic arm collision. To accomplish this, all arms should be positioned having at least a 30-degree angle between the camera and instrument arms, with a 45-degree angle being most ideal [9]. Following docking of the Si surgical system, the operative table cannot be further adjusted or moved, and one must undock the robot before any adjustments in position can be made.

The da Vinci® Xi robotic system has unique features that work to facilitate robot docking. These include an overhead rotating boom, thinner robotic arms with longer reach instruments, and an integrated laser docking system (Figure 28.8). These enhancements over the previous platform offer an easier and more efficient docking process. Additionally, the Xi platform features table movement technology, which permits simultaneous movements of the operative table and the robotic arms as needed throughout the procedure, thereby saving time and improving efficiency.

With the newer platform, we prefer side docking with either a 45- or 90-degree angle to the operative table (Figure 28.9). The endoscope arm is affixed first and a 30-degree endoscope is gradually inserted to point to the target anatomy. Next, while stabilizing the cannula at the patient's body wall, the targeting button on the endoscope is pressed. The targeting process positions the boom over the initial endoscope port, and further orients and positions the boom in order to maximize range of motion. The remaining arms are docked once the targeting process is completed.

Regardless of robotic system used, all instruments should be placed under direct visualization while aiming towards the target pelvic anatomy. The choice of instruments will vary depending on the planned surgical procedure and the surgeon's preference. Cost-effectiveness may play a role with instrument selection and this may vary among surgeons. For a robotic sacrocolpopexy with or without a hysterectomy, we place a monopolar scissor in the robotic right arm (1 for Si or 4 for Xi), a fenestrated bipolar instrument in the left arm (2 for Si or Xi), and an atraumatic grasper in the assistant arm (3 for Si or 1 for Xi).

Even though the camera can be placed on any robotic port when using the Xi platform, our preference is to place the camera in arm 3, followed by placement of the instruments as mentioned above. For suturing, a SutureCut™ needle driver is placed in the right arm (1 for Si or 4 for Xi), a needle driver in the left arm (2 for Si and Xi), and the atraumatic grasper is kept in assistant arm. When suturing is indicated, we utilize 15–20 cm long sutures that are tied with intracorporeal suturing technique. Suture kits inserted into the abdomen, which contain multiple needles, are

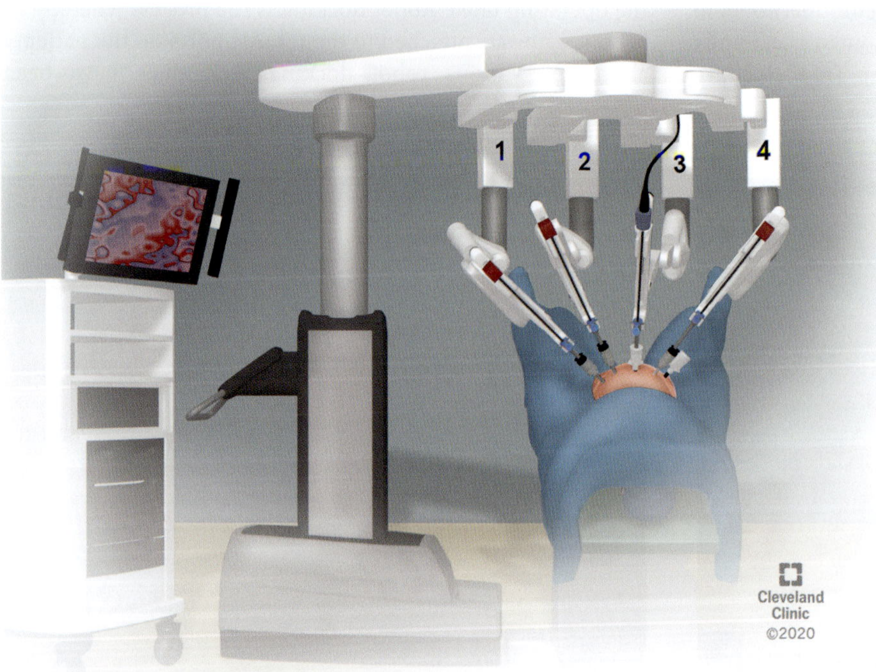

Figure 28.8 'Anterior port view'.

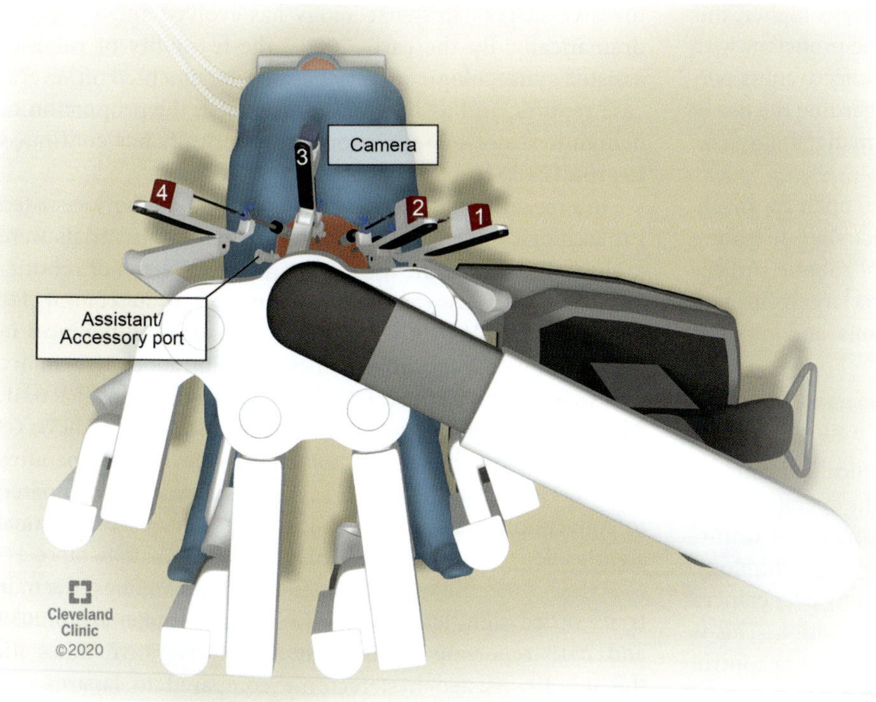

Figure 28.9 Docking 'top port view'.

also commercially available. Hysterectomy and sacrocolpopexy procedure steps and technique essentially mirror those performed with conventional laparoscopy. Refer to Chapters 14 and 20 for a detailed description of surgical techniques.

Learning Curve

The learning curve associated with robotic technology can be measured either by procedure-related factors, such as the robotic set-up and operative times, or surgeon-related factors, such as the surgeon's expertise, skillset, and complications [10]. Based on limited data, the combination of improved precision, visualization, and instrument control with the robotic platform may facilitate learning and adoption of minimally invasive robotic surgery by less experienced surgeons, compared to conventional laparoscopy. Learning curves are reported to vary according to the surgical procedure, and while data has shown improvements in robotic surgical technique within the first 100 cases, proficiency with robotic-assisted hysterectomy has been shown to be attained after 20 to 30 procedures [1,11].

Previous work on the validation of various laparoscopic simulation programmes has consistently shown improvements in surgeon's skills and performance of minimally invasive gynaecologic surgery [12]. Unlike conventional laparoscopic simulation testing, recently made a requirement among trainees of various surgical specialties, robotic simulation training has not yet become mandatory [1]. Furthermore, despite the exponential growth and utilization of robotic technology in gynaecology, exposure and access to the robotic platform continues to vary on a national level. For inexperienced surgeons, various robotic-assisted surgery web-based and on-site robotic training curricula exist, which allow the surgeon to become familiar with the technology, and practice robotic surgical skills on models or simulators without compromising patient safety [13].

Cost

Cost modelling studies on robotic-assisted hysterectomy for benign conditions have demonstrated increased equipment expense and longer operating room times compared with laparoscopic surgery [14–16]. Depending on the model, the robotic platform costs between $0.5 to $2.5 million. Each instrument is limited to 10 uses, with pricing ranging from $220 to $320. Additional expenses include those for training, equipment maintenance, and repair [17].

In a population-based analysis by Wright et al, which included 264,758 women who underwent hysterectomy for benign indications, the median total cost of robotic-assisted laparoscopic hysterectomy was $2,189 (95% CI, $2,030–$2,349) more per case than for conventional laparoscopic hysterectomy [5]. Of note, costs reported in this study represented direct expenses for the operative procedure and did not reflect capital or societal costs. The most recent Cochrane review on robotic-assisted gynaecologic surgery by Lawrie et al reported significant heterogeneity in cost reports, making it difficult to draw any conclusions on differences between minimally invasive hysterectomy approaches [6].

It has been suggested that robot-associated expenses may be offset by the indirect benefits for the surgeon through the improved ergonomics, and possible decreased healthcare costs due to shorter patient hospital stays. A recent analysis of the National Inpatient Sample compared the costs between all robotic and conventional laparoscopic surgeries performed between 2012 through 2014 [18]. In this study, hysterectomy was the only procedure found to be primarily performed with robotic assistance (60%). Compared to other surgeries, hysterectomy showed the narrowest percent cost change, at 5.9%, with laparoscopic hysterectomy averaging $9,368, and robotic-assisted hysterectomy averaging $9,923. These findings suggest even though the overall cost of robotic surgery is higher, this difference may be offset once surgeons become proficient with the robotic technique. However, from a cost-effectiveness perspective, significant controversy still exists regarding the use of robotic technology for the treatment of non-malignant gynaecologic conditions.

Regarding comparison with the traditional open approach, cost-effectiveness analyses in the urogynaecologic literature have, not surprisingly, shown an advantage of robotic surgery compared to open abdominal approach. This is largely through the prevention of perioperative complications and reduced length of hospital stay [19,20].

Advantages of Robotic Surgery

The robotic platform provides many technical advantages including three-dimensional visualization of the operative field, improved dexterity with the use of wristed instruments featuring seven degrees of freedom, and tremor-filtering technology. Additionally, the surgeon has complete autonomy over camera control thereby optimizing surgical field visualization. This is in contrast to conventional laparoscopy where camera control and image stability is highly dependent on both the surgical assistant's hand–eye coordination and the patient's breathing pattern. Such advancements inherent to the robotic technology are also thought to facilitate deep pelvic dissection and intracorporeal knot tying, skills known to have a prolonged learning curve when performed by conventional laparoscopy [21]. Additionally, the robotic console can be electronically adjusted to each surgeon's height and comfort level, which has shown to improve ergonomics while minimizing surgeon fatigue and physical strain [22].

Disadvantages of Robotic Surgery

One of the main disadvantages of robotic technology is the absence of haptic or tactile feedback. To overcome this limitation, the surgeon must rely on visual cues in order to judge the appropriate amount of tension or force being applied to tissues. Learning the intricacies of robotic set-up takes time and requires training. Also, the ability to clutch, exchange instruments, focus the camera, and use monopolar and bipolar energy modalities can vary between the generations of the da Vinci® Robotic Surgical System, which requires the surgical team be familiar with and adapt to these differences [9]. Lastly, the most commonly cited disadvantage of robotic technology is the increased cost of the surgical system.

Applications of Robotic Surgery in Benign Gynaecology

Hysterectomy

Hysterectomy is one of the most commonly performed surgeries in women, with 400,000 hysterectomies performed annually in the US [5]. Historically, hysterectomy was performed either by the abdominal or vaginal routes. In 1989, Reich published the first laparoscopic-assisted vaginal hysterectomy [23]. Since that time, the application of minimally invasive surgery in gynaecology has evolved and improved dramatically. By the early 2000s, the feasibility of robotic-assisted gynaecologic surgery became documented on several case reports, and as previously discussed, the proportion of benign hysterectomies performed robotically has continued to grow [24,25].

In a recently published Cochrane review on robotic-assisted gynaecologic surgery, four randomized controlled trials were evaluated to determine the safety and effectiveness of robotic-assisted versus conventional laparoscopic hysterectomy for benign gynaecologic disease [6]. There were no differences in perioperative complications, including intraoperative injury (RR 1.62, 95% CI 0.20, 12.91), bleeding complications (RR 0.41, 95% CI 0.10, 1.66), or surgical site infection (RR 0.62, 95% CI 0.13, 2.88) between surgical routes. The mean total operative time was longer in the robotic-assisted surgery arm compared to conventional laparoscopy, but this did not reach statistical significance (mean difference of 41.18 minutes, 95% CI, 6.17, 88.53). Of note, the reported operative times amongst the four trials varied significantly, with two earlier studies from 2012 and 2013 reporting significantly longer operative times for the robotic-assisted hysterectomy compared to laparoscopy (29 minutes versus 77 minutes mean difference, respectively) [16,26]. These findings may be explained by surgeons practicing early in their robotic learning curve or due to larger specimen weights in the robotic-assisted group [27,28]. Conversely, Deimling and colleagues found similar operative times between robotic-assisted and conventional laparoscopic hysterectomy (73.9 minutes versus 74.9 minutes) [29]. The aforementioned studies also found similar rates in conversion to an alternative approach, blood loss, pain, and quality of life between the two groups. As such, the Cochrane review conveyed low-certainty evidence to support comparable outcomes between surgical modalities [6].

Several retrospective studies have sought to compare clinical outcomes between robotic and conventional laparoscopic routes for benign hysterectomy. Using the Michigan Surgical Quality Collaborative (MSQC) database, Swenson et al explored the clinical outcomes of 8,313 women who underwent hysterectomy for benign indications including vaginal, laparoscopic, and robotic-assisted surgery [28]. The authors found similar perioperative complication, re-admission, and re-operation rates between the groups. The robotic-assisted group, however, had lower rates of superficial surgical site infection and blood transfusion as compared to the conventional laparoscopy group. These findings should be interpreted with caution, given the overall low incidence of outcomes within their cohort. A retrospective study by Lim et al comparing outcomes of 32,118 women who underwent either a robotic, laparoscopic, vaginal, or open hysterectomy found a shorter length of hospital stay in the robotic cohort (1.37 days) as compared to other routes, despite a higher rate of adhesive disease, uteri >250 grams, and morbid obesity in this group [30]. The clinical significance of these findings is unclear as a similar trend in length of stay was also observed in the laparoscopic group. Additionally, despite greater case complexity in the robotic group, there was no difference in conversion rates between the robotic and laparoscopic routes when performed by highly experienced surgeons.

Sacrocolpopexy

Sacrocolpopexy is widely recognized as the gold standard treatment for vaginal vault prolapse [31]. Traditionally, sacrocolpopexy was performed by the open or conventional laparoscopic routes, with steeper learning curves described when utilizing the laparoscopic approach, likely due to the more technically challenging dissection, suturing, and increased ergonomic strain. Over time, there was a rapid rise in the utilization of the robotic platform for sacrocolpopexy, starting in 2008. This was likely due to the benefits offered by minimally invasive surgery, increasing concerns associated with transvaginal mesh placement for pelvic organ prolapse, and in the setting of emerging robotic technology [32].

Data on minimally invasive sacrocolpopexy are limited mostly to retrospective studies with only two randomized controlled trials comparing laparoscopic and robotic-assisted techniques [33,34]. These trials showed longer operative times in the robotic arm compared with conventional laparoscopy (202 minutes versus 178 minutes, p=<0.03; 227 minutes versus 162 minutes, p<0.001). However, robotic experience among surgeons in both studies varied significantly as compared to conventional laparoscopy, ranging from 10 to 50 robotic cases to as high as 400 to 500 laparoscopic procedures. Both studies reported higher postoperative pain scores and greater cost in the robotic group, with no differences in anatomic, functional, quality of life, or mortality outcomes at six to twelve months.

A recent Cochrane review of all randomized trials suggested very low-certainty evidence for little to no difference in the rates of intraoperative and postoperative complications between women undergoing robotic or laparoscopic sacrocolpopexy (RR 0.82, 95% CI 0.09–7.59 and RR 0.95, 95% CI 0.21–4.2, respectively) [6]. Furthermore, low-certainty evidence suggests there may be higher postoperative complications in the robotic group (RR 3.54, 95% CI 1.31–9.56), with little to no difference on postoperative length of hospital stay. None of the included studies reported death at up to 30 days postoperatively [6].

Enhanced Recovery after Surgery Protocol Application in Minimally Invasive Surgery

Enhanced recovery after surgery (ERAS) pathways are an important part of delivering high-quality surgical care. Initially developed in the 1990s in Europe for colorectal surgery, the goal of ERAS protocols were to challenge longstanding, non-evidence-based perioperative care. As surgery creates a catabolic state, the goal of ERAS pathways is to maintain a physiologic state, thereby attenuating the impact of surgical stress. To do so, these protocols incorporate multiple evidence-based perioperative patient interventions. These include preemptive analgesia, measures to reduce postoperative nausea and emesis, maintain fluid balance with the goal of euvolaemia, and encourage both early ambulation and oral intake. Together, the ultimate goal is to improve patient outcomes without increased complications or re-admissions. Indeed, ERAS pathways have been consistently shown to shorten recovery time, decrease hospital stay, reduce complications/nosocomial infections, and conserve resources.

There are multiple excellent resources available, including a publication by the American College of Obstetricians and Gynecologists, which outlines the pre-, intra-, and postoperative interventions recommended as part of an ERAS protocol [35].

Same Day Discharge (SDD) has increasingly become a central component of ERAS pathways. To date, numerous studies have investigated the feasibility and safety of SDD after minimally invasive hysterectomy. With careful patient selection and planning, nearly 80% of patients can achieve SDD, with no increase in complications or re-admissions when compared to discharge on or after postoperative day 1 [36]. Lastly, after hysterectomy, there is high patient satisfaction and less cost associated with SDD [37,38].

Fewer studies have evaluated the role of ERAS pathways and SDD in pelvic reconstructive surgery. A retrospective study of patients undergoing pelvic organ prolapse repair before and after implementation of an ERAS protocol found high SDD rates, over 90%, with no increase in 30 day postoperative complications, but a higher rate of re-admission [39]. Two prospective studies of women undergoing pelvic organ prolapse repair found no differences in healthcare resource utilization, high patient satisfaction, reduced length of hospital stay, and no differences in 30-day outcomes [40,41]. For women undergoing minimally invasive sacrocolpopexy, multiple studies have demonstrated feasibility, efficacy, and safety with no increase in postoperative adverse events or readmissions, and high associated patient satisfaction [42,43].

Taken together, ERAS protocols play an important role in the perioperative management of women undergoing minimally invasive surgery in benign gynaecology, including robotic-assisted hysterectomy and prolapse repairs. Consideration should be given to the implementation of ERAS pathways to facilitate SDD given the evidence supporting a lack of increase in healthcare resource utilization or serious adverse events, high patient satisfaction, and reduced cost.

Future Considerations/Conclusions

Robotic surgery may help to facilitate more technically challenging procedures due to improved visualization, precision, dexterity, and ergonomics compared to traditional laparoscopy. These advantages, however, should continue to be weighed against the cost of this technology. Over the last decade, there has been a significant increase in the utilization of the robotic platform for the treatment of benign gynaecologic conditions, despite low evidence in the literature to justify its use over conventional laparoscopy. Proponents of robotic surgery tout a greater ability to perform complex cases with improved ergonomics with this technology. However, in the setting of benign gynaecologic conditions, it is unclear whether robotic technology affords clear advantages over the conventional laparoscopic route, given comparable safety and efficacy outcomes between techniques. Further comparative studies are needed to identify specific subgroups of patients who would potentially benefit from robotic-assisted surgery as compared to other approaches.

References

1. American College of Obstetricians and Gynecologists' Committee on Gynecologic Practice, The Society of Gynecologic Surgeons. Robot-assisted surgery for noncancerous gynecologic conditions: ACOG Committee Opinion, Number 810. Obstet Gynecol 2020; 136(3): e22–e30. https://doi.org/10.1097/AOG.0000000000004048
2. Tarr M, Paraiso, MF. Laparoscopic and robotic surgery for pelvic organ prolapse and stress urinary incontinence. In: Mark D. Walters MMK (ed), *Urogynecology and Reconstructive Pelvic Surgery*, 4th edn. Elsevier: 2015; 295–317.
3. Payne TN, Dauterive FR. A comparison of total laparoscopic hysterectomy to robotically assisted hysterectomy: surgical outcomes in a community practice. J Minim Invasive Gynecol 2008; 15(3): 286–91. https://doi.org/10.1016/j.jmig.2008.01.008
4. Childers CP, Maggard-Gibbons M. Estimation of the acquisition and operating costs for robotic surgery. JAMA 2018; 320(8): 835–6. https://doi.org/10.1001/jama.2018.9219
5. Wright JD, Herzog TJ, Tsui J, et al. Nationwide trends in the performance of inpatient hysterectomy in the United States. Obstet Gynecol 2013; 122(2 Pt 1): 233–41. https://doi.org/10.1097/AOG.0b013e318299a6cf
6. Lawrie TA, Liu H, Lu D, et al. Robot-assisted surgery in gynaecology. Cochrane Database Syst Rev 2019; 4: CD011422. https://doi.org/10.1002/14651858.CD011422.pub2
7. Paraiso MF. Robotic-assisted laparoscopic surgery for hysterectomy and pelvic organ prolapse repair. Fertil Steril 2014; 102(4): 933–8. https://doi.org/10.1016/j.fertnstert.2014.08.010
8. Das D, Propst K, Wechter ME, Kho RM. Evaluation of positioning devices for optimization of outcomes in laparoscopic and robotic-assisted gynecologic surgery. J Minim Invasive Gynecol 2019; 26(2): 244–52 e241. https://doi.org/10.1016/j.jmig.2018.08.027
9. Unger CA, Paraiso MF. Robotic management of pelvic organ prolapse and incontinence. In: Jon Ivar Einarsson AW (ed.), *Minimally Invasive Gynecologic Surgery: Evidence-based Laparoscopic Hysteroscopic and Robotic Procedures*. JP Medical Ltd: 2016; 205–20.
10. Varghese A, Doglioli M, Fader AN. Updates and controversies of robotic-assisted surgery in gynecologic surgery. Clin Obstet Gynecol 2019; 62(4): 733–48. https://doi.org/10.1097/GRF.0000000000000489
11. Lin JF, Frey M, Huang JQ. Learning curve analysis of the first 100 robotic-assisted laparoscopic hysterectomies performed by a single surgeon. Int J Gynaecol Obstet 2014; 124(1): 88–91. https://doi.org/10.1016/j.ijgo.2013.06.036
12. Badash I, Burtt K, Solorzano CA, Carey JN. Innovations in surgery simulation: a review of past, current and future techniques. Ann Transl Med 2016; 4(23): 453. https://doi.org/10.21037/atm.2016.12.24
13. Chen R, Rodrigues Armijo P, Krause C, et al. A comprehensive review of robotic surgery curriculum and training for residents, fellows, and postgraduate surgical education. Surg Endosc 2020; 34(1): 361–7. https://doi.org/10.1007/s00464-019-06775-1
14. Jonsdottir GM, Jorgensen S, Cohen SL, et al. Increasing minimally invasive hysterectomy: effect on cost and complications. Obstet Gynecol 2011; 117(5): 1142–9. https://doi.org/10.1097/AOG.0b013e3182166055
15. Pasic RP, Rizzo JA, Fang H, et al. Comparing robot-assisted with conventional laparoscopic hysterectomy: impact on cost and clinical outcomes. J Minim Invasive Gynecol 2010; 17(6): 730–8. https://doi.org/10.1016/j.jmig.2010.06.009
16. Sarlos D, Kots L, Stevanovic N, von Felten S, Schar G. Robotic compared with conventional laparoscopic hysterectomy: a randomized controlled trial. Obstet Gynecol 2012; 120(3): 604–11. https://doi.org/10.1097/AOG.0b013e318265b61a
17. Lim CS, Griffith KC, Travieso J, As-Sanie S. To robot or not to robot: the use of robotics in benign gynecologic surgery. Clin Obstet Gynecol 2020; 63(2): 327–36. https://doi.org/10.1097/GRF.0000000000000491
18. Khorgami Z, Li WT, Jackson TN, Howard CA, Sclabas GM. The cost of robotics: an analysis of the added costs of robotic-assisted versus laparoscopic surgery using the National Inpatient Sample. Surg Endosc 2019; 33(7): 2217–21. https://doi.org/10.1007/s00464-018-6507-3
19. Elliott CS, Hsieh MH, Sokol ER, et al. Robot-assisted versus open sacrocolpopexy: a cost-minimization analysis. J Urol 2012; 187(2): 638–43. https://doi.org/10.1016/j.juro.2011.09.160
20. Leitao MM, Jr., Bartashnik A, Wagner I, et al. Cost-effectiveness analysis of robotically assisted laparoscopy for newly diagnosed uterine cancers. Obstet Gynecol 2014; 123(5): 1031–7.. https://doi.org/10.1097/AOG.0000000000000223
21. Stefanidis D, Wang F, Korndorffer JR, Jr., Dunne JB, Scott DJ. Robotic assistance improves intracorporeal suturing performance and safety in the operating room while decreasing operator workload. Surg Endosc 2010; 24(2): 377–82. https://doi.org/10.1007/s00464-009-0578-0
22. Stefanidis D, Hope WW, Scott DJ. Robotic suturing on the FLS model possesses construct validity, is less physically demanding, and is favored by more surgeons compared with laparoscopy. Surg Endosc 2011; 25(7): 2141–6. https://doi.org/10.1007/s00464-010-1512-1
23. Reich H. Laparoscopic hysterectomy. Surg Laparosc Endosc 1992; 2(1): 85–8.
24. Diaz-Arrastia C, Jurnalov C, Gomez G, Townsend C, Jr. Laparoscopic hysterectomy using a computer-enhanced surgical robot. Surg Endosc 2002; 16(9): 1271–3. https://doi.org/10.1007/s00464-002-8523-5
25. Nezhat C, Saberi NS, Shahmohamady B, Nezhat F. Robotic-assisted laparoscopy in gynecological surgery. JSLS 2006; 10(3): 317–20.
26. Paraiso MF, Ridgeway B, Park AJ, et al. A randomized trial comparing conventional and robotically assisted total laparoscopic hysterectomy. Am J Obstet Gynecol 2013; 208(5): 368 e361–7. https://doi.org/10.1016/j.ajog.2013.02.008
27. Lonnerfors C, Reynisson P, Persson J. A randomized trial comparing vaginal and laparoscopic hysterectomy vs robot-assisted hysterectomy. J Minim Invasive Gynecol 2015; 22(1): 78–86. https://doi.org/10.1016/j.jmig.2014.07.010
28. Swenson CW, Kamdar NS, Harris JA, et al. Comparison of robotic and other minimally invasive routes of hysterectomy for benign indications. Am J Obstet Gynecol 2016; 215(5): 650 e651–650 e658. https://doi.org/10.1016/j.ajog.2016.06.027
29. Deimling TA, Eldridge JL, Riley KA, Kunselman AR, Harkins GJ. Randomized controlled trial comparing operative times between standard and robot-assisted laparoscopic hysterectomy. Int J Gynaecol Obstet 2017; 136(1): 64–9. https://doi.org/10.1002/ijgo.12001
30. Lim PC, Crane JT, English EJ, et al. Multicenter analysis comparing robotic, open, laparoscopic, and vaginal

hysterectomies performed by high-volume surgeons for benign indications. Int J Gynaecol Obstet 2016; 133(3): 359–64. https://doi.org/10.1016/j.ijgo.2015.11.010

31. Oliver JL, Kim JH. Robotic sacrocolpopexy - Is it the treatment of choice for advanced apical pelvic organ prolapse? Curr Urol Rep 2017; 18(9): 66. https://doi.org/10.1007/s11934-017-0715-6
32. Wang LC, Al Hussein Al Awamlh B, Hu JC, et al. Trends in mesh use for pelvic organ prolapse repair from the medicare database. Urology 2015; 86(5): 885–91. https://doi.org/10.1016/j.urology.2015.08.022
33. Anger JT, Mueller ER, Tarnay C, et al. Robotic compared with laparoscopic sacrocolpopexy: a randomized controlled trial. Obstet Gynecol 2014; 123(1): 5–12. https://doi.org/10.1097/AOG.0000000000000006
34. Paraiso MF, Jelovsek JE, Frick A, Chen CC, Barber MD. Laparoscopic compared with robotic sacrocolpopexy for vaginal prolapse: a randomized controlled trial. Obstet Gynecol 2011; 118(5): 1005–13. https://doi.org/10.1097/AOG.0b013e318231537c
35. Committee on Gynecologic Pathways. ACOG Committee Opinion No. 750: Perioperative Pathways: Enhanced Recovery After Surgery. Obstet Gynecol 2018; 132(3): e120–e130. https://doi.org/10.1097/AOG.0000000000002818
36. Korsholm M, Mogensen O, Jeppesen MM, et al. Systematic review of same-day discharge after minimally invasive hysterectomy. Int J Gynaecol Obstet 2017; 136(2): 128–37. https://doi.org/10.1002/ijgo.12023
37. Bruneau L, Randet M, Evrard S, Damon A, Laurent FX. Total laparoscopic hysterectomy and same-day discharge: satisfaction evaluation and feasibility study. J Gynecol Obstet Biol Reprod (Paris) 2015; 44(9): 870–6. https://doi.org/10.1016/j.jgyn.2015.02.003
38. Schiavone MB, Herzog TJ, Ananth CV, et al. Feasibility and economic impact of same-day discharge for women who undergo laparoscopic hysterectomy. Am J Obstet Gynecol 2012; 207(5):382 e381–389. https://doi.org/10.1016/j.ajog.2012.09.014
39. Carter-Brooks CM, Du AL, Ruppert KM, Romanova AL, Zyczynski HM. Implementation of a urogynecology-specific enhanced recovery after surgery (ERAS) pathway. Am J Obstet Gynecol 2018; 219(5): 495 e491–495 e410. https://doi.org/10.1016/j.ajog.2018.06.009
40. Kalogera E, Bakkum-Gamez JN, Jankowski CJ, et al. Enhanced recovery in gynecologic surgery. Obstet Gynecol 2013; 122(2 Pt 1): 319–28. https://doi.org/10.1097/AOG.0b013e31829aa780
41. Liu L, Yi J, Cornella J, et al. Same-day discharge after vaginal hysterectomy with pelvic floor reconstruction: pilot study. J Minim Invasive Gynecol 2020; 27(2): 498–503 e491. https://doi.org/10.1016/j.jmig.2019.04.010
42. Lloyd JC, Guzman-Negron J, Goldman HB. Feasibility of same day discharge after robotic assisted pelvic floor reconstruction. Can J Urol2018; 25(3): 9307–12.
43. Kisby CK, Polin MR, Visco AG, Siddiqui NY. Same-day discharge after robotic-assisted sacrocolpopexy. Female Pelvic Med Reconstr Surg 2019; 25(5): 337–41. https://doi.org/10.1097/SPV.0000000000000573

Chapter 29

Unique Advantages of Robotics in Urogynaecology

Siri Drangsholt, Patrick Culligan

Introduction

Laparoscopic urogynaecology is a challenging technique that requires a unique skillset compared to open surgery. As a result, this limits the implementation of this technique to a select cohort of surgeons. In contrast, robotic-assisted techniques have the potential of enabling a greater number of surgeons to perform minimally invasive surgery. The da Vinci Surgical System® (Intuitive Surgical, Sunnyvale, California) has many of the same advantages of open surgery without the limitations of straight laparoscopy. Advantages of robotic assistance include the three-dimensional stereoscopic view with 10 times magnification, tremor attenuation, and articulating arms with seven degrees of freedom. These advantages work to further the surgeon's inherent skill and ability rather than requiring him/her to learn a different technique such as laparoscopy. Inherent to new technology, literature on robotic gynaecologic surgery is limited to observation and retrospective studies. It has been a challenge to impartially evaluate and compare robotic surgery to more traditional surgical methods where there is an abundance of data. We acknowledge that there are criticisms of robotic surgery, but having made it through the learning curve, and being pleased with those results, we transitioned to robotic assistance for multiple reasons, as we will highlight.

Advantages of Robotics in General

Minimally invasive laparoscopic surgery was first reported in the 1980s and has since transformed the surgical landscape. The advantages of minimally invasive surgery included improved cosmesis, small incisions, decreased length of stay, lower blood loss, decreased postoperative pain, and shorter convalescence. However, there are inadequacies with laparoscopy including a loss of tactile feedback, reduction in dexterity, loss of three-dimensional visualization, and difficulty accessing anatomical structures, particularly deep in the pelvis. It is because of these technical limitations that the efficacy of laparoscopic surgery is being challenged. Robotic surgery does not share these shortcomings and thus appears to be replacing conventional laparoscopic approaches due its perceived advantages.

The introduction of any new surgical technique invariably has a learning curve. In urology, it was found that the learning curve for robotic prostatectomy is faster than for open radical prostatectomy; when comparing number of cases for each and having equivalent outcomes [1,2]. Similarly, for experienced laparoscopic colorectal surgeons, the formal learning process for robotic total mesorectal excision (TME) may be short (15 cases) to reach a similar performance level as obtained in conventional laparoscopy [3]. The authors suggest that skills obtained during laparoscopic TME surgery may translate to faster robotic skill acquisition.

The accelerated achievement of skill may be due to the unique dual console platform which allows for safe and dynamic teaching of trainees. This was verified at an academic institution where they compared the first 10 dual console resident-performed procedures in colorectal surgery to matched cases on a single console with an experienced professional attending. They found patient outcomes were equivalent, with no difference in length of stay, morbidity and mortality, or total operative time [4]. Even without the second console, robotics gives the surgeon greater autonomy with the addition of the 'fourth' surgical arm and a stable camera. This allows him/her to be less reliant on team members knowledge and skill which may translate into more efficient and safer surgery.

One of the true benefits of robotics is ergonomics. While laparoscopic surgery has advantages for the patient, it appears to increase physical and mental strain on the surgeon. With a seated position and brow and arm rests, robotic surgery greatly modifies the laparoscopic and open surgeons working environment. Studies have found robotic-assisted surgery appears to decrease physical and mental strain compared to laparoscopy. Both heart rate, heart rate variability, and physical strains in surgeons were significantly decreased when comparing laparoscopic and robotic cholecystectomies [5,6]. Kuo et al used hand dexterity and grip strength test as objective measures to compare the difference in surgeon fatigue with robotic and laparoscopic colorectal surgery. They found resultant fatigue of both surgeon hands after laparoscopic surgery, but no difference in dexterity or muscle fatigue in surgeon hands after operating using the robot [7]. Robotics may be a way to optimize surgeon performance by reducing fatigue, which would be expected to help reduce iatrogenic injuries and mistakes.

The addition of three-dimensional imaging has become a cornerstone in the benefit of robotic-assisted surgery and translates to both greater accuracy and precision. Laparoscopy has seen a reduction in error rate and performance time with three-dimensional compared to two-dimensional displays with both novice and expert surgeons [8,9]. When comparing laparoscopic three-dimensional versus robotic three-dimensional in a validated head-to-head for surgical tasks, robotics showed significant decreases in median error rate and performance time for novice surgeons [10]. These results further suggest that improved visualization translates to precise surgery.

In addition to improved ergonomics and image quality, robotic-assisted surgery allows a platform of continual improvement. The unique ability to uniformly record cases and share with a community allows for feedback and development of video assessment techniques for evaluating surgical skills among both training and experienced surgeons. C-SATS (Crowd-Sourced Assessment of Technical Skills group) uses 'lay-people' and experts to perform video analysis of clinical activities. Crowd workers are paid a small fee for each video clip they rate and are trained to use an assessment tool of robotic surgery. Crowdsourcing has indicated that it can be used to reliably differentiate skill levels [11–13] and that skill levels are associated with postoperative complications [14]. This platform is being used for surgical quality improvement during intraoperative steps to increase quality of care provided to patients.

The continual adoption and rise of robotic surgery in nearly every surgical field speaks to real advantages. In gynaecology alone, there has been growth from less than 100,000 cases per year in 2009 to over 300,000 in 2018 [15]. Robotic surgery is established within urologic surgery with robotic prostatectomy now the standard of care and the most common route of surgery [16]. There is level one evidence that robotic prostatectomy is associated with lower estimation of blood loss (EBL), blood transfusions, OR time, LOS, intraoperative adverse events, pain relief, and greater lymph node yield [17]. Once surgeons switch over to the robotic platform they tend to stick with it. The use of robotic surgery across all fields increased from 1.8% in 2012 to 15.1% in 2018 at 73 Michigan hospitals and this trend was associated with a concomitant decrease in laparoscopic surgery [18].

Amongst general surgery, robotic assistance is the fastest growing modality, not because they weren't facile at laparoscopy, but because surgeons are happy with their results. Following FDA approval, robotic-assisted colorectal surgery has increased in prevalence, case complexity, severity of illness score, volume, and number of centres [19]. Comparative studies have suggested improved TME grade following robotic TME, which is thought to be due to improved precision, which allows easier visualization of surgical planes [20,21]. As surgeons become more comfortable with the robotic platform, they are able to take on more complex cases and can thus offer MIS to a wider range of patients across all surgical fields. Although there may not be specific evidence for this, it is self-evident.

Specific Advantages of Robotics in Urogynaecology

Urogynaecologic procedures have quickly been adapted to the robot platform because of the aforementioned advantages of improved visualization, ease of suturing deep within the pelvis, increased dexterity, and ergonomic positioning. Urogynaecologic procedures completed with the robot are reproducible, and highly 'teachable' with the dual console. Because of this, some centres have noticed an increase in robotic surgeries and a simultaneous decline in open and 'straight stick' laparoscopy [22]. Institutions have found that robotic hysterectomy rates increased significantly with the addition of a comprehensive robotics training programme [23]. Gynaecologists appear to have incorporated this platform into their armamentarium at a much greater rate than traditional laparoscopic approaches were adopted.

The robotic technology has been incorporated into the field in almost every surgery. Both urologists and gynaecologists have extrapolated their robotic success with prostatectomy and hysterectomy into other robotic pelvic surgeries for reconstructive purposes. The surgical steps and principles for robotic surgery remain the same as for laparoscopy. While there are case reports for how to perform robotic Burch colposuspension, vesicovaginal fistula repair, neovagina creation, uterosacral ligament suspension, and mesh removal, the essential steps are the same. Benefit has not been measured in terms of outcomes but the advantages remain, namely improved visualization and fine motor control. Robotics excels for precision surgery within confined spaces such as the pelvis and therefore continues to be adapted for challenging cases.

Robotics in gynaecology appears to have a shorter learning curve than laparoscopic surgery. Because it is more intuitive, this allows surgeons without advanced laparoscopic skills to perform a complex procedure with a minimally invasive approach. The learning curve for robotic sacrocolpopexy is estimated to be 10 to 20 cases whereas laparoscopic has been thought to be as high as 60 cases [24,25]. We found that the learning curve for robotic supracervical hysterectomy was eliminated by completion of a rigorous training protocol. A group of credentialed gynaecologic surgeons naïve to robotics practised simulator skills until they performed as well as experts; they then completed a robotic supracervical hysterectomy during a pig lab and then performed the same surgery as their first ever live human robotic surgery [26]. Comparisons of EBL and blinded video assessment of skill yielded similar differences between the novices and experts. This study established true expert benchmarks for the surgical simulator and incorporated real life surgical outcomes to establish predictive validity. The seamless ease of these trainers does not exist for laparoscopic training.

Surgical Steps where Robotics Excels in Urogynaecology

Using robotic assistance, we have found excellent objective and subjective long-term outcomes for robotic-assisted laparoscopic sacrocolpopexy using very lightweight polypropylene Y-mesh. Our five-year data showed a surgical success rate of 89.3% with patient satisfaction rates of 90–97% [27]. Our unique technique for each specific step is contained in videos (www.youtube.com/channel/UCWTyK7tNj6M6xDONCCOlhcA) thus we won't spend time detailing technique as this is covered in other chapters. However, we highlight several steps where the robot excels during sacrocolpopexy.

1. Our posterior dissection is completed at the level of the perineum. The robot allows for deep dissection in the pelvis with excellent visualization. While many surgeons are wary of creating defaecatory dysfunction, we have found the

opposite to be true. At 12 months after sacrocolpopexy for women with preoperative defaecatory dysfunction, 70% reported a complete resolution of splinting. Performing concomitant perineorrhaphy did not result in any differences in 12-month colorectal anal distress inventory short form 8 or colorectal-anal impact questionnaire short form 7 scores; we therefore have largely dropped this from our practice [28]. Along similar lines, the robot is ideal for the delicate dissection of the pre sacral space. There are considerable variations in anatomy that may require a surgeon to avoid major vessels and nerves. The robot allows for this safe and careful dissection.
2. Many women with symptomatic pelvic organ prolapse (POP) experience sexual dysfunction and have improved sexual function after successful POP repair. We found that our specific technique improves post-operation sexual function. Total sexual experience questionnaire (SEX-Q) scores for male partners improved after surgery for many, driven by very significant improvement in the individual satisfaction subscale. Our female patients postoperative PISQ scores also improved significantly [29].
3. With recent controversies involving the use of synthetic mesh for reconstructive surgeries that has led to a withdrawal of products from the market, we feel that very lightweight mesh is a safe and proven product for women. We base this on having no mesh erosions in a five-year cohort of 253 patients. We attribute this to using supracervical hysterectomy rather than total hysterectomy and taking split thickness bites for vaginal suturing [27].

As with all surgery, some patients will fail sacrocolpopexy and need mesh removal either for pain or for surgical failure. One of the main advantages is the ease to remove it the way it went in. Using the same principles for mesh removal, such as 'stay on the mesh', the robot allows for fine motor control to remove only the graft. When the graft is removed, the surgical dissection is identical to a primary case; this allows for repeat sacrocolpopexy when indicated. Our technique highlights the superiority of a mesh-augmented repair without coming at the price for mesh-related complications.

The Da-Vinci Robotic System® dominates the worldwide market, however its patents have started to expire since 2019. There are several other robotic systems being developed or in use in other markets. Senhance is the first abdominal platform since 2000 to received FDA approval; it is approved in the US for laparoscopic colorectal, gynaecologic, inguinal hernia, and cholecystectomy surgery. The Versius from CMR Surgical in the UK is approved in Europe and Australia for general surgery, urological and gynaecological surgery, and is a modular system comprised of individual robotic arms on wheeled base units. Several others are expected in the next five years, including the Medtronic robot, Corpath, Monarch, and Avatera, many with their unique selling point of single-use instruments, open console design, or console-based parts. We anticipate some of these new systems and new versions such as the Da-Vinci Single Port to capitalize on the benefits of the robotic platforms and reach narrower spaces with precision.

Conclusion

In conclusion, over the past two decades, robotic approaches to urogynaecology have spread, with almost all of the open and laparoscopic approaches being performed with robotic assistance. Patients benefit from this minimally invasive surgical approach without the ergonomic strain and a shorter learning curve for surgeons.

References

1. Fossati N, et al. Robotic and open radical prostatectomy: the first prospective randomised controlled trial fuels debate rather than closing the question. Eur Urol 2017; 71: 307–8.
2. Martini A, Gandaglia G, Briganti A. What is new in robot-assisted radical prostatectomy: a narrative review. Curr Opin Urol 2019; 29: 14–18.
3. Odermatt M, et al. Prior experience in laparoscopic rectal surgery can minimise the learning curve for robotic rectal resections: a cumulative sum analysis. Surg Endosc 2017; 31: 4067–76.
4. Bolger JC, et al. Initial experience with a dual-console robotic-assisted platform for training in colorectal surgery. Tech Coloproctology 2017; 21: 721–7.
5. Heemskerk J, et al. Relax, it's just laparoscopy! A prospective randomized trial on heart rate variability of the surgeon in robot-assisted versus conventional laparoscopic cholecystectomy. Dig Surg 2014; 31: 225–32.
6. Hubert N, et al. Ergonomic assessment of the surgeon's physical workload during standard and robotic assisted laparoscopic procedures. Int J Med Robot Comput Assist Surg 2013; 9: 142–7.
7. Kuo L-J, et al. A pilot study comparing ergonomics in laparoscopy and robotics: beyond anecdotes, and subjective claims. J Surg Case Rep 2020; 2020: rjaa005.
8. Smith R, et al. Advanced stereoscopic projection technology significantly improves novice performance of minimally invasive surgical skills. Surg Endosc 2012; 26: 1522–7.
9. Smith R, et al. Effect of passive polarizing three-dimensional displays on surgical performance for experienced laparoscopic surgeons. Br J Surg 2014; 101: 1453–9.
10. Shakir F, Jan H, Kent A. 3D straight-stick laparoscopy versus 3D robotics for task performance in novice surgeons: a randomised crossover trial. Surg Endosc 2016; 30: 5380–7.
11. Kowalewski TM, et al. Crowd-sourced assessment of technical skills for validation of basic laparoscopic urologic skills tasks. J Urol 2016; 195: 1859–65.
12. Ghani KR, et al. Measuring to improve: peer and crowd-sourced assessments of technical skill with robot-assisted radical prostatectomy. Eur Urol 2016; 69: 547–50.
13. Powers MK, et al. Crowdsourcing assessment of surgeon dissection of renal artery and vein during robotic partial nephrectomy: a novel approach for quantitative assessment of surgical performance. J Endourol 2016; 30: 447–52.
14. Birkmeyer JD, et al. Surgical skill and complication rates after bariatric surgery. N Engl J Med 2013; 369: 1434–42.
15. Intuitive. *Annual Report*. Available from: www.intuitive.com. Published 2019.
16. Mazzone, E. et al. Contemporary national assessment of robot-assisted surgery rates and total hospital charges for major surgical uro-oncological procedures in the United States. J Endourol 2019; 33: 438–47.

17. Dell'Oglio P, Mottrie A, Mazzone E. Robot-assisted radical prostatectomy vs. open radical prostatectomy: latest evidence on perioperative, functional and oncological outcomes. Curr Opin Urol 2020; 30: 73–8.
18. Sheetz KH, Claflin J, Dimick JB. Trends in the adoption of robotic surgery for common surgical procedures. JAMA Netw Open 2020; 3: e1918911.
19. Damle A, et al. Diffusion of technology: trends in robotic-assisted colorectal surgery. Am J Surg 2017; 214: 820–4.
20. Baik SH, et al. Robotic tumor-specific mesorectal excision of rectal cancer: short-term outcome of a pilot randomized trial. Surg Endosc 2008; 22: 1601–8.
21. Erguner I, et al. What have we gained by performing robotic rectal resection? Evaluation of 64 consecutive patients who underwent laparoscopic or robotic low anterior resection for rectal adenocarcinoma. Surg Laparosc Endosc Percutan Tech 2013; 23: 316–19.
22. Wright JD, et al. Robotically assisted vs laparoscopic hysterectomy among women with benign gynecologic disease. JAMA 2013; 309: 689–98.
23. Papalekas E, Fisher J. Trends in route of hysterectomy after the implementation of a comprehensive robotic training program. J Minim Invasive Surg 2018; 2018: 7362489.
24. Geller EJ, Lin F-C, Matthews CA. Analysis of robotic performance times to improve operative efficiency. J Minim Invasive Gynecol 2013; 20: 43–8.
25. Akl MN, et al. Robotic-assisted sacrocolpopexy: technique and learning curve. Surg Endosc 2009; 23: 2390–4.
26. Culligan P, et al. Predictive validity of a training protocol using a robotic surgery simulator. Female Pelvic Med Reconstr Surg 2014; 20: 48–51.
27. Culligan PJ, et al. Long-term outcomes of robotic-assisted laparoscopic sacrocolpopexy using lightweight Y-mesh. Female Pelvic Med Reconstr Surg 2020; 26: 202–6.
28. Lewis C, et al. Prospective cohort study of bowel function after robotic sacrocolpopexy. Female Pelvic Med Reconstr Surg 2014; 20: 87–9.
29. Culligan PJ, et al. Sexual satisfaction changes reported by men after their partners' robotic-assisted laparoscopic sacrocolpopexies. Female Pelvic Med Reconstr Surg 2019; 25: 365–8.

Chapter

30 Troubleshooting for Robotic Laparoscopic Urogynaecological Surgery: Tips and Tricks

Matt Hewitt

Introduction

The introduction of minimally invasive surgical technology has revolutionized a huge number of surgical specialties in recent years. Despite further refinements in the quality and scope of equipment, there are limitations to a minimally invasive approach. These have, at least in part, been overcome with the introduction of robots into theatre, the first widespread commercially available of which was the da Vinci® robot made by Intuitive Surgical [1] (see Figure 30.1).

The introduction of any new technology brings new challenges, and the content of this chapter is to help surgeons who are considering or have just purchased a robot.

The author has used the da Vinci S and daVinci X since 2009. Therefore, the contents of the chapter are based on the author's personal experience of this platform, but Intuitive Surgical have had no part in the production of this chapter.

Other systems have been introduced recently including the Versius® platform made by Cambridge Medical Robotics.

Setting Up a Programme

Arguably, the most challenging aspect of setting up a robotic surgery programme is actually acquiring a robot in the first place. No amount of enthusiasm will purchase a robot without the appropriate finances being in place.

To spread the cost of a robot, and justify its purchase, it is important that it is used as much as possible, as this dilutes the significant service cost over a larger number of cases. All specialties and subspecialties need to come together in a unified group to create a business plan to purchase a robot. Having one specialty 'owning' the robot builds up restrictions and resentment between the specialties and will reduce its use. However, the urology and gynaecology specialties are generally the largest users of the robot and thus a partnership between these two specialties may be the most cost-effective route to financing a robotic programme.

How multispecialty use of the robot works day to day will depend on the set-up of an individual hospital. Some centres have a designated robot theatre and robotic trained nurses who work across the specialties whilst others use the robot theatre with their own specialty nurses. Other centres move the robot between the theatres depending on which specialty is working on a particular day. Whatever system is in place, it's important to establish some ground rules before starting a programme, e.g. day of usage, informing other specialties when the robot is not being used, and open and timely reporting of accidental damage and malfunctions.

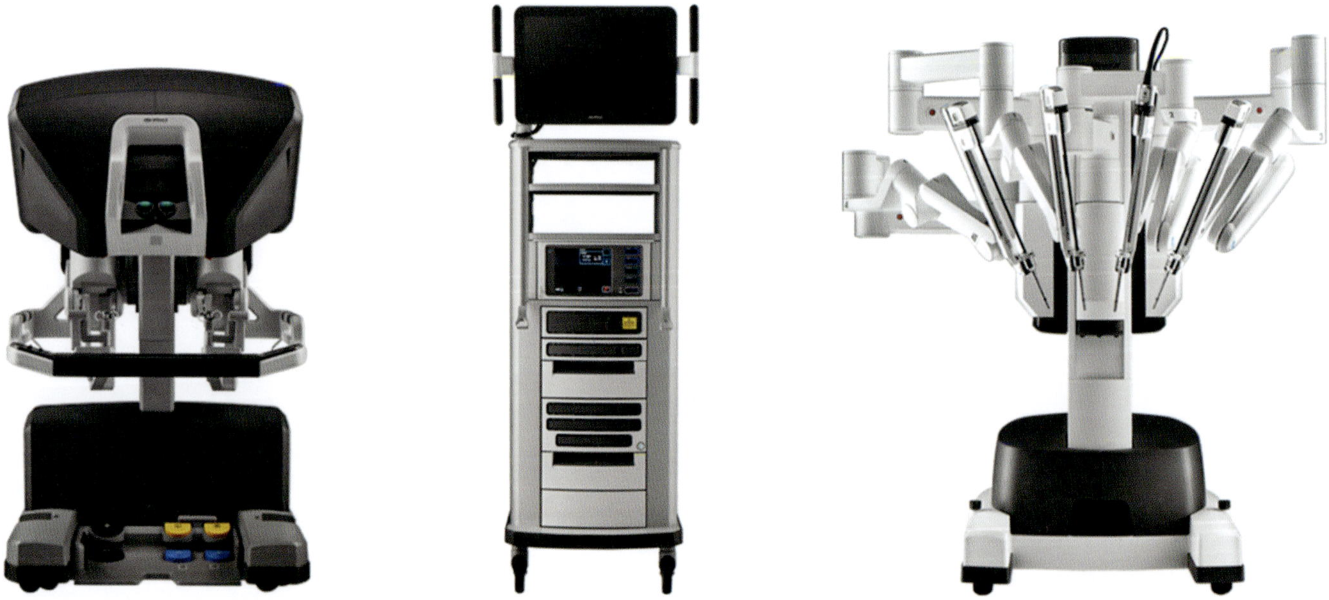

Figure 30.1 Components of the da Vinci X. Left to right: console, stack, cart.

Data

It is critically important to collect accurate, comprehensive, contemporaneous data on the use of the robot to facilitate appropriate audit and research. A suggested minimal data set should include:

- Patient demographics
- Indication for the operation
- Blood loss/transfusion rates
- Conversion to open
- Major complications
- Instruments used to enable comparisons between surgeons, with the possibility of surgeons changing instrument usage to decrease costs, e.g. using one needle holder instead of two with a Maryland bipolar.
- Surgical times – this should initially include set-up, docking, and theatre clearance times to demonstrate how the team is improving in the use of the robot. In the longer-term, the operating times are important to demonstrate increased efficiency of the robot.

This data set should be able to be linked or integrated into the urogynaecology database to enable detailed monitoring of patient outcomes.

First Cases

On the first day of operating, it is important that the entire team are fully briefed including the nurses, anaesthetists, and theatre assistants. A representative from da Vinci will be present in theatre together with a proctor funded by Intuitive Surgical. The role of the proctor is to guide and advise and not to operate but they can occasionally adjust instruments during surgery and help to dock.

Case selection for the commencement of the programme is critical. The anticipated surgery should be technically easy, e.g. a simple hysterectomy and in an appropriate patient who is slim and fit without previous surgeries. In addition, the author recommends that the procedure itself must be one that the surgeon is very familiar with. It is recommended that no more than two cases are undertaken on the first day as this will take longer than a usual procedure. However, it is equally important that the first few weeks of the programme have regular robotic cases, so the team has an intensive introduction to robotic surgery. Ideally more than one day per week for the first few weeks should be set aside to train the team. Having three days in the first week with six cases and the same robotic representative and proctor would be ideal.

In a large unit, it is recommended two surgeons per speciality are initially trained to allow them to become fully competent before more surgeons join the robotic team. These initial surgeons, if possible, should train together, one assisting the other and then swapping, to enable the most efficient learning environment. Much can be learnt from being the bedside assistant as well as the operating surgeon. If this is not possible, then a senior trainee should be assigned to act as the robot bedside assistant, who can then become familiar with use of the robot.

It is important, wherever possible, that the same nursing team should also be used so they too become familiar and efficient in the set-up of the robot.

Finally, prior to surgery, there should be local discussion and agreement regarding the consent process. The first few patients need to be fully informed that new equipment is being used.

Previous Laparotomies and Potentially Difficult Surgeries

In complex patients who, for example, have had multiple previous laparotomies or who have a very high BMI, there may be a significant chance that robotic surgery may not be possible. In this case, consideration can be given to not draping the robot, but instead having it positioned in theatre ready and switched on. A conventional 5 mm camera can be inserted to perform an initial inspection of the abdominal cavity and assess the feasibility of the approach. If a robotic surgical approach is deemed possible, the robot can then be draped. This may increase operating time but potentially can save significant money on consumables by avoiding unnecessary draping of the robot.

The older versions of the robot, da Vinci S and Si, use non-proprietary trochars for the camera. This enables 'donut' ports to be used in the event of pneumoperitoneum being made by a cut down approach. The newer versions of the robot, the daVinci X and Xi, have a proprietary trochar without donut capability. Therefore, it can be more difficult to maintain pneu moperitoneum if this is made by the 'cut down' method. The author suggests using a Veress needle to create a pneumoperitoneum and then inserting the proprietary trochar. This will avoid unnecessary air leakage. However, when first using the robot, the pneumoperitoneum should be created as per how the surgeon normally performs insufflation. In situations where the patient has had a previous midline laparotomy, a Veress needle can be inserted at Palmer's point (left subcostal midclavicular line) which is the area least likely to have intraabdominal adhesions. A conventional 5 mm port can be inserted at this point and then a conventional 5 mm endoscope inserted. This endoscope can be used to inspect the peritoneal cavity, guide insertion of the robot trochars and, if necessary, adhesions can be divided initially using conventional endoscopic instruments. This trochar can then act as the fee assistant port (see Figure 30.2a,b,c,d).

Safety

It is important to be safety aware when using the robot. Although any surgery is potentially dangerous, the robot has its own unique risks. However, many of these can be mitigated with appropriate training and preparation.

Junior doctors, scrub assistants, and nurses rotate through most hospitals on a regular basis. It is ultimately the surgeon's responsibility to make sure that all personnel are appropriately trained in handling of cables, cameras, and associated equipment. It is a good idea to provide floor markings for consistent docking and ensure all external cabling is covered on the theatre floor and safely protected from creating a hazard to

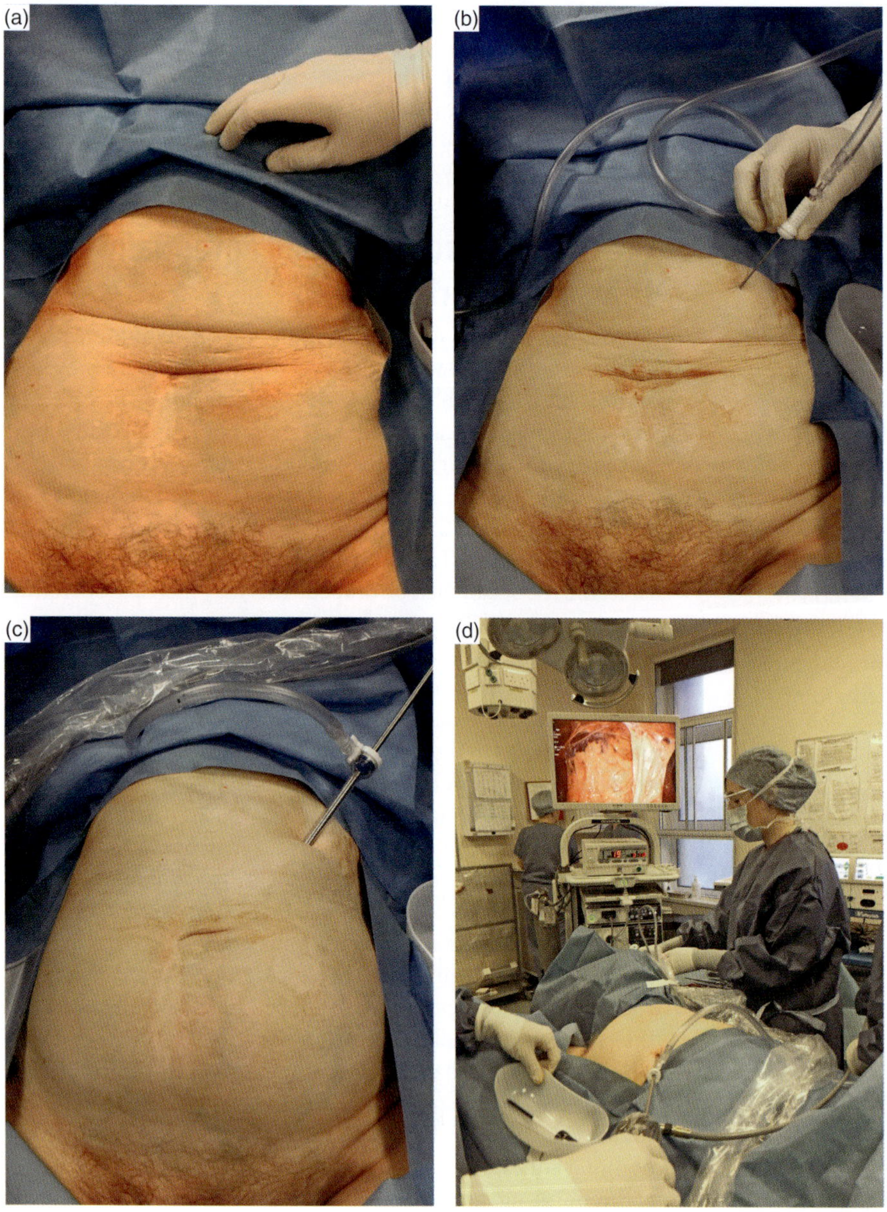

Figure 30.2 (a) Patient with midline laparotomy. (b) Palmer's point insufflation with Veress needle. (c) 5 mm trochar inserted with standard 5 mm endoscope. (d) Screen view of anterior wall adhesions over previous laparotomy scar. Robot trochars can be inserted safely under direct vison and adhesions divided before docking of the robot cart. The 5 mm trochar is then suitably placed to act as the assistant's trochar.

circulating staff. The first assistant should be able to remove and replace instruments appropriately and safely. In particular, the first assistant should be able to remove and clean the camera (in the event of this becoming blurred, having touched tissue or blood) and reinsert it. Finally, the first assistant should be able to undock the robot smoothly and efficiently in the event that an emergency undock is required (see below). This a procedure that all theatre staff should be rehearsed and competent in as part of a team.

Some of the robot's instruments have separate energy cables that need attaching to the instruments before they can be used. It is recommended that these are connected to the instruments before they are attached to the robot arms and inserted into the peritoneal cavity. Attaching these cables after the instruments are in place could result in inadvertent, sudden, and unguided advancement of the instruments further into the peritoneal cavity that can damage an intraabdominal viscus.

Removing instruments and replacing them is easier with the robot than with conventional straight-stick surgery, but care still needs to be taken. The surgeon is distant from the first bedside assistant, who could inadvertently remove the wrong instrument. If the wrong instrument is removed and this is still attached to tissue or a suture, this can result in tissue trauma. It is therefore recommended that the surgeon not only names the instrument to be removed but they also number the arm that the instrument is still attached to; for example, 'remove bipolar forceps from arm number 3'. To further lower the risk, it is recommended that no other instrument is attached to tissue or holding a suture when a request is made to remove an instrument and that all instruments are in the surgeon's field of view. The author personally performs the above measures, but in addition he also gently performs a rocking movement of the instrument to be removed and this guides the assistant to the correct one quickly.

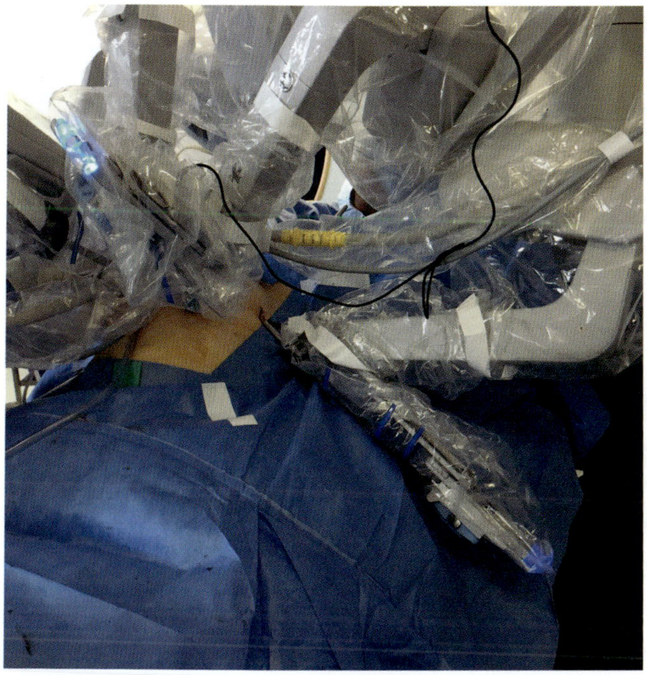

Figure 30.3 The robot arm on the right can be seen to be pointing at the anterior abdominal wall. This would be a usual location for the arm to be positioned and is likely being used to divide anterior abdominal wall adhesions. Note that the robot arm in this position is at risk of pressing on the patient's right arm, which is positioned by the patient's side.

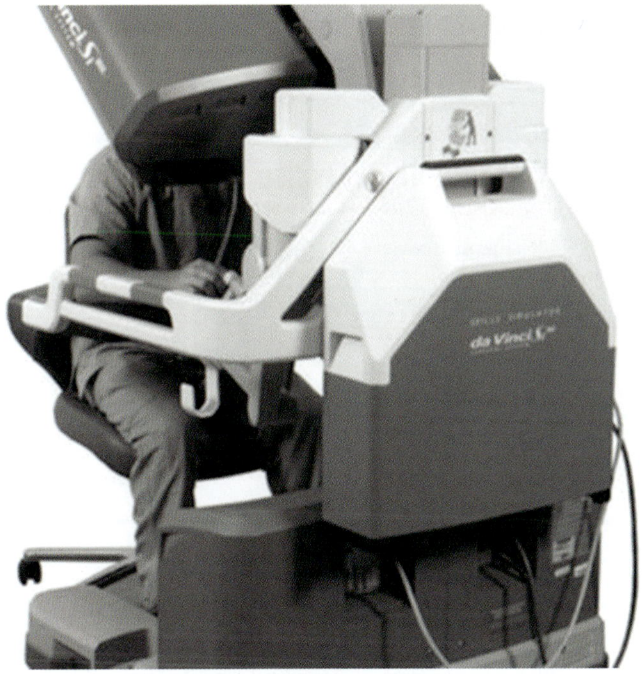

Figure 30.4 The simulator attached to the back of the console.

As previously mentioned, the use of a suture cut needle driver avoids reinsertion of scissors, be they robotic or straight-stick, and this reduces potential tissue damage. Although the robot is specifically designed with 'memory', such that when one instrument is replaced with another it will return to exactly the same point as the previous one, there is still the potential of tissue damage. A loop of bowel may move into the instrument pathway, so no assumption should be made about safe passageway of a newly inserted instrument even under 'memory' and this must be done under direct vision.

After docking and insertion of the instruments and before sitting at the console, the author recommends performing a secondary survey of the surgical field and theatre [2]. The purpose of this is to check for dangerously placed cables, potential areas where the robot may come into contact with the patient, and any other potential risks to the patient or theatre staff (see Figure 30.3).

Simulator

The da Vinci system has the additional option of a simulator (see Figure 30.4). This is a device that attaches to the back of the console and allows a surgeon to practice using the robot without the need to have the cart in operation and connected to a patient. A virtual reality environment is created, and the surgeon can use all the controls on the console. This is very useful in training a new surgeon on how to use the robot in a safe environment [3]. There are many exercises that are available which come with the simulator, and these differ in range of complexity. A personalized log-in system allows the trainee surgeon to undertake the exercises in their own time and record their progress. Each exercise is measured by the simulator and a score given at the end. Parameters measured include time to complete the exercise, economy of movement, instrument collisions, excessive instrument force, instruments out of view, master workspace range, misapplied energy time, blood loss volume and broken vessels (see Figure 30.5). A portfolio of exercises can be assigned to each trainee/new surgeon, and they can then record successful completion of the exercises before they move on to the next one and ultimately complete the assigned programme before they are allowed to operate on a patient. In the author's experience, surgeons who have had access to a simulator before using the robot are much more fluid, efficient, and safe than those who have not.

Newer software is becoming available that allows a trainee surgeon to practise specific procedures, e.g. a hysterectomy (see Figure 30.6).

Anaesthetic, Set-up, and Theatre Turnaround

There has been a trend in recent years for induction of anaesthesia to take place in the operating theatre rather than the anaesthetic room. In robotic surgery, this practice slows down the theatre process, as set-up and draping of the robot are delayed until the patient is asleep. If the anaesthetic room is used to anaesthetize the patient, then the robot can be set-up and draped ready for use, so the two processes are occurring at the same time thus increasing time efficiency.

At the end of the case there are a lot of tasks for the nurses to complete before the next surgery can take place. Although some tasks are nurse specific, it is recommended that the surgical team assist in this process as much as possible. This can involve such tasks as undraping the robot and helping to transfer the patient.

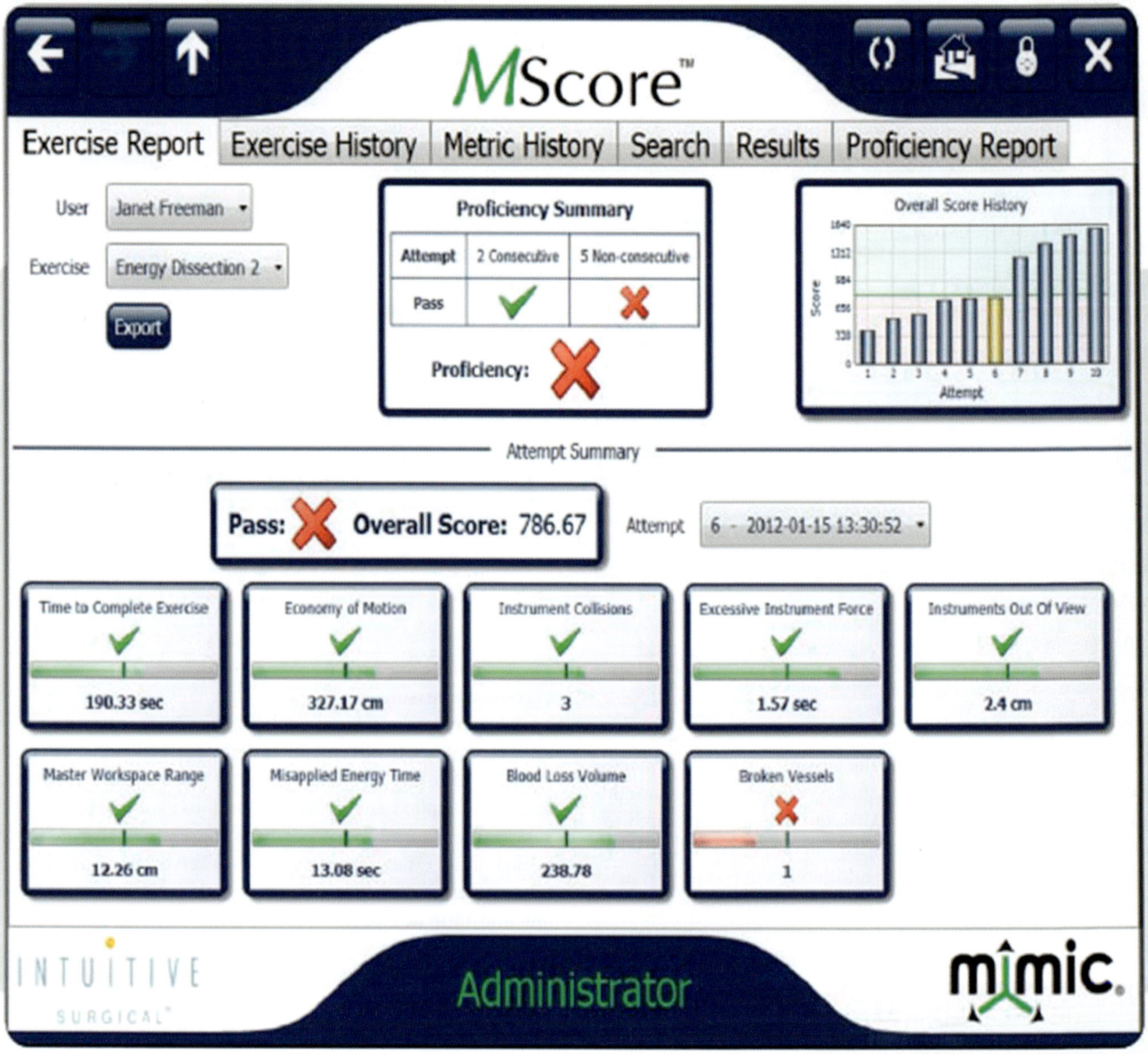
MScore™
Exercise Report
Exercise History
Metric History
Search
Results
Proficiency Report
User
Janet Freeman
Exercise
Energy Dissection 2
Export
Proficiency Summary
Attempt
2 Consecutive
5 Non-consecutive
Pass
Proficiency:
Overall Score History
Score
Attempt
Attempt Summary
Pass:
Overall Score: 786.67
Attempt
6 - 2012-01-15 13:30:52
Time to Complete Exercise
190.33 sec
Economy of Motion
327.17 cm
Instrument Collisions
3
Excessive Instrument Force
1.57 sec
Instruments Out Of View
2.4 cm
Master Workspace Range
12.26 cm
Misapplied Energy Time
13.08 sec
Blood Loss Volume
238.78
Broken Vessels
1
INTUITIVE SURGICAL
Administrator
mimic

Figure 30.5 Screenshot of an exercise score undertaken on the simulator. Note the different parameters measured and the score history.

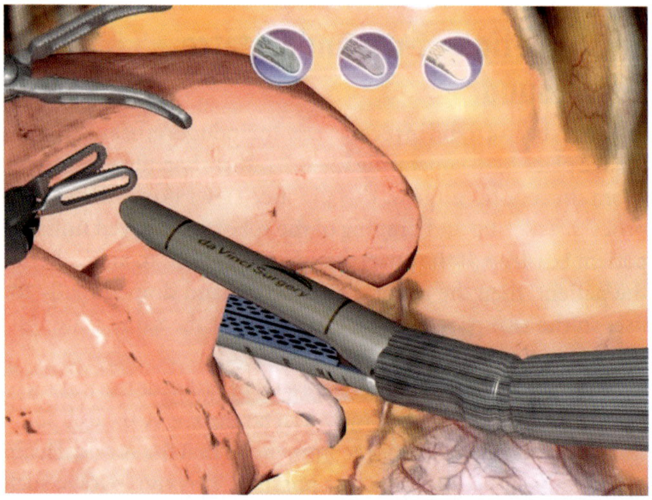

Figure 30.6 Screenshot of a simulated surgery available on the simulator.

The author believes none of the surgical team should leave the theatre until the patient is transferred to the bed and has left the theatre. Not only does this increase theatre turnaround it also increases team moral.

Docking

With the older models (da Vinci S and Si) and with the newer da Vinci X, consideration needs to be given to which side of the patient to dock the robot cart from. The da Vinci Xi does not require any such consideration, as the cart adjusts accordingly wherever it is positioned next to the patient.

When operating in the pelvis, there is an option to dock between the legs. However, this means that access to the vagina is limited. Furthermore a 'between-the-legs assistant' can feel claustrophobic, so it has become the norm to dock from the left or right of the patient at approximately 45 degrees to the midline

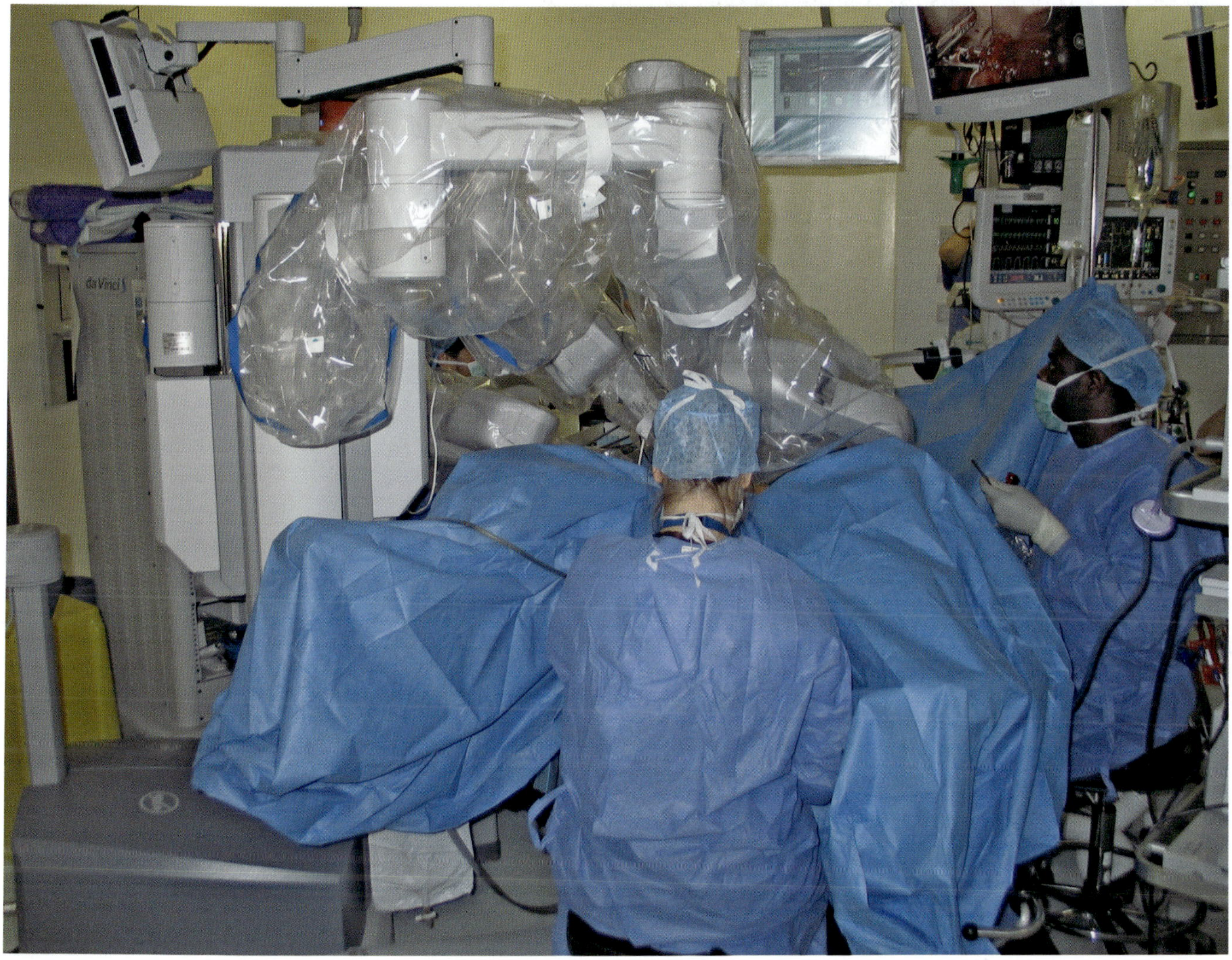

Figure 30.7 A 'between-the-legs view' of a patient right side dock approach. This allows easy access to the vagina.

(see Figure 30.7). Most right-handed surgeons will dock from the right-hand side of the patient, which results in two robot arms being on the patient's right and one on the left. Some surgeons, even when right-handed, prefer to have two robot arms on the left in order to use the arm to retract from right to left when pulling the sigmoid to the left to expose the sacral promontory during a sacrocolpopexy.

When docking from either side, there is more of a chance of clashing of arms as the symmetry of the 'between-the-legs dock' has been lost. It is important to have the robot arms pushed in towards the central column to reduce clashing and to increase the movement available in the robot arm (see Figure 30.8a and b).

The most difficult part of learning how to use the robot is the process of docking. Familiarizing oneself with the robot arms and the position of the various buttons before the first case will make the process easier. A team-based approach to this rehearsal is highly recommended.

It is usual for the surgeon and assistant to be scrubbed while the robot cart is being pushed towards the patient and docked. Verbalizing clear, precise, and constant instructions at an appropriate volume to the person pushing the cart is essential. The author recommends that the automatic drive on the cart is disabled, and the cart is pushed manually, as with an inexperienced operator, the automatic drive can be difficult to control.

Dual Console

Dual consoles are available. A dual console is very useful for teaching new surgeons and for assisting in complicated cases with trained surgeons [4]. It negates the need for the trainee surgeon to unseat themselves from the console to allow the trainer to take over. The second console can be set up in various ways. Firstly, it can be used simply by the trainer to control two pointers that can be seen on the trainee's screen and these are moved by the trainer to point and guide the trainee. Secondly, the dual console can allow the teaching surgeon to immediately take over control of all instruments from the trainee if needed. The control can be handed back to the trainee at any point. Alternatively, the teaching surgeon can just take control of one of the instruments while the trainee controls two instruments. All three robot arms can thus be used simultaneously. The dual console is useful but is expensive and adequate training on a simulator significantly negates the need to purchase one.

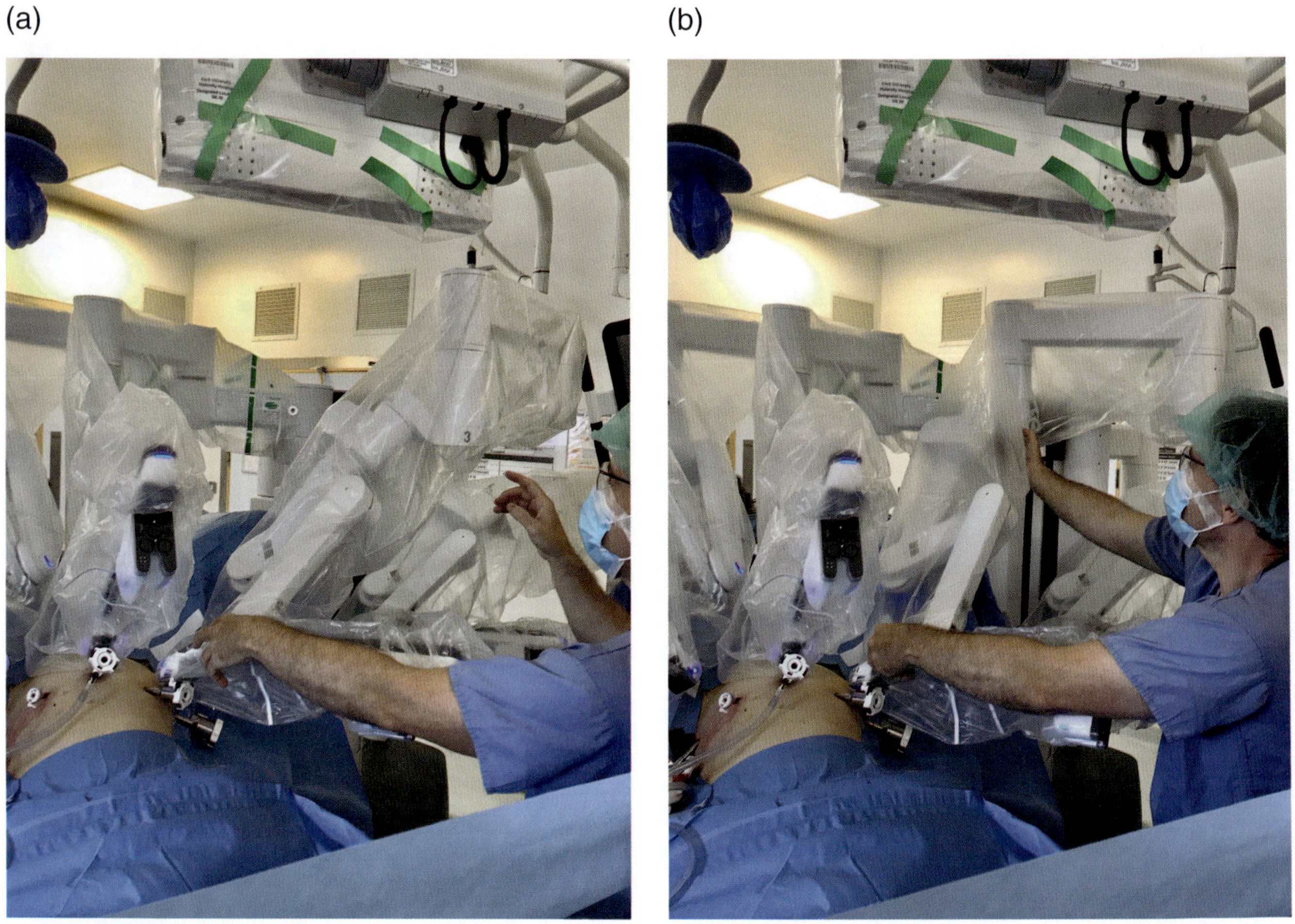

Figure 30.8 (a) Robot arm 3 is in an incorrect position away from the central column. (b) The arm is pushed towards the central column, reducing potential clashing with the ipsilateral arm and increasing the movement available to the instrument attached to this arm.

Instrument Usage

The author recommends that in centres where there is multispecialty use of the robot, each department uses their own instruments. This enables monitored use of instruments and will reduce the number used and thus the overall cost. Any damages that do occur can be traced more easily, which is particularly important in the case of the endoscopes, which are more expensive to replace.

Cost savings can be made using less instruments during a procedure. In the author's centre, a hysterectomy would typically involve using four instruments; Monopolar Scissors, Bipolar Maryland, Fenestrated Grasper, and a Needle Driver with suture cut. It can be seen that only one needle driver is used. It is only in very fine suturing, e.g. suturing the urethra, that using two needle drivers may be necessary. Closing the vagina with the robot only needs one needle driver in the dominant hand and the bipolar instrument can be used in the non-dominant hand, saving the cost of a second needle driver. This can also apply to suturing mesh in urogynaecological cases, where only one needle driver may be required.

Furthermore, in easy cases, such as an uncomplicated simple hysterectomy, it's unnecessary to use a fourth instrument. The Fenestrated grasper can be made redundant and not used if the needle driver is used to safely manipulate tissue.

The author uses a suture cut needle driver, as although this is slightly more expensive than a needle holder, it is safer than reinserting the robot scissors or free hand scissors to cut a suture.

There is an array of instruments available and more are coming on stream. The Intuitive vessel sealer is a single use instrument that coagulates and then cuts in the same device. This is a very quick and easy way of operating; however, this instrument is more expensive than standard instruments. The author therefore reserves it for use in obese patients, where access is difficult. In this situation, using bipolar to coagulate and then swapping over to the scissors to cut the tissue may involve spillage of bowel into the operating field. This simultaneous vessel sealing property then negates swapping instruments.

Patients with Extremes of Body Composition

The obese patient presents problems for the entire team. Everything from surgery and anaesthesia to handling the patient presents an additional risk. However, the robot is particularly useful in the obese patient; studies have shown that the conversion rate is lower with robot surgery compared with traditional laparoscopic surgery [6].

It is important to become experienced in robotic surgery on non-obese patients before attempting the same procedure in a patient who is either obese or very slim.

With the obese patient it is vitally important to have the full support of the anaesthetist, as the surgeon is reliant on their ability to achieve a satisfactory Trendelenburg. In the author's experience, a good relationship between the surgeon and anaesthetist is key, as is the shared understanding that the duration of the operation is inversely proportional to the degree of Trendelenburg. It is therefore better to have the patient at the limit of the airway pressure and have a shorter surgery time than have lower airway pressures and have a prolonged surgery [5].

The author recommends performing a 'practice' Trendelenburg position before draping the patient to check the patient's position is stable and that the anaesthetist can monitor the patient adequately.

Where possible, lower the insufflation pressures to 10 mm Hg rather than the standard 13 mm Hg during the surgery which lowers the airway pressures needed. Excessive Trendelenburg for a short amount of time, before docking, can facilitate removing the bowel from the pelvis and then the Trendelenburg can be reduced slightly to help with ventilating the patient. Some centres will give full bowel preparation the night before surgery to reduce the volume of bowl contents and to increase its ability to fall out of the pelvis into the upper abdomen.

Having a free or 'non robot port' is not essential but recommended during robotic surgery to enable free passage of the suction device sutures or pass tape or mesh into the pelvis. In the obese patient we recommend using two free ports so the first assistant can have two conventional instruments in the pelvis to help retract the bowel (see Figures 30.9 and 30.10).

Very slim patients provide different challenges. Spacing the trochars sufficiently apart may require the standard port placement to be adapted. In this situation, it may be necessary to place the camera port higher than usual to enable the operating ports to be placed sufficiently far apart from both the camera and each other to avoid clashing of instruments. Most centres will have the patient's arms down by their sides while operating. In doing so there is a tendency to push the patient's arms anteriorly, i.e. to become level with the patient's anterior abdominal wall. This is dangerous as this can result in the robot arms clashing with the patient's arms.

Emergency Undocking Protocol

Rarely an emergency can develop during robotic surgery. This could be an anaesthetic issue or major vessel damage associated with uncontrolled haemorrhage. In these situations, an emergency undock needs to be employed to flatten the patient, if this is an anaesthetic issue, or to perform laparotomy on a surgical complication. It is advisable to have an emergency undock protocol in place. The author recommends running through the emergency undocking drill after docking and before the surgeon sits at the console. This involves the surgeon assigning each person in the team a job to perform in the event of an emergency undock. On hearing the words 'emergency undock', the first assistant and the scrub nurse remove the instruments and trochars and the between-the-legs assistant joins the first assistant to commence the laparotomy. The surgeon drives the robot away from the surgical field and is free to issue instructions including giving permission to the anaesthetist to flatten the table, and is then free to scrub if necessary. The scrub nurse, having helped undock, then hands the scalpel to the first assistant and then opens the laparotomy set, which should be easily accessible [7]. Each centre will have a different array of staff with different experience so it's important to develop your own protocol.

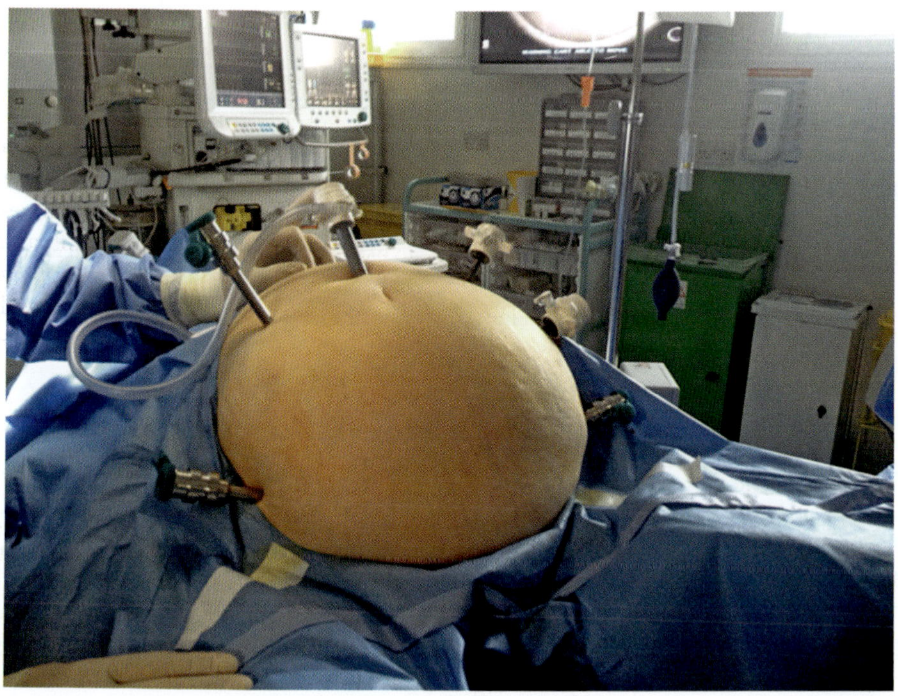

Figure 30.9 Picture taken caudally looking cranially. Port position with an obese patient showing the two assistant ports on the patient's left-hand side.

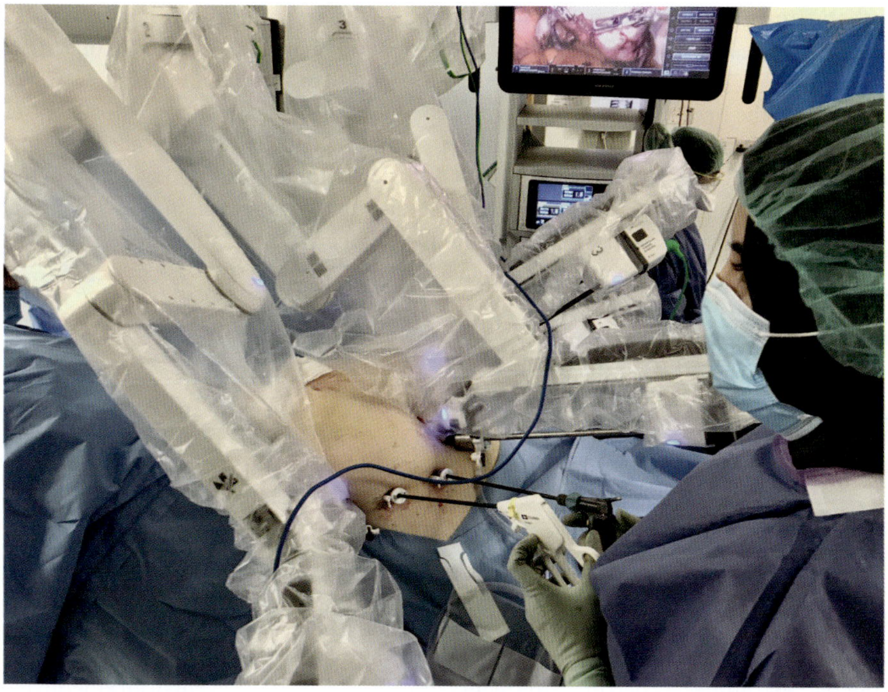

Figure 30.10 There are two assistant ports in use for the surgery on an obese patient. Note how they are positioned.

Assistant Port

It is possible to operate without a free or assistant port but this is not recommended. A free port allows quick and easy access to insert a sucker, swab, mesh, or suture. The size of such a port depends on the surgical procedure. Inserting a suction device can be done through a 5 mm port. Some sutures can also be inserted through a 5 mm port, but some larger needles may require a larger port. In the author's experience, passing the needle through the vagina for suturing is not linked with an increase in vault infections and thus this could also be considered for insertion of mesh into the abdominal cavity.

Experience will lead to each surgeon having a preference as to where the assistant port is placed, but most surgeons will place it between the camera port and the robot port on the side where only one robot arm is in place.

It is important that it is placed such that the assistant can easily access the port and still be able to see a screen. Having the assistant port between the camera port and the 'single sided' robot arm gives more access for the assistant than having the assistant port lateral to the robot arm.

Burping

The trochars have a black mark positioned down the shaft. This is the 'fulcrum point' of the trochar and it is around this point that the arm will rotate and thus this is the depth to which the trochar should be inserted, positioning the black mark at the abdominal wall. This will result in the minimal movement of the abdominal wall during the surgery and thus potentially less postoperative pain for the patient. It is therefore essential to ensure that the trochar in inserted perpendicular to the patient's abdominal wall.

It is important that prior to insertion of the instruments, the arm is positioned such that it is pointing towards the surgical field. If the trochar and robot arm indent the skin, the arm and trochar can be gently lifted off the skin while still keeping the trochar at the appropriate depth on the abdominal wall (see Figure 30.11). This author terms this 'burping'.

Use of the 'Third Arm'

It is possible to use just two of the robot arms and instruments in addition to the camera arm. This will save money. However, in the majority of situations, particularly in difficult surgeries, the third robot arm and instrument will be used. It's important to use this to maximum benefit for retraction of tissue to expose the surgical field. It can be particularly useful to push a large or 'boggy' uterus into acute anteversion or retroversion to gain access to the pouch of Douglas or uterovesical pouch (see Figure 30.12). In addition, the third instrument can be used to pull the uterus to the left or right using the articulation features of the instruments.

Use of the third arm can cause clashing of the ipsilateral instrument and experience will reduce the incidence of this occurring. Using the head of the third arm at a right angle to the instrument shaft will create more space for the ipsilateral instrument to work in (see Figure 30.13).

Summary

A robot can transform the surgical experience for both patient and surgeon. The most important factors to take from this chapter are to consider patient safety and to practice as much as possible before using the robot to operate.

Conflict of Interest

The author is a proctor for Intuitive surgery.

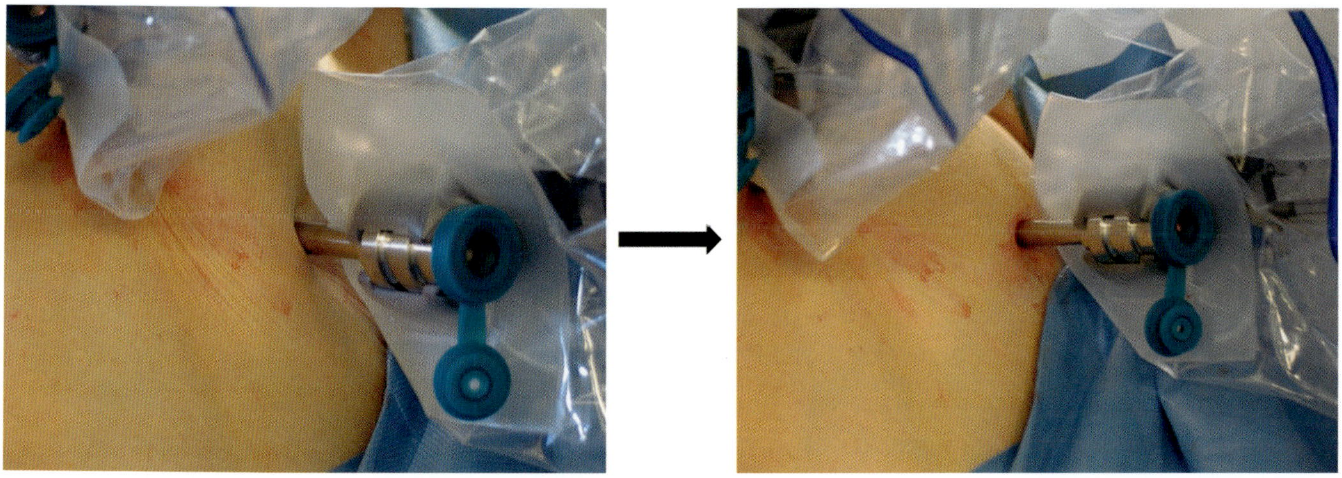

(a) (b)

Figure 30.11 a,b The left-hand picture shows puckering of the skin and abdominal wall. Following a minor adjustment or 'burp' of the arms they can be moved to a more natural position on the abdominal wall and thus potentially reduce pain. If arms are clashing the reverse can be undertaken to separate the robot arms to reduce clashing.

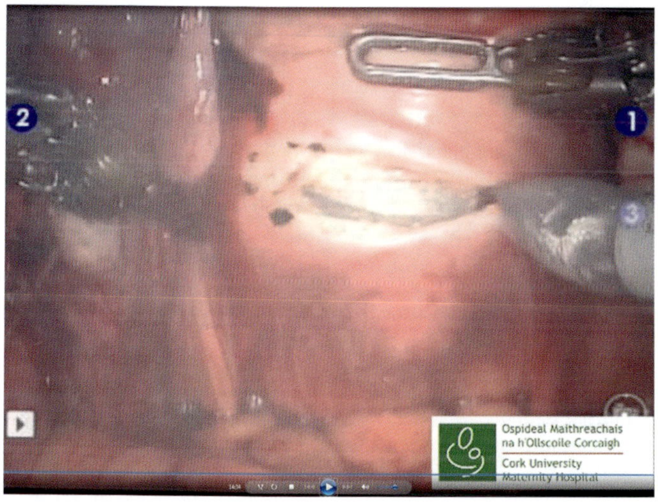

Figure 30.12 Use of the third arm to keep the uterus in acute anteversion, which enables the posterior colpotomy to be undertaken. This is particularly useful in a large boggy uterus.

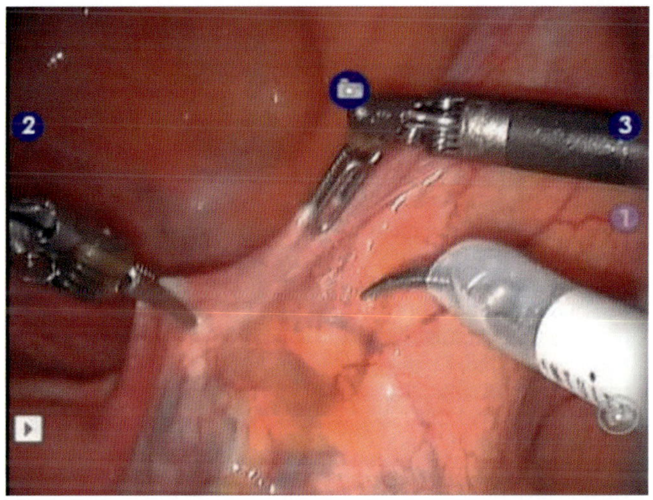

Figure 30.13 The fenestrated grasper in arm 3 is grasping the round ligament while articulated to near 90 degrees and pointing posteriorly. This allows increased space beneath this instrument in which the scissors in arm 1 can work.

References

1. Lim S, Mowers EL, Mahnert N. Risk factors and outcomes for conversion to laparotomy of laparoscopic hysterectomy in benign gynecology. Obstet Gynecol 2016; 128(6): 1295–305
2. Mills JT, Burris MB, Warburton DJ, et al. Positioning injuries associated with robotic assisted urological surgery. J Urol 2020; 190(2): 580–4.
3. Patel A, Patel M, Lytle N, et al. Can we become better robot surgeons through simulator practice? Surg Endosc 2014; 28(3): 847–53.
4. Smith AL, Scott EM, Krivak TC, et al. Dual-console robotic surgery: a new teaching paradigm. Robot Surg 2013; 7(2): 113–18.
5. Daskalakis M, Scheffel O, Weiner RA. High flow insufflation for the maintenance of the pneumoperitoneum during bariatric surgery. Obes Facts 2009; 2(Suppl 1): 37–40.
6. Lindfors A, Heshar H, Adok C, Sundfeldt K, Dahm-Kähler P. Long-term survival in obese patients after robotic or open surgery for endometrial cancer. Gynaecol Oncol 2020; 158(3): 673–80.
7. O'Sullivan OE, O'Sullivan S, Hewitt M, O'Reilly BA. Da Vinci robot emergency undocking protocol. J Robot Surg 2016; 10(3): 251–3.

Index